Handbook of
Rural Health

Handbook of
Rural Health

Edited by

Sana Loue

Case Western Reserve University
Cleveland, Ohio

and

Beth E. Quill

University of Texas, Houston
Houston, Texas

Kluwer Academic / Plenum Publishers
New York, Boston, Dordrecht, London, Moscow

Library of Congress Cataloging-in-Publication Data

Handbook of rural health/edited by Sana Loue and Beth E. Quill.
    p.   cm.
    Includes bibliographical references and index.

    1. Rural health—Handbooks, manuals, etc. 2. Public health—Handbooks, manuals, etc.
3. Rural health services—Handbooks, manuals, etc. I. Loue, Sana. II. Quill, Beth E.

RA771 .H26 2000
362.1′04257—dc21

00-062191

ISBN 978-1-4419-3347-8

© 2010 Kluwer Academic / Plenum Publishers, New York
233 Spring Street, New York, New York 10013

http://www.wkap.nl/

10 9 8 7 6 5 4 3 2 1

A C.I.P. record for this book is available from the Library of Congress

Printed in the United States of America

Contributors

Neva Abbott • Monroe, North Carolina 28110

Lu Ann Aday • University of Texas School of Public Health, Houston, Texas 77225

Keith B. Armitage • Division of Infectious Diseases, Case Western Reserve University, Cleveland, Ohio 44106-4984

Guadalupe X. Ayala • San Diego State University, Graduate School of Public Health and SDSU–UCSD Joint Doctoral Program in Clinical Psychology, San Diego, California 92123

Roberta D. Baer • Department of Anthropology, University of South Florida, Tampa, Florida 33620-8100

John B. Conway • College of Health Sciences, University of Texas at El Paso, El Paso, Texas 79968-0581

Leslie K. Dennis • Department of Epidemiology, College of Public Health, University of Iowa, Iowa City, Iowa 52242-1008

John P. Elder • San Diego State University, Graduate School of Public Health and SDSU–UCSD Joint Doctoral Program in Clinical Psychology, San Diego, California 92123

Christine A. Gehrman • San Diego State University, Graduate School of Public Health and SDSU–UCSD Joint Doctoral Program in Clinical Psychology, San Diego, California 92123

Bruce W. Goldberg • Department of Family Medicine, Oregon Health Sciences University School of Medicine, Portland, Oregon 97201

Jeffrey J. Guidry • Department of Health and Kinesiology, Texas A & M University, College Station, Texas 77843-4243

Helena Hansen • School of Medicine, Yale University, New Haven, Connecticut 06510

Ardis Hanson • Louis de la Parte Florida Mental Health Institute Library, University of South Florida, Tampa, Florida 33612-3807

Robert Isman • California Department of Health Services, Office of Medi-Cal Dental Services, Rancho Cordova, California 95670, and University of California at San Francisco, San Francisco, California 94143

Bruce Lubotsky Levin • Louis de la Parte Florida Mental Health Institute, College of Public Health, University of South Florida, Tampa, Florida 33612-3807

Sana Loue • Department of Epidemiology and Biostatistics, School of Medicine, Case Western Reserve University, Cleveland, Ohio 44106-4945

Hal Morgenstern • Department of Epidemiology, School of Public Health, University of California at Los Angeles, Los Angeles, California 90095-1772

Keith J. Mueller • Center for Rural Health Research, University of Nebraska Medical Center, Omaha, Nebraska 68198-4350

Susan Murty • School of Social Work, University of Iowa, Iowa City, Iowa 52242

Marie Napolitano • Department of Primary Care, Oregon Health Sciences University School of Nursing, Portland, Oregon 97201

Janice Nichols • Department of Anthropology, University of South Florida, Tampa, Florida 33620-8100

Karen Olness • Department of Pediatrics, Case Western Reserve University, and Rainbow Center for International Child Health (RCIC), Rainbow Babies and Children's Hospital, Cleveland, Ohio 44106-6003

Stacie L. Pallotta • Department of Epidemiology and Biostatistics, School of Medicine, Case Western Reserve University, Cleveland, Ohio 44106

Judith J. Prochaska • San Diego State University, Graduate School of Public Health and SDSU–UCSD Joint Doctoral Program in Clinical Psychology, San Diego, California 92123

Beth E. Quill • University of Texas School of Public Health, Houston, Texas 77225

L. A. Rebhun • Department of Anthropology, Yale University, New Haven, Connecticut 06520-8277

Cielito C. Reyes-Gibby • University of Texas School of Public Health, Houston, Texas 77225

Everett R. Rhoades • Native American Prevention Research Center, University of Oklahoma College of Public Health, Oklahoma City, Oklahoma 73104

James Robinson III • Department of Social and Behavioral Health, School of Rural Public Health, Texas A & M University System, Health Science Center, College Station, Texas 77843-1266

Gary I. Sinclair • School of Medicine, Case Western Reserve University, Cleveland, Ohio 44106-4984

Gail E. Souare • Alliance Healthcare Foundation, San Diego, California 92123

Lorann Stallones • Colorado Injury Control Research Center, Department of Environmental Health, Colorado State University, Fort Collins, Colorado 80523-1676

Elizabeth Wheeler • School of Nursing, University of Vermont, Burlington, Vermont 05405

Patricia Winstead-Fry • School of Nursing, University of Vermont, Burlington, Vermont 05405

Marion F. Zabinski • San Diego State University, Graduate School of Public Health and SDSU–UCSD Joint Doctoral Program in Clinical Psychology, San Diego, California 92123

Preface

This book integrates the expertise of professionals from a broad array of disciplines—anthropology, health services research, epidemiology, medicine, dentistry, health promotion, and social work—in an examination of rural health care and rural health research. This investigation includes an inquiry into issues that are universal across rural populations, such as public health issues and issues of equity in health care. Several chapters explore the health care issues that confront specified subpopulations including, for instance, migrant workers and Native Americans, while others provide a more focused approach to diseases that may disproportionately have an impact on residents of rural areas, such as specific chronic and infectious diseases.

Several common themes emerge, despite the variation in the disciplines from which the authors hail and the substantive areas of their inquiry. The development of additional mechanisms for the provision of care by health care professionals and an increase in the accessibility of that care to rural consumers constitute major challenges. This task is rendered even more difficult by the relative dearth of information available on the various health concerns and subpopulations and by the numerous methodological complexities in compiling the necessary data. Recognition of the nuances within and across rural populations, as recommended here, will allow us to provide care more efficiently and effectively and to prevent disease or ameliorate its effects. Reliance on some of the newer technologies and approaches discussed here, such as distance learning and broad-based, community-wide health initiatives, will facilitate disease treatment and prevention in relatively isolated areas. Ultimately, all of us must work to ensure the availability of adequate health care to even the most isolated communities, for "as we all know, it is we collectively who are responsible for allocating and reallocating responsibilities . . . we who appoint the judges" (Baier, 1995).

References

Baier, A. (1995). *Moral prejudices*. Cambridge, MA: Harvard University Press.

Contents

1

Rural Health Policy

Past as a Prelude to the Future

KEITH J. MUELLER

"You've come a long way, baby." This well-known slogan comes from advertisements for Virginia Slims cigarettes, introduced with great fanfare as cigarettes for women. Seeing women smoke was one more indication in the 1960s and 1970s of the cracking of societal barriers to equal treatment for women. Some progress. As we know now better than in the 1960s and 1970s, getting more women to smoke was to confuse apparent equity and the best interests of the target population. Is the same thing true of striving for equity in health care services? Is it in the best interests of rural residents to have the same system as that available to urban residents? Are we making the cigarette example mistake of confusing equal access to the same delivery system with the ultimate goal of improved quality of life?

Public policy is easily driven by simple, easily understood paradigms. In the 1990s the paradigm driving much of health policy was one of expanding consumer choice among a host of competing health plans. Hence, all national policies were crafted based on that approach and applied to rural health care systems, regardless of appropriateness of fit. As the decade ended, specifically in the Medicare, Medicaid, and State Child Health Insurance Program (SCHIP) BBA Refinement Act of 1999 (Refinement Act), policies began to recognize that circumstances might warrant different approaches in rural areas. Because rural delivery systems were different than their urban counterparts at an earlier time, reflecting on that time might inform future policy choices.

This chapter will begin with the premise that the past can inform the future in an opening section articulating the historical perspective. A second section will examine some threads in public policy concerning rural health care delivery that weave through the various policies and across time. The third section will look at the current dominance of payment as the driving force behind public policy, including an examination of Medicare policies. The fourth section offers scenarios for the future of rural health policy, and the final section looks at the mechanisms available to influence the direction of those policies.

Historical Perspective on Rural Health

One town, one doctor, health care for all . . . fond memories of a time gone by in rural America? Perhaps so, but the stereotype of frontier life permeated federal policy from the 1940s through the 1960s, in that an implicit policy objective was to get resources located

KEITH J. MUELLER • Center for Rural Health Research, University of Nebraska Medical Center, Omaha, Nebraska 68198-4350.

Handbook of Rural Health, edited by Loue and Quill. Kluwer Academic/Plenum Publishers, New York, 2001.

wherever there were settlements of people. An overarching goal during those decades was to assure that people had access (defined as proximity) to essential health care services. During the 1970s policymakers became concerned about the costs of providing health care services, which was related to increased use of expensive resources to provide specialized services. As a result, the implicit direction of policy shifted, from bringing resources to the people, to bringing the people to the resources. A clear indication of this shift was the discussion, in the mid-1990s, of establishing "centers of excellence" for various clinical treatments. Table 1 offers a chronology of federal legislation since 1946.

Some policymakers argue in favor of bringing people to resources in order to achieve economies of scale and introduce competitive pressures to health care delivery. Others would argue that in order to assure appropriate use of health services and to establish equity among people who pay for health care, services need to be available locally. Debates about the quality of health care services influence thinking about where to locate services. Some policymakers believe there is a strong relationship between volume and quality, an argument favoring centralizing services. Others believe quality is more a function of patient–physician relationships, which could argue for locally available resources.

Bringing Resources to the People

Two stories about primary care physicians illustrate the imagery of one town, one doctor. The first is about medical care in Collbran, Colorado, a town of 350 in the western mountains of that state. During the late 1800s and until the 1920s, the town was served by "pioneer physicians" (Rollins, 1999). In 1926 Dr. Henry Ziegel arrived and staffed the local hospital, a building donated by a local church. He was the only physician in the community for 50 years, until he died in 1976 (Rollins, 1999). The second story is from McGregor, Iowa. This town and the surrounding area in northeastern Iowa and southwestern Wisconsin has been served by Dr. Clifford Smith since 1962. Dr. Smith was a solo practitioner until 1987. During those 25 years of practice he accepted bartering in exchange for medical services, and (today he remains an active practitioner) he continues to make house calls (Talbott, 1998).

Those same two stories help illustrate the

TABLE 1. Chronology of Federal Legislation Affecting Rural Health

Year	Legislation	Rural Provisions
1946	Hospital Survey and Construction Act	Funding for capital expenses
1970	National Health Service Corps	Financial assistance for health care professionals locating in shortage areas
1974	Health Planning and Resources Development Act	Certificate-of-need program created and provided funding for regional health systems agencies
1976	Health Professions Education Assistance Act	Funding for health professions training
1982	Tax Equalization and Fiscal Responsibility Act	Established prospective payment system to pay for inpatient services in Medicare
1995	Health Insurance Portability and Affordability Act	Allowed for creating purchasing cooperatives for health insurance; requires offering continuous insurance coverage to persons changing jobs
1997	Balanced Budget Act (BBA)	Created the Medicare Rural Hospital Flexibility program (Critical Access Hospitals); reduced expenditures in the Medicare program; created the State Child Health Insurance Program (SCHIP); created the Medicare+Choice Program
1999	Medicare, Medicaid, and SCHIP BBA Refinement Act	Modified the Hospital Flexibility Program; reduced size of expenditure reductions; modified the Medicare+Choice Program

transitions that have taken place in rural health care delivery—some things change and others stay the same. In Colorado, a two-physician practice and community-owned clinic have been developed. The community-based values that characterized Dr. Ziegel's practice are continuing, but the model has changed to reflect needs for physician downtime (the two-person practice allows for this), and the reality of what services can be delivered locally (the change from a hospital to a clinic). The solo practice model in McGregor became a group practice model in 1987, affiliated with the Gundersen Lutheran–McGregor Clinic. In addition to making house calls, Dr. Smith travels one day a week to an outreach clinic, maintaining the philosophy of bringing the care to the people, but within a different context of group practice based in a local clinic.

The Colorado story was about a local hospital as well as the physician. In the 1950s, the image was that every community should have a hospital. The federal government, through the Hospital Survey and Construction Act of 1946 (known as the Hill-Burton Act), encouraged this philosophy by making funds available for hospital construction in communities with populations as low as 1,000 (Bauer, 1987). Providing convenient hospital services has remained a policy objective, modified over time to focus on a more narrow range of hospital services needed in rural communities. A special project, funded by the Robert Wood Johnson Foundation in the Northwest in the 1970s, included an emphasis on services appropriate in an isolated rural hospital:

> The basic assumption underlying scope-of-service planning is that rural residents should have access to all available hospital services, but that rural hospitals could expect to provide only a certain subset of those services in the local facility. The crux of scope-of-service planning was the development of explicit criteria to decide whether a specific service should be provided in the rural hospital or in a remote urban hospital, through a regional inter-hospital agreement (Rosenblatt, 1991, p. 477).

This philosophy of the 1970s is the same as that driving a federal program that began in 1997, the Medicare Rural Hospital Flexibility Program (in the Balanced Budget Act of 1997 [BBA]).

If physicians and hospitals could be consid-ered as building blocks for a system of delivering care in local communities, a third block would be emergency medical services. Local hospital emergency departments provide those services at the site of the hospital. Getting emergency services to the site of the emergency is problematic in rural areas, given great travel distances. Staffing rural emergency services has required recruiting and training volunteer providers (Pullum, Sanddal, & Obbink, 1999). A heavy dose of neighbor-helping-neighbor is also required, particularly in isolated areas, and use of small local clinics. Maintaining these services requires commitment by the volunteers, a supply of replacement volunteers, training programs, and connection to broader delivery systems. As is true for physicians and hospitals in isolated communities, continuing to take the services to people becomes expensive and difficult to sustain.

Bringing People to the Resources

Because much of rural America is only sparsely populated, one method of delivering health care services would be to bring the people to the resources. This is especially true for those services that require minimum volumes of patient business to be viable, both financially and as a quality program. Public policy in the United States has encouraged regionalization of medical services, sometimes explicitly, as in the regional medical program and comprehensive health planning efforts of the 1960s and the successor Health Planning and Resources Development Act of 1974 (Starr, 1982). The Health Planning Act was an attempt to rationalize the delivery system both by preventing excessive growth in facilities and by adopting local and statewide plans to coordinate the delivery of services. Certificate-of-need (CON) laws in the states were intended to force providers to justify capital expansion and deny expansions when not justified. Regional and state planning agencies, which included consumer representation, were to integrate CON actions into rational plans for optimal configuration of health care delivery services. While these efforts were not targeted explicitly at rural systems, the implications were obvious. If a minimum number of hospital beds and limited purchase of expensive equipment are the policies in place, then those resources will not be distributed widely in sparsely populated areas.

The increasing reliance on physicians with specialty training, and on equipment that is expensive to purchase and maintain, leads to increased concentration of those resources where population is also concentrated. For example, oncologists will see only those patients diagnosed with cancer and use diagnostic equipment and procedures applicable to only those cases. Although cancer is a leading cause of death and a disease of concern to all, only a limited number of us at any one time will need the services of oncologists. Turning this thinking around, an oncology practice will need a large population base from which to draw the number of patients required to keep the practice viable. The lower the percentage of persons expected to need a particular service, the larger the population base needed to support the service. This logic precludes locating most specialty services in multiple rural sites. Another reason to concentrate services is evidence that quality for many specialty procedures improves as the specialists gain more experience. For those services for which this is true, the logical approach to develop a health care delivery system is to get the people to those places that have maintained sufficient volume to assure high-quality services.

The principal means by which public policy can promote getting people to resources in health care is to stay out of the way. The philosophy that "bigger is better" is a powerful force in health care, and people can be convinced to bypass local health care services based on a perception of better care elsewhere. Without incentives to do otherwise, providers and citizens alike would support the concentration of medical care resources. As with most generalizations, there would be exceptions of course. Persons without the means to travel for care would continue to patronize local providers, and some providers would locate in sparsely populated areas due to a preference for other amenities available there (including outdoor activities, small community cultural life, being near family).

A more deliberate approach in public policy supporting centralized care is to direct public resources to the providers practicing in larger communities. Some of the same policies that helped build health care facilities in small rural communities, such as the Hill-Burton Act, have been used to build larger facilities in larger communities. Public investment in transportation systems, including rural highways, facilitates travel to centrally located providers (although these investments were not necessarily made with health care in mind). Payment policies based on the costs reported by providers favor higher-cost care that is associated with larger communities, particularly when adjusted for cost of labor. Finally, policies that promote centers of excellence favor large facilities.

Critique

Neither approach—resources to people or people to resources—is the one best way to provide high-quality services to rural residents. Perhaps there was a time when the state of the art in medical care was such that clinicians could set up practice virtually anywhere. That is no longer true. However, much of the practice of medicine can be done effectively by primary care practitioners in settings without large, well-equipped facilities. Indeed, effective, convenient delivery of primary care services may be more important, in many instances, than state-of-the-art specialty care. Getting health care services to where the people live remains an important objective in public policy, while recognizing that this applies to the range of services that can be delivered effectively (including with high-quality outcomes) in sparsely populated areas.

The concept of centers of excellence could be helpful in clarifying what might appear to be a conundrum—how to blend assurance of high quality with local access. Primary care centers of excellence can and should be established in rural communities. Rural hospitals can be centers of excellence for a limited range of surgical procedures. For example, a study of readmissions to hospitals in Washington State found no differences in hospital readmissions based on urban or rural location for appendectomy, cesarean section, cholecystectomy, or transurethral prostatectomy (Welch, 1991). These and other procedures do not require the same volume of patient work to generate high-quality outcomes as, for example, cardiac bypass surgery.

Rural residents need access to specialized services as well. So getting the people to the service remains an important objective in health care delivery and public policy. Policies that promote effective exchange of information between primary care and specialty care are a step in this direction. The need to be addressed is one of assuring continuity in care for the rural resident.

Policy Threads

Health policy in the United States does not follow a blueprint that integrates all actions into a fabric guided by a coherent set of goals and objectives. Policy in health care has been reactive, as elected officials respond to specific problems. In the 106th Congress (1999–2000), for example, policy issues included the rights of patients enrolled in managed care plans, Medicare payment for health care providers, and extending insurance benefits to particular groups such as children. There have been attempts to be more comprehensive in health policy, most recently in 1993–94 when President Clinton tried to get Congress to pass the Health Security Act. Thus far those attempts have failed, leaving policymaking firmly anchored in the "crisis du jour" mode of tackling one highly visible issue at a time: "The development of a comprehensive and consistent health care policy is made difficult, if not impossible, by the shotgun approach followed by many policymakers, such as the President and Congress" (Patel & Rushefsky, 1999, p. 1). Nevertheless, policy initiatives do seem to cluster into collective, if disjointed, strategies. Patel and Rushefsky identify historical periods in health policy: transformation of American medicine (1900–1935), expansion of health facilities and services (1930–1960), increasing access to health care (1960s), and cost containment (1970–1980s). We are currently in a cycle when issues of access, quality, and cost containment are arising simultaneously. Our "shotgun" strategy in public policy is struggling to deal with all three at once, and the resulting policy confusion, and at times, contradiction, can be seen in policies affecting health care services in rural areas.

As the following paragraphs put forward some themes in rural health policy, we will see that each new effort adds to what is already under way; rarely do policymakers abandon previous efforts (a notable exception was comprehensive health planning, for which federal legislation was actually repealed [Mueller, 1988]). Despite the resulting confusion, we are witnessing the early signs of policy efforts to push health care providers into systems of health care delivery, pulling away from the "lone ranger" approach of the past.

Committing Resources to Rural Areas

The Hill-Burton Act led to a substantial federal investment in rural health care facilities. During a 30-year period the federal government spent $3.7 billion, matched by $9.1 billion in state and local funds. Over half of those funds were spent on facilities in communities with fewer than 25,000 people. By 1986, thanks to this program, the number of hospital beds per 1,000 population evened out between rural and urban areas—4.0 in rural (nonmetropolitan) and 4.1 in urban areas (Ricketts, 1999). Rural hospitals benefitted from a grant program targeted to meet their needs to establish new services or coordinate their services with others—the rural Transition Grants Program that existed from 1987 to 1991. Hospitals received up to $50,000 per year for up to three years. The first year of the program saw $8 million awarded to 182 rural hospitals in 45 states (Office of Technology Assessment, 1990). Another grant program for small rural hospitals was created in the Refinement Act, this one to fund equipment and software to assist hospitals in their conversions to new Medicare payment systems (Mueller, 1999).

The federal government has also invested in facilities designed to serve the poor and uninsured in rural areas. Community health centers provide services to low income persons, based on a sliding fee schedule. As of 1995 approximately 60% of the 623 federally funded community health centers were located in rural areas (Harriman, 1999). Migrant health centers provide primary care and other services to migrant populations, which are predominantly located in rural areas. In 1998, 118 migrant health center clinics served over 500,000 people (Office of Technology Assessment, 1990, p. 80). Currently, the migrant health center and migrant health programs provide services to about 600,000 migrant and seasonal farm workers per year, in about 390 facilities (Bureau of Primary Health Care, U.S. Department of Health and Human Services, 1999).

A related investment is the federal government's expenditures through the National Health Service Corps, created in 1970. The National Health Service Corps provides loans and scholarships to students in the health professions in exchange for a commitment to practice for specified lengths of time in underserved areas (originally focused exclusively on rural areas, but later amended to include urban underserved areas). More than 21,000 health professionals have served with the National Health Service Corps, and current field strength is more than 2,200 persons (National Health Service Corps, 1999).

The health center and service corps programs are both consistent with the federal government's emphasis on access to care, which as Patel and Rushefsky (1999) argued, was a dominant theme of federal policy in the 1960s. The fact that both programs have grown is an indication that the commitment to access continues and that the federal government recognizes a continuing problem in getting appropriate services into many rural communities.

More recent federal investments are consistent with another general theme in health policy: the organization of health care services needs to adapt to a changed environment. As was argued in the opening sections of this chapter, advances in medical care technology have combined with changes in finance and organization to favor larger delivery systems. Federal grant programs consistent with this trend support development of rural health care delivery networks. The Federal Office of Rural Health Policy (ORHP) administers a Network Development Grant Program, which began in federal fiscal year (October 1 to September 30) 1997. In the first cycle of this program health providers in 34 communities were funded; another $5.7 million was awarded in the second year of the program (Ricketts, 1999). There have been 41 networks funded by this program (Federal Office of Rural Health Policy, 1999). These net-

work projects are designed for an array of purposes, including better serving the uninsured in their communities, competing with other providers for managed care contracts, improving the quality of care in their communities, and enhancing the availability of services in local communities. The specific projects and networks are developed by the applicants, making this a program through which the government seeks to support initiatives, not create new systems of delivering care that are responsive to federal requirements (the latter type of federal program will be discussed later).

Network development grants have also been awarded by the Bureau of Primary Health Care, U.S. Department of Health and Human Services, to participating community and migrant health centers. Much like the grants awarded by the ORHP, these grants facilitated locally developed plans to integrate services, either within centers, or more typically, between centers and other providers in their service areas. Programs designed to enhance economic development, funded by the U.S. Department of Agriculture, could be used to enhance rural health care delivery networks, given their contributions to the economies of their communities.

In recent years, the federal government has invested very directly in local rural health projects through the Outreach Grant Program, administered by the ORHP. The program began in 1991 with funding provided to 100 projects (National Rural Health Association, 1992). As of awards made for fiscal year 1998, over 365 projects have been funded through this program (Federal Office of Rural Health Policy, 1999). The program required that at least three distinctly different organizations participate in the projects, which are targeted to meet specific community needs. Projects funded by this program in 1998 included:

- a program targeting high-risk, emotionally disturbed youth in rural Alaska;
- health education for youth in five isolated counties in rural Idaho;
- an occupational health and safety program in rural Iowa; and
- a program to improve delivery of services related to mental health in rural Kentucky (Federal Office of Rural Health Policy, 1999).

The nearly 10-year commitment to communities through the Outreach Grant Program is the most direct evidence of the continuing interesting in bringing resources to populations.

Creating Incentives to Induce Providers to Rural Areas

Physicians practicing in underserved rural areas receive bonus payments from Medicare, equal to 10% of the normal payment. While some would argue that this program is ineffective in attracting and retaining health care professionals to shortage areas, much of the criticism is related to the expenditures made in urban areas (U.S. General Accounting Office, 1999). Others are less critical of the bonus payment policy and especially supportive of it for rural areas (Physician Payment Review Commission, 1994).

In addition to the National Health Service Corps and bonus payments for providers in underserved areas, the federal government supports specific programs in health professions training that are designed to increase the number of professionals locating practices in underserved areas. The 1976 Health Professions Education Assistance Act created Title VII of the Public Health Service Act, originally to increase the supply of primary care physicians. The range of programs funded has grown to include area health education centers (AHECs), rural interdisciplinary grants, dentistry, pubic health workforce development, and student assistance scholarship, loans, and programs (Ricketts, 1999). Title VIII of the Public Health Service Act supports programs for nurse training, including nurse anesthetists, who provide 65% of anesthetics administered annually and are the sole providers in 85% of rural hospitals (Ricketts, 1999). These health professions programs are intended to produce the types of professionals needed in underserved areas, especially for primary care services. Some programs are directly linked to rural health care delivery, such as family medicine training programs with rural rotations and rural training tracks, and the rural interdisciplinary training program. The AHEC program, started in 1972, is intended to expand geographic access to services by involving local education centers directly in training

health care professionals in their communities. The program also supports special initiatives AHECs may undertake, including improving services for particular populations. In 1996 AHEC programs provided community-based training experiences at 1,400 urban and rural areas (Ricketts, 1999).

A final example of federal dollars used to attract providers to rural areas is the designation of rural health clinics (RHCs). Under both Medicare and Medicaid regulations RHCs are paid for their services based on the costs they incur (as of 1999, states can pay 95% of cost). RHCs must be located in underserved areas and include either nurse practitioners, physician assistants, or nurse midwives on their staffs. In 1980 there were 285 clinics; by 1997 that number had increased to 3,538 (Ricketts, 1999). In the case of RHCs, dollars have attracted providers to underserved areas, although the net effects are difficult to measure. Many RHCs represent providers who were already working in those communities but achieved designation as RHCs, which enhanced their payment. Would they still be in those communities if not for the enhanced payments? There is no clear answer. Federal policymakers have assumed an impact in continuing to support this and other programs.

Programs Targeted to Specific Needs

The policy threads discussed so far have been efforts to support, in general, delivery of essential health care services in rural areas. A different policy thread is to fund programs that meet very specific needs. For example, in the 1970s Congress created and funded grant programs designed to improve the provision of emergency health care services in America, including rural areas. Grants were used to purchase equipment and to develop regional plans for trauma services. There have been efforts, since 1992, to develop a second generation of these grant programs, because much of the capital equipment purchased in the first round needs to be replaced and emergency medical care providers need assistance to maintain and improve their skills.

The Indian Health Service is an illustration of programming for a specific population, as are services provided through the Department of Veterans Affairs. Migrant health centers also target a specific population. Policymakers have, apparently, been able to conceive of the needs of particular populations more readily than they can the general population or larger subsets, such as all households with incomes below the median income in the community. Programs targeted to low-income households, Medicaid, and the new SCHIP, focus on "deserving poor"—primarily children and the elderly.

Other programs may target a specific need in rural health care. For example, the regional planning programs (comprehensive health planning and its successors) of the 1960s and 1970s funded efforts to introduce economic rationality into the distribution of resources. In the case of rural health, this meant integrating different services, such as emergency care to hospitals. Grants to fund research related to rural health care delivery are also examples of funding specific needs. Examples include placement and retention of appropriate health care professionals, access to services for the uninsured, appropriate distribution of mental health services, effects of changes in health care finance and organization on the delivery of services in rural areas, and development and functioning of rural health provider networks.

Pushing Toward Integrated Delivery Systems

The final policy thread to consider is a current emphasis on building systems of health care providers, under the implicit assumption that current financing and delivery philosophies require both minimum numbers of persons to serve and the ability to influence the spectrum of services provided throughout any episode of care. Providers are expected to share the financial risk associated with caring for patients enrolled in their practice, which requires spreading that risk across a large number of persons and managing patient care in a cost-effective manner. Proponents of risk-sharing believe provider networks are required, perhaps in all urban areas, and certainly in all rural areas.

The mantra of "managed competition," which was used in support of systemic reform in 1993 and 1994, continued beyond the failure of national health reform. The 1995–1999 iteration of managed competition, though, dropped

"managed" from consideration. For providers in rural America, networks are means of protecting their "turf" from "hostile takeover" by urban-based health care systems. Rural provider networks may be in a better position strategically to negotiate with urban-based networks. The faith in policies based on the benefits of competition combines with a contrasting fear of adverse consequences of competition to produce current federal health policies. The Medicare program has undergone significant change in pre-set payments, driven in recent years by a political philosophy that favors mimicking market-based strategies for saving money while improving choice among providers.

Policies that are intended to accelerate the development of competitive rural networks of health care providers include the network grants programs described earlier, administered by the ORHP and the Bureau of Primary Health Care. Another major grant program, the State Rural Hospital Flexibility Grant Program, was started in 1999. This new program is linked closely with the designation of a new category of hospital—the critical access hospital (CAH). Designated CAHs must have agreements with at least one other hospital for the purposes of referring and transporting patients and to enhance the quality of services provided by the network of at least two hospitals. In a background paper prepared for the ORHP, which administers the new program, its primary goal is said to be development of rural health networks, with grant funds to be used for information systems, quality assurance programs, and other activities to develop those networks (Wellever, 1999). The report also states the purpose of rural health networks: "Rural health networks are commonly used to reduce fragmentation of health services in a community, improve access to health services, eliminate unnecessary services, and support clinical and administrative services" (Wellever, 1999, p. 1).

A component part of the networks being supported by this latest federal grant program is a particular type of hospital, the CAH, for which the parameters are set forth in federal legislation. The attraction of being designated as a CAH is cost-based reimbursement from Medicare, which is likely to have a significant fiscal impact on those hospitals with high volumes (as a percent of total business) of outpatient visits from Medicare beneficiaries. The carrot, then, is a rather large one, and the result is widespread interest in this program. However, one simple principle underlying this program is inescapable: central policymakers and planners know what is best. The program, ironically, both creates new flexibility for rural health care providers (ability to qualify for Medicare payment as a different classification of hospital) and compels them to accept federally drafted parameters of what they do as providers. Examples include length-of-stay limitations (96 hour per patient annual average), limits on the number of acute care beds (15), and the requirement for an agreement with a larger hospital. Some of the parameters are optional, but likely to be used by CAHs, such as a staffing requirement for emergency room services that does not require that a physician be on call. These become the 'conditions of participation" in Medicare for CAHs, as compared to the more exhaustive and elaborate conditions for larger, full-service acute care hospitals.

Both the new program and continuing network grant programs illustrate a policy theme of supporting access to services by strengthening the financial condition and competitiveness of rural providers. A nuance to this policy, though, is that the federal government has committed its support to a favored model for delivering services locally—that local providers are linked with providers in other locations in a network configuration.

Summary

The historical examination of rural health policy reveals a change in emphasis from investments in a rural health infrastructure to investments in rural health care delivery systems. Some programs continue to focus on building infrastructure by inducing health care professionals to practice in rural underserved areas. Grant programs to support extending telemedicine into rural areas can also be characterized as building infrastructure, although they do not provide sufficient funds to finance the construction of a complete system. The funds that once flowed for building rural institutions such as hospitals have dried up. Transition grants, which could have been helpful in paying costs of converting

to differently configured providers, were available to rural hospitals for a few years, but those too have ended. The new Rural Hospital Flexibility Grant Program could be used to help with some of the costs of converting hospitals from full-service acute care to CAHs, including some capital expenses related to the network connections that would be needed. However, those funds are insufficient to provide significant capital grants to multiple hospitals in a given state (the largest first-year grant to any state was less than $600,000).

The move away from building an infrastructure is predicated on the implicit assumption that, with the exception of remaining needs for health care professionals, the infrastructure is in place. By the end of the 1990s, the emphasis in public policy shifted to making the best use of the providers we have in rural areas. Another way of expressing this change is to say that government grant programs in rural health are now directed toward sustaining what the earlier grant programs helped to build. Given that philosophical shift in public policy, the parallel shift from minimal influence on how dollars were used to more prescriptive grant programs is not surprising. Current investments in health care delivery systems are related to what health care policy analysts are saying is the environment within which those systems must survive. This favors supporting integrated systems serving large rural areas, sufficient to generate critical masses of persons to have clout in insurance contract negotiations. Larger networks are also thought to have an easier time supporting new systems of quality assurance and service delivery that require large capital investments. In short, the new federal programs are not designed to support small, solo providers. However, as will be seen in the next section, payment policies are not always consistent with this approach.

Payment Policy

Health policy analysts do not need "Deep Throat" to tell them to 'follow the money." Grant programs and other initiatives can be rendered meaningless by changes in payment policies controlled by public policy—Medicare, Medicaid, and insurance for public employees. The impact of payment policy in rural areas is most easily illustrated by focusing on Medicare policies. Medicare is the single most significant payer for patient services rendered by rural providers, accounting for over 40% of patient revenues for rural hospitals and 60% of inpatient acute care days; over 30% of patient revenues for rural physicians are generated by Medicare payments (Frenzen, 1997). Providers must be responsive to changes in payment policy and the incentives created to alter their practice styles and organizational configuration. In the most extreme cases, rural providers can be forced out of business by policies that reduce sharply their Medicare payments.

Medicare payments can be used to sustain rural delivery systems even when other sources of revenue are depleted. Policymakers, being responsive to the demands of their constituents for local access to essential services, may decide that Medicare will pay most of the full cost of sustaining rural providers, such as hospitals and primary care practices. Conversely, if policymakers are convinced that there are too many providers in rural communities they could use sharply reduced Medicare payment policies to force those providers unable to attract sufficient volume of other business to cease their operations. Medicare payments have become an even more important source of revenue for providers who have experienced the effects of signing agreements with commercial health plans to accept lower than historical charges and for those who are treating increasing numbers of persons without any health insurance. Instead of being able to recoup any shortfalls from public payers like Medicare through revenues from privately insured patients, providers in many areas are reversing the direction and looking to Medicare to recoup losses from other lines of business. In fiscally tight times, which most rural providers would say includes the present day, small changes in payment from a major source of revenue (Medicare) can influence major decisions.

Medicare policies (and Medicaid and employee insurance) are driven by two sometimes inconsistent imperatives. The first imperative is to pay a fair price for services so that Medicare beneficiaries have the same financial access to services as privately insured persons. The second imperative is to be fiscally prudent with public dollars and pay only a fair price for Medicare services. As discussed earlier in this chapter, since the 1970s public policies in general have been driven by concerns about levels of health expenditures. This has been especially true for Medicare, with an eye cast on the solvency of the trust fund that pays for Part A services (institutional care, including hospital services). The tension between these two policy objectives has been evident in policies since the early 1980s, as will be illustrated in the two subsections that follow.

Discrimination in Payment Policies: Prospective Payment and Risk Contracts

In 1982 Congress established a new system for Medicare payment to hospitals for inpatient services—the prospective payment system (PPS), based on diagnostic-related groups (DRGs). The PPS is based on the law of averages—that hospitals could be paid on the average length of stay among all hospitals for each of the 494 DRGs. The payment is based on a formula that includes the DRG, adjustments for wage differences across regions of the country, teaching status of the hospital, and the case mix of the hospital. When the hospital's costs exceed the predetermined payment, losses are incurred, but they are, in theory, balanced by the cases in which hospitals are able to keep costs below those used to calculate the payment. The expectation in 1982 was that hospitals could become more efficient providers and thus do at least as well under PPS as they had been doing under payment based on reasonable and allowable costs. Indeed, the early experience with inpatient PPS supported this notion, as hospital profit margins under PPS were initially positive by over 10% (Ricketts & Heaphy, 1999).

The experience for rural hospitals under PPS, though, has been less favorable since the inception of the new payment system. In an example of inequitable policy, rural hospitals were paid less than urban hospitals simply because they were rural. The cost data used to establish PPS rates indicated lower costs among rural hospitals, even after accounting for all other explanations. Therefore, Congress set two different rates, one rural and one urban. Consequently, in what should not be surprising, rural Medicare PPS margins have been consistently lower than those for all hospitals, and have been negative for several years of the PPS experience (Ricketts & Heaphy, 1999). The initial difference has been eliminated by congressional action, after a lawsuit was filed claiming discrimination against rural beneficiaries.

Another difference, though, is keeping rural inpatient hospital payments considerably lower than urban payments for the same DRGs. Part of the formula used to pay hospitals is an adjustment for the wages paid to health care workers in the area. A wage index is used as a multiplier in the formula; for urban hospitals it is 1.02, and for rural it is 0.79 (1997 data). As a result, the base payment per admission to urban hospitals in 1997 was $3,935, and for rural hospitals it was $3,416. After further adjustments for case mix, outliers (cases that exceed expected length of stay by two standard deviations) and medical education–disproportionate share (Medicaid and uncompensated care accounts for large percentage of business), the respective payments in 1997 were $7,281 for urban hospitals and $4,392 for rural hospitals (Medicare Payment Advisory Commission, 1998). A critical problem with the wage index is that it does not adjust appropriately for the mix of health care professionals (occupational mix) in the various hospitals. Hospitals use different complements of professionals to treat patients with exactly the same conditions. Rural hospitals use fewer professionals than do large teaching hospitals, creating the largest disparities that account for an index of 0.70 in rural areas of Mississippi and South Dakota versus 1.40 in urban areas of California and New York (Size, 1998). The wage index, calculated in this manner, is in effect double-paying hospitals for some expenses—for medical education (a positive multiplier for medical education and a higher wage index multiplier) and for treating high intensity cases (case mix multiplier and higher payment for certain DRGs, combined with the wage index multiplier). Further, because the wage index applies to an area and not to individual hospitals, hospitals with lower intensity cases and no teaching mission are benefitting from being in the same geographic area.

Both the problem of PPS separately classifying rural hospitals and the discrimination built into the wage index are illustrations of unintended consequences of public policy and the ease with which rural health delivery concerns are overlooked. The intent of both practices was, and is, to pay providers fairly but in a way that lowers Medicare expenditures from previous levels. The payment systems are developed in the context of all Medicare expenditures and achieve the desired results. However, since rural beneficiaries are only approximately 25% of the total, disproportionate effects on rural providers are not evident in the initial calculations. As they become evident, they are difficult to remedy because of continued focus on the more global policy decisions. For example, calling attention to low hospital margins, even negative margins, falls on deaf ears when the overall margin for all hospitals is increasing. Similarly, arguments about the wage index are difficult to raise to highly visible levels when the focus of the policy debates is on lowering expenditures and the approach to doing so is to force providers to be ever more efficient. A lawsuit helped to force the issue with regard to PPS base payments, and the issue of the wage index is high on the priority list for several major advocacy associations, including the National Rural Health Association and the Federation of Hospitals and Health Systems. There are proposals to deal with the wage index issue by removing teaching physicians and certified registered nurse anesthetists from the occupational mix, which have been supported by the Medicare Payment Advisory Commission. Nevertheless, the salience of the wage index issue continues to pale in comparison to the debates about levels of overall expenditures.

The tension between wanting to move the entire delivery system in the direction of more efficient provision of care and the desire to maintain whatever system exists in some rural areas has been apparent in PPS policy decisions. Special categories of hospitals were created that would receive exemption from the PPS, continuing to be paid based on their costs. These were sole community hospitals (more than 25 miles from nearest similar institution) and Medicare dependent hospitals (over 59% of inpatient days or discharges are accounted for by Medicare beneficiaries). Rural referral centers became another category of hospital, in their case eligible for the same base payment as comparable urban hospitals. Federal policy in the late 1980s and early 1990s recognized a need for special treatment of essential rural hospitals that provided only limited services in remote areas. The initial foray into this arena was approval of a special demonstration project, the Montana Medical Assistance Facility Program. Remote rural hospitals were permitted to meet Medicare conditions of participation by staffing with physician assistants or nurse practitioners and contracting out for some of their services. They were limited in what they could do, using a length-of-stay determination. This was the predecessor to the Essential Access Hospital (EACH)/Rural Primary Care Hospital Program (RPCH) in seven states, which included a provision that the small limited service hospital (RPCH) needed an agreement with a full service acute care hospital (EACH). The present-day iteration of this effort is the previously discussed critical access hospital (CAH) program.

Another source of disparity in urban and rural payments has been the Medicare payment to risk contracts (managed care, health maintenance organizations [HMOs]). These are payments to managed care organizations, an option begun in earnest with the 1982 Tax Equalization and Fiscal Responsibility Act Medicare provisions. Payment is calculated for each county in the United States and was initially based on the previous expenditures by Medicare on behalf of the beneficiaries living in that county. Of course, this meant that the payments have reflected the biases discussed above that favor urban over rural providers. In addition, they reflect differences in use of health care services by rural and urban beneficiaries that may be an issue of access to services and not of actual need for care. The county payment rate was recalculated annually, based on a three-year average. The net result of this system has been an extraordinary variation in rates across counties and volatility in rates from year to year. In 1997 the rates ranged from a low of $221 per member per month in two rural Nebraska counties to $767 in Richmond County (Staten Island), New York. Not surprisingly, there have been few plans offered in rural areas and very little enrollment of Medicare beneficiaries into managed care plans in rural counties. Researchers have pointed to the variation and volatility in rates as major reasons for differences in enrollment (Serrato, Brown, & Bergeron, 1995; McBride, Penrod, & Mueller, 1997). Once again, payment becomes a major incentive (or disincentive) for action. In counties with high-risk contract payment, managed care organizations have an economic incentive to seek Medicare enrollment, assuming they will have a net positive return on investment. In low payment counties the reverse is true; there is little reason to even establish a managed care plan. The discussion of payment changes in the BBA will illustrate the difficulty Congress has had in dealing with this issue.

The Balanced Budget Act of 1997

In 1997 Congress was faced with a large budget deficit and a political imperative to balance the budget by 2002. In addition, the Medicare Part A Trust Fund was forecasted to become insolvent by about 2008. To deal with both issues, the Balanced Budget Act of 1997 passed and was signed into law by President Clinton in August 1997. The BBA had mixed consequences for rural health care delivery, including in the same legislation some victories for rural health advocates and some major problems that would become even more obvious later.

Much of the initial reaction to the BBA focused on its first subtitle, the Medicare+Choice Program. The program would pay, on a prepaid capitated basis, any of the following types of health plans: HMOs, Preferred Provider Organizations, fee-for-service plans, provider sponsored organizations (PSOs), and medical savings accounts. The basis of payment was changed from the old system of annual per-county calculation to annual increases from the 1997 base, adjusted by establishing a minimum payment. Both the new array of choices and the new calculation of payment were perceived to be at least potentially beneficial for rural health systems (Mueller, 1997b). In the end, expectations would prove to be wide of the mark, in part because policies were enacted to address one or two considerations, such as payment, but did not (perhaps could not) address other contextual circumstances such as readiness to offer risk-bearing contracts.

The new option of most interest to rural health advocates and systems was the PSO. It was not immediately available in late 1997 because regulations were needed to determine such basic requirements as minimum solvency standards. A negotiated rule-making process was used, which meant that the advocates for PSOs were involved in developing the new regulations under the condition that they would support the outcome. PSO is a special Medicare designation, applying to health plans that are owned and operated by health care providers and that are unable to be licensed as HMOs by their states but do meet federal requirements as PSOs. After the regulations were published, it was apparent that the designation would be operative in only about half of the states. Hence, there can be provider-sponsored HMOs in the other states, but they would not be designated as PSOs. Therefore, while the current count of PSOs (as of the end of 1999) is two (in Albuquerque, New Mexico, and Bend, Oregon), there may be other provider-sponsored HMOs participating in Medicare+Choice. Having recognized that possibility, it is still easy to conclude that this particular option has not been as attractive as perhaps thought. A principal reason has been that rural providers have not been ready with the necessary capital to invest and business plans to operate an insurance plan (Kelly, 1998). There are, though, a few provider-based plans in the early stages of development, including Central Oregon Independent Health Services of Bend, Oregon and Gundersen Lutheran Health Plan of La Crosse, Wisconsin ("Clear Choice PSO," 1999). So, although not the promising vehicle for rapid movement into Medicare managed care some may have hoped, PSOs remain an option to consider for rural areas.

The changes in Medicare payment to risk contracts illustrate an important point in understanding public policy—to recognize the constraints imposed on significant change. In this instance the constraint is the requirement that change be budget-neutral. Obviously, increasing payment in rural counties requires getting the dollars from somewhere. The hope was that there would be sufficient increases in total spending for Medicare managed care so that the county payment increases would come from a disproportionate share of the increases in overall expenditures. However, Medicare spending has slowed since the BBA became law, leaving only enough resources to fund the two minimum payments guaranteed by the BBA—the new floor payment ($367) and the guaranteed minium 2% increase in all other counties. The promised blending of national and area rates was not started until January 1, 2000.

The changed payment rates illustrate another lesson in public policymaking: the importance of persistence and presence. Attention was first focused on the payment issue in 1995, in a broader context than just rural interests (urban rates vary by over $200 per member per month). During the debates preceding the BBA enactment in 1997, advocates for payment change worked with policy analysts to craft language changing the calculations, including simulations of various proposals (Rural Policy Research Institute Rural Health Panel, 1997). The team of analysts and staff worked on language throughout the process, up until immediately preceding final markup by the Senate Finance Committee. Final simulations showed that if the blended rates were fully implemented, in the year 2004 approximately 83% of all counties would be paid according to the blended formula, which would increase payment in rural counties, and 15% of all counties would be receiving the floor payment (McBride, 1997). In the closing stages of writing the final legislation, nuances of the formula were simulated. One critical concern was the ordering of steps involving removing payment for graduate medical education from the payment and calculating the 2% minimum increase. Basing the 2% on the payment prior to withholding graduate medical education payment would benefit the urban-based plans at the expense of rural plans. Because the total payments cannot change (budget neutrality), and because the 2% increases were guaranteed, payments in other counties would be reduced.

As was true for PSOs, the change in payment policy has proven to be insufficient to induce a lot of new activity in Medicare+Choice in rural areas. However, enrollment of rural beneficiaries into managed care plans has increased since the advent of the BBA, this despite the pullout of several plans from rural counties (McBride & Mueller, 1999). Two issues of context were not fully considered when the new payment policy was enacted and expectations were raised about enrollment. First, the payment levels represent increases from the previous amounts but may still be insufficient. The previous payments were based on what Medicare paid for care provided to beneficiaries, not the total cost of that care. Therefore, if health plans provide any benefits beyond the basic Medicare package, they are incurring costs not factored into the Medicare payment. Included in costs to plans but not Medicare are administrative expenses associated with medical management, advertising or marketing the plan, developing actuarial tables to facilitate calculating member premiums, and general administration. The second reality of the environment is that appropriate payment is a necessary, but not sufficient, condition to induce managed care plans into new territories. Other factors include: a system for medical management, a plan for marketing the plan, a financial plan leading to solvency and positive return on investment, a system for handling member grievances, a network of providers and a business plan for maintaining that network, and a reinsurance plan for high-cost cases. In short, changing Medicare payment was important for developing options for rural beneficiaries, but much other work is also needed.

The BBA included other measures important to advances in rural health care delivery systems. The Medicare Rural Hospital Flexibility Program and associated CAH designation was created by this legislation. The Medicare-dependent small rural hospital program was restored and extended to 2001. Medicare payments were established for telemedicine services (in shortage areas only) and for services rendered by physician assistants and nurse practitioners as payments independent of physician payment. These policies are examples of modest gains for rural health delivery that can be secured as part of much more comprehensive legislation.

The most significant payment changes made in the BBA were ones not sought by rural health advocates—reductions in future payment to providers paid through "traditional" Medicare, fee-for-service. Because rural providers do not have much, if any, Medicare business through any other payment, the reductions affect them "full force." Further, because rural hospitals are more dependent than urban hospitals on Medicare payments for their total revenues, any reduction in payment will have a disproportionate impact on them. For example, Medicare outpatient payments account for 9.5% of revenues for rural hospitals, compared with 7.1% for urban hospitals (Mohr, Blanchfield, Chen, Evans, & Franco, 1998). The original Congressional Budget Office estimate of savings achieved through these changes was $100 billion during the years 1998–2002. At the time the BBA passed, most analysts and advocates were aware there would of course be some impact from the reductions, but in late 1997 the very dramatic impact on rural providers had not yet been documented.

The potential for the BBA to cripple the rural health infrastructure because of its impact on already precarious financial conditions became the focus of BBA dialogue in 1999. For rural hospitals, the important point made in policy analysis was that of the cumulative impact of a number of reductions in payment:

> The impact of the changes in inpatient prospective payment can account for as little as only approximately 1/3 of the reduced Medicare revenue predicted for rural hospitals. . . . The net impact on rural hospitals is the sum of a number of different payment changes that affect PPS hospitals. (Mueller & McBride, 1999, p. 4)

As many as 12 different payment changes made by the BBA could affect the same rural hospital. In a February 1999 report on this issue (Mueller & McBride, 1999), the Rural Policy Research Institute's Rural Health Panel cited the following estimated effects: $32 million in Missouri rural hospitals in 1998, $45.3 million in 1999; $598.7 million (7.4% of anticipated revenues) for the years 1998–2002 in eight rural California congressional districts; and for one rural hospital in Wisconsin, 6.1% of Medicare reimbursement, 17.3% of net income on an annual basis. Nor are hospitals the only rural providers affected. Independent home health agencies have been affected by sharp reductions in payment during two years of an interim payment system before a new prospective payment system is put in place. Federally qualified health centers (including community and migrant health centers) and RHCs could see drops in their revenues if the BBA provision allowing states to discontinue cost-based payment for Medicaid services is fully implemented.

By late 1999, the adverse effects of the BBA were very apparent. Projections completed by two different accounting firms under contract with trade associations (American Hospital Association and Federation of Hospitals and Health Systems) indicated operating margins for small rural hospitals would be negative at the time the BBA is fully implemented, with the most dramatic effects coming from changes in outpatient payment (Rural Policy Research Institute Rural Health Panel, 1999). Even though staff of the Medicare Payment Advisory Commission found analytical problems with the work of one of the accounting firms, their memo of May 17, 1999, echoed the now-familiar theme: "Policymakers should consider the combined effects of all Medicare payment policies on hospitals' financial performance, rather than payment policies for inpatient care alone" (Rural Policy Research Institute Rural Health Panel, 1999, p. 6). A special campaign by the American Hospital Association provided specific examples of decisions being made by rural hospitals affecting access to services, such as closing skilled nursing facilities, reducing services in rural health clinics, and reducing home health visits (Rural Policy Research Institute Rural Health Panel, 1999). A special study of six rural hospitals with reputations for sound business management found (through independent analysis of cost reports) that in five of the six hospitals net profitability declined sharply from 1997 to 1999, by as much as 515%, and that losses in four of the hospitals for the years 1999–2002 would range from $438,000 to $1,278,000 (WWAMI, 1999).

Two important lessons in policy development should be learned from the experiences of financial difficulties triggered by the BBA. First, ways should be found to convert unanticipated consequences into anticipated consequences. In this instance, Congress acted to reduce Medicare spending by cutting projected expenditures in areas where the aggregate data indicated there was room to reduce (because of high net margins in Medicare PPS). What was not known was that the cuts that looked reasonable in the aggregate were not tolerable for a subset of hospitals. The second lesson is related: reliable in-

formation is needed before the policy is enacted. In this instance the consequences were unknown because the analysis had not been completed to indicate the problems. Further, even in 1999 as the pressure intensified to provide relief from the BBA reductions, information was not readily available about the outcomes of the changes. Instead, the information being used was, for the most part, either projections of what would happen or information about actions by providers that could have been due to a variety of circumstances, including the BBA payment reductions.

The BBA RefinementAct of 1999

In November 1999 President Clinton signed into law the Medicare, Medicaid, and SCHIP Balanced Budget Refinement Act of 1999. Congress and the President acted to restore approximately $17 billion, over five years, of what would otherwise be reduced payments to providers. In doing so, the Refinement Act reaffirms a policy choice to keep providers in place in rural communities (resources to people) but also continues the theme of developing larger systems for delivering care and matching payment incentives to a general fiscal environment in which providers are not paid based on charges they submit.

Policies to slow the implementation of conversions to new payment systems will mean continuation of cost-based reimbursement for many rural providers. Small rural hospitals (100 or fewer beds), for example, will be paid based on costs for outpatient services (assuming that payment is more than what would be paid under prospective payment) until January 2004. The Medicare Dependent Hospital program, which includes cost-based payment, is extended to fiscal year 2005, and sole community hospitals will see their inpatient payment rebased to more recent hospital cost-reporting periods (which for most will increase inpatient payment). In addressing the issue of cumulative impact of cuts in multiple payment streams, the Refinement Act restores some cuts in payment for hospice care, durable medical equipment, and therapy services. A 15% reduction in payment for home health services, scheduled to take effect in 2000, is delayed until one year after the implementation of a new prospective payment system. The scheduled phaseout of the requirement that states, in their Medicaid programs, reimburse health centers and rural health clinics based on costs, is also delayed.

Changes were made in the Medicare Rural Hospital Flexibility Program that make CAH designation a more attractive option to small rural hospitals. The previous rule that inpatient stays could not exceed 96 hours was changed not to exceed an annual 96-hour average, and eligibility to participate in the program was expanded to include for-profit hospitals and hospitals that have closed or converted to a health clinic or health center within the past 10 years. CAH designation brings with it cost-based reimbursement for both inpatient and outpatient services.

The net effect of the Refinement Act alterations of payment polices set by the BBA is to offer choices to rural hospitals for at least the next four years, all of which include cost-based reimbursement: CAH designation, sole community hospital status, Medicare Dependent Hospital status, or full-service acute care hospital (the last choice would mean PPS for inpatient care) (Mueller, 1999). However, that same Refinement Act clearly continues on the path of changing Medicare payment systems to reach perceived conformity with more general practices in health care finance. Studies are mandated to examine the appropriateness of categories of special payments for rural hospitals and evaluate the effects of phasing out cost-based reimbursement for federally qualified health centers and RHCs (Mueller, 1999). Once those studies are completed, cost-based reimbursement will likely end for most of the affected rural providers.

The Refinement Act also continued the congressional push toward establishing managed care as a choice for all Medicare beneficiaries, including those living in rural areas. Changes designed to encourage more plans to market to rural beneficiaries included a two-year extension of cost-based contracts, bonus payments for entering previously unserved counties, flexibility to tailor benefits for distinct services, and changing quality assurance requirements for preferred provider organization plans. Although these changes are in most instances targeted to rural areas, they are rather modest and unlikely,

by themselves, to induce entry of plans into new areas (Mueller, 1999).

Summary

Medicare is sometimes fondly (or not so fondly) called "the big gorilla" affecting rural health delivery. Because Medicare payment is a significant percentage of patient income for rural providers, changes in Medicare payment policies do influence the actions of those providers. Used in a constructive, targeted manner, payment policies can help develop a rural health care delivery system that assures local access to appropriate services. Conversely, if Medicare payment policies are designed to wield a heavy club to force providers to "be more efficient" and survive with less than expected revenues, the consequences for small rural providers can be devastating. Recent major policy initiatives, the BBA and the Refinement Act, are the products of a legislative struggle to balance the need for access to rural services and the policy objective of containing Medicare expenditures.

No one can say with any certainty what the Medicare payment policy of the future will be. What is becoming apparent, though, is that the cost-based systems of the past are just that—from the past and not characteristic of the future. That said, payment policies are likely to lead to a reconfiguration of the delivery system. If proponents of Medicare+Choice are correct in their assumptions and successful in continued legislative policy designed to induce more beneficiaries into new health plans, rural beneficiaries will have choices, whether wanted or not.

Payment policies do seem to be evolving in a manner consistent with the threads of public policy presented earlier. Initially, payment was determined by the charges of the provider, an approach of having finances support the location of health care providers. However, since the overwhelming majority of providers would not of their own choosing locate in rural areas, this approach could be labeled "benign neglect." That is, the policy itself is neutral vis-à-vis getting resources to the people or people to the resources, but the consequence, at best, is to do nothing to improve the situation for rural residents. As the problems of sustaining a health care delivery infrastructure in rural areas have become more obvious, payment policies were altered to create special categories of providers who would be paid differently. For example, sole community hospital became a special category under the prospective payment system, and now critical access hospital is another special category. Rather than devising payment formulas that can differentiate types of providers in a manner to account for issues of low volume, geographic isolation, and higher than average dependency on Medicare payment, a path of "policy by exception" has been chosen. That trend in policy is now in conflict with the newest approach, to favor large systems that can treat a range of conditions throughout any episode of illness. Resolving the tension between sustaining the financial viability of essential rural providers and creating incentives to develop larger systems of care is the policy dilemma of the next few years.

The Future of Rural Health Policy

The short-term future in rural health policy is likely to be characterized by considerable confusion. The roles of local hospitals, physicians, clinics, health centers, and long-term care providers will evolve into something other than what they have been historically. During the evolution different models may be tried, and in some rural settings the roles may not change all that much but will probably be labeled differently than they were in 1999. Public policies will influence the directions taken in health care delivery in rural communities, ideally, in a manner that is consonant with those overall changes that optimize the health of rural residents.

Healthy Providers, Healthy Communities

Public policies can be expected to continue supporting essential providers in local communities, bringing resources to the people. However, in doing so, policies will also continue the emphasis implicit in the Medicare Rural Hospital Flexibility Program that the federal government is willing to support only those institutional providers who fit a predetermined mode of what is appropriate for the types of communities they serve. This policy direction is im-

plicit in the studies required by the Refinement Act, to assess the appropriateness of paying different classifications of hospitals (such as sole community hospitals, Medicare dependent hospitals, and rural referral centers) differently and to define the roles of rural health care providers.

Steps taken in the BBA and the Refinement Act indicate a move toward health professions policies also directed to support local providers, but in the mold deemed appropriate. Nonphysician primary care providers, including physician assistants, nurse practitioners, and certified nurse midwives, are now eligible for direct payment from Medicare. These professions are also the ones that will staff the emergency rooms of CAHs and will continue to be used in RHCs. Public support for health professions training programs is taking a turn toward supporting those programs that meet the need for health care professionals in underserved, including rural, areas. The BBA set limits on the number of graduate medical residents that the Medicare program would continue to support, and the Refinement Act modified those rules to favor training programs based in, or serving, rural areas. The next steps in health professions policies will be ones that challenge the role of Medicare in supporting graduate medical education and ones that redefine the roles of various professionals. Through 1999 there has been a proliferation of medical specialties, including specialization among nurses and physician assistants. The appropriate roles for all of these professionals, especially as health care expenditures continue to be a concern, will become issues for state governments (licensure and certification), courts (antitrust) and the federal government (payment) to resolve. The debates should include concern for securing the appropriate professionals as practitioners in rural communities.

Policies should be based on what services are needed locally for rural residents, and how those can best be provided. To illustrate, consider general surgery. Many procedures do not require extensive hospitalization (indeed, many are now done with no hospitalization) and can be performed by general practitioners. Health professions policies affecting this include licensing and certifying the appropriate personnel, including general surgeons, primary care physicians who can complete many procedures, medical anesthesiologists, and certified nurse anesthetists. In much of rural America certified nurse anesthetists are more likely to be used than medical anesthesiologists (Cromwell, 1999). For health care institutions, limited service hospitals (CAHs) should be capable of supporting general surgery. They need not have a full-time 24-hour medical staff to do so; nor would they need extensive capacity in equipment associated with more extensive procedures. If the limited number of inpatient beds (15) becomes an issue, that may be an indication that volume is sufficient to support a full-service hospital accepting prospective payment instead of cost-based reimbursement. Payment policies will be very important if cost-effective general surgery is to be offered in rural communities. Cromwell (1999) identified problems in the Medicare payment policies that favor use of medical anesthesiologists rather than certified nurse anesthetists, despite the recognition that the two are interchangeable for most procedures, and certainly for those that would be provided by small rural hospitals. Public policy would need to facilitate, rather than inhibit, using the less costly professional in appropriate settings.

In addition to structuring payment and other policies to support the appropriate health care providers for rural communities, public policies will continue to evolve in a manner to provide the resources those providers need. In the 1940s, the need was for capital to build hospitals and other facilities. In the 1960s to the 1980s, the need was for incentives for health professions training programs to train, in greater quantity, professionals for underserved areas. In the 1990s, the need was for the initial investment capital to adjust to changes in health care finance delivery, as in preparing to participate in health care delivery networks and comply with the claims-reporting and other administrative practices associated with managed care. That need will continue, now combined with a need to link directly with providers in remote locations. Management information systems and other communications can link the work of tracking a patient throughout an entire episode of care, facilitating the job of the primary care provider. In addition, advances in telemedicine will facilitate delivering an increasing array of services locally, such as counseling for families with children with attention deficit disorder.

Policies supporting local providers will also be enhancing the health of local residents. This will be evident in any measures of quality of life, which include both physical condition and ability to function at the highest possible level of independence. Local providers of community-based services (such as meals on wheels programs) and long-term care services (such as assisted living) will be part of the mix that should be supported by public policy. In the case of assisted living facilities and home health services, payment policies in Medicare and Medicaid would need to be designed to allow for adequate payment to low-volume providers. When primary care, limited surgical services, long-term care, and other services are provided locally, residents should be more likely to obtain preventive and consistent care associated with treating maladies at early stages and enhancing their daily lives.

Appropriate Systems of Care, Optimum Health Outcomes

Health care providers, insurance plans, and policymakers all recognize the need to care for people rather than illnesses. Doing so first requires explicit recognition of the objectives of policies, in this instance improved health outcomes. Further, health outcomes are not defined simply as clinical recovery from specific episodes of illness but instead as improvements in quality of life. The operational definition of health outcomes includes measures of ability to return to normal routines or to a routine the person affected finds at least satisfactory. In addition to this focus on outcomes for individuals, another objective in public policy, and for many health insurance plans, is improvement of the health of communities. For some purposes the community is defined as the people enrolled in a particular health plan, and it is measured by applying indicators developed by the National Committee for Quality Assurance. In public policy, the community is more broadly defined to include all residents of a certain geographic area, whether or not they are enrolled in a particular health plan.

What are the implications of these objectives for rural health care delivery? Achieving acceptable results requires coordinated activities of several levels of medical care with other services that also contribute to the quality of life of affected persons. Initially, services need to be coordinated throughout the spectrum of medical care, including primary care, specialty care, and postacute care (such as therapy services). A high-quality result could occur following a surgical procedure, but the outcome could be in jeopardy without adequate postsurgical therapy or medication. For example, knee surgery will not improve outcomes without appropriate physical therapy, and heart surgery may require appropriate medication to sustain an improved outcome. In both instances lasting improvements in quality of life may require paying attention to the lifestyles of affected persons beyond the medical attention as they learn to adjust daily activities. As considerations of health care broaden beyond what is done through specific medical procedures to what contributes to the overall health of populations, nonmedical services such as community outreach programs become important parts of the total system of health care delivery in any community. The rural implication, then, is to focus on systems of health care delivery, not individual pieces (such as having a primary care physician in town).

There are two approaches that will continue to be used in public policy to address the need to develop systems of health care delivery. The first approach is to focus on the weak links in the present system. Although having a local physician is not sufficient to meet the health care needs of a community, access to primary care is a necessary condition. Therefore, policies focused on delivering services in shortage areas continue to be high priorities in many rural areas. Similarly, if communications between the local primary care provider and referral physicians elsewhere are inadequate, a policy initiative will address that link. However, this example also illustrates the reason for rapid transition to the second approach—supporting integrated systems of health care delivery. Public policies will increasingly favor investments in systems of health care, rather than incremental improvements in component parts. Even

when parts of the system are addressed, the precedent set by the CAH program can be expected to continue, and be strengthened. That is, specific programs that will continue to include local hospital services will be supported only if they are part of health care networks.

Public policies will continue to promote the development of rural networks, both directly and indirectly. The direct efforts are represented by network grant programs, including the one administered by ORHP. Those programs may evolve in three directions. First, the length of grants may stretch to as much as five years. Developing integrated networks in rural areas has proven to be quite challenging. Providers in multiple communities have to learn first to trust each other and then to work together. This can prove more difficult than integrating providers who are in the same metropolitan area. Often, all of the rural providers involved also have to learn how to function as a system, with new uses of information and new ways of thinking about coordinating services. The second direction will be to bring urban-based partners into rural health care network projects. Doing so will address needs to provide care throughout the entire continuum of services and provide capital from urban-based providers to adopt new systems of care management. The third direction will be to encourage networks to include service providers outside of the medical care community. As the focus continues to be on community health, other service providers will play a key role in the success of networks.

Influencing the Future of Rural Health Policy

The appropriate close to this discussion of rural health policy is to address the question: "How do we improve on what we have?" Policy objectives, as described in the previous section, are important, but actions are needed to realize the best of those alternatives. For action, both analysis and advocacy are needed.

Researchers and analysts need to be engaged in the policy process, helping to define problems and find alternative solutions. Analysis can make a difference in policy development, but only if those producing the analysis are in close, constant contact with policymakers. This will include assistance in drafting legislative alternatives and forecasting the effects of those alternatives (Schauffler & Wilkerson, 1997). As new payment systems are developed and implemented, research and analysis relevant to rural health delivery is especially important. Claims of special problems in financing rural health care delivery need to be supported by results of empirical research. The studies required by the Refinement Act are opportunities for research findings specific to rural health to make a difference. They are also potential examples of the failure of rural health researchers and policy advocates should they be executed without any consideration for application to rural facilities and delivery systems. That some of the studies already require rural research is a testament to the growing recognition of policy advocates and allies in the legislative process that research results unique to rural circumstances are necessary to inform policy. With advance research, policymakers can act proactively to promote the interests of rural health delivery instead of reacting to protect those same interests from excessive damage.

With the help of research and analysis, rural health advocates enter the next decade in the best position they have had in national politics for some time. With a renewed strength in the U.S. Senate Rural Health Caucus and the U.S. House Rural Health Coalition, members of Congress acted in behalf of rural health with many of the provisions of the Refinement Act. Advocacy associations, led by the National Rural Health Association, have built their strength in recent years and their presence is obvious in national policies. The future is promising for national policy in rural health care delivery, thanks to improvements in research and use of the resulting analysis, responsiveness of the organized interests in Congress, and the activities of the advocacy associations (Mueller, 1997a).

As this chapter is written, the 106th Congress is entering its final year, a time during which major health care policy issues will be debated but probably not resolved. Because these issues are not likely to be resolved in this Congress, they are the ones that should be gaining the attention of researchers now and for which advocates should be prepared to argue the rural perspective. Three issues are dominating the health policy debates, and each presents the difficult problem of balancing competing political pressures.

One of the issues is determining the future of the Medicare program. In the BBA of 1997 Congress created the Bipartisan Commission on the Future of Medicare, which while unable to reach the required supermajority to support a specific proposal, did develop a plan that would redesign the Medicare program. That proposal, using an approach characterized as premium support (as compared to defining benefits and paying any premium) has been introduced by several U.S. senators (Breaux, D-LA; Frist, R-TN; Hagel, R-NE; Kerrey, D-NE) for consideration in the second half of the 106th Congress. President Clinton introduced a competing proposal, and others are likely to follow. A debate has developed about the approaches that should be used to guide the Medicare program. The alternatives are defining a set of health care benefits and paying whatever a reasonable cost is for those benefits (the current system is characterized this way), or the "fixed benefits" approach; determining what government can afford for Medicare and offering all eligible persons a stipend (voucher) to purchase whatever services they can with that amount of money, or the "fixed contribution" approach; or allowing a market place of competing insurance plans to develop, under rules defining minimum benefits and other guarantees related to quality of care, and have government pay either the lowest premium charged in any given area or some other amount based on the range of premiums charged—the "premium support" approach. Regardless of the approach that gains favor, any comprehensive legislative action regarding Medicare creates an opportunity to bolster the rural health care delivery system through changes in Medicare payment policies. As was made obvious by previous discussion in this chapter, Medicare can influence the location of health care providers, the nature of services offered by institutional providers (such as hospitals), and the ability to sustain services in sparsely populated rural areas.

A second policy debate, which may result in some legislation as early as 2000, but not reach resolution, is to assure Americans that medical decisions are made based on quality of care considerations first, and economics later. During 1999 this issue revolved around the quality of care provided by HMOs, and in particular whether care suffered because of zeal to save costs. So-called patient protection legislation has been developed and debated. The larger issue, though, is using public policy as a means of monitoring quality and enforcing standards applicable to any delivery of care. In late 1999 the Institute of Medicine issued an early release of a study of errors that occur in U.S. hospitals, and the rate astounded many. In the next few years the concern for quality of care will likely broaden to include all settings. As that occurs there will be opportunities to support research into the quality of care in rural areas and to advocate for rural health centers of excellence in primary care.

The third major issue is a recurring theme in recent years: providing financial access to care for the uninsured. The number of uninsured in the United States has increased every year during the 1990s, despite a growing economy and shrinking unemployment rate, to over 41 million by the end of 1998. The presidential election campaigns of 2000 include proposals to deal with this problem, and proposals are being prepared for introduction as legislation in the second half of the 106th Congress. Given the previous attempts and failures to develop comprehensive approaches to health care reform in the United States, most recently with the fall of the Health Security Act proposal by President Clinton in 1994, there may be some tendency among policy advocates to devote little energy to this next round of debates. However, general policy debates can present opportunities for modest legislative victories. Earlier health reform debates preceded the development of SCHIP as part of the BBA of 1997, and the Health Insurance Portability and Affordability Act of 1995. In the early stages of the debates about extending insurance coverage to the currently uninsured population, research results will be needed to inform policymakers about any particularly rural problems in securing insurance (for example, problems related to small business in rural areas and seasonal employment). The task of advocates then becomes one of being sure that any policy remedies to the problem of uninsurance address those rural concerns.

Two final thoughts close this chapter on developments in rural health policy, one reflective and one prescriptive. The reflection: the 1990s have been the best of times and the worst of times in rural health delivery. They have been the best of times because the influence of rural health advocates on policy development has never been stronger. The community of analysts and advocates has more breadth (numbers) and depth (solid information and analysis) than ever before. Conversely, these have been the worst of times because the emphasis of the last 15 years on cost containment has resulted in actions that threaten the financial viability of rural providers. Policies enacted to apply to all providers, based on aggregate examinations of effects, have had a disproportionate impact on rural providers. The strength of the rural advocacy has blunted some of the impact, but the scars remain. The balance of best and worst remains uncertain as of the time this chapter is written.

The prescription: rural health policy needs to "put people first." Many of the concerns in rural health policy have been cast in terms of the delivery system and health care providers. As we move into the next round of policy discussions that emphasis needs to be recast to start with the interests of the people being served, and then the institutions and practitioners providing that service. Only by thinking of the people served can policymakers, advocates, and providers get past thinking about protecting interests and into thinking about the health outcomes of individuals and communities. Hospitals may need to be reconfigured, not because Medicare payment drives them unwillingly to do so but because the communities are best served by a different type of provider. A different institution might be able to sharpen its focus on what it does well without trying to maintain services better performed elsewhere. Integrated systems are needed to promote community interests, and only incidentally to protect the financial interests of participating providers and organizations. Policies based on the needs of the people will be more easily advocated and defended in future debates than those based on sustaining a delivery system only for the purposes of keeping existing providers where they are. As debates based on how to finance an increasingly expensive Medicare program intensify, policy must be based on the needs of beneficiaries; any other basis will be insufficient. Of course we should expect close linkage between the welfare of the rural populace and the welfare of rural providers, but the starting point of the policy dialogue has to be the people.

References

Bauer, J. C. (1987). The prospects for rural health. *HealthSpan, 4,* 14–17.

Bureau of Primary Health Care, U.S. Department of Health and Human Services. (1999). Migrant health center program. Washington, DC: Author (December 27, 1999); http://www.bphc.hrsa.dhhs.gov.

Clear Choice PSO expands in high desert, other provider plans entering program. (1999, December 20). *News and Strategies for Managed Medicare & Medicaid, 5,* 1–3.

Cromwell, J. (1999). Barriers to achieving a cost-effective workforce mix: Lessons from anesthesiology. *Journal of Health Politics, Policy and Law, 24,* 1331–1363.

Federal Office of Rural Health Policy. (1999). *Rural health outreach grantee directory, 1998.* Washington, DC: Author (January 4, 2000); http://www.nal.usda.gov/orhp/orgrante.htm.

Frenzen, P. D. (1997). How will measures to control Medicare spending affect rural communities? *Issues in Rural Health 734.* Washington, DC: United States Department of Agriculture, Agriculture Information Bulletin.

Harriman, J. (1999). *Facts about the rural population of the United States.* Beltsville, MD: Rural Information Center Health Service, National Agricultural Library (November 23, 1999); http://www.nalusda.gov:80/ric/richs/stats.htm.

Kelly, M. P. (1998). Is your organization operationally ready to be a Medicare PSO? *Healthcare Financial Management, June,* 39-41.

McBride, T. D. (1997). Implementation of the Balanced Budget Act of 1997: Impact on Medicare capitation rates and issues for policy consideration. (Rural Policy Brief 1[4]). Columbia, MO: Rural Policy Research Institute.

McBride, T. D., & Mueller, K. J. (1999). *The Medicare+Choice Program: Tracking the response to the Balanced Budget Act through fall 1999.* Manuscript currently under review, available from the Nebraska Center for Rural Health Research, Omaha.

McBride, T. D., Penrod, J. D., & Mueller, K. (1997). Volatility in Medicare AAPCC rates: 1990–1997. *Health Affairs, 16,* 172–180.

Medicare Payment Advisory Commission. (1998, March). *Report to the Congress: Medicare payment policy. Volume I: Recommendations.* New York: Author.

Mohr, P. E., Blanchfield, B. B., Chen, C. M., Evans, W. N. & Franco, S. J. (1998, July). *The financial dependence of rural hospitals on outpatient revenue.* (Working paper). Bethesda, MD: Project Hope Walsh Center for Rural Health Analysis.

Mueller, K. (1988). Federal programs do expire: The case of health planning. *Public Administration Review, 48,* 719–725.

Mueller, K. (1997a). Rural health care delivery and finance: Policy and politics. In T. J. Litman & L. S. Robins (Eds.), *Health politics and policy* (pp. 402–418). Albany, NY: Delmar Publishers.

Mueller, K. (1997b). *Rural implications of the Balanced Budget Act of 1997: A rural analysis of the health policy provisions.* (Policy paper P97-10). Columbia, MO: Rural Policy Research Institute.

Mueller, K. (1999). *Rural implications of the Medicare, Medicaid, and SCHIP Balanced Budget Refinement Act of 1999.* (Policy paper P99-11). Columbia, MO: Rural Policy Research Institute. December 8.

Mueller, K., & McBride, T. (1999). *Taking Medicare into the 21st Century: Realities of a post BBA world and implications for rural health care.* (Policy paper P99-2). Columbia, MO: Rural Policy Research Institute. February 10.

National Health Service Corps. (1999). *Our history.* Bureau of Primary Health Care, U. S. Department of Health and Human Services. Washington, DC: Author. (December 27, 1999); http://www.bphc.hrsa.dhhs.gov/nhsc/Pages/about_nhsc/3A5_history.htm.

National Rural Health Association. (1992). Rural health: The story of outreach. Kansas City, MO: National Rural Health Association.

Office of Technology Assessment. (1990). *Health care in rural America.* (OTA-H-434). Washington, DC: U.S. Government Printing Office.

Patel, K., & Rushefsky, M. E. (1999). *Health care politics and policy in America* (2nd ed.). New York: M. E. Sharpe.

Physician Payment Review Commission. (1994). *Annual report to Congress.* Washington, DC: U.S. Government Printing Office.

Pullum, J. D., Sanddal, N. D., & Obbink, K. (1999). Training for rural prehospital providers: A retrospective analysis from Montana. *Prehospital Emergency Care, 3,* 231-8.

Ricketts, T. C. III. (1999). Federal programs and rural health. In T. C. Ricketts III (Ed.), *Rural health in the United States* (pp. 61–69). New York: Oxford University Press.

Ricketts, T. C. III, & Heaphy, P. E. (1999). Hospitals in

rural America. In T. C. Ricketts III (Ed.), *Rural health in the United States* (pp. 101–112). New York: Oxford University Press.

Rollins, S. (1999). Keeping the country in rural medicine. *Rural Health FYI, 21,* 26–29.

Rosenblatt, R. A. (1991). Part 1: Historical and theoretical underpinnings. *The Journal of Rural Health, 7,* 473–591.

Rural Policy Research Institute Rural Health Panel. (1997). *The rural implications of Medicare AAPCC capitation payment changes: Background assessment and simulation results of key legislative proposals.* (Congressional Briefing Document P97-8). Columbia, MO: Rural Policy Research Institute.

Rural Policy Research Institute Rural Health Panel. (1999). Implementation of the provisions of the Balanced Budget Act of 1997: Critical issues for rural health care delivery (Policy paper P99-5). Columbia, MO: Rural Policy Research Institute.

Schauffler, H. H., & Wilkerson, J. (1997). National health care reform and the 103rd Congress: The activities and influence of public health advocates. *American Journal of Public Health, 87,* 1107–1112.

Serrato, C., Brown, R. S., & Bergeron, J. (1995). Why do so few HMOs offer Medicare risk plans in rural areas? *Health Care Financing Review, 17,* 85–97.

Size, T. (1998). Medicare sausage from rural road kill.

RWHC eye on health. Sauk City: Rural Wisconsin Health Cooperative (December 29, 1999); www.rwhc.com.

Starr, P. (1982). The social transformation of American medicine. New York: Basic Books.

Talbott, T. H. (1998, September-October). Dr. Smith stays home and makes a world of difference in the lives of his patients. *Rural Health FYI, 5,* 20–21.

U.S. General Accounting Office. (1999). *Physician shortage areas: Medicare incentive payments not an effective approach to improve access.* (Report to Congressional Requesters. GAO/HEHS-99-36). Washington, DC: U.S. General Accounting Office.

Welch, H. G. (1991). Readmission following surgery in Washington State rural hospitals. *Rural Health Working Paper Series* (Working paper #10). Seattle: WAMI Rural Health Research Center.

Wellever, A. (1999). *Organizing for achievement: Three rural network case studies.* Background paper prepared for the Medicare Rural Hospital Flexibility Grant Program. Washington, DC: Federal Office of Rural Health Policy (January 4, 2000); www.nal.usda.gov/orhp/complete.htm.

WWAMI Rural Health Research Center. (1999). *An initial report on the impact of the Balanced Budget Act on small rural hospitals.* Seattle: University of Washington.

2

Methodological Issues in Rural Health Research and Care

SANA LOUE AND HAL MORGENSTERN

Numerous calls have been made to increase the quantity and the quality of research on rural health and rural health care (Cohen, Braden, & Ward, 1993). A cogent response to this plea necessarily mandates greater attention to various methodological issues and objectives. We examine three general issues. The first is the estimation of disease parameters, such as disease frequency or exposure effects in rural populations—that is, focusing attention on people who live in rural areas and on the important health problems of these populations.

The second is the comparison of disease frequency or health indicators for rural and urban populations, whereby rural–urban is treated as the main exposure (independent) variable and urban–rural differences are explained in terms of specific risk factors for the health conditions under study—that is, treating these risk factors as covariates.

The third is the comparison of the "exposure" effects for rural and urban populations—that is, treating rural–urban as a potential modifier of the exposure effect (also called interaction).

SANA LOUE • Department of Epidemiology and Biostatistics, School of Medicine, Case Western Reserve University, Cleveland, Ohio 44106-4945. **HAL MORGENSTERN** • Department of Epidemiology, School of Public Health, University of California at Los Angeles, Los Angeles, California 90095-1772.

Handbook of Rural Health, edited by Loue and Quill. Kluwer Academic/Plenum Publishers, New York, 2001.

Defining Rural Health

Perhaps one of the most critical methodological issues in rural health is the lack of consensus about what constitutes "rural." Using varying definitions across studies may result in inconsistent findings that are not easily compared or translated into policy or practice. As Hewitt (1989, p. 1) noted, "It is difficult to quantify rural health problems and to make informed policy decisions without a clear definition of what and where 'rural' areas are." The Task Force of the Rural Elderly of the House of Representatives' Select Committee on Aging (U.S. House of Representatives, 1983) took note of the inability to interpret research on rural populations due to the lack of a consistent definition of what constitutes a rural population.

Lack of a uniform definition may impede not only our understanding of the research findings related to rural health but also our ability to design studies to address the issues identified. For instance, if our operational definition of rural–urban is inappropriate to the research question under investigation, or if it is not applied uniformly across the total population, we may unknowingly introduce misclassification bias into our study, resulting in an over- or underestimation of disease frequency. The following discussion provides an overview of the inconsistencies that have characterized the designation of rural–urban over time.

The United States Census Bureau essentially

defines rural as nonurban. However, the definition of urban has changed over time. Before the 1950 census, for instance, the term urban encompassed all territory, persons, and housing units in (1) incorporated places of 2,500 or more persons and (2) areas categorized as urban pursuant to special rules dealing with population size and density. This definition resulted in the exclusion of densely settled unincorporated areas.

In an attempt to address some of the deficiencies resulting from the urban designation, the Census Bureau created the concept of "urbanized area" and "delineated boundaries for unincorporated places." These latter areas are now termed "census-designated places." The definition of urban was expanded to include all territory, persons, and housing units in (1) urbanized areas and (2) areas with 2,500 or more persons that were outside of urban areas, regardless of whether they were incorporated.

Several modifications to the definition of urban have since been made. For example, the 1960 census identified the following as urban: Arlington County, Virginia, certain townships in New Jersey and Pennsylvania, and some towns in New England. These designations were not repeated in the 1970, 1980, or 1990 censuses.

The concept of "extended cities" was introduced in the 1970, 1980, and 1990 censuses. The extended city concept reflects states' extension of city boundaries to include territories that would otherwise be considered rural.

The 1990 census defines urban as encompassing (1) places of 2,500 or more persons incorporated as cities, villages, boroughs, or towns, with certain exceptions, but excluding the rural portions of extended cities; (2) census-designated places of 2,500 or more persons; and (3) other territory, whether incorporated or unincorporated, that is included in urbanized areas (U.S. Census Bureau, 1995). The definition of an urbanized area has also changed since the 1970 census, so that such areas are now defined around smaller centers. Urbanized area (UA) is defined by the Census Bureau as follows:

> A UA comprises one or more places ("central place") and the adjacent densely settled surrounding territory ("urban fringe") that together have a minimum of 50,000 persons. The urban fringe generally consists of contiguous territory having a density of at least 1,000 persons per square mile. The urban fringe also includes outlying territory of such density if it was connected to the core of the contiguous area by road and is within 1-1/2 road miles of that core, or within 5 road miles of the core but separated by water or other undevelopable territory. Other territory with a population density of fewer than 1,000 people per square mile is included in the urban fringe if it eliminates an enclave or closes an indentation in the boundary of the urbanized area. The population density is determined by (1) outside of a place, one or more contiguous census blocks with a population density of at least 1,000 persons per square mile or (2) inclusion of a place containing census blocks that have at least 50 percent of the population of the place and a density of at least 1,000 persons per square mile. (U.S. Census Bureau, 1995).

Because the boundaries of urban and urbanized areas are based on settlement size and density, these areas can cross county and state lines (U.S. Census Bureau, 1985). Urban and rural territories may be in either metropolitan or nonmetropolitan areas. This has implications for research because it complicates data management and analysis.

Even at the level of the federal government, the usage of "rural" is inconsistent. The General Accounting Office's (GAO) definition of rural area excludes nonmetropolitan counties that have populations of more than 20,000 or more urban residents, a scheme that resulted in the classification in 1980 of two-thirds of U.S. counties as rural. These counties, however, contained only 16 percent of the U.S. population (Cohen *et al.*, 1993).

State definitions of rural are not always consistent with those of the federal census. For instance, North Dakota defines as rural those communities with fewer than 5,000 persons that are located at least 30 miles away from a larger center. Communities having 10,000 or more residents are not considered rural (Talley, 1990). New York law defines rural counties as those with fewer than 200,000 people. Accordingly, New York State has 18 metropolitan counties and 44 rural counties (Crosby, Ogden, Kerr, & Heady, 1996).

Various other conceptualizations of "rural" have been used. Many rely on population density as a defining criterion. In formulating a four-part taxonomy of rural mental health services,

Perlman and Hartman (1983) defined rural as a county or counties without a population center of 10,000 or more residents and in which less than 50% of the population lived in towns with 2,500 or more residents. Ebert's (1994) has formulated three additional criteria to refine the categorization of an area as rural: (1) the extent to which people live in places with fewer than 2,500 residents, (2) the size of the largest place in the county, and (3) the extent to which people commute outside of the county for employment. Coward, McLaughlin, Duncan, and Bull (1994) have emphasized three factors in determining the rural character of a location: (1) the total number of persons resident in the target geographic area, (2) the distance of the location from a major metropolitan service area in terms of the time needed to move between them, and (3) the population size and space. Mata and Castillo (1986) characterize an area as rural by reference to the size of its population and the presence or absence of an agricultural economy.

Other criteria have also been used to define what is rural. For instance, rurality has been defined with reference to the environmental, interpersonal, and intrapersonal characteristics of an area. Compared with the environmental characteristics of an urban area, a rural area has a lower population density, fewer buildings, fewer service facilities, fewer mass-media outlets, and less congestion, pollution, and crime. In an interpersonal context, rural areas are characterized by a slower pace of life, strictly defined norms governing behavior, and limited privacy and anonymity. From an intrapersonal perspective, a rural environment may be more likely to foster adherence to conservative religious norms, resistance to change and innovation, and emphasis on hierarchical social relations, well-specified gender roles, and a present-time orientation.

Area of residence has also been viewed on a continuum, with very large cities such as New York and Los Angeles at one end and small, remote locales at the other. Reliance on the continuum concept requires the delineation of points along the continuum and the criteria to be used to define such points (U.S. Census Bureau, 1995). Chavez, Beauvais, and Oetting (1986) also rely on isolation as a distinguishing feature of rurality.

Unlike the Bureau of the Census, the federal Office of Management and Budget (OMB) designates metropolitan statistical areas (MSAs) and nonmetropolitan statistical areas (non-MSAs). The OMB relies on census data to classify an area as an MSA if it includes either a city with 50,000 or more residents or is an urbanized area that is part of a county or counties with a population of 100,000 or more (Beale, 1984; U.S. Department of Commerce, 1981; Hewitt, 1989). Rural areas are counties that are non-MSAs. Census-defined urbanized areas are usually smaller in size than MSAs (Cohen et al., 1993). The Department of Commerce (1990) estimated that by 1989, 40% of the rural population as defined by the census lived in metropolitan areas, while 16% of the MSA population lived in rural areas as defined by the census.

The National Rural Health Association has advocated reliance on the concept of "frontier area." These are areas that have population densities of fewer than 6 persons per square mile. In 1980, a total of 3 million people lived in the 38 rural frontier counties in the United States. Residents of these areas often had to travel for more than an hour to access health care providers and facilities (Patton, 1989).

Hays and colleagues (1994) have argued that additional factors must be considered in defining "rural doctors," as distinct from rural areas. In addition to relying on geographical area, the definition of rural doctor or rural medical practice must consider the distance from the closest large city, the self-perception of rurality, the requirements for what the physician must do, and the physician's access to support services.

A multidimensional approach to assessing of the rural–urban nature of an area is the most cogent. In operationalizing this assessment, we urge researchers to consider the following indicators:

1. Population density; that is, the number of residents per square mile. However, a determination must be made about what areas should serve as the reference—counties, census tracts, census blocks, and so forth.
2. Land use; that is, the percentage of land in the area that is devoted to agricultural uses, the percentage of buildings that are

single-family homes or commercial operations. And again, which areas serve as the reference point?

3. Distance in feet or miles of an individual dwelling unit to the nearest residential neighbor.

4. Distance in minutes of an individual dwelling unit to the nearest urban or commercial center. The question then raised is as to how such centers should be defined.

Statistical Issues in Estimating Parameters and Indicators

There are numerous difficulties in estimating parameters and indicators, such as incidence or prevalence of disease in a population and availability of health care providers in a region.

Estimating Incidence and Prevalence

The validity and precision of incidence and prevalence estimates of disease in rural areas may be diminished due to uncertainty about both the number of persons included in the numerator (the incident or prevalent cases of disease) and the number of individuals in the population (the denominator) from which cases in the numerator are identified. (It should be noted that this is also a concern with research in urban areas, albeit for different reasons.) It is critical in estimating the rates of disease in populations that appropriate numerators be matched with appropriate denominators. Our goal is to identify all new cases or changes in health status that occur in a particular population during a given period (incidence) or to identify all cases that exist in a particular population at a given time (prevalence). Failure to do this will result in invalid and misleading results, such as when estimating the frequency of a disease in a population or when estimating exposure effect by comparing exposed with unexposed populations. The estimation of valid rates is made more difficult when rural boundaries do not correspond to common census-based areas.

It is difficult for a number of reasons to detect all health events of interest (the numerator). First, accurate data on the morbidity and mortality of individuals employed as migrant farmworkers are lacking. Agriculture has been rated as one of the three most hazardous occupations (Rust, 1990). Although injuries have been reported as the leading cause of mortality and morbidity among agricultural workers (U.S. Department of Labor, 1988; Wilk, 1986), there is no comprehensive surveillance system for such injuries and the data sources currently available have limitations. For example, workmen's compensation data, which are widely used to estimate rates of injury, are often inaccurate with respect to injuries in agricultural employment because of various state laws' exemptions and exclusions (Mobed, Gold, & Schenker, 1992).

Second, it is extremely difficult to conduct surveillance and follow-up studies because the population of a rural area may vary considerably on a seasonal basis with the migration of farmworkers between areas. Approximately 40% of farmworkers are migratory, often employed as harvesters. It is estimated that two-thirds of them come from Mexico to the United States to follow crops for a while and then return to Mexico, whereas one-third remain in the United States to follow crops (Mines, Gabbard, & Boccalandro, 1991). In addition, population data on the migrant population are often inadequate. This is the result, to some extent, of investigators using varying definitions of "migrant farmworker" (Rust, 1990; Napolitano & Goldberg, 1998). For instance, the Office of Migrant Health defines a migrant farmworker as one "whose principal employment is in agriculture on a seasonal basis, who has been so employed during the past 24 months and who establishes for the purpose of such employment a temporary abode" (United States Department of Health and Human Services, 1980). Seasonal farmworkers are those who work cyclically but do not change their residence. Yet the term "migrant farmworker" may often be used to refer to both migrant and seasonal farmworkers (Napolitano & Goldberg, 1998).

When investigating injuries, identifying the denominators of rates is particularly problematic. How, for example, do we define the population and times (person-time) at risk of being injured with farm equipment? Relying on census data for geographic areas to define the denominator, as we generally do for estimating disease rates, is not accurate because not everyone living in a rural area, or even living on a farm, is at risk of such injuries, and no one is at risk all of the time. We would need to know how often each person in a population uses or is near each type of farm equipment. Thus, to estimate injury rates by exposure status requires additional information that is not usually available to the investigator; indeed, there is no recognized correct method for doing this in practice.

Even assuming that we are able to identify the denominator, additional statistical issues may be present. Small denominators in rural areas make estimates of disease rates unstable (imprecise), especially if the health event of interest is rare.

Estimating Risk and Rate (Incidence) of Disease

Issues relating to risk of disease may arise in a number of contexts in the rural setting. First, certain exposures may be more common in rural areas than in urban settings—including occupationally related exposures such as uranium and radium deposits in mines and nitrate contamination resulting from agricultural practices (Checkoway, Pearce, & Crawford-Brown, 1989; Matthew, 1992). Understanding the effects of such exposures is critical to the development of disease prevention mechanisms and may prove vital to clinicians' efforts to diagnose and treat their patients. Issues of disease risk may also arise in connection with perceived clusters of adverse health events, where a concerned citizen or a group believes that the risk of a specified disease may have increased among a particular group due to a specific exposure (Rothenberg & Thacker, 1992). Such clusters are usually localized in a community or neighborhood.

Assessing Exposures

Estimating the risk of disease may be difficult because of uncertainties about exposure status. For example, an assessment of the relation between a particular substance and the development of specified forms of cancer necessarily depends not only on the accurate classification of those who were environmentally exposed or not exposed to the substance under investigation but also on the accurate measurement of the effective biological dose among those who were exposed. Measurement requires data relating to the route of exposure; the burden, or the amount of the substance residing in the body or organ at a particular time; and retention, or the persistence of the substance in the body, resulting from rates of uptake, metabolism, and clearance (Checkoway et al., 1989).

The burden may vary over time and is, consequently, a function of the temporal pattern of exposure and retention. The dose, which refers to the amount of substance that persists in the biological target during a specified time interval, is a function of both the burden and the time interval during which the substance is present at the target. Because of the difficulties associated with ascertaining estimates of burden and dose, research often relies instead on measures of exposure concentration, duration, and accumulation (Checkoway et al., 1989).

Where the exposure of concern is occupationally related, the researcher must first identify the potentially toxic exposures and establish the most likely routes of exposure. Exposure data may be obtainable in a variety of forms, including quantified personal measurements of exposure, quantified area- or job-specific data, an ordinal ranking of jobs or tasks based on the level of exposure, data pertaining to employees' duration of employment in the relevant occupation, and information about whether the individual ever worked in the occupation of interest. The first two sources of data generally provide better estimates of the dose (Checkoway et al., 1989). This procedure might be relevant, for instance, in situations in which agricultural workers are exposed to multiple potentially toxic substances.

Investigating Clusters

The Centers for Disease Control (1990) has recommended a four-step approach to the investigation of a reported cluster of cases: initial contact with the individual reporting the health concern, an initial assessment, a major feasibility study, and an etiological investigation. Each of these stages includes numerous procedures, described as follows.

The initial contact generally requires that contact information be gathered from the individual. This individual might be a staff person at the local department of health, a community official, a person afflicted with a chronic condition, or another concerned citizen. The individual's name, address, telephone number, and so on should be gathered, as well as preliminary data on the potential cluster and the suspected cases. These preliminary data include the suspected health events and exposures, the number of cases, the geographic area and time period of concern, how the contact person learned about the cluster, and information about the suspected cases, such as their names, sex, ages, diagnoses, addresses, and physician contacts. A log of these contacts should be maintained. If further inquiry is indicated, an assessment should be conducted.

The initial assessment consists of confirmation of the cases, a preliminary determination that there is an excessive number of cases, and an "occurrence evaluation," which includes a literature review, the definition of time-space boundaries, and an assessment of the community's response. If both excess in the number of cases and the biological plausibility of a causal relation between the exposure and an adverse health event are confirmed, the investigation should proceed to stage 3.

The major feasibility study requires a re-review of the relevant literature and an examination of logistical, economic, political, and social feasibility of conducting a study. If the study indicates that additional investigation is warranted, an etiological investigation should be conducted to assess the relation between exposure and disease. (Centers for Disease Control, 1990).

Assessing the Level of Provider Need and Availability

Various strategies have been used to assess the numbers of physicians needed in a specific geographic area. These methods, however, may be somewhat problematic in rural areas. Research has found that rural residents are no more likely than nonrural residents to lack a usual source of care. However, rural residents are more likely to cite a lack of local resources as the reason (Hayward, Beynard, Freeman, & Corey, 1991), and they are less likely to have employment-based health insurance (Frenzen, 1991), which may bear on whether they use the services of their regular source of care. Consequently, if having a regular source of care is the only indicator of a physician need, and rural populations are no less likely to lack a regular source than urban populations, then the need for physicians in the rural area may be underestimated.

The physician-to-population ratio has also been used as a measure of medical care availability. This ratio compares the number of physicians in a specified geographic region to the size of the population in that area (Makuc, Haglund, Ingram, Kleinman, & Feldman, 1991).

There are numerous weaknesses associated with the use of the physician-to-population ratio. First, researchers frequently use the county as the geographic unit of analysis because data are more easily available for counties. However, this measure may provide limited insight into actual availability because many people obtain their medical care outside of their county of residence (Kleinman & Makuc, 1983), so that the actual availability of providers may be greater. Second, reliance on a ratio fails to consider other provider-related factors that may be critical in evaluating access to care, such as provider work hours, provider time allocated to nonclinical functions, and provider location in the county (U.S. Department of Health, Education, and Welfare, 1980). Third, a ratio that relies on the estimated total population as the denominator cannot accurately portray the availability of providers because the formula fails to weigh greater and lesser health care needs of subpopulations within the larger total. For instance, research has shown that rural populations tend to include a higher proportion of elderly individuals than do more urban areas. A physician-to-population ratio for a geographic area that includes a large proportion of elderly individuals with intensive health care needs would reflect the same level of (non)availability as a second geographic area that had the same ratio, but whose residents were primarily of working age or younger, with significantly fewer health care needs (U.S. Department of Health, Education, and Welfare, 1980). In addition, rural residents have been reported to have higher infant and maternal mortality rates than urban residents, and often rural residents have a higher prevalence of serious chronic health conditions (Burke, 1990). Again, an assessment of access between specified rural and urban areas that considers only the physician-to-population ratio for those areas might find no disparity in the level of (non)availability of providers, but would have failed to consider the possibly heightened need for medical care in the rural areas due to the higher prevalence of morbidity. Finally, reliance on a physician-to-population ratio presumes a relatively static population. But in rural areas a significant proportion of the population may be migrants, so that the population requiring medical care may vary seasonally.

The needs-based approach has been used to assess the number of physicians required in a specific geographic area in relation to the region's health needs. The needs-based approach is methodologically more complex than the physician-to-population approach. The needs-based approach requires (1) a definition of the target population whose need for physicians is to be assessed, including age distribution, and so on; (2) a listing of relevant disease categories; (3) an estimate of the incidence and prevalence of these diseases; (4) a determination of the number of physician encounters per acute disease episode, encounters per year for chronic diseases, and physician time per encounter; (5) a determination of the recommended number of annual medical encounters to detect or prevent these diseases; and (6) a determination of the number of hours worked by physicians in each specialty (Pathman, 1991). Projections of future need for physicians are based on (1) population growth and decline, (2) changes in disease prevalence, (3) recognition of new diseases, (4) changes in the frequency of physician visits and the amount of physician time required per visit, and (5) changes in physician work hours (Pathman, 1991).

This approach permits the estimation of the number of required physicians on the basis of a variety of assumed conditions. Because the data are disaggregated, these assumptions can be modified as appropriate. For instance, the rate of HIV infection in rural areas has been steadily increasing over time (Beltrami, Vermund, Fawal,

Moon, Von Bargen, & Holmberg, 1999; McCoy, Metsch, McCoy, & Weatherby, 1999). Utilization of the needs-based approach permits the estimate of the number of physicians required to treat patients with AIDS to be adjusted based on the projected increase or decrease in the numbers of persons who have the disease. However, this approach represents a theoretical model of need for physician services, which may poorly approximate patient demand due to variances between what is professionally defined as a need for disease treatment and patient self-perception of need (Cordes & Lloyd, 1979; Kleinman, Eisenberg, & Good, 1978), as well as barriers to accessing health care.

The demand-based approach offers another alternative to estimating the number of physicians needed. This approach relies on past patient service utilization as an indicator of future physician needs. Additional factors to be considered in deriving the estimate include the projected effects of potential changes in demographics, ability to pay, health insurance coverage, and disease status. This approach is able to address seasonal variation in population, which the physician-to-population ratio approach cannot do. It incorporates actual utilization, rather than theoretical utilization, which is a component of the needs-based approach. However, it fails to account for either unmet need or the proportion of the population's desired utilization of services that is not accommodated due to existing barriers (Pathman, 1991).

Various writers have recommended that multiple methodologies be used to estimate provider need (Kindig & Rickets, 1991; Pathman, 1991). Where these estimates diverge, researchers and policymakers may find it advisable to consider a range within which the need may fall, rather than a single-point estimate of need (Bureau of Health Planning and Resources Development, 1976; Pathman, 1991).

Sampling

Sampling has been characterized as "the weakest aspect of data collection" in the conduct of rural health research (Stokes & Miller, 1985, p. 546). For example, a review of 50 years of empirical research published in *Rural Sociology* found that only 34% of the published studies used probability sampling (Stokes & Miller, 1985).

However, even when probability sampling is used, the manner in which the sampling frame is constructed may introduce bias or limit the generalizability of the findings. Gilbert and colleagues (1997) conducted a study to evaluate bias and logistical issues in a survey of adults' oral health. The research group conducted a telephone survey that relied on both listed numbers and random-digit dialing to identify dentate persons 45 years of age or older and to oversample blacks, the poor, and residents of nonmetropolitan communities. In order to assess the bias that resulted from the inclusion of only households with telephones, they relied on county-level census data to compare households with telephones to households without them. Persons residing in households without telephones, and therefore excluded from the study, were more likely to be residents of nonmetropolitan areas, poor, black, middle-aged, limited in instrumental activities of daily living, and limited in activities of daily living. The authors concluded that the results of a telephone survey could not be generalized to the portion of the population not having telephones because of the large variation in sociodemographic characteristics relevant to dental health, but that appreciable bias in the estimation of parameters of interest was unlikely because of the small proportion of households without telephones.

Recommendations

Our ability to conduct rural health research and the quality of that research can be greatly improved if various strategies are adopted. First, we strongly urge authors to provide explicit details about the operationalization of "rural" and "rurality" in published papers. This will facilitate understanding the methodology and the results, as well as making comparisons across studies. Second, we recommend that researchers use a multidimensional schema to classify areas as rural or nonrural. This approach recognizes the heterogeneity of rural areas by requiring that the classification be based on

multiple dimensions. Third, we encourage researchers to consider the heterogeneity of the rural population in the design of studies, the conduct of analyses, and the reporting of study findings. This focused approach facilitates an understanding of where resources are most needed and how prevention and intervention efforts can be enhanced.

References

Beale, C. L. (1984). Poughkeepsie's complaint or defining metropolitan areas. *American Demographics,* January, 29–48.

Beltrami, J. F., Vermund, S. H., Fawal, H. J., Moon, T. D., Von Bargen, J. C., & Holmberg, S. D. (1999). HIV/AIDS in nonurban Alabama: Risk activities and access to services among HIV-infected persons. *Southern Medical Journal, 92,* 677–683.

Bureau of Health Planning and Resources Development. (1976). *Methodological approaches for determining health manpower supply and requirements.* Vol. II. (DHEW Publication No. HRA 76-14512). Washington, DC: United States Government Printing Office.

Burke, M. (1990). Policymakers struggle to define essential access. *Hospitals, 64,* 38, 40, 42.

Centers for Disease Control. (1990). Guidelines for investigating clusters of health events. *Morbidity and Mortality Weekly Report, 39,* 1–23.

Chavez, E., Beauvais, F., & Oetting, E. R. (1986). Drug use by small town Mexican American youth: A pilot study. *Hispanic Journal of Behavioral Science, 8,* 243–258.

Checkoway, H., Pearce, N. E., & Crawford-Brown, D. J. (1989). *Research methods in occupational epidemiology.* Oxford: Oxford University Press.

Cohen, S. B., Braden, J. J., & Ward, E. P. (1993). Enhancing the representation of rural areas in the National Medical Expenditure Survey. *Journal of Rural Health, 9,* 188–203.

Cordes, S. M., & Lloyd, R. C. (1979). Recent social science research on rural health services: A critique and directions for the future. *American Journal of Rural Health: Rural Health Communications, 5,* 1–19.

Coward, R. T., McLaughlin, D. K., Duncan, R. P., & Bull, C. N. (1994). An overview of health and aging in rural America. In R. T. Coward, C. N. Bull, G. Kukulka, & J. M. Galliher (Eds.), *Health Services for Rural Elders* (pp. 1–32). New York: Springer.

Crosby, F. S., Ogden, A. B., Kerr, S. L., & Heady, J. (1996). Focus groups describe rural nursing in New York State. *Journal of the New York State Nurses Association, 27,* 4–8.

Eberts, D. (1994). *Socieconomic trends in New York*

State: 1950-1990. Albany, NY: Report to New York State Legislative Committee.

Frenzen, P. D. (1991). The increasing supply of physicians in U.S. urban and rural areas, 1975 to 1988. *American Journal of Public Health, 81,* 1141–1147.

Gilbert, G. H., Duncan, R. P., Heft, M. W., Dolan, T. A., Vogel, W. B. (1997). Oral disadvantage among dentate adults. *Community Dentistry and Oral Epidemiology, 25,* 301–313.

Hays, R. B., Craig, M. L., Wise, A. L., Nichols, A., Mahoney, M. D., Adkins, P. B., Sheehan, M., & Siskind, V. (1994). A sampling framework for rural and remote doctors. *Australian Journal of Public Health, 18,* 273–276.

Hayward, R. A., Beynard, A. M., Freeman, H. E., & Corey, C. R. (1991). Regular sources of ambulatory care and access to health services. *American Journal of Public Health, 81,* 434–438.

Hewitt, M. (1989). *Defining rural areas: Impact on health care policy and research.* Washington, DC: United States Government Printing Office.

Kindig, D. A. & Ricketts, T. C. (1991). Determining adequacy of physicians and nurses for rural populations: Background and strategy. *Journal of Rural Health, 7,* 313–326.

Kleinman, A., Eisenberg, L., & Good, B. (1978). Clinical lessons from anthropologic and cross-cultural research. *Annals of Internal Medicine, 88,* 251–258.

Kleinman, J. C. & Makuc, D. M. (1983). Travel for ambulatory medical care. *Medical Care, 21,* 543–557.

Makuc, D. M., Haglund, B., Ingram, D. D., Kleinman, J. C., & Feldman, J. J. (1991). The use of health service areas for measuring provider availability. *Journal of Rural Health, 7,* 347–356.

Mata, D. G., & Castillo, V. (1986). Rural female adolescent dissatisfaction, support, and helpseeking. *Free Inquiry Creative Sociology, 14,* 135–138.

Matthew, G. K. (1992). Health and the environment: The significance of chemicals and radiation. In P. Elliott, J. Cuzick, D. English, & R. Stern (Eds.), *Geographic and Environmental Epidemiology: Methods for Small Area Studies* (pp. 22–33). New York: Oxford University Press.

McCoy, C. B., Metsch, L. R., McCoy, H. V., and Weatherby, N. L. (1999). HIV seroprevalence across the rural/urban continuum. *Substance Use and Misuse, 34,* 595–615.

Mines, R., Gabbard, S., & Boccalandro, B. (1991). *Findings from the National Agricultural Workers' Survey (NAWS). 1990: A demographic and employment profile of perishable crop farm workers* (U.S. Department of Labor, Office of Program Economics Research Report No. 1). Washington, DC: United States Government Printing Office.

Mobed, K., Gold, E., & Schenker, M. (1992). Occupational health problems among migrant and seasonal farm workers. *Western Journal of Medicine, 157,* 367–373.

Napolitano, M., & Goldberg, B. W. (1998). Migrant health. In S. Loue (Ed.), *Handbook of Immigrant Health* (pp. 261–276). New York: Plenum.

Pathman, D. E. (1991). Estimating rural health professional requirements: An assessment of current methodologies. *Journal of Rural Health, 7,* 327–346.

Patton, L. (1989). Setting the rural health services agenda: The congressional perspective. *Health Services Research, 23,* 1005–1051.

Pearlman, B., & Hartman, E. A. (1983). The community health care administrator project: Characteristics and problems of rural administrators. *Journal of Mental Health Administration, 10,* 15–18.

Rothenberg, R. B. & Thacker, S. B. (1992). Guidelines for the investigation of clusters of adverse health events. In P. Elliott, J. Cuzick, D. English, & R. Stern, (Eds.), *Geographic and environmental epidemiology: Methods for small area studies* (pp. 264–277). New York: Oxford University Press.

Rust, G. S. (1990). Health status of migrant farmworkers: A literature review and commentary. *American Journal of Public Health, 80,* 1213–1217.

Stokes, C. S. & Miller, M. K. (1985). A methodological review of fifty years of research in rural sociology. *Rural Sociology, 50,* 539–560.

Talley, R. C. (1990). Graduate medical education and rural health care. *Academic Medicine, 65,* S22–S25.

U.S. Census Bureau. (1985). Census and geography concepts and products. Factfinder (CCF No. 8). Washington, DC: United States Government Printing Office.

U.S. Census Bureau. (1995, October). Urban and rural definitions; http://www.census.gov/population/censusdata/urdef.txt.

U.S. Department of Commerce. (1981). *Census of Population, 1980: Volume 1, Characteristics of the Population: General Social and Economic Characteristics.* Washington, DC: U.S. Government Printing Office.

U.S. Department of Commerce. (1990). *Residents of Farms and Rural Areas: 1989. Current Population Reports* (Series p-20, No. 446). Washington, DC: U.S. Government Printing Office.

U.S. Department of Health, Education, and Welfare. (1980). *Evaluation of health manpower shortage area criteria* (DHEW Publication No. HRA 80-20). Washington, DC: Health Resources and Services Administration.

U.S. Department of Health and Human Services. (1980). *Migrant health program target population estimates.* Rockville, MD: Author.

U.S. Department of Labor. (1989). *Occupational injury & illnesses, 1989.* Washington, DC: National Bureau of Labor Statistics.

U.S. House of Representatives, Select Committee on Aging. (1983). *Status of the rural elderly.* (Vols. I, II). Washington, DC: United States Government Printing Office.

Wilk, V. A. (1986). *Occupational health of migrant and seasonal farmworkers in the United States* (2nd ed.). Washington, DC: Farmworker Justice Fund.

3

Public Health Issues

JOHN B. CONWAY

According to Reynolds, Banks, and Murphree (1976), rural America includes people living on farms or in nonfarm communities of less than 2,500 residents. Twenty-five years ago such areas were home to 55 million people in the United States and that number had remained essentially stable for the previous five decades. The most recent census (U.S. Census Bureau, 1995) numbered the rural population of this country at more than 61 million people or 24% of the total population.

The percentage of the total population living in rural America has declined since the turn of the century. We have gone from a rural agrarian population to an urban population; Table 1 illustrates this trend. In 1990, the state with the highest percentage of its population living in a rural area was Vermont at 67%. Other states where the rural population was more than 50% were West Virginia, Maine, Mississippi, and South Dakota. However, although the percentage of the total United States population living in rural areas has steadily decreased over the past 100 years, the actual number of people living in these areas has increased by 25%. This fact certainly has ramifications for the health care delivery system and the quality of care available to this segment of the U.S. population.

Before discussing specific public health issues, it is beneficial to look at a list of public

JOHN B. CONWAY • College of Health Sciences, University of Texas at El Paso, El Paso, Texas 79968-0581.

Handbook of Rural Health, edited by Loue and Quill. Kluwer Academic/Plenum Publishers, New York, 2001.

TABLE 1. Rural Population in the United States

Year	Rural Population	Rural Percentage of Total Population
1900	45,997,336	60%
1930	54,042,025	43%
1960	54,054,425	30%
1990	61,656,386	24%

Note: From *Urban and Rural Population: 1900 to 1990*, 1995, Washington, DC: U.S. Census Bureau.

health services offered by national, state, and local health departments. Last (1998) conveniently lists all levels of governmental services in his recent book. Table 2 lists the national public health services; Table 3 specifies services supplied by the state of New York; and Table 4 itemizes services supplied by a local health department. Table 3 lists only those services offered or administered by the New York State Department of Health. The original table shows 11 other agencies in New York State with various public health responsibilities. Clearly, not every state is similar to New York, but for purposes of discussion it is representative of state-level public health programs. Last's (1998) example of a local health department is very comprehensive and the services listed probably exceed what is offered by most rural health departments.

All three levels of government have public health programs in communicable disease control, environmental health, and health education. Trained public health professionals are needed to administer these programs. Contact with the

TABLE 2. National Public Health Services

Protect the nation's health
  Quarantine
  Communicable disease control
  Other diseases of importance (Cancer; birth defects;
    heart disease; injury control; etc.)
Health promotion
  National food policies
  Fitness policies
  Health education
Enviromental protection
  Workers' health and safety
  Food safety
Health care of special groups
  Armed services
  Government employees
  Native people
  Remote communities
  Aged, indigent, etc.
Medical research
Health statistics
Standard setting, licensure, etc.

Note: From *Public Health and Human Ecology* (2nd ed.), by J. M. Last, (1998), Stanford, CT: Appleton and Lange.

public is at the state and local level, and this is where individuals with specific public health training should be actively employed. State health departments have academically trained individuals in most of their programs, and the same is true in the larger urban health departments. Hiring and retaining trained and quali-

fied public health workers has become problematic in many local health departments and this is especially true in rural areas.

A discussion about trained public health workers in rural areas should start with physicians. If the state of New York is used as an example, then 13 local health departments list physicians as commissioners or public health directors of county health departments (New York State Association of County Health Officials, 1999). Other commissioners or public health directors are nurses, environmental health specialists (sanitarians), professional engineers, and so on. The degrees held include B.S., B.S.N., M.P.H., M.P.A., M.B.A., M.D., and Ph.D. Many of the commissioners or public health directors that are not physicians are well qualified to direct a health department but must contract for their department's medical services.

With one exception (Chautauqua County), the New York State health departments headed by physicians are in urban areas or suburban counties near New York City. Operating without a full-time physician on staff is not a fatal flaw, but it does complicate delivery of services, especially in times of emergency. Many rural counties not only in New York but in other states have no licensed practicing physician living in the county. This means that for access to basic public health care involving the services of a

TABLE 3. Services Commonly Provided and Administered by the State of New York Department of Health

Maternal and child health, including prenatal and postnatal services, family planning, immunization, and well-baby care

Public and personal health education

Communicable disease control, including immunization, tuberculosis and disease control, epidemiology, and laboratory services

Handicapped children's services

Chronic disease screening

Mental health, mental retardation, and alcohol and drug abuse services

Enviromental health, including consumer protection and sanitation, air and water quality management, occupational health and safety, and radiation control

Health professions licensure

Health resources management, including planning, development, and regulation of health services, facilities, manpower, and health statistics activities

Laboratory, including analytic services and laboratory improvement to assist in efforts to prevent, detect, and treat disease

Note: From *Public Health and Human Ecology* (2nd ed.), by J. M. Last, 1998, Stanford, CT: Appleton and Lange.

TABLE 4. Services Supplied by a Local Health Department

Health needs assessment, using all available health
   information systems
Control of communicable disease
   Immunizations
   Special clinics (STDs, tuberculosis, etc.)
   Environmental Sanitation
   Pest control
   Surveillance of cases, contacts
Environmental health
   Waste disposal
   Noise abatement
   Nuisance control
   Water, air pollution monitoring
   Hazardous waste disposal
Food hygiene
   Inspection of food producing, processing
   Restaurant Inspection
Health education
   School health
   Public campaigns
Special health-related clinic services
   Family planning
   Dental health
   Maternal and child health
   Geriactric health
   STDs
Preventive screening programs
   Hypertension
   Pap smears
   Chest x-rays surveys for invalids, pensioners
Home care plans
   Visiting services for invalids, pensioners
Disaster planning
   Coordinated with other services (poloce, fire
   department, hospital, etc.)
Coordination of voluntary service agencies
   Meals on wheels
   Aid to dependent, handicapped, etc.

Note: From *Public Health and Human Ecology* (2nd ed.), by J. M. Last, 1998, Stamford, CT: Appleton and Lange.

physician, a family may have to travel over a considerable distance. A major issue is how to attract and retain board-certified physicians to practice medicine in rural areas.

Nurses make up the largest number of employees in health departments. They are trained at several levels—that is, they have a master's degree in public health nursing or community health, a bachelor's degree in nursing, or a two-year associate degree in nursing, or are licensed practical nurses. These individuals are the backbone of any health department and perform myriad tasks, from performing immunizations and staffing special clinics to providing family planning, preventive screening programs, home care programs, coordination of voluntary programs, aid to dependent families, disabled programs, and so on. Nurses frequently perform other tasks in a health department too, such as health education and sanitation surveillance. It would be ideal for all nursing employees to have their B.A. degrees, but in reality most rural health departments rely heavily on those with associate degrees, licensed practical nurses, and aides. The workload for these individuals is diverse and demanding, and they would benefit from additional education and training.

Another personnel problem for rural health departments is hiring and keeping trained environmental health specialists. The benefit of having environmental health specialists on staff can't be emphasized enough. These individuals are responsibile for maintaining the quality and sanitation of food handling establishments in the county. They must understand time-temperature relationships, food handler training, and the Hazard Analysis and Critical Control Point (HACCP) system. They also are responsible for oversight of public water systems, installation of on-site wastewater systems, and other environmental tasks. Specific education and training are necessary for these public health workers to carry out their responsibilities effectively.

Some rural health departments have no personnel serving as environmental health specialists or sanitarians. They use state health department personnel to carry out environmental health tasks. The state employees operate out of regional offices and generally cover several counties. Obviously this is not as efficient as having trained environmental health personnel in the local county.

A bigger problem is the employment at the local level of individuals without any professional training as environmental health specialists. In some instances untrained individuals have been put in the position of environmental health specialist and have learned how to do various tasks or inspections on the job. Many of these people have become proficient, but they lack the training necessary to effectively perform the wide variety of tasks the position requires.

Environmental health specialist training is available at both the undergraduate and graduate level in accredited programs at many universities. These programs vary, and specialization is possible at the graduate level. The biggest obstacle to hiring these graduates in rural health departments is the salary. It is an even greater problem when it comes to hiring individuals with graduate degrees.

Another important position in a health department is the public health educator, who serves as a link between the health department and the community. Knowledge of intervention strategies is an important skill these individuals possess. The public needs to be made aware of a particular health problem or concern and the appropriate action to take to correct the problem.

There are many other public health issues for populations in rural areas in addition to the need for adequately trained public health professionals in their local public health agencies. Each of these issues will be discussed briefly on the following pages.

Access to Public Health Clinics and Programs

It is important to the success of any public health program for the services offered to be accessible to the target population. It is easy to overlook ease of access when trying to find a suitable site or building for a clinic or other public health program. An inexpensive building in a deteriorating warehouse district may be attractive from a financial standpoint, but a disaster in terms of accessibility.

This is especially true in rural areas where visits to the community containing the clinic or program are limited or inconvenient. The author remembers well the establishment of a clinic in an urban area in a structurally sound building located in a low socioeconomic neighborhood. The building was renovated, provided with state-of-the-art equipment, and well staffed. Everyone felt that it would be a positive influence in the neighborhood and would provide much needed screening and immunization services. The clinic doors were opened and almost no one took advantage of the services. When those who did come were ques-

tioned, they indicated difficulty in finding and accessing the facility. Transportation was a major barrier; the clinic was 10 blocks from the nearest bus stop. In addition, it wasn't near any shopping area and had limited parking. Transportation has frequently been identified as a problem for low-income families and a major barrier. When the clinic was moved nearer to public transportation, more people began taking advantage of the services.

People living in a rural area make infrequent trips into town to buy groceries and other supplies. The trip can involve an hour or more on the road, especially in the western United States. If public health clinics or services are located in a remote or inaccessible area, the likelihood that they will be used is reduced. In contrast, if the site of the clinic or services is near the farmers' co-op or the grocery store, then it becomes "one-stop shopping" and the likelihood of use is increased.

Dental Health

Preventing dental caries and providing restorative work are important components of public health. Last (1998) indicates that many local health departments operate dental clinics for low-income families. These clinics are staffed by dentists and offer preventive dental care, such as fluoride mouth rinses to all children. Many local health departments work with the school nurse to provide an educational program promoting good oral hygiene.

In many communities, fluoride is added to potable water supplies at a level of 1 ppm to prevent dental caries and strengthen the brittle bones of older people (Koren, 1991). Last (1998) discusses the opposition to fluoridation of drinking water and states that it is "based in part on the unfounded fear that fluoride can cause cancer or some other dread disease" (p. 375). Epidemiological evidence has shown that this fear is unfounded and that opposition is more political than a public health issue. The bottom line is that for infants and small children fluoridated drinking water makes the difference between healthy and carious teeth. A comprehensive public health program includes preventing dental caries, and this service should be available to people living in the rural areas of the United States.

Disaster Planning

Disaster planning is an often overlooked but important public health issue. Every part of the United States is prone to natural or anthropogenic disasters. Flooding or heavy snow storms in the Northeast, hurricanes in the South, tornados and flooding in the Midwest, volcanic eruptions in the Northwest, and earthquakes and fires in the Southwest all make disaster planning necessary. All of these incidents can cause human suffering and property damage.

All local health departments should participate with appropriate agencies in preparing for such disasters. Other appropriate agencies include law enforcement, fire departments, ambulance transportation companies, local hospitals, local communication stations (radio, television, etc.), voluntary agencies (the Red Cross), and local and state emergency services. One agency should be designated as the "lead agency," and all communication and response and recovery efforts should be coordinated through this agency.

It is very important in the aftermath of flooding or a tornado that people know where to go for food and shelter and how to get in touch with family members. A county disaster or emergency response plan should be in place and all participating agencies should know the role they are expected to perform. Many counties have been negligent in defining their role in a disaster or major emergency and the result has been chaos, including unnecessary pain and suffering by those affected. This important public health issue involves extensive planning.

Health Needs Assessment and Program Evaluation

Local entities must from time to time evaluate the programs they are providing their constituents. This is true for all public programs and especially true for public health. It is easiest to continue to offer the same public health programs that have always been offered because someone in the past decided that these were the best programs for the community. Keeping the status quo takes essentially no planning and reduces the expectation that a program will be evaluated.

The old adage, "We have always done it this way" no longer works. In an era of diminishing resources, it is necessary to evaluate public health programs constantly and strengthen those that are effective and necessary and revise or eliminate those that are neither.

Needs assessment and program evaluation require continual effort and trained personnel. Individuals trained in epidemiological investigation, health statistics (data collection and analysis), and evaluations are especially important in carrying out these tasks. These individuals are usually trained at the graduate level and require higher salaries than many other public health workers, but the benefit derived from the work they do should more than offset their increased compensation.

Injury Control (with Emphasis on Farm Machinery)

The National Safety Council (1997) lists the five leading causes of death in 1996 due to unintentional injuries as: motor-vehicle accidents, falls, poisoning by solids and liquids, drowning, and burns and deaths associated with fires. The death rate per 100,000 persons was 35.2 for all causes, and the total number of disabling injuries was estimated at 20.7 million. The total cost of all unintentional injuries in 1996 was estimated to be $444.1 billion.

Injury control is an important public health issue from both a human health and economic standpoint. Many local communities have few or no programs designed to prevent unintentional injuries. There are several reasons for this: lack of trained personnel, cost, and lack of incident reporting. Clearly, a program designed to prevent unintentional injuries is important and should be part of any public health plan, including in rural areas.

The five leading causes of unintentional injuries suggest several approaches to implementing preventive programs. Motor vehicle accidents occur most frequently among the 15 to 24 and 75 and over age groups. Falls occur most often in the 65 to 75 and over age group. Poisoning by solids and liquids is most prevalent in the 25 to 64 year age group. Drowning occurs most frequently in the 0 to 4 age group, and burns and deaths associated with fires occurs most often in the very young (0 to 4) and the old (75 and older) age groups. This information can be effectively used to design and direct educational programs for the affected populations.

In rural counties, much of the workforce is often involved in farming. The National Safety Council (1997) reported the age group most affected, the source of injury, and fatalities associated with farming in 13 states. Two hundred and fifty deaths occurred in these 13 states, and the major source of injury involved a tractor. The median age of those affected was 50 to 55. The agricultural work fatalities by source in the 13 states were: tractor (42%), agricultural machinery (14%), animal (6%), ground/floor (5%), truck (4%), other vehicle (3%), chemical (2%), and other (24%). Tractor overturns had the highest fatality rate for unintentional injuries according to revised reports from 13 states (National Safety Council, 1997).

A surveillance and intervention safety program involving farm machinery was conducted from 1990 to 1996 (National Safety Council, 1997). Results of the survey indicate that much work remains to be done in rural communities. Occupational health nurses are one group of health professionals that has the training and expertise needed to deal with fatal and nonfatal unintentional injuries.

Preventive Public Health

Preventive public health presumes identification of potential public health problems and implementing the necessary steps to prevent them from occurring. Also assumed is that someone or some agency has the experience and expertise to recognize potential public health problems. Time to devote to preventive programs has always been at a premium, and many health workers and health departments spend much of their time "fighting fires." They are reacting to a health problem, usually after it has

occurred. The *cryptosporidium* outbreak that occurred in Milwaukee, Wisconsin, in 1993 is an example of a problem that could have been avoided. The actual cause of the outbreak has never been conclusively established, but officials suspect that heavy spring rains washed large amounts of animal manure into reservoirs, rivers, and Lake Michigan, increasing turbidity levels (*cryptosporidium* oocysts can survive in moist soil for two to six months, increasing the danger posed by erosion into these waterways). Nadakavukaren (1995) states that the city of Milwaukee has taken the following steps to ensure against a repeat of the outbreak: setting stringent new effluent goals for turbidity; discharging, rather than recycling, filter backwash waters; and testing for the presence of *cryptosporidium* on a bimonthy basis. *Cryptosporidium* has been identified as a potential waterborne human health problem for some time. If preventive practices had been in effect before the spring runoff, they could have prevented the problem or, at least, the inhabitants of Milwaukee could have been warned to boil their water before using it.

Last (1998) defines the three levels of prevention as primary, secondary, and tertiary. Primary prevention maintains health by removing the precipitating causes and determinants of departure from good health. Examples are eliminating disease agents such as smallpox, pasteurizing milk, wearing seatbelts in automobiles, and eating a diet high in fiber. Secondary prevention means early detection of disease, before it has time to produce irreversible damage. Secondary prevention uses screening as the tool of choice to detect birth defects, hypertension, breast and colon cancer, and so on. Tertiary prevention means preventing deterioration and complications from occurring when disease and disability are already established. Tertiary prevention can minimize complications in seriously ill or injured patients.

Public Health Planning

Planning is the keystone of a good public health prevention program. Planning implies that the population at risk is well known and knowledge is available about specific public health problems. Planning involves setting goals and periodically evaluating whether the goals have been met. Strategic public health planning for all programs offered should take place in three- or five-year cycles and must include evaluation to be effective.

Planning is frequently overlooked or placed on the "back burner." Planning is especially important in many rural areas where resources and trained public health personnel are scarce.

Sex Education

Teen pregnancy is a major public health problem throughout the world (Zero Adolescent Pregnancy, 1991). The United States has the highest teenage pregnancy rate among Western developed countries, and it is the single most reliable predictor of welfare dependency in this country. A child born to a teen mother is at greater risk of lower intellectual and academic achievement and behavioral and self-control problems (Hayes, 1987). Girls born to teen mothers are much more likely to become teen parents themselves (Fustenberg, Levine, & Brooks-Gunn, 1990); boys are more likely to serve jail terms. Public monies pay for the delivery of at least half of all children born to teens (Alan Guttmacher Institute, 1987).

Teen pregnancy is a public health issue that affects all of us. A good example of what can be accomplished by a small rural community in combating this problem is the Zero Adolescent Pregnancy (ZAP) program started in Cortland County, New York, in 1991. Cortland County had high teen pregnancy rates throughout the 1980s. The program set a 10-year goal of reducing tthe rate in the county by one-third by the year 2000. The objectives (ZAP, 1991) were to:

- Reduce the occurrence of unintended pregnancy among never-married teens to 100 per year or less by the year 2000.
- Help never-married teens and pre-teens postpone initial sexual intercourse.
- Promote the consistent use of contraception among sexually active teens.

Cortland County's teen pregnancy rate decreased by 30% in the first six years and the number of unintended teen pregnancies was reduced from 152 to 108—two striking examples of the success of the program. The success of this program can be attributed to information dissemination, enthusiasm, energy, and a can-do attitude. This is a good example of what planning, implementation, and evaluation can accomplish in a rural area.

Substance Abuse

Substance abuse is prevalent in our society and the rural areas of the country are not excluded. Cycles of substance abuse change rapidly. Last (1998) states that the high prevalence of heroin addiction in the 1960s was replaced by cocain addiction in the mid-1980s. Bearman (1985, personal communication), a former director of the Student Health Services at San Diego State University, listed the "drug of the year" for the period from 1964 to 1980. He states, "Each year, it seems, over the past 15 years or so, the media have seemed to focus primarily on one particular drug. (In fact since 1971 there has been very little change in drug-taking behavior among college students of a number of substances, including barbiturates, amphetamines, hallucinogens, tobacco, and alcohol.)" Bearman's "recreational drug of the year" is specified in Table 5. In the period discussed by Bearman, marijuana use in college

TABLE 5. Recreational Drug of the Year

1964	Tobacco
1965	Glue
1966	LSD
1967	Marijuana
1968	Amphetamines
1969	Heroin
1970	Angel dust (Phencyclepine)
1971	Quaalude
1972	Cocaine
1973	Poly-drug abuse
1974	Alcohol
1975	Alcohol
1976	Valium
1977	Cocaine
1978	Propoxyphene (Darvon)
1979	Phencyclepine (PCP)
1980	Marijuana

students increased from 50 to 66%. In recent years, Last (1988) states that marijuana use has remained about the same. Overall, the kinds of drugs used continues to increase and change.

Alcohol has been a problem in our society for centuries. Cook and Abreu (1998) state that alcohol abuse is more common than any other form of drug abuse in the world. They further state that alcohol is consumed by roughly half of the adult U.S. population and that the number of individuals directly affected by alcohol use disorders is at least 20 to 30 million at any given time. Alcohol use disorders are seen across all socioeconomic groups. Drinking is most prevalent in urban America, and geographically in the Northeast. Again, the rural parts of the United States are not exempt.

Substance abuse continues to be a major public health problem in the United States. There are no easy solutions to this problem and qualified public health professionals and agencies must constantly seek new and innovative programs to bring about behavioral change among those affected. Rural areas are included in these programs, and efforts there must be taken to offset the isolation that increases the difficulty of effective program delivery in these areas.

Violence Prevention

Violence is another major public health problem in all geographic and socioeconomic areas of the United States. Violence affects all segments of our population. The major categories are domestic violence, spousal violence, child abuse, and sexual assaults against children. Although violence is not a new problem, it has only recently been embraced by the public health community. Not too many years ago it was thought to be the exclusive domain of police departments and the courts.

A recent example of violence is the fatal shooting of a 6-year-old girl by a classmate, a 6-year-old boy, in February 2000 in Mount Morris Township, Michigan. The boy brought a loaded handgun to his first-grade classroom. He told authorities that the shooting was an accident; he was only trying to scare the girl. He told police that he had found the gun under blankets in a bedroom at a dilapidated wood-frame

house where he resided with his 8-year-old brother and an uncle. The boy's father was in jail at the time of the incident.

A youth risk behavior surveillance conducted in the United States in 1997 (Kann et al., 1998) found that 4% of students missed at least one day of school during the preceding month because they felt unsafe at school or when traveling to and from school. Hispanic and black students were significantly more likely than white students to feel unsafe. Nearly one in five students (18.3%) admitted to having carried a concealed weapon within the preceding month, while 8.5% of students admitted to having carried a concealed weapon to school during the preceding month. Male students were significantly more likely (12.5%) than female students (3.7%) to have carried a weapon on school property. Being threatened or injured with a weapon on school property one or more times in the preceding 12 months was reported by 7.4% of the students. Physically fighting on school property one or more times during the preceding 12 months was reported by 14.8% of the students. Approximately one-third (32.9%) of students nationwide had had property stolen or deliberately damaged on school grounds one or more times during the preceding 12 months.

All the signs have been there for some time, and conventional wisdom dictates that the shooting in Michigan could have been prevented. This is just one example of violence, and there are many others in all age groups and among both genders. Substance abuse is a contributing factor in violence. Public health workers must include violence prevention among their high-priority programs in both urban and rural areas.

Summary and Conclusions

The public health issues are many and varied for residents of rural areas. Several important problems have been briefly mentioned here. Traditional public health programs in both rural and urban areas should include programs in dental health, disaster and emergency planning, injury control, program needs assessment, program planning and evaluation, sex education, substance abuse, and violence prevention.

Unique problems for rural areas include access to services and hiring and retaining qualified, trained public health workers. If all public health agencies work together and use innovative ideas and methodologies, it will go a long way toward solving many of the public health problems today and those that will occur in the future.

References

Alan Guttmacher Institute. (1987). *The financing of maternity care in the United States.* New York: AGI.

Cook, B. L., & Abreu, J. A. (1998). Alcohol-related health problems. In R. B. Wallace & B. N. Doebbeling (Eds.), *Public Health and Preventive Medicine* (pp. 847–860). Stamford, CT: Appleton and Lange.

Fustenberg, E. F., Levine, J. A., & Brooks-Gunn, J. (1990). The children of teenage mothers: Patterns of early childbearing in two generations. *Family Planning Prospectives, 22*(2).

Hayes, C. C. (Ed.). (1987). *Risking the future: adolescent sexuality, pregnancy, and childbearing.* Washington, DC: National Research Council, National Academy Press.

Kann, L., Kinchen, S. A., Williams, B. I., Ross, J. G., Lowry, R., Hill, C. V., Grunbaum, J. A., Blumson, P. S., Collins, J. L., & Koble, L. J. (1998). *Youth Risk Behavior Surveillance—United States, 1997.* Rockville, MD: Chronic Disease Prevention and Health Promotion; www.cdc.gov/nccdphp/dash/MMWRFile/ss4703.htm

Koren, H. (1991). *Handbook of environmental and safety, principles and practices* (Vol. II, 2nd ed.). Chelsea, MI: Lewis Publishers.

Last, J. M. (1998). *Public health and human ecology* (2nd ed.). Stamford, CT: Appleton and Lange.

Nadakavukaren, A. (1995). *Our global environment: A health prospective* (4th ed.). Prospect Heights, IL: Waveland Press.

National Safety Council. (1997). *Accident Facts.* Itasca, IL: National Safety Council.

New York State Association of County Health Officials. (1999). *1999 Directory.* Albany, NY: New York State Association of County Health Officials.

Reynolds, R. C., Banks, S. A., & Murphree, M. A. (1976). *The health of a rural county.* Gainesville: University Presses of Florida.

U.S. Census Bureau. (1995). *Urban and rural population: 1900 to 1990.* [www.census.gov/population/censusdata/urpop].

Zero Adolescent Pregnancy. (1991). *Winning the war against teen pregnancy.* Cortland, NY: Zero Adolescent Pregnancy, Jacobus Center for Reproductive Health.

4

Equity in Rural Health and Health Care

LU ANN ADAY, BETH E. QUILL, AND
CIELITO C. REYES-GIBBY

This chapter assesses the equity of rural health and health care delivery. It presents a conceptual framework and normative and empirical criteria for measuring equity; reviews major federal and state policy initiatives to enhance equity; assembles current evidence regarding the extent to which equity has actually been achieved; and presents alternative models of rural health care programs and policy for enhancing equity.

The perspective assumed in this chapter is that equity is concerned with health disparities between and within rural as well as between rural and urban communities and the fairness and effectiveness of the procedures for addressing them. The ultimate test of the equity of health policy is the extent to which disparities or inequalities in health persist among subgroups (by rural or urban place of residence, race, income, and insurance coverage, for example). *Substantive equity* is reflected in minimizing subgroup disparities in health. *Procedural equity* refers to the extent to which the structure and process (or procedures) for achieving these outcomes may be judged to be fair. The normative relevance of variations in the structure and pro-

cess of rural health care can, however, ultimately be judged empirically by their contributions to predicting inequalities in health across subgroups and communities.

A Framework for Studying Equity in Health and Health Care

Three philosophical traditions that have focused primarily on individuals, institutions, or the community in judging justice may be used to illuminate the correlates and indicators of equity in rural health and health care (Aday, Begley, Lairson, & Slater, 1998; Daly, 1994; Habermas, 1996; Mulhall & Swift, 1992).

The distinctions between the individual and community perspectives are most deeply lodged in the debate between liberal and communitarian values (Mulhall & Swift, 1992). The liberal political tradition focuses on the norms of personal well-being and individual freedom. Policies grounded in this tradition have been concerned with protecting or assuring individual rights, and the underlying distributive justice paradigm. Rights are those benefits to which one has a claim, based on assessing what might be a fair distribution of benefits and burdens. This encompasses a consideration of both negative and positive rights—that is, noninterference and freedom of choice as well as a positive conferring of specific material or nonmaterial benefits.

LU ANN ADAY, BETH E. QUILL, AND CIELITO C. REYES-GIBBY • University of Texas School of Public Health, Houston, Texas 77225.

Handbook of Rural Health, edited by Loue and Quill. Kluwer Academic/Plenum Publishers, New York, 2001.

The question of equity posed from this point of view is, "What can *I* justly *claim*?" This perspective has focused most notably on the availability, organization, and financing of rural health care services.

Communitarian sentiments are based on norms of the common good, social solidarity, and protecting the public welfare (Daly, 1994). The concept of justice on which this perspective is based is concerned with the social, economic, and environmental underpinnings of inequity. Rather than focusing on conferring or assuring positive or negative rights (or benefits) to individuals, this paradigm encompasses a broader consideration of public health and social and economic interventions required to enhance the well-being of groups or communities as a whole. The essential question of justice posed from this perspective is, "What is *good* for *us*?" Health policy ultimately directed toward improving the health of individuals and of populations demands investments in more comprehensive, integrated, and effective medical and nonmedical interventions to improve the health of rural populations.

Contemporary social theorists, and most notably the German philosopher Jürgen Habermas, have argued for a new synthesis of these competing foundations for fairness based on a theory of deliberative democracy (Habermas, 1996). Policies attuned to this perspective address the extent to which norms of participation appear to guide decision making. The question of justice posed from this point of view is, "*Who* decides and *how*?" This deliberative justice paradigm recognizes and attempts to resolve conflicts rooted in the other dominant paradigms of fairness through posing the need for rational discourse on the part of affected groups and individuals. Habermas argues that strategic or technical-rational aims of decision makers at either the macro or micro level (such as negotiating contract provisions for a state Medicaid rural health care managed care program or achieving patient adherence to therapeutic regimens) are unlikely to be orchestrated and achieved unless affected stakeholders (providers, payers, and patient advocates, for example) have the opportunity to present and have their points of view heard and respected in the process.

Figure 1 displays a conceptual framework of equity integrating the deliberative, distributive, and social justice paradigms. The access framework begins with the role of health policy in influencing the characteristics of the health delivery system and the population to be served by it. The *deliberative* justice character of health policy focuses on the institutions and procedures through which policy is formulated and implemented. Placing the governing norm of deliberative justice above health policy in the expanded framework is intended to convey that conflicts between the disparate paradigms of distributive justice and social justice that have tended to guide medical care and public health policy, respectively, must be effectively addressed if the health and well-being of rural communities and individuals are to be enhanced. Assuring that those most affected by health policy decisions at both the macro and micro levels are involved in shaping them constitutes the means for doing so. The deliberative paradigm has not been explicitly explored as a basis for the equity of health policy. It is, however, implicit in the focus on consumer involvement and community participation in the design and implementation of private and public health programs in the United States and other countries (Green, 1986; Wallerstein, 1992; Wallerstein & Bernstein, 1994).

The unshaded boxes in Figure 1, encompassing the delivery system, population at risk, and realized access, define the major components of the conceptual framework that has guided much of health services research on access to medical care, grounded in the *distributive justice* paradigm developed by Andersen, Aday, and their colleagues (Aday & Andersen, 1981; Aday, Andersen, & Fleming, 1980). Relevant characteristics of the health system include the availability, organization, and financing of services. Predisposing characteristics of the population at risk include those that describe the propensity of individuals to use services—including basic demographic characteristics (e.g., age, sex), social structural variables (e.g., race and ethnicity, education, employment status, and occupation), and beliefs (e.g., general beliefs and attitudes about the value of health services, or knowledge of disease). Enabling characteristics include the means individuals have available to them for the use of services. Both finan-

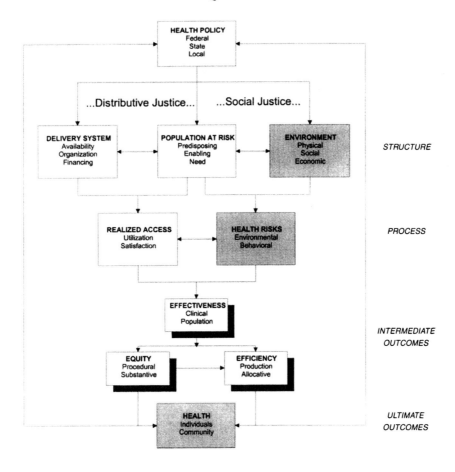

FIGURE 1. An expanded conceptual framework of equity. From Aday, Begley, Lairson, and Slater (1998), copyright 1998 Health Administration Press. Reprinted with permission.

cial resources (such as family income or insurance coverage) and organizational resources (such as having a regular source or place to go for care), specific to the individuals and their families, are relevant here. Need refers to health status or illness as a predictor of health service use. The need for care may be perceived by the individual and reflected in reported disability days or symptoms, for example, or evaluated by a provider in terms of actual diagnoses or complaints.

Realized access refers to objective and subjective indicators of the actual process of care seeking. These are, in effect, indicators of the extent to which the system and population characteristics predict whether or not or how much

care is used (or the demand for care), and how satisfied potential or actual consumers are with the health care system.

As implied by the shaded boxes in Figure 1, in the expanded *social justice* component of the model, there is, first, an explicit acknowledgment of the ultimate outcome of interest that was only implicit or assumed in the original model: the health and well-being of individuals and communities. Second, the model acknowledges that the physical, social, and economic environment of the rural areas in which individuals live and work can also have consequences for their access to health and health care. Third, it indicates that the environment directly influences the likelihood of exposures to significant environmental and behavioral health risks.

The social justice component of the model may be viewed as focusing on the community level of analysis. It primarily examines the characteristics of the physical, social, and economic environment, the population residing within it, and the health risks they experience as a consequence.

The distributive justice component of the model relies on individuals as the ultimate unit of analysis. Their attributes and behavior may, however, be aggregated to reflect the characteristics of patients in a given health system or delivery organization or of the population resident in a designated geographic area. The distributive justice paradigm has led to an emphasis on the equity of the medical care delivery system, whereas the social justice paradigm is reflected in public health and social and economic policy directly or indirectly related to health.

TABLE 1. Criteria and Indicators of Equity

Dimensions	Criteria	Indicators
PROCEDURAL EQUITY		
Deliberative Justice		
Health policy	Participation	Type and extent of affected groups' participation in formulating and implementing policies and programs
Distributive Justice		
Delivery system	Freedom of choice	
• Availability		Distribution of providers
• Organization		Types of facilities
• Financing		Sources of payment
Realized access	Cost-effectiveness	
• Utilization		Type and volume of services used
• Satisfaction		Public opinion, patient opinion
Distributive & Social Justice		
Population at risk	Similar treatment	
• Predisposing		Age, sex, race, education, etc.
• Enabling		Regular source, insurance coverage, income, etc.
• Need		Perceived, evaluated
Social Justice		
Environment	Common good	
• Physical		Toxic, environmental hazards
• Social		Social capital (family structure, voluntary organizations, social networks)
• Economic		Human and material capital (schools, jobs, income, housing)
Health risks	Need	
• Environmental		Toxic, environmental exposures
• Behavioral		Lifestyle, health promotion practices
SUBSTANTIVE EQUITY		
Health	Need	
• Individuals		Clinical indicators
• Community		Population rates

Note: From Aday, Begley, Lairson, and Slater (1998), copyright 1998 Health Administration Press. Reprinted with permission.

The goal of health policy, implied in the expanded equity framework, is to contribute to improving the health of individuals and communities. The ultimate test of the equity of health policy from the social justice perspective is the extent to which disparities or inequalities in health between rural and urban areas and among subgroups of the rural population are minimized (Whitehead, 1992).

Indicators and Data Sources

Indicators

Table 1 summarizes empirical indicators of equity in relationship to the primary dimensions of the framework for assessing equity (see again Figure 1) and the related criteria of justice underlying them. Data may be gathered to assess dimensions of procedural and substantive equity descriptively, and to conduct analytic or evaluative research, exploring those factors that are most predictive of persistent substantive inequities—mirrored in subgroup variations in health. The challenge to analytic and evaluative research is how best to design studies and gather data to assess the factors that are most likely to influence this endpoint and the health policy interventions suggested as a consequence.

Participation

Empirical indicators of deliberative justice attempt to express the type and extent of involvement of affected groups' participation in formulating and implementing policies and programs. This is manifest, for example, in the extent to which community residents or patient advocacy groups are involved in influencing the assessments of needs in rural communities, and the design of programs and services to address those needs (Hornberger & Cobb, 1998).

Freedom of Choice

Empirical indicators of access, based on the freedom-of-choice norm, are the distribution and availability of health care resources to consumers. For example, personnel (e.g., primary care physicians or specialists) and facility (e.g., inpatient and outpatient services) to population

ratios and related inventories of rural health care personnel or providers (e.g., nonphysician providers, managed care plans, and contractors) in a given target area are indicators of the basic supply of providers and delivery sites available to community residents. The index of medical underservice (IMU) and health professions shortage area (HPSA) indicators have been used to identify rural communities most in need of expanded health care services (Office of Rural Health Policy, 1997a).

Cost-Effectiveness

Components of the costs and benefits of care are reflected in the type and comprehensiveness of services received and how satisfied patients and families are with them relative to some standard. Studies comparing the costs and outcomes of rural health care services delivered in alternative delivery system arrangements (essential access community hospitals/rural primary care hospitals [EACH/RPCH], rural health clinics) or through different providers (physician and nonphysician practitioners) would, for example, provide useful guidance in terms of how best to invest limited health care dollars (Agency for Health Care Policy and Research, 1991; Cheh & Thompson, 1997).

Similar Treatment

The similar treatment criterion emphasizes that age, sex, race, income, or whether a person is covered by Medicaid, private insurance, or has no insurance should not dictate that people with similar needs enter different doors (e.g., private versus public providers) or be treated differently (in terms of the type or intensity of services provided). This criterion is a defining tenet of the egalitarian concept of justice. A primary concern in rural health and health care delivery is that certain groups (minorities, the elderly, low-income individuals, and the uninsured) may be particularly disadvantaged in their ability to obtain needed care (Office of Technology Assessment, 1990).

Common Good

Empirical indicators related to the common good would encompass a look at the array of social status, social capital, and human and material capital resources available to the population at risk in a given area, as well as the significant physical environmental exposures that are likely to exist. The focus of interventions is not on altering individual actions and motivations, but on the more distal but foundational roots of health problems, such as the social–structural correlates of health and health care inequalities rooted in the physical, social, and economic environments in which individuals live and work. Health risks in the physical environment include toxic and environmental contaminants or stressors (e.g., exposure to agricultural chemicals) in a given community. The social environment encompasses the social resources (or social capital) that may be available to the individuals who live there, associated with the family structure, voluntary organizations, and social networks that both bind and support them. The economic environment encompasses both human and material capital resources, reflected in the schools, jobs, income, and housing that characterize the community (Aday, 1993). The economic well-being of rural communities that are heavily dependent on single-source industries, such as agriculture, mining, or oil, is, for example, greatly affected by downturns in those major sources of income and employment in the community (National Association of Community Health Centers, 1988).

Need

Indicators of equity from the perspective of need attempt to assess the magnitude of health risks and health disparities in a population. Procedural equity is reflected in minimizing population groups' differential exposure to health risks. The ultimate test of substantive equity of health policy is the extent to which disparities or inequalities in health outcomes are minimized in rural areas or among subgroups of the rural population.

Data Sources

As implied in the conceptual framework of equity (Figure 1), studies of equity could focus on the rural health care delivery system as a whole, particular institutions within it, groups of patients, or the communities that are the target of health policy initiatives, or various combinations of these levels and their interrelationships. Such studies may entail collecting new (primary) data as well as make use of data collected for other purposes (secondary data). Both quantitative and qualitative data may be needed to capture fully the array of factors reflected in the expanded framework of equity. The sources of primary and secondary data that are particularly relevant for examining the various dimensions of equity in rural areas are reviewed in the discussion that follows (Aday *et al.*, 1998).

Environment

Environmental indicators focus on the community itself or definable geographic areas within it as the unit of analysis. They are explicitly intended to reflect the structural or environmental context in which residents live and work that significantly affect health risks and health. One of the challenging issues in rural health care research is how precisely to define "rural" communities and the relevant indicators for assaying their health and health care needs.

The World Health Organization Healthy Cities and Healthy Communities movement has identified a range of community-level variables related to air and water quality, housing availability and quality, and economic development, among others, that can be used in profiling the health and well-being of communities (U.S. Health Corporation, 1994; World Health Organization Healthy Cities Project, 1988). These data are available from planning agencies, business censuses, U.S. census data on household characteristics, and local public health environmental surveillance systems. Qualitative studies using participant or nonparticipant observation methods may also be useful for profiling the social and environmental context that may affect the health or health care of individuals in designated communities or subgroups.

Population

Population-based studies look at individuals who do not use a given delivery system or institution as well as those who do. The denominator for population-level analyses represents individuals residing in a designated geographic area. Surveys are particularly useful in measuring the attitudes or barriers that preclude targeted individuals or subgroups from seeking care. State or local agencies may lack the resources and expertise for conducting such studies. Qualitative or semistructured interviews and focus groups may also be instructive in profiling the health and health care experiences of a population at risk, as well as informing the design or interpretation of more structured surveys of a representative sample of the target population.

Public health population surveillance systems, disease registries, census or vital statistics data, and synthetic estimates based on national sources are some of the major types of secondary data used in profiling the health and health care of a population at the state or local level. Small area estimation procedures make use of data gathered at the national level (on utilization rates for certain age–sex–race groups) to impute what the estimates are likely to be at the state or local level (given the age–sex–race composition of the state or community) (National Center for Health Statistics, 1979). Managed care plan enrollment files also provide data on the denominator of individuals residing in a given geographic area who are eligible to use plan services.

System

Descriptors at the system level focus on the availability, organization, and financing of services as aggregate, structural properties. Secondary data sources are most often used for this type of analysis. The Bureau of Health Professions, within the Health Resources and Services Administration, has, for example, compiled a computerized area resource file that has an array of health and health care data by county or metropolitan statistical area. The American Medical Association and the American Hospital Association, as well as other provider groups, routinely publish directories, and in some instances have computerized data available on the characteristics and distribution of medical personnel. The National Center for Health Statistics (NCHS) collects data on the characteristics and utilization of hospitals, nursing homes, and outpatient medical care practices. The Health

Care Financing Administration and the Health Insurance Association of America also periodically publish information on the amount and distribution of expenditures by major public (Medicare and Medicaid) and private third-party payers (NCHS, 1997).

Public health departments or private providers (such as national HMO firms considering entering a market) may want either more current or more detailed information on the types of services being provided or the profile of clients seen by facilities in a given area than is available from existing sources. In this case, the interested agencies or organizations could collect primary data, based on interviews with key community informants, telephone requests to providers for brochures describing their services, or full-fledged surveys of providers to gather data on the programs and services being offered and who is being served.

Institutions

Secondary data used most often by institutions (or organizations) for assessing access to the facility include enrollment, encounter data, claims, and medical records. Financial records provide an indication of the level of uncompensated or undercompensated care the facility provides, and for what types of patients and services. Other institutional sources (such as clinic logbooks or emergency room referral records) are used in conducting studies of the magnitude and profile of unscheduled walk-in visits, and nonmedically motivated transfers within an institution. Surveys might also be conducted of administrators, providers, or patients to provide data on the operation of the institutions relevant to access or availability issues.

Patients

Patient surveys are the major sources of primary data for evaluating access at the institutional level. Patient surveys tap individuals' subjective perceptions of their experiences at a given facility (how long they had to wait to be seen), which may or may not agree with more objective institutional records or data sources (average clinic waiting time estimates, for example). These subjective perceptions are, however, more reflective than are objective, records-based indicators of the extent to which people actually are satisfied and loyal users of a facility. Focus groups and ethnographic interviews conducted with patients may also help explain problems providers have encountered in dealing with certain types of patients or help them design more culturally sensitive or consumer-oriented services.

Patient origin studies use patient address and zip code information to determine the areas from which most patients are drawn. Patient record data can also serve as the basis for generating profiles of the demographic composition (age, sex, and race) or the major presenting complaints of patients seen at the facility.

The next section highlights major federal and state policy initiatives to improve the equity of health and health care delivery in rural areas, followed by a review of the evidence regarding the success of these initiatives.

Health Policies to Address Equity

Federal Policies

The federal government has developed a number of initiatives over the past 30 years to support the delivery of health care in rural areas. Most of these, not surprisingly, have attempted to address issues of distributive justice. Policies focused on medical providers have included specific workforce initiatives such as medical education (Public Health Service Act, Section 780), educational loans for primary care physicians and other health professionals, including midlevel practitioners. The National Health Service Corps, a federal program to provide health professionals to underserved areas, most of them rural, has been instrumental in recruiting and retaining physicians in remote rural areas. In addition, federal policy has supported the ongoing education of health professionals through Area Health Education Centers and the use of telemedicine to enhance primary care in rural areas. Special projects such as the Rural Medical Education Demonstration Projects (1987 Omnibus Budget Reconciliation Act) complemented the federal government's efforts to place family medicine providers in rural communi-

ties. Recognizing that lack of specialists is also a dramatic need in rural areas, programs to support OB/GYN and pediatricians were established. Designating selected rural areas as health professions shortage areas and MUAs (medically underserved areas) permitted federal funds to be used to recruit physicians. The federal government also developed the Rural Health Clinics and the Community Health and Migrant Health Centers, primary sites for delivery of care in rural areas. Rural Health Care Transition grants and Primary Care Cooperative agreements continue to offer support as mechanisms to provide resources to local communities for primary care. Programs that provided loans, scholarships and other incentives to health care providers and facilities were viewed as a major policy thrust to address the inadequacy of resources in rural areas.

The financial underpinning of these policies is a significant factor in their success in reconciling the inequity of health care services distribution in rural areas. Modifying such programs as Medicare, Medicaid, and reimbursement to physicians acknowledges the differential costs to operate facilities and provide medical care in rural areas. Further, rural residents are far more likely than urban residents to have no health insurance.

In summary, federal policy has been challenged to define and designate areas and populations in need, enhance the capacity of those areas to provide specified care, ensure that policies respect the diversity of rural areas, and work collaboratively with states to develop effective and efficient mechanisms to deliver care to rural residents.

State Policies

The declines in utilization of inpatient hospital care, diminishing federal resources, and changing demography (i.e., age and racial or ethnic composition and migration patterns) have placed a burden on states to undertake further innovative policies to ensure the care of rural citizens. Although states remain highly dependent on federal funding, they have established offices of rural health to define specific state needs and identify rural health issues. They have actively engaged legislative action to modify professional licensure and health facility regulations, emergency service requirements and certificate of need (CON). In addition they have complemented loan programs to recruit and retain needed health professionals to their state. One critical state action has been to increase the payments to hospitals, and providers, especially Medicaid payments, that have been notably low and a disincentive to practice in rural areas. Several states have also undertaken initiatives to develop their own models of rural hospital care, based on the federally funded EACH/RPCH programs.

In summary, states have effected change by modifying legislation, supporting recruitment and retention efforts, expanding reimbursement for hospitals and providers, and controlling licensure of professionals and facilities. In the section that follows, the current evidence on the extent to which both state and federal policy initiatives have been successful in achieving equity in rural health and health care delivery will be reviewed.

Evidence Relating to Equity

Evidence on the extent to which equity of rural health and health care has been achieved by these various state and federal policy initiatives will be reviewed. The review will be presented first, from the perspective of the social justice paradigm, focusing in particular on rural–urban disparities in health; second, from the distributive justice paradigm, looking at the adequacy of health services provision in rural areas; and last, from the deliberative justice paradigm, emphasizing the nature of the policy and program design process to address rural health care needs. Major empirical findings, based on the equity framework introduced here, are summarized in Tables 2 through 7.

As discussed in Chapter 2, there is a wide variation in the definition and consequent measurement of what is rural. In the following review, "rural" will refer to areas or residents outside metropolitan statistical areas (MSAs), unless noted otherwise.

Social Justice

The social justice dimension of equity encompasses a broad look at health disparities between urban and rural areas or between groups (by age, gender, and race, for example) within rural areas and the underlying physical, social, and economic environment in which individuals live and work. Overall, evidence suggests that disparities in health status between urban and rural populations exist. Although mortality rates are lower in rural areas, chronic illness and disability affect a larger proportion of rural than urban residents (Office of Technology Assessment, 1990). For example, data from the National Medical Expenditure Survey (Braden & Beauregard, 1994) and the U.S. Bureau of the Census and the NCHS (1999a) show that rural adult residents reported their health status less favorably and had more activity limitation because of their health than their urban counter-

Table 2. Availability: Distribution of Providers–Physicians (American Medical Association, 1999): Distribution of Nonfederal Physicians in Metropolitan and Nonmetropolitan Areas, 1997

Type	Total	Metropolitan		Nonmetropolitan	
		Number	Percent	Number	Percent
Office-based practice	458,209	402,848	88.0	55,361	12.0
a. General/family	62,022	46,448	74.9	15,574	25.0
b. Medical specialty	157,359	142,887	90.8	14,472	9.2
c. Surgical specialty	117,362	103,454	88.1	13,908	11.9
d. Other specialty	121,466	110,059	90.6	11,407	9.4
Hospital-based practice	145,318	135,767	93.4	9,551	6.6
Other professional activity	41,519	39,408	94.9	2,111	5.1
Not classified	20,046	18,278	91.2	1,768	8.8
Inactive	71,015	60,424	85.1	10,591	14.9
TOTAL	736,107	656,725	89.2	79,382	10.8

TABLE 3.   Availability: Distribution of Providers–Nurses (Stratton, Dunkin, and Juhl, 1995): Size and Demographic Classification of US Counties with a Shortage of Nurses, 1990

Type	Description	Percent of shortage counties within each demographic region[a]	
		Number	Percent
Metro Counties			
Large metropolitan core counties	Core counties of greater MAs[b] of 1,000,000 or more population	1	0.2
Fringe counties	Noncore counties of metro areas of 1,000,000 or more population	10	1.6
Medium metropolitan	Counties of metro areas of 250,000 to 999,999 population	24	3.9
Lesser metropolitan	Counties of metro areas of less than 250,000 population	12	1.9
Subtotal (metropolitan)		47	7.6
Nonmetro Counties			
Urbanized			
Adjacent[c] to MA	Counties contiguous to metropolitan areas that have 20,000 or more urban residents	16	2.6
Not adjacent to MA	Counties not contiguous to MA that have 20,000 or more urban residents	20	3.2
Less urbanized			
Adjacent[c] to MA	Counties contiguous to MA with < 20,000 but > 2499 urban residents	136	22.0
Not adjacent to MA	Counties not contiguous to MA but with < 20,000 but > 2499 urban residents	206	33.3
Thinly populated			
Adjacent[c] to MA	Counties having 2500 urban residents, contiguous to MA	48	7.7
Not adjacent to MA	Counties having < 2500 urban residents, not contiguous to MA	146	23.6
Subtotal (Non-metropolitan)		572	92.4
TOTAL		619	100.0

[a]Total N=3080; counties designated as shortage counties = 619 (20.1%).
[b]MAs—metropolitan areas
[c]Counties physically adjacent to one or more MAs and having at least 2% of the employed labor force in the nonmetropolitan county commuting to central metropolitan counties.
Note: From Stratton, Dunkin, & Juhl (1995), copyright 1995 Mosby, Inc. Reprinted with permission.

parts. Rural residents (> 18 years old) were more likely to report that they had been diagnosed with a chronic condition compared with residents of other areas in the United States. In particular, in 1996, heart disease was reported by 72.6 per 1,000 urban adults compared to 98.8 per 1000 rural adults. Further, 101.3 urban compared to 128.8 per 1,000 rural adults reported having hypertension (NCHS, 1999a).

Braden and Beauregard (1994) also report that 22.6% of rural adults as opposed to 18.8% of adults in core metropolitan areas received medical treatment in 1987 for life-threatening conditions, and 36% of rural adults versus 30.2% of adults in core metropolitan areas received medical treatment in 1987 for degenerative or chronic conditions. Life-threatening conditions include malignant neoplasms, heart disease, and cardiovascular disorders and liver disorders. Degenerative or chronic conditions include diabetes, kidney disease, arthritis and rheumatism, and chronic diseases of the blood, the nervous system, the respiratory system, and the digestive system.

TABLE 4. Enabling: Regular Source of Care (National Center for Health Statistics, 1999b). Percentage of persons without usual source of care according to age and location of residence, United States, average annual 1995–1996

	Under 6 years of age	6–17 years of age	18–64 years of age
MSA	4.3	7.3	13.6
Non-MSA	3.9	6.8	11.6

Age continues to be a factor associated with increased morbidity in rural areas. Traumatic injuries are higher among rural children (Hwang, Stallones, & Keefe, 1997; Svenson, Spurlock, & Nypaver, 1995) compared with urban children, and rural elders (age > 65) were found to have significantly poorer health status than urban elders (Mainous & Kohrs, 1995).

Urban–rural disparities in the prevalence of infectious diseases also exist. In particular, data from various surveillance reports from the Centers for Disease Control and Prevention (CDC) on Acquired Immune Deficiency Syndrome (AIDS) show that the average annual percent increase of cumulative AIDs cases for the years 1992 to 1995 in nonmetropolitan areas was 30% compared to 25.8% in metropolitan areas (Fordyce, Thomas, & Shum, 1997). Increasing rates of primary and secondary syphilis were also observed in North Carolina's rural population, for example, with the highest increase between the years 1985 and 1993 occurring among nonwhite rural women (Thomas, Kulick, & Schoenbach, 1995).

Environment

Physical (Indicator: Environmental Hazards)

Environmental hazards in rural areas include lack of clean water, wastewater services, and paved roads. Rural residents, particularly in the border region (e.g., Texas, Arizona, and California), are exposed to polluted waters like the New River (California–Mexico border), which is estimated to carry more than 280 million gallons a day of industrial waste and sewage, and the Rio Grande (Texas–Mexico border), which is also one of the most polluted waters in the United States (Powers & Byrd, 1998).

Exposure to agricultural chemicals is also a concern for residents in rural areas. Pesticides, which are used extensively in agriculture, are known to be harmful to the environment, and although toxicity data are not complete in all pesticides many are known to be toxic to humans (Napolitano & Goldberg, 1998).

Social (Indicator: Family Structure; Voluntary Organizations; Social Networks)

Rural households are generally larger than those in urban areas, include multigenerational living arrangements, and offer greater access to

Table 5. Enabling: Insurance Coverage (National Center for Health Statistics, 1999b)
a. Percentage of persons under 65 years of age according to type of health coverage and location of residence: United States, 1996

	Private Insurance	Private Insurance through workplace	Medicaid or other public assistance	Not Covered
MSA	72.5	66.5	11.1	15.3
Non-MSA	65.8	58.6	13.9	19.2

b. Percentage of persons 65 years of age or over according to type of health coverage and location of residence: United States, 1996

	*Private Insurance	*Private Insurance through workplace	Medicaid or other public assistance	Medicare only
MSA	72.2	40.5	7.7	18.7
Non-MSA	71.3	32.2	10.4	15.9

*Almost all persons 65 years of age and over are covered by Medicare also.

TABLE 6. Need: Respondent-assessed Health Status, Chronic and Acute Conditions (National Center for Health Statistics, 1999a), Selected Health Status Indicators for Adults by Place of Residence: United States, 1996

Selected Health Status Indicators	MSA	Non-MSA
Respondent-assessed Health Status		
(Percent of persons)		
Excellent	38.6	33.2
Very good	29.8	28.2
Good	22.6	25.2
Fair	6.8	9.5
Poor	2.2	3.8
Reported Chronic Condition		
(per 1,000 persons)		
Hypertension	101.3	128.8
Arthritis	121.0	150.5
Diabetes	28.9	28.7
Heart disease	72.6	98.8
Number of Acute Conditions		
(per 100 persons per year)		
Injuries	21.2	23.4
Infective/parasitic diseases	19.2	25.4
Acute musculoskeletal conditions	2.9	4.3

kinship support systems (Bushy, 1998). Further, rural communities are community-oriented and have a tendency to be resistant to accepting services from "outsiders" (Bushy, 1998; Long & Weinert, 1989). Thus, efforts designed to build a healthy community that assure community participation and draw on existing expertise in the community are most likely to be successful.

Economic (Indicator: Human and Material Capital)

The rural as compared to the urban labor force is reported to be less educated than urban residents: only 42.4% of rural residents had greater than a high school education versus 56.2% of urban residents. It is estimated that 10% of rural residents 16 years and older are employed in two of the most hazardous occupations—farming and underground mining (Maningas, 1991).

Rural areas also generally have higher unemployment rates than urban areas (Economic Research Service, 1998). Although the U.S. Census Bureau reports that the proportion of people living below poverty level (for a family of four in 1997 the threshold was $16,400; for a family of three, $12,802) decreased nationwide from 13.7% in 1996 to 13.3% in 1997, this improvement was not observed for rural area residents. For the years 1989, 1996, and 1997, 15.9% of rural area residents lived below poverty level. In addition, median income in rural areas (outside metropolitan areas) is 76% ($30,057) of urban areas ($39,381).

Homelessness continues to be a problem in both urban and rural communities. Estimates of the homeless population widely vary. The proportion representing the "rural" homeless ranges from 6.9% to 11% or even 14% (National Rural Health Association, 1996). The 1990 U.S. census showed 240,140 rural homeless whereas other studies show even up to millions (National Rural Health Association, 1996). The wide variation arises from the operational definitions used for homelessness as well as difficulties associated with accessing the homeless population (i.e., transient homeless).

In contrast to their urban counterparts, the

TABLE 7. Use of Services (National Center for Health Statistics, 1999b)

a. Number of physician contacts per person according to location of residence: United States, 1990–1996

	1990	1991	1992	1993	1994	1995	1996
Within MSA	5.6	5.8	6.0	6.1	6.0	5.9	5.8
Outside MSA	4.9	5.1	5.6	5.6	5.7	5.3	5.7

b. Percent distribution of physician contacts according to place of contact and location of residence: United States, 1996

	Doctor's office	Hospital outpatient	Telephone	Home	*Other
MSA	56.2	11.9	13.3	3.3	15.4
Non-MSA	54.1	13.8	12.4	3.2	16.5

c. Percent distribution of time-interval since last physician contact, according to location of residence: United States, 1996

	Less than 1 year	1 year-less than 2 years	2 years or more
MSA	80.4	9.4	10.2
Non-MSA	78.8	10.1	11.1

d. Percentage of children under 6 years of age without physician contact within the past 12 months according to location of residence: United States, average annual 1995–1996

MSA	8.9
Non-MSA	10.9

* Includes clinics or other places outside a hospital.

profile of the rural homeless suggests that they include more women, more whites, and more recently employed, and are less likely to have spent time in penal institution and less likely to have abused drugs and alcohol. Also, the men are less likely to have been in the military or to have served in Vietnam (National Rural Health Association, 1996).

Health Risks

Environmental (Indicator: Environmental Exposures)

Children in rural areas have increased lead exposure (Norman, Bordley, Hertz-Picciotto, & Newton, 1994) whereas migrant and seasonal farmworkers, a subset of the rural population, are typically exposed to poor living conditions. Napolitano and Goldberg (1998) report that migrant farmworkers live in substandard housing such as shacks and barns or in overcrowded bungalows, dormitories, apartments, or hotel rooms lacking in electricity, plumbing, cooling or heating, and adequate ventilation. In addition, the work of migrant fieldworkers exposes them to environmental risks (and associated illnesses) such as injuries (machine-related fatalities, electrocution, falls from ladders, neck–shoulder–back pain, amputations, eye injuries); crowded living conditions (tuberculosis); pesticide exposure (cancers, limb reduction, birth defects, dermatitis); lack of field sanitation (acute gastroenteritis); and unfavorable climate conditions (heat stroke).

Behavioral (Indicator: Health Promotion Practices)

Research suggests that improvement in health promotion efforts is needed in rural areas. For example, Michielutte, Dignan, Sharp, Boxley, and Wells (1996) found that prevention and early-detection behaviors for skin cancer were low among rural women. Also, Hoyt, Conger, Valde, and Wiehs (1997) found that persons living in rural areas were more likely to hold stigmatized attitudes toward mental health care, thereby preventing them from seeking needed services.

Further, data on preventive health behaviors from a survey of Otsego County, New York, suggest that rural residents tend to be late adopters (Pearson & Lewis, 1998). Late adopter behavior in the rural population may be influenced by different levels of exposure to health messages on video, audio, and print media; less visibility or absence of health promotion organizations, health care providers, and work site health promotion programs; higher rates of poverty; and lower rates of educational attainment.

Distributive Justice

The distributive justice dimension of equity encompasses availability, organization, and financing of health care services; the populations they are intended to serve; and the utilization of and satisfaction with those services. The prevailing concern is the adequate provision of health services. This paradigm, in particular, has dominated the conceptualization and measurement of the equity of the U.S. health care system (Aday et al., 1998).

Delivery System: Availability (Indicator: Distribution of providers)

A persistent problem in rural areas is the shortage of health care providers. Even though roughly 23% of Americans live in rural areas, only 12% of physicians practice there and as many as 25% of these physicians were expected to retire by the year 2000 (McDowell, 1997). Despite the National Health Service Corps (NHSC) program established by the federal government in 1970 to place physicians and other health care providers in underserved areas, the American Medical Association (1999) reports that although physician supply increased in rural areas during the 1970s and 1980s, the urban–rural gap remained about the same. For example, the percentage of (total) physicians in metropolitan areas increased from 86.9% in 1980 to 89.2% in 1997; conversely, the percentage of nonmetropolitan areas physicians decreased during the same period.

The Office of Rural Health Policy estimates that over 20 million rural residents live in areas that have a shortage of physicians to meet their basic needs. In addition, persons living in rural areas are more than four times more likely to live in a health professions shortage area (HPSA) as compared to urban residents (Office of Rural Health Policy, 1997b). The smallest rural counties (population <5,000) have on average, only 41 primary care physicians per 100,000 population compared to 77 in metropolitan areas and 54 in all nonmetropolitan areas (U.S. Department of Health & Human Services, 1991).

The shortage is not limited to physicians alone. Analysis of the area resource file of the Bureau of Health Professions also shows that nursing shortage (92.4%) is most acute in nonmetropolitan counties (Stratton, Dunkin, & Juhl, 1995). Further, the numbers of nurse practitioners, nurse midwives, and physician assistants who also serve as providers of primary care in rural areas are decreasing. By 1989, their numbers in the National Health Service Corps had decreased dramatically from 319 nurse practitioners, 68 nurse midwives, and 111 physicians assistants to 17, 1, and none, respectively (U.S. Department of Health & Human Services, 1991).

Reasons for the shortage of health personnel in rural areas include: (1) economic instability especially in those areas that are not adjacent to a metropolitan center (Stratton, Dunkin, & Juhl, 1995); (2) lack of rural background and rural experiences among the practitioners and their spouses (Moscovice & Nestegard, 1980); and (3) social isolation (Brooks, Bernstein, DeFriese, & Graham, 1981).

Organization (Indicator: Types of facilities and models)

Several types of facilities and models of health care services in rural areas have been developed in response to changes in federal legislation, financing sources and mechanisms, and the changing demographics of the rural population. To date, the needs of the rural population remain largely unmet despite several initiatives over the past 30 years by the federal government and the private sector to support the delivery of health care in rural areas.

Stationary Ambulatory Care. Several federal and private-sector initiatives were undertaken to improve the provision of primary care and preventive health services in rural areas. Federal-sector initiatives include community health centers, migrant health centers, and rural health centers.

Migrant health centers are designated health centers for the migrant populations concentrating on primary care needs whereas community health centers (CHCs) provide primary care to both urban and rural residents including the establishment of outreach activities and linkages with hospitals. CHCs, which are federally subsidized and locally governed, differ from private medical practice by their community governance, provision of a broader range of services, nonprofit status, and obligation to serve all patients regardless of their ability to pay. As reported by Kolimaga, Konrad, and Ricketts (1994), CHCs provide care to the poorest and most underserved populations.

In 1977, the U.S. Congress also passed the Rural Health Clinic Services Act, which mandated the following: (1) cost-based reimbursement and (2) utilization of midlevel practitioners by providing reimbursement for their services to Medicare and Medicaid patients, even in the absence of a full-time physician (Travers, Ellis, & Dartt, 1995).

A report by the General Accounting Office, however, stated that although there was an increase in the number of rural health clinics, many clinics did not reduce travel time or increase the availability of providers for Medicare or Medicaid beneficiaries. In addition, the program was not being implemented in underserved areas. In contrast, Cheh and Thompson (1997) in their study of 18 RHCs in the states of Texas, California, Kansas, Michigan, Maine, and North Carolina state that the RHC program has increased access to care among Medicare and Medicaid beneficiaries at a substantial but reasonable cost.

Private-sector initiatives include the Robert Wood Johnson Foundation's Rural Practice Project (RPP) and W. K. Kellogg Foundation's Community Oriented Primary Care (COPC) program.

The RPP was aimed at building new health care organizations by pairing highly motivated

physicians with professional administrators; encouraging self-sufficiency by requiring significant community contributions through legal sponsorship of the practice by in-kind and out-of-pocket contributions; and emphasizing comprehensive health services (Moscovice & Rosenblatt, 1982), whereas the focus of COPC was to provide a framework for identifying and addressing the health care needs of the community it serves.

Assessment of RPP showed that after four years of operation, practices were still in operation with most retaining community sponsorship, salaried physicians, and a commitment to comprehensive care (Moscovice & Rosenblatt, 1982).

The COPC National Rural Demonstration Program was implemented in 13 rural sites across the United States. Evaluation of the COPC National Rural Demonstration Program showed that at most sites, staff and physician turnover and the extensive demands on the time of the rural primary care physician limited the ability to incorporate COPC activities in clinical practices (Kukulka, Christianson, Moscovice, & DeVries, 1994).

Mobile Ambulatory Care. Telemedicine, defined as a practice of medicine at a distance, involves the use of telecommunication and information technologies to provide clinical care to individuals. Rural communities in particular benefit from telemedicine by being able to access health services—that is, consultation with specialists, among others—through telecommunications. The Office of Rural Health Policy (1997c) reported that the most common clinical uses of telemedicine are diagnostic consults and medical data transmissions with radiology and cardiology, followed by orthopedic, dermatology, and psychiatry applications.

Cost, however, remains a major barrier to the use of telemedicine in rural areas. Although telecommunications equipment costs are decreasing, the costs of using the equipment (i.e., transmissions costs, maintenance, staffing, and so on) remain high (Puskin, 1995).

Mobile vans and mobile clinics provide health care services to clients who are hard to reach due to geographic isolation and lack of financial resources. Garrett (1995) cites how mobile vans in rural areas have been successful in serving the needs of farmworkers (Migrant Health Outreach Program in rural Arizona); improving immunization levels (southeastern Idaho); providing nutrition training, research, and development (Penn State Nutrition Program); and providing pre-natal care (Northeast Indiana's HealthQuest).

Provisions of emergency medical services (EMS) or the lack thereof is cited as a contributing factor to the higher incidence of deaths from motor vehicle accidents in rural versus urban areas (Maningas, 1991). Rural communities are widely dispersed, making it more difficult to reach them in emergency situations. In addition, limited financial resources, physician shortages, declining number of volunteers, hospital closings, and outdated equipment also face EMS in rural communities throughout the country.

Acute Institutional Care (Hospitals). Since the early 1980s, many rural hospitals have been threatened with closure. It is estimated that between 1980 and 1988, the number of rural community hospitals dropped by 235 (9%). The U.S. Department of Health and Human Services (1987) reported that the following changes in health system trends created pressures on rural hospitals: (1) restricted reimbursement by public and private payers (which resulted in conflict between cost-containment and access goals); (2) shift of locus of care from inpatient to outpatient settings; (3) rapid advances in medical technology; (4) inadequate supply of health personnel in rural areas; (5) aggressive competition from urban-based providers; and (6) rapid advances in medical technology with increased consumer expectation. Further, poor economic growth and higher unemployment levels contributed to increased indigent care and bad debt, which further reduced opportunities for public support through tax revenues and donations (Moscovice, 1989).

In response, federal programs were initiated to keep rural hospitals from closure: the Rural Health Care Transition Program, which helps hospitals to change their type and mix of services; the Essential Access Community Health Program, which encourages states and hospitals to experiment with alternatives to full-service hospitals and to develop regionalized rural health networks and a downsized facility called a rural primary care hospital; and the Sole Community Hospital Provision, which provides favorable Medicare payments to hospitals isolated from other hospitals.

Long-Term Care. Based on a 1991 survey of nursing homes and board-and-care homes by the NCHS (1994), there were approximately 46,942 long-term care facilities nationwide (excluding 8,578 that did not respond). Of those, 31,431 were board-and-care homes (18,262 not for the mentally retarded and 13,169 for the mentally retarded) and 15,511 were nursing homes (14,744 freestanding and 767 hospital-based).

In addition, the survey showed that for every 1,000 people age 65 and over, approximately 77 people were either in nursing homes (42 people), in board and nursing homes (6 people), or receiving home health care (29 people). Broken down by region, the need for nursing homes was shown to be similar in all regions. However, data showed that some regions relied more on board-and-care homes, which may be due to lack of facilities or higher cost of nursing home care. For example, the West relied relatively little on nursing homes and home health care while relying more than any other region on board-and-care homes (in 1990, the Office of Technology and Assessment reported that frontier counties are predominantly located in the West); the Midwest relied heavily on nursing homes, little on board and care, and moderately on home health care; the Northeast relied heavily on all three with more reliance on nursing homes than other regions; and the South had rates near the national average, with moderate usage of all types.

Data from the Nursing Home Component of the Medical Expenditure Panel Survey (Agency for Health Care Policy and Research, 1998), conducted among nursing home residents, also showed that overall, only 30.9% of the nursing home population was in nursing homes in rural areas. From the perspective that rural residents are more likely to be at greater risk for placement in a nursing home at a younger age and more likely to have greater functional limitation (Coward & Cutler, 1989), the need for long-term care facilities in rural areas needs to be emphasized.

Integrated Service Delivery Models. Casey, Wellever, and Moscovice (1997) define rural health networks as a formal organizational arrangement among more than one type of rural health care provider (i.e., physician groups, hospitals, long-term care providers, and public health agencies), using the resources of more than one member organization, to perform functions or activities according to an explicit plan of action. To date, rural health networks have not been widely implemented in rural areas. For example, an evaluation of the Robert Wood Johnson Foundation's (RWJF) Hospital-Based Rural Health Care Program (which provided grant support to rural hospital networks from 1988 to 1992) showed that although almost half of all the rural hospitals in the country participated in a rural hospital network, very few members were integrated networks with shared decision making (Moscovice, Cristianson, Johnson, Kralewski, & Manning, 1995).

In 1995, more than 80% of all rural counties were within the service area of at least one health maintenance organization (Rural Health Research Center, 1997). Increased competition among urban-based HMOs, expansion of Medicaid managed care through Section 1115 and 1915b waivers, desire to increase Medicare beneficiary enrollment in HMOs as part of Medicare reform, and the reliance on managed care by state health care reform initiatives have all contributed to the expansion of managed care in rural areas. However, despite the substantial increase in potential access to HMOs in rural areas, rural HMO enrollment is still comparatively low to that of its urban counterpart. It is estimated that at best, the national rural commercial HMO enrollment rate is 7.8%, whereas enrollment in rural Medicaid HMOs and prepaid health plans is 10.5% of Medicaid recipients (Rural Health Research Center, 1997).

Wysong, Bliss, Osborne, Graham, and Pikuzinski (1999) assert that if managed care activity in rural areas continues to depend primarily on market-driven, urban-based HMO expansion, rural markets that are less attractive and include more high-risk groups are likely to fall behind more affluent and healthy urban and rural markets.

Financing (Indicator: Sources of Payment)

Health care in the United States is financed through a complex mechanism of public payers (federal, state, and local government) as well as private insurance and individual payments. Since there is no single nationwide system of health insurance, the United States primarily relies on employers voluntarily to provide health insurance coverage to their employees and dependents and on government programs for the elderly (Medicare), the disabled (Medicare), and some of the poor (Medicaid). However, persons without insurance either through Medicare, Medicaid, or employers can still receive health services either through public clinics or hospitals, state and local health programs, or private providers that finance care through shifting costs to other payers (De Lew, Greenberg, & Kinchen, 1992).

Medicare. Medicare is a national health insurance program administered by the federal government for the elderly and the disabled. Financed through a combination of payroll taxes, federal revenues, and premiums, it is reported to be the single largest insurer in the country. Medicare has two components: Part A, which covers hospital, nursing home, hospice, and home health care, and Part B, which covers physician services, laboratory and diagnostic tests, and other outpatient care. Part A coverage is financed through the Hospital Insurance Trust Fund, which is funded by the Social Security hospital insurance payroll tax on workers and employers. Part B is financed by general federal revenues and a monthly premium paid by enrollees. Beneficiaries are also liable for deductibles, copayments, and physician charges in excess of standard Medicare fees.

Because rural areas have a higher proportion of the elderly (14.3% versus 11.3% in urban) and the disabled (7.4% versus 5.6% in urban), Medicare coverage in 1992 was 16.2% among rural residents as compared to 12.7% among urban residents. However, although Medicare covered a higher proportion of rural residents, the average Medicare expenditure per rural beneficiary was 20% less than their urban counterpart (Frenzen, 1997).

Medicaid. Medicaid is a health insurance program administered by states under broad federal guidelines for certain groups of the poor. Jointly financed by the federal and state governments, Medicaid outlays by the states are matched by the federal government and vary by state personal income levels (i.e., poorer states receive a higher match). Aside from being poor, Medicaid recipients must be either aged, blind, pregnant, or the parent of a dependent child. Expansions in eligibility criteria in recent years have included two-parent families based on income. The services covered by Medicaid include preventive, acute, and long-term care services.

NCHS (1999b) reports that Medicaid (or other public assistance) coverage in 1996 was approximately 13.9% for rural residents compared with 11.1% for urban residents. For the same year, Medicaid coverage for those who are over age 65 was 10.4% for rural residents compared with 7.7% for urban residents, suggesting that older rural residents are relatively poorer compared with their urban counterparts.

Child Health Insurance Program (CHIP). CHIP is a federal program designed to extend health insurance to uninsured children with family incomes up to twice (200% of) the federal poverty level who are ineligible for other insurance coverage, including Medicaid. States are tasked to implement and run the program so that states decide on eligibility rules and strategies to find and enroll children. An analysis of the March 1997 Current Population Survey by Thorpe and Florence (1999) showed that approximately 9 million of the 11.3 million children without health insurance lived in families with incomes at or below twice (200% of) the federal poverty line.

Current estimates show that 21% of rural children are without insurance compared with 14% of urban children. Further, approximately 4.6 million children below twice (200% of) poverty are uninsured (Weil, 1997), making them likely to be eligible for CHIP.

Private Insurance. In 1996, private insurance companies provided health insurance coverage to an estimated 71.4% of the U.S. population (NCHS, 1999b). With coverage varying as to benefit structures, premiums, and rules for paying the medical care providers, private insurance is obtained either through the individual's employers or direct purchase of nongroup health insurance.

In 1996, 65.8% of rural residents under 65 years of age had private insurance compared with 72.5% of urban residents in the same age group. Because there is a higher percentage of small business economies in rural areas, private insurance obtained through the workplace was approximately 58.6% for rural residents as compared with 66.5% for urban residents (NCHS, 1999b).

Uninsured. Despite efforts to improve access to health care, the United States continues to have a high number (approximately 40 million in 1996) of individuals without any type of health coverage. In 1996, 19.2% of rural residents did not have health coverage compared with 15.3% of urban residents (NCHS, 1999b).

Population at Risk

Predisposing (Indicator: Age, Sex, Race, Education)

The age profile of the rural population includes the following: median age, 30.2; 29.4% under age 18; and 13% over age 65 (Office of Technology Assessment, 1990). In terms of racial distribution, 88.2% are white (3.2% of whom are Hispanic) and 11.8% are nonwhites. The nonwhites include blacks (8.8%); American Indians (1.3%); and Asians/Pacific Islanders (0.6%). With respect to educational experience, 83.1% of the rural population graduated from high school, with only 9.2% having had some college education.

These characteristics suggest that risks among rural residents include those associated with the young (i.e., traumatic injuries, teenage pregnancy, substance abuse) and the old (i.e., chronic diseases) as well as with a blue-collar labor force (i.e., job-related injuries) and minority populations (i.e., cardiovascular diseases, diabetes).

Enabling (Indicator: Regular Source of Care)

Overall, there is not a wide gap between the proportion of rural and urban children with a usual source of care. Approximately 94.9% of rural children under 6 years have a usual source of care compared with 95.9% of urban children for 1993–94, which improved in 1995–96, with 96.1% of rural children having a usual source of care compared with 95.7% of urban children (NCHS, 1999b). The same is true among the 6 to 17 age group, with 92.3% of rural children having a usual source of care compared with 91.8% of urban children for the period 1993–94. The trend continued with 93.2% of rural children compared with 92.7% of urban children having a usual source of care in 1995–96 (NCHS, 1999b).

With respect to the adult population, data from the National Medical Expenditure Survey (Braden & Beauregard, 1994) showed that rural adults were more likely to identify a usual source of medical care compared with urban adults (85.0% versus 80.4%).

Need (Indicator: Perceived Health)

As noted earlier, rural adults (> 18 years old) perceived their health status less favorably than urban adults. In 1996, 86.6% of rural adults rated their health as good or better (i.e., good, very good, excellent) compared with 91% of urban adults who did so (NCHS, 1999a). Further, in 1987, selected health status indicators (work limitations, physical activity limitations, mobility, and self-care limitations) showed that 78.6% of rural adults as opposed to 82.9% of urban adults reported having no work limitations; 63.6% of rural as opposed to 68.76% of urban adults reported having no serious limitations; and 73.6% of rural adults as opposed to 79.23% of urban adults reported having no mobility and self-care limitations (Braden & Beauregard, 1994).

Realized Access

Utilization (Indicator: Type and Volume of Services Used)

NCHS (1999b) reports a similar distribution for the number of physician contacts per per-

son for the year 1996 between rural and urban residents (i.e., 5.7 for rural residents and 5.8 for urban residents). Further, during the same year, rural residents had 54.1% of these contacts at physicians' offices, 13.8% at hospital outpatient departments, 12.4% by telephone, 3.2% at home, and 16.5% in "other" places. Among urban residents, 56.2% of these physician contacts were made at physicians' offices, 11.9% at hospital outpatient departments, 13.3% by telephone, 3.3% at home, and 15.4% in "other" places.

Although the trend improved from the years 1964 to 1995 in terms of the interval since last physician contact for rural residents, the rural–urban gap remains. The time interval since last physician contact for total rural and urban residents for 1996 was as follows: 78.8% of rural and 80.4% of urban residents for the <1 year interval; 10.1% of rural and 9.4% of urban residents for the >1–2 year interval; and 11.1% of rural and 10.2% of urban residents for the ≥2 year interval (NCHS, 1999b).

The percentage of rural and urban children < 6 years without a physician contact within the past 12 months increased between the years 1993 and 1996. Approximately 10.8% of rural children had no physician contact within the past 12 months (1993–94) which worsened to 11.3% in the subsequent 12 months (1994–95). In contrast, only 7.6% of urban children had no physician contact within the past 12 months (1993–94), which worsened to 8.2% in the subsequent 12 months (1994–95).

Satisfaction (Indicator: Public Opinion and Patient Opinion)

Although there are limited data on patient satisfaction among rural residents, research suggests that overall, rural patients are satisfied with the health care services they receive. For example, a national survey of 1,784 patients in 46 community and migrant health centers found that patient satisfaction with quality of care is high (National Association of Community Health Centers, 1994). Similarly, Blazer, Landerman, Fillenbaum, and Horner (1995) found that rural adults living in North Carolina were as satisfied with their health care as their urban counterparts. Client satisfaction in a rural nurse practitioner–managed health center was also found to be high (Ramsey, Edwards, Lenz, Odom, & Brown, 1993).

Deliberative Justice

Health Policy (Indicator: Type and Extent of Participation in Formulating and Implementing Programs)

Studies show that the extent of rural citizen participation ranges from designing community education and health promotion programs (Cook, Goeppinger, Brunk, Price, Whitehead, & Sauter, 1985) to providing nonmedical interventions (Heins, Nance, & Ferguson, 1987) and emergency medical services (Myrick, Bonnie, Kishbaugh, Pittman, & Sayford, 1983; Perlstadt & Kozak, 1977).

However, evidence is lacking of "effective" and "meaningful" citizen participation wherein policy or development of activities are oriented toward gaining a reasonable consensus about the definition of the problem and the best possible ways to address it on the part of those most likely to be affected by the resulting policy. Zimmerman (1990) suggests that this has been hampered by the lack of confidence among consumers to influence the policy process effectively. Further, he suggests: a) the need for laypersons to develop decision-making and problem-solving skills as well as knowledge of health care systems to enhance their impact and to be considered as equal partners by providers; and (b) the need for providers to develop incentives and training to improve their capacity to work with consumers in a collaborative and noncontrolling fashion.

In the concluding section of the chapter, models that are likely to be most successful in enhancing the equity of access to health and health care in rural areas are presented.

Alternative Models

Developing alternative models to address the concerns about the delivery of health services in rural areas is not a new phenomenon. As early as the 1940s with the establishment of health service areas, the limited-service rural hospitals of the 1970s, and the alternative models of the 1980s, both federal and state governments recognized their role in reshaping the rural health care system (Wellever & Rosenberg, 1993a). The Omnibus Reconciliation Act of 1989, for example, marked a major legislative initiative to address rural health care needs through structural change. The act required the establishment of essential access community hospitals (EACH) or rural primary care hospitals (RPCH) through a grant program to states. These grants stimulated the development of nontraditional models, including the creation of rural health networks, regionalization of rural health services, improved access to hospitals and other services, and enhancement of rural emergency and transportation systems (Agency for Health Care Policy and Research, 1991).

States used these models and others to fashion alternative models that suited their specific needs. Although states have varied in the implementation of the models, all have been constructed to include: (a) reduction or elimination of in-patient beds; (b) discontinuation of costly and complicated services; (c) focusing on providing emergency care, primary care, and long-term care; (d) cross-training of personnel to perform multiple tasks; and (e) development of referral relationships and linkages with other hospitals (Agency for Health Policy and Research, 1991; Wellever & Rosenberg, 1993a).

In an effort to evaluate best practices and understand the evolution of these nontraditional models, researchers and policymakers have attempted to describe the characteristics of and classify the different types of models. Generally, all alternative models can be characterized in terms of their scope of service, and whether they have linkages with one or more other hospitals and with one or more local nonacute providers. Further, alternative models emerge from environments that have: (a) a rural health policy infrastructure; (b) willing provider organizations and practitioners; (c) flexible regulatory environment; (d) emergency medical services; and (e) other linkage systems that support the system (data, and so on) (Wellever & Rosenberg, 1993a).

The classification of the models begins by distinguishing acute and nonacute hospital beds and describing those that employ institutional

TABLE 8. Nontraditional Rural Health Care Delivery Model Taxonomy

Model Types	Dimensions (Factors)				Example
	Service Role	Hospital Linkage	Other Provider Linkage	Waiver Status	
Fully integrated primary care hospital	Inpatient	Network	Integrated	Waiver	Federal RPCH; Community clinic/ emergency center (Colorado)
Fully integrated hospital	Inpatient	Network	Integrated	No Waiver	Rural medical centers (Wisconsin); Hill Center model (Alabama)
Long-linked primary care hospital	Inpatient	Network	Nonintegrated	Waiver	Medical assistance facility (Montana)
Long-linked hospital	Inpatient	Network	Nonintegrated	No waiver	Consortia/alliances
Short-linked primary care hospital	Inpatient	Freestanding	Integrated	Waiver	None
Short-linked hospital	Inpatient	Freestanding	Integrated	No waiver	Provider-based rural health clinic; diversified hospital
Primary care hospital	Inpatient	Freestanding	Nonintegrated	Waiver	None
Hospital	Inpatient	Freestanding	Nonintegrated	No waiver	Alternative rural hospital model (California)
Fully integrated ambulatory care system	Ambulatory	Network	Integrated	—	Roanoke Amaranth Community Health Group (North Carolina)
Long-linked ambulatory care system	Ambulatory	Network	Nonintegrated	—	Cle Elum Family Medical Center (Washington); Caney Clinic (Kansas)
Short-linked ambulatory care system	Ambulatory	Freestanding	Integrated	—	Freestanding rural health clinics with "other ambulatory services"
Ambulatory care system	Ambulatory	Freestanding	Non-integrated	—	Physician office

Note: From Wellever & Rosenberg (1993a), copyright 1993 Anthony Wellever. Reprinted with permission.

or networking approaches. Institutional approaches tend to focus on the changing regulations that govern hospitals, viewing hospitals as the central actor in rural health care. Networking approaches concentrate on establishing relationships among providers of essential rural health services to assure efficiency and access to services (Wellever & Rosenberg, 1993b). The taxonomy in Table 8 identifies different types of models and the dimensions of these models (Wellever & Rosenberg, 1993a). Examples are noted for 10 of the 12 models.

Twelve model types are characterized, as follows. Fully integrated primary care hospital is a downsized rural hospital that is part of a network with a single local point of entry. Services include primary care, acute care and long-term care. Fully integrated hospital is a hospital that provides inpatient diagnostic and therapeutic services for which staff is trained and the facility is equipped. The hospital has a formal linkage with other hospitals. Long-linked primary care hospital is a downsized rural hospital connected to a larger hospital through a formal arrangement. The purpose is to provide basic low-intensity acute care and assure a referral pathway for patients who leave the area because there are insufficient patient services. Long-linked hospital is a Medicare-recognized hospital with a formal agreement with other hospitals. These arrangements are usually consortium or alliances focused on information sharing and administrative issues. Short-linked primary care hospital is a downsized rural hospital that has a formal agreement with other community providers to coordinate and share services. Short-linked hospital is a Medicare-recognized hospital that has formal agreements with other community providers to coordinate and share services. A diversified hospital with a range of services is a common example. Primary care hospital is a freestanding, downsized rural hospital. To date, every state and federal statute has required that primary care hospitals have at least a linkage with a full-service hospital to accept transfers and provide services beyond their scope. Hospital is a freestanding acute care facility without externally imposed limitations. This meets Medicare requirements and fits the definition of the traditional rural hospital. Fully integrated ambulatory care system includes ambulatory primary care providers with formal relationships with a hospital for the provision of acute care services and linkages to providers of nonacute services. Long-linked ambulatory care system is a formal relationship between a primary care practice and a hospital. Short-linked ambulatory care system is a system of primary care providers that is linked with other nonacute provider organizations (home health, mental health, dental health services). Finally, ambulatory care system is an unaffiliated physician office or group practice or clinic with no formal linkages, but informal referrals do exist (Wellever & Rosenberg, 1993a).

Table 8 further details the characteristics of these alternative models. *Service role*: This is expressed as a choice between inpatient and ambulatory services. Facilities offering inpatient care will most likely offer outpatient services. The reverse may not be true, however. *Hospital linkages* refers to the extent to which hospitals have established network linkages (networks) with other hospitals or do not have linkages (are freestanding). Formal relationships are considered "long-linked." *Other provider linkages* denotes those models that have linkages with other

providers (integrated) and those that do not (non-integrated). Models that have linkages with other nonhospital providers are called "short-linked." Models that include hospital and others are "fully integrated." *Waiver status* refers to those models that require waivers of sections of the Social Security Act and its accompanying regulations and those that do not require waivers. Models that change the operation or organization may become a different kind of facility subject to different licensure and reimbursement regulations. This may specifically affect payment by Health Care Financing Administration for Medicare patients.

Second to hospital conversions, the most prevalent model is the networking model. "Network providers can include hospitals, private providers, primary care clinics, local health departments, emergency medical services, agencies, specialty service providers. These entities choose to work together for a variety of reasons, the most prevalent being to provide care most cost-effectively, share costly administrative and technological services, eliminate duplication of services, and maintain some competitive edge in the market" (Orloff & Tymann, 1995, p. iii). A study by the National Governors' Association in 1995 revealed that 29 states were developing rural health networks and 17 states were preparing these networks to function in a managed care environment (managed care–related networks) (Orloff & Tymann, 1995).

Seven states had EACH/RPCH programs and one state, Montana, developed a Medical Assistance Facilities Program (Orloff & Tymann, 1995). This model was the first alternative one to be established by law in 1987. The Montana medical assistance facility (MAF) falls within the long-linked primary care hospital model and is defined as a health care facility that: provides inpatient care to ill or injured persons prior to their transportation to a hospital or provides inpatient medical care to persons needing care for a period no longer than 96 hours, and is either located in a county with less than six residents per square mile or is located more than 35 road-miles from the nearest hospital (Wellever & Rosenberg, 1993b). The states of Wyoming and Florida have tailored this model to their specific needs.

Alternative models have also included attention to the critical need for specialized services in rural areas. Perinatal, pediatric, and emergency services have been long-standing needs in many states. Thus, networking models have achieved some success in including specialty services. A study conducted by the National Governors' Association noted that 14 states had developed specialty programs in perinatal/obstetrics/pediatrics, and 8 states in emergency medical services. In addition, 8 states had rural health or health clinic transition projects, and 11 had mental health/substance abuse services. Other states had also developed programs for specialized populations (Orloff & Tymann, 1995). These specialized services emphasize the individual variation inherent in state rural health models.

Characterization of the models has been difficult due to state variation in regulatory requirements, health status of residents, and resources available. How well the alternative models might address prevention, treatment, and long-term care needs provides another perspective on the contributions of the alternative models and how the needs of rural residents might be met.

Preventive Services

The restructuring of the traditional rural hospital to emphasize primary care is fundamental to the building of the alternative models. Alternative models include ambulatory care, and networks specifically include payers, governmental networks (finance and delivery), and providers (Weisgrau & Rosenberg, 1993a). These network participants may include public health, HMOs (private), and providers. The Community Solutions for Rural Health Project funded by the Office of Rural Health (DHHS) focused on improving health status and economic development through leadership, community involvement, and health service development, suggesting that community investment in the system design and implementation will remain a critical component. This project included 14 states that committed to develop expanded community capacity and leadership in rural health. The project documented the inadequacy of community involvement in determining what services are needed and desired and what the community is willing to financially

support (National Rural Health Association, 1997). Although local variation is inherent in the application of the models, preventive services in rural areas may be achieved through alternative models.

Treatment Services

Hospitals, long the locus of health services in rural areas, remain the primary focus of system restructuring. The Rural Hospital Flexibility Program initiated in August 1999 by the Department of Health and Human Services, as well as the earlier EACH and RPCH programs, are designed to bring together key stakeholders to determine how local care can be delivered more effectively. The grant program allows more than 40 states to designate certain hospitals as "critical" and help communities develop primary care and emergency services (American Public Health Association, 1999). This example and the congressional action in the past decade suggest that hospitals will remain a focus of the restructuring of rural health care. The need for states and federal governments to collaborate in minimizing the barriers to the evolving configurations of hospitals and networks to achieve appropriate tertiary (inpatient) care will likely create ongoing tension. The alternative models do offer frameworks sufficient to develop adequate tertiary services, and several institutional prototypes in California, Colorado, Florida, Kentucky, Montana, and Wyoming provide the evidence (Weisgrau & Rosenberg, 1993a).

Long-Term Care

An aging population and changing migration patterns challenge the provision of long-term care services. The networking alternative models offer an approach to linking institutional care with home and community services—a linkage with both hospital and nonacute service providers specific to the needs of the elderly. The Montana MAF program has been successfully implemented because a waiver to permit reimbursement of inpatient services to Medicare beneficiaries was granted. Since a large percentage of the inpatients in the MAF communities are elderly, Medicare reimbursement plays a substantial role in the financial viability of this model (Weisgrau & Rosenberg, 1993b). Institutional models (modified MAF) in Florida and Kentucky include skilled nursing facilities and home health care. Network models in Washington also include these services, as well as mental health services (Weisgrau & Rosenberg, 1993a). The evidence of models that include long-term care services appears related to the modification of regulatory requirements and Medicaid and Medicare reimbursement policies by changing the services or facility type. The prototypes do present a method for providing services to the elderly population, although the number of prototypes is limited.

Summary of Alternative Models

Several questions arise in considering the progress made in changing the status of rural health service systems. First, to what extent do alternative models improve access to health care and how are the dimensions of equity realized? Second, which characteristics suggest sustainability and which are required to sustain the success? And last, how well will the alternative models meet future challenges in rural health care? Research on the models has been limited by their prolific development, their complexity, and local variation in their design. There is a clear impetus for evaluation research to assist in understanding the successes and failures of these models. Although they offer the promise of success, evidence is limited and likely to emerge incrementally as states gain experience and as regulatory and reimbursement policies change.

Implications for Future Policy and Program Design

In conclusion, the existing evidence reviewed in this chapter, which is based on the three justice paradigms—distributive justice (access to health care), social justice (health disparities), and deliberative justice (effective participation in policy and program design)—reveals that there continues to be inequity in health and health care for rural residents along each of these dimensions. Policies and programs have attempted to remedy these inequities through federal, state, and local and private efforts. Historically, the approaches have emphasized the availability of providers and facilities, the organization and systems of delivery of medical care, and the financing of health services by rural providers and institutions.

Though substantial investments in both the organization and financing of medical care services have been made at federal, state, and local levels, wide variations in access to care and coverage persist across regions and subgroups of the U.S. population, and both the costs and effectiveness of the care provided continue to present challenges to policymakers in deciding what rights should be assured, and at what cost to whom, within this framework.

The Public Health Service's Objectives for the Nation provide a template for examining the extent to which the social justice goals of minimizing health risks and health disparities have been achieved, based on indicators and evidence of subgroup variations in achieving desired health promotion, health protection, and preventive services goals. The data routinely gathered to monitor progress toward these objectives show progress on some, as well as persistent or widening disparities on others, for rural populations.

Though there is emerging evidence of the importance of the participation of affected parties in health policy and program design, the deliberative justice paradigm has been largely unexamined and implemented as a component of the fairness of the policy formulation process. The challenge to the public health and health services research community is how best to conceptualize and measure norms of deliberative justice so that its impact can be more explicitly assessed.

An innovative framework for the design of new models for improving equity of access to health and health care in rural areas would encompass programs and services that focus on how best to improve the health of rural populations through a comprehensive, coordinated continuum of care, grounded in principles derived from the deliberative, distributive, and social justice paradigms (see Figure 2).

Such a continuum of rural health care delivery would seek to enhance the continuity and integration over time and between components

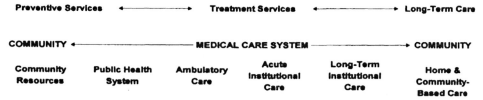

FIGURE 2. Continuum of health services. From Aday (1993), copyright 1993 Jossey–Bass, a subsidiary of John Wiley & Sons, Inc. Reprinted with permission.

in the context of promoting and protecting the health of individuals and populations in three ways: primary prevention to inhibit the onset of health problems, secondary prevention to restore a person who is already affected to maximum functioning in the least restrictive environment, and tertiary prevention to minimize the deterioration of functioning for those experiencing chronic conditions. Ambulatory and acute institutional care within the conventional clinical care system would encompass the treatment-oriented center of the continuum (secondary prevention). Community social and economic resources, as well as public health programs, define the primary prevention-oriented beginning of the continuum. Long-term institutional, home, and community-based care extend the continuum toward enhancing the quality of life and maximizing functioning of those with chronic illness. The prevention-oriented and long-term care poles encompass an array of clinical, as well as nonclinical, programs and services directed at promoting or protecting the physical, mental, and social health of rural populations (Aday, 1993; Aday *et al.*, 1998).

A beginning point for developing such a continuum can be found in the Integrated Service Network Development Initiative (Casey *et al.*, 1997). Rural health networks have great appeal for local providers to cut their costs and provide services more efficiently. Integrated rural networks are formal organizational arrangements among more than one type of rural health care provider (physician groups, hospitals, long-term care providers, and public health agencies). These networks also allow the group to compete with larger purchasing groups to secure managed care contracts. These arrangements present significant challenges to states that must consider antitrust and antikickback legislation and regulatory implications. Although research on their performance is limited, such networks

represent an alternative model that holds promise in the current health care environment.

For these and other innovative models to address the issues of deliberative, distributive, and social justice in rural health and health care delivery what is needed is the evolution of broader partnerships between managed care, public health, and other health-oriented sectors and a corollary focus on the community-wide health effects of these initiatives.

Acknowledgments

The authors gratefully acknowledge permission to adapt or reprint selected text from the following: excerpts from Chapters 1 and 6, Figure 6.1, and Table 6.2 from *Evaluating the Healthcare System: Effectiveness, Efficiency, and Equity* (2nd ed.) by Aday, Begley, Lairson, & Slater (1998); Figure 5.1 from *At Risk in America: The Health and Health Care Needs of Vulnerable Populations in the United States* by Aday (1993); Table 1 from "Redefining the Nursing Shortage: A Rural Perspective" by Stratton, Dunkin, & Juhl (1995); and Table 2 from "A Taxonomy of Model Types" by Wellever and Rosenberg (1993a).

References

Aday, L. A. (1993). *At risk in America: The health and health care needs of vulnerable populations in the United States.* San Francisco: Jossey-Bass.

Aday, L. A., & Andersen, R. (1981). Equity of access to medical care: A conceptual and empirical overview. *Medical Care, 19* (Supplement) 4–27.

Aday, L. A., Andersen, R., & Fleming, G. (1980). *Health care in the U.S.: Equitable for whom?* Beverly Hills: Sage.

Aday, L. A., Begley, C. E., Lairson, D. R., & Slater C. H. (1998). *Evaluating the healthcare system: Effectiveness, efficiency, and equity* (2nd ed.). Chicago: Health Administration Press.

Agency for Health Care Policy and Research. (1991). *Delivery of essential health care services in rural areas: An analysis of alternative models.* Rockville, MD: U.S. Department of Health and Human Services.

Agency for Health Care Policy and Research. (1998). *Characteristics of nursing home residents, 1996. MEPS Research Findings No. 5.* (AHCPR Pub. No. 99-0006). Washington, DC: U.S. Government Printing Office.

American Medical Association. (1999). *Physician characteristics and distribution in the U.S.* Chicago: American Medical Association.

American Public Health Association. (1999, October). Rural hospitals receive means to improve care. *The Nation's Health, 29*(9), p. 24.

Blazer, D. G., Landerman, L. R., Fillenbaum, G., & Horner, R. (1995). Health services access and use among older adults in North Carolina: Urban vs. rural residents. *American Journal of Public Health, 85*(10), 1384–90.

Braden, J. J., & Beauregard, K. (1994). *Health status and access to care of rural and urban populations.* Rockville, MD: U.S. Public Health Service.

Brooks, E. F., Bernstein, J. D., DeFriese, G. H., & Graham, R. M. (1981). New health practitioners in rural satellite health centers: The past and future. *Journal of Community Health, 6*(4), 246–56.

Bushy, A. (1998). Health issues of women in rural environments: An overview. *Journal of American Medical Women's Association, 53*(2), 53–56.

Casey, M. M., Wellever, A., & Moscovice, I. (1997). Rural health network development: Public policy issues and state initiatives. *Journal of Health Politics, Policy, and Law, 22*(1), 23–49.

Cheh, V., & Thompson, R. (1997). *Rural health clinics: Improved access at a cost.* Baltimore, MD: Office of Research and Demonstrations, Health Care Financing Administration.

Cook, H. L., Goeppinger, J., Brunk, S. E., Price, L. J., Whitehead, T. L., & Sauter, S. V. (1985). A reexamination of community participation in health: Lessons from three community health projects. *Family and Community Health, 11*(2), 1–13.

Coward, R. T., & Cutler, S. J. (1989). Informal and formal health care systems for the rural elderly. *Health Services Research, 23*(6), 785–806.

Daly, M. (Ed.). (1994). *Communitarianism: A new public ethics.* Belmont, CA: Wadsworth.

De Lew, N., Greenberg, G., & Kinchen, K. (1992). A layman's guide to the U.S. health care system. *Health Care Financing Review, 14*(1), 151–169.

Economic Research Service. (1998). Appendix Table 2: Metro and non-metro labor force and unemployment by demographic group. *Rural Conditions and Trends, 8*(2), 97.

Fordyce, E. J., Thomas, P., & Shum, R. (1997 April—June). Evidence of an increasing AIDS burden in rural America. *Statistical Bulletin–Metropolitan Insurance Companies, 78*(2), 2–9.

Frenzen, P. (1997). How will measures to control Medicare spending affect rural communities? *Agriculture Information Bulletin, 734,* 1–10.

Garrett, D. K. (1995). Mobile access: Opening health care doors. *Nursing Management, 26,* 29–33.

Green, L. W. (1986). Theory of participation: A qualitative analysis of its expressions in national and international health policies. In W. B. Ward, Z. T. Salisbury, S. B. Kar, & J. G. Kapka (Eds.), *Advances in health promotion, Vol. 1* (pp. 215–240). Greenwich, CT: JAI Press.

Habermas, J. (1996). *Between facts and norms: Contributions to a discourse theory of law and democracy* (W. Rehg, Trans.). Cambridge, MA: MIT Press.

Heins, H. C., Nance, N. W., & Ferguson, J. E. (1987). Social support in improving perinatal outcome: The resource mothers program. *Obstetrics and Gynecology, 70*(2), 263–6.

Hornberger, C. A., & Cobb, A. K. (1998). A rural vision of a healthy community. *Public Health Nursing, 15*(5), 363–369.

Hoyt, D. R., Conger, R. D., Valde, J. G., & Wiehs, K. (1997). Psychological distress and help seeking in rural America. *American Journal of Community Psychology, 25*(4), 449–70.

Hwang, H. C., Stallones, L., & Keefe, T. J. (1997). Childhood injury deaths: Rural and urban differences in Colorado 1980–1988. *Injury Prevention, 3,* 35–37.

Kolimaga, J., Konrad, T., & Ricketts, T. (1994). Does subsidizing rural community health centers hurt private practice physicians? *Journal of Health Care for the Poor and Underserved, 5,* 121–141.

Kukulka, G., Christianson, J. B., Moscovice, I. S., & DeVries, R. (1994). Community oriented primary care in a brave new world. *Archives of Family Medicine, 3,* 493–494.

Long, K. A., & Weinert, C. (1989). Rural nursing: Developing the theory base. *Scholastic Inquiries in Nursing Practice, 3*(2), 113–27.

Mainous, A. G., & Kohrs, F. P. (1995). A comparison of health status between rural and urban adults. *Journal of Community Health, 20*(5), 423–431.

Maningas, P. A. (1991). *Emergency medical services in rural America: New solutions to urgent needs.* Rockville, MD: Federal Office of Rural Health Policy, 3–7.

McDowell, S. H. (1997). *Market reform and managed care: Implications for rural communities.* Rockville, MD: Federal Office of Rural Health Policy.

Michielutte, R., Dignan, M. B., Sharp, P. C., Boxley, J., & Wells, H. B. (1996). Skin cancer prevention and early detection practices in a sample of rural women. *Preventive Medicine, 25*(6), 673–83.

Moscovice, I. (1989). Rural hospitals: A literature synthesis and health services research agenda. *Health Services Research, 23*(6), 891–930.

Moscovice, I., & Nestegard, M. (1980). The influence

of values and background on the location decision of nurse practitioners. *Journal of Community Health, 5*(4), 244–53.

Moscovice, I. S., & Rosenblatt, R. A. (1982). Rural health care delivery amidst federal retrenchment: Lessons from the Robert Wood Johnson Foundation's Rural Practice Project. *American Journal of Public Health, 72*(12), 1380–1385.

Moscovice, I., Cristianson, J., Johnson, J., Kralewski, J., & Manning, W. (1995). *Building rural hospital networks.* Ann Arbor, MI: Health Administration Press.

Mulhall, S., & Swift, A. (1992). *Liberals and communitarians.* Oxford, UK: Blackwell.

Myrick, J. A., Bonnie, B. J., Kishbaugh, D., Pittman, J. V., & Sayford, N. F. (1983). Acceptance of a volunteer first-responder system in rural communities: A field experiment. *Medical Care, 21*(4), 389–99.

Napolitano, M., & Goldberg, B. W. (1998). Migrant health. In S. Loue (Ed.), *Handbook of Immigrant Health* (pp. 261–276). New York: Plenum.

National Association of Community Health Centers. (1988). *Health Care in Rural America: The Crisis Unfolds.* Washington, DC: National Association of Community Health Centers.

National Association of Community Health Centers. (1994). *A National Survey of Patient Experiences in Community and Migrant Health Centers: Key points.* Washington, DC: National Association of Community Health Centers.

National Center for Health Statistics. (1979). Small area estimation: An empirical comparison of conventional and synthetic estimators for states. (DHEW Publication No. PHS 80-1356). *Vital and Health Statistics Series 2, No. 82.* Washington, DC: U.S. Government Printing Office.

National Center for Health Statistics. (1994). *Advance Data 244: Nursing Homes and Board and Care Homes.* (DHHS Publication No. PHS 94-1250). Hyattsville, MD: Public Health Service.

National Center for Health Statistics. (1997). *Health, United States, 1996–97, and Injury Chartbook.* Hyattsville, MD: Public Health Service.

National Center for Health Statistics. (1999a). Current estimates from the National Health Interview Survey, 1996. (DHHS Publication No. PHS 99-1528). *Vital and Health Statistics Series 10, No. 200.* Hyattsville, MD: Public Health Service.

National Center for Health Statistics. (1999b). *Health, United States, 1999, with Health and Aging Chartbook.* Hyattsville, MD: Public Health Service.

National Rural Health Association. (1996). *The rural homeless: America's lost population.* Kansas City: National Rural Health Association.

National Rural Health Association. (1997). *Community solutions for rural health: An empowerment initiative for rural communities.* Kansas City: National Rural Health Association.

Norman, E. H., Bordley, W. C., Hertz-Picciotto, I., &

Newton, D. A. (1994). Rural-urban blood lead differences in North Carolina children. *Pediatrics, 94*(1), 59–64.

Office of Rural Health Policy. (1997a). *Rural health dictionary of terms, acronyms, and organizations, 1997.* Rockville, MD: Office of Rural Health Policy.

Office of Rural Health Policy. (1997b). *Facts about rural physicians.* Rockville, MD: Office of Rural Health Policy.

Office of Rural Health Policy. (1997c). *Exploratory evaluation of rural applications of telemedicine.* Rockville, MD: Office of Rural Health Policy.

Office of Technology Assessment. (1990). *Health care in rural America.* Washington, DC: Congress of the United States.

Orloff, T. M., & Tymann, B. (1995). *Rural health: An evolving system of accessible services.* Washington, DC: National Governors' Association.

Pearson, T. A., & Lewis, C. (1998). Rural epidemiology: Insights from a rural population laboratory. *American Journal of Epidemiology, 148*(10), 949–57.

Perlstadt, H., & Kozak, L. J. (1977). Emergency medical services in small communities: Volunteer ambulance corps. *Journal of Community Health, 2*(3), 178–88.

Powers, J. G., & Byrd, T. (1998). *U.S.–Mexico border health: Issues for regional and migrant populations.* Thousand Oaks, CA: Sage.

Puskin, D. S. (1995). Opportunities and challenges to telemedicine in rural America. *Journal of Medical Systems 19*(1), 59–67.

Ramsey, P., Edwards, J., Lenz, C., Odom, J. E., & Brown, B. (1993). Types of health problems and satisfaction with services in a rural nurse-managed clinic. *Journal of Community Health Nursing, 10*(3), 161–70.

Rural Health Research Center. (1997). *Rural managed care patterns and prospects, 1997.* Minneapolis: University of Minnesota School of Public Health.

Stratton, T. D., Dunkin, J. W., & Juhl, N. (1995). Redefining the nursing shortage: A rural perspective. *Nursing Outlook, 43*(2), 71–7.

Svenson, J. E., Spurlock, C., & Nypaver, N. (1995). Factors associated with the higher traumatic death rate among rural children. *Annals of Emergency Medicine, 27*(5), 625–632.

Thomas, J. C., Kulick, A. L., & Schoenbach, V. J. (1995). Syphilis in the South: Rural rates surpass urban rates in North Carolina. *American Journal of Public Health, 85*(8), 1119–1122.

Thorpe, K. E. & Florence, C. S. (1999). Covering uninsured children and their parents: Estimated costs and number of newly insured. *Medical Care Research and Review, 56*(2), 197–214.

Travers, K. L., Ellis, R. B., & Dartt, L. A. (1995). *Comparison of the rural health clinic and federally qualified health center programs.* Rockville, MD: Office of Rural Health Policy.

U.S. Department of Health & Human Services. (1987). *Work group on rural hospitals. Executive summary of final report on rural hospital strategies.* Rockville, MD: Health Resources and Services Administration.

U.S. Department of Health & Human Services. (1991). *Health personnel in the United States: Eighth report to Congress.* (DHHS Pub. No HRS-P-OD-92-1). Rockville, MD: Health Resources and Services Administration.

U.S. Health Corporation. (1994). *U.S. Health Corporation's healthy community initiative: The healthy community assessment process.* Columbus, OH: U.S. Health Corporation.

Wallerstein, N. (1992). Powerlessness, empowerment, and health: Implications for health promotion programs. *American Journal of Health Promotion, 6,* 197–205.

Wallerstein, N., & Bernstein, E. (1994). Introduction to community empowerment, participatory education, and health. *Health Education Quarterly, 21,* 141–48.

Weil, A. (1997). *The new children's health insurance program: Should states expand Medicaid?* Washington, DC: The Urban Institute, Series A, No. A-13.

Weisgrau, S., & Rosenberg, S. (1993a). *Independent networks. Vol. 4 of Alternative models for organizing and delivering health care services in rural areas.* Princeton, NJ: Robert Wood Johnson Foundation.

Weisgrau, S., & Rosenberg, S. (1993b). *State-sponsored alternative models: Experiences of participating providers. Vol. 3 of Alternative models for organizing and delivering health care services in rural area.* Princeton, NJ: Robert Wood Johnson Foundation.

Wellever, A., & Rosenberg, S. (1993a). *A taxonomy of model types. Vol. 1 of Alternative models for organizing and delivering health care services in rural area.* Princeton, NJ: Robert Wood Johnson Foundation.

Wellever, A., & Rosenberg, S. (1993b). *State-sponsored alternative models: The state government perspective. Vol. 2 of Alternative models for organizing and delivering health care services in rural areas.* Princeton, NJ: Robert Wood Johnson Foundation.

Whitehead, M. (1992). The concepts and principles of equity and health. *International Journal of Health Services, 22,* 429–45.

World Health Organization Healthy Cities Project. (1988). *A guide to assessing healthy cities.* (WHO Healthy Cities Paper No. 3). Copenhagen: Association of Danish Medical Students Publishing House.

Wysong, J. A., Bliss, M. K., Osborne, J. W., Graham, R. P., & Pikuzinski, D. A. (1999). Managed care in rural markets: Availability and enrollment. *Journal of Health Care for the Poor and Underserved, 10*(1): 72–84.

Zimmerman, M. A. (1990). Citizen participation in rural health: A promising resource. *Journal of Public Health Policy, 11*(3), 323–340.

5

Ethnic Issues

ROBERTA D. BAER AND JANICE NICHOLS

Introduction

Rural areas of the United States were once more homogeneous than more urban areas, which were the destination of incoming immigrants. This pattern is changing for several reasons. One is the increased number of immigrants in general. The second is the growing number and diversity of migrant farmworkers, who bring to rural areas cultural practices quite different from those of the majority population. Increasingly, health care workers in these areas will encounter this diversity and be forced to adapt their approaches to deal effectively with these new and different populations. This chapter will examine the situation in one of the areas of the United States that remains the most rural, the South.

New ethnic groups join the two dominant populations that have lived in this region for centuries—southern Anglo Americans and southern African Americans. Although these groups represent the majority of inhabitants of the rural areas, their beliefs about health and illness and their approaches to health care are not always those recognized by biomedically trained providers. The more recent groups, many of which are part of farmworker streams (Mexican Americans, Guatemalans, Mixtecs, and Haitians), bring even more divergent views and approaches to heath care. This chapter is de-

signed to provide the background information necessary for health care practitioners to deal more effectively with the perspectives, practices, and needs of these ethnic groups. Each subsection of this chapter will cover one of these groups, and will provide an overview of its historical background, health beliefs, specific health problems, and diet and will offer recommendations for effectively dealing with members of these ethnic groups.

A key topic that must be considered is that of differing worldviews. Worldview includes a deeply rooted, ethnically based understanding of causality of illness, as well as of other life events. Since worldview is so deeply rooted and covers such basic ideas about life, it is rarely questioned and nearly impossible to change. Biomedical explanations are based on a scientific perspective or worldview of illness causality. One becomes ill because of the actions of germs and viruses. Advocates of this perspective explain other events in life using similar types of scientific explanation; it rains because of the forces of evaporation and condensation. In contrast, members of many ethnic groups hold perspectives or worldviews that see causality of much in life, including illness, as due to nonscientific forces, that are often in the spiritual realm. Illness may be due to the actions of a person, spirit, or ancestor, or to the breach of social rule.

Worldviews are resistant to change. Therefore it is unlikely that attempts to "re-educate" scientifically oriented biomedical practitioners to a more spiritual sense of causality will be at all successful. Similarly, explanations of illness causality based on science will seem unreal to

ROBERTA D. BAER AND JANICE NICHOLS • Department of Anthropology, University of South Florida, Tampa, Florida 33620-8100.

Handbook of Rural Health, edited by Loue and Quill. Kluwer Academic/Plenum Publishers, New York, 2001.

those holding more spiritual worldviews. And current approaches to health education and prevention based on scientific causality will be equally incomprehensible. Because neither group is likely to change their worldviews, successful health care will be dependent on the ability of the health care provider to recognize that unresolvable differences exist, to understand the worldview of the patient, and given that the patient is unlikely to "lose" or be "educated out of" his or her worldview, to find a way to bridge the differences. It is hoped that the material in the remainder of the chapter and references will be useful in that endeavor.

Southern Anglo Americans

Historical Background

Unlike many of the other ethnic groups discussed in this chapter, southern Anglo Americans (sometimes referred to as southern whites), have lived in the region for hundreds of years, with many families having lived in the same locale for several generations. Although a number of European ethnic groups and religions are represented, this population predominantly derives from Anglo-Saxon Protestant roots. Whites are the dominant ethnic group, but not all whites are in a privileged position. From early in their history there has been a distinction between poor whites and the slave-owning landed gentry, which has resulted in class divisions among whites that are sometimes equated with a caste system (Flynt, 1979). In some cases, poor whites suffered a more meager existence than did slaves, which served to exacerbate racial tensions. Most of the poor whites lived on farms, practicing one-crop agriculture with poor farming methods, and were not able to take advantage of assistance programs due to their isolation. Social programs in the mid-20th century have attempted to bring about some parity, but with limited results. Their poverty eventually forced many of the poor whites into grueling work in mill towns and mining camps.

Southern culture has its roots in a rural way of life, with agriculture being the economic backbone of the region. It is only in recent decades that manufacturing and industry have played a major role in the economy. The sizable low-wage labor pool, abundant natural resources, and strong resistance to unionization that characterized the South initially were attractive features for northern industrialists (Cobb, 1984). Following rapid expansion in the post–World War II years, however, the northerners were more interested in other amenities that would increase the appeal of southern living. It was in response to this that much of the social, educational, and political reform in the South came about, along with increased attention to public facilities and living conditions (Cobb, 1984). The reforms that took place reflected a strong white middle-class bias, however. For example, slums were cleared to enhance the attractiveness of the cities, but large numbers of poor African Americans were displaced in the process. Programs benefitting the middle class were embraced, while the response to programs for African Americans was not so enthusiastic. The reforms and changes improved the reputation for backwardness that had long been held by the southern states. However, the intolerance and inequities that characterized race relations remained. Following the 1954 Supreme Court desegregation decision, the 1950s and 1960s were marked by racial conflict and social upheaval, with repercussions persisting into the present time. The civil rights movement did, however, bring about grudging progress in race relations. Increased industrialization has not solved all of the South's problems. It has not brought general prosperity to the region; a significant number of southerners continue to live in poverty. There is significant outmigration from areas in the South that have not industrialized, while other areas have experienced rapid population growth that has strained their institutions and services (Cobb, 1984). The 20th century in the South brought a movement from simplicity to complexity. People now practice a wider variety of lifestyles, earn their living in more ways, and are subjected to more diverse influences than ever before (Scott, 1970).

Worldview and Health Beliefs

Some southern whites are proud of their ethnic roots and claim their ethnic heritage, while others may ignore them in an effort to fit more quickly in with American society. By the second and third generation, most European American immigrants acculturate and become upwardly mobile; achievement and progress are highly valued. These values perhaps have served to moderate the stress of the rapid changes that the region has undergone in a relatively short period of time.

Religion is of central importance to many southern white families with the emphasis on seeking salvation and reward in the hereafter rather than on earth, although southerners typically are not as apt to deny themselves earthly pleasures as are their Protestant neighbors to the North. There is also a strong faith in the family as the focal institution of society (McGill & Pearce, 1982). In the South, extended families are more likely to live in close proximity and to be involved in the family than is the case in other regions of the country. Traditionally patriarchal, southern families have assumed a more egalitarian complexion in recent history. Still, a premium tends to be placed on manliness in males and modest, ladylike demeanor in women (Scott, 1970).

A key belief is that people can control nature through science and technology. In terms of health beliefs, this suggests that interventions will be sought out and accepted, although there may be cultural variation in terms of which type of practitioner will be sought out for health care intervention. On the other hand, autonomy, independence, and competence are highly valued among southern whites. These values may stand in the way of acknowledging symptoms and seeking or accepting help until a health condition is well advanced. In rural areas, noninterference in the lives of neighbors is a widely held value (McGill & Pearce, 1982). From a public health standpoint, this may create problems in case finding and follow-up. Outside major metropolitan areas the immediate locale is very meaningful to people, particularly for families that have been in the same location for several generations. The outside world is usually regarded with suspicion. This may be problematic if it becomes necessary to go outside the community for health care.

The classism that has persisted in the South since antebellum times may affect health beliefs and practices in myriad ways. Access to health care may be related to class, as may be the basic understanding of health, disease, and its symptoms, and expectations about the outcome of health care intervention. In addition, racism, anti-Semitism, and other prejudices have played a significant role in European history; these views have been transplanted and thrived in the American South, even though, in general, they may have become less overt over time. There are an increasing number of racial incidents and bias-related crimes, and there is almost complete separation between Anglos and African Americans in housing (Giordano-McGoldrick, 1996). These biases may threaten the therapeutic relationship if the people involved are of differing backgrounds.

Most rural areas are characterized by separation of sex roles and a high value placed on the family, particularly on children. Neighborliness and reciprocity and exchange of goods and services are common attributes in the rural South. When illness strikes a family, friends and neighbors will likely be inclined to help out, but this may place a burden on the recipients if they are not able to return the kindness in a meaningful way.

Beliefs about health maintenance include practices such as good diet, sufficient sleep, daily exercise, fresh air, cleanliness, and keeping warm and dry. Popular home remedies include chicken soup, tea with honey, lemon, or whiskey, and hot milk. Less common remedies today than they were in the past are sulfur and molasses, cod liver oil, mustard packs, and oatmeal plasters.

Specific Health Problems

In the many small towns and rural areas of the South, medical facilities are frequently absent, thereby raising problems of access to biomedical health care. Although advances in public health have decreased their impact in recent times, maladies of the poor—such as malaria, hookworm, and clay-eating (Flynt, 1979)—have been debilitating to poor whites and are still occasionally reported.

Diet

The southern diet relies heavily upon pork and corn products and fresh vegetables, particularly greens, sweet potatoes, and peas. With the proximity to ocean, lakes, and rivers, fish also make a significant contribution to the diet. Other meats and poultry are frequently eaten, with fried chicken being a regional favorite. Milk is consumed at mealtimes; another popular beverage is sweetened iced tea. Southern whites typically follow a three-meal-a-day pattern, with a substantial breakfast, lighter lunch, and larger dinner; the exception is on Sunday, when the major meal often is served midday. Foods are usually cooked thoroughly. The traditional southern diet is high in fat, sodium, and sugar. Fried foods, vegetables, and beans prepared with pork fat, the liberal use of butter, syrup, molasses, and honey, and sweetened beverages are characteristic. As a result of exposure to other cuisines and concerns about health, many southerners have made dietary changes in recent years, decreasing meat and fried foods, salt, and cooking fat, and consuming more salads (Stans, 1990).

Recommendations to Practitioners

1. Although the majority of white Southerners are of Anglo-Saxon origin, it cannot be assumed that everyone is. Other European groups are represented and there may be other ethnic beliefs and practices evident in a person's health practices and responses to illness and treatment. These may assume particular significance during periods of health crisis. It is important to be aware of these factors in order to avoid misunderstanding.
2. Practitioners should use appropriate religious beliefs and support systems that may give a sense of comfort and meaning in times of illness.
3. Illness and forced dependency may be particularly difficult for this population to accept. Be alert to the possibility that symptoms are being ignored or minimized. Encourage as much autonomy for the sick individual as is appropriate given his or her condition.
4. Encourage health care screenings and early intervention as a way of taking responsibility for one's own well-being and survival.

5. Attempt to develop an understanding of the origins of biases based on class, race, and other prejudices and find common ground upon which to facilitate trust and acceptance in the health care setting.
6. When planning community-based care for a sick individual, be cognizant of the social support from friends and neighbors that can realistically be expected and of the burden that home care may place on the family, particularly the women.
7. It is important not to mistake stoicism in the face of illness and death for lack of emotion on the part of patients and their loved ones.

Southern African Americans

Historical Background

During the sixteenth and seventeenth centuries, West Africans were torn from their communities and forcibly transported to North and South America and the Caribbean. There they experienced centuries of slavery, during which they suffered the indignity of being owned by others, being subjected to forced menial labor and long hours, and being dependent on their "masters." Families were often torn apart on a whim, and the slaves had no control over their own lives. During the Civil War, some slaves were compelled to support the Confederacy, fighting for the very system that enslaved them. Others joined federal troops. Following the Civil War, the former slaves were thrust unprepared into freedom and responsibility for themselves. Many in the South did not fare any better with freedom than they did under slavery.

African Americans were subject to so-called Jim Crow laws, which restricted their use of public facilities. Schools were segregated, with those for African Americans being markedly inferior to those for other children. Decades passed before African Americans were guaranteed full rights as members of American society as a result of the civil rights movement (Dressler, 1991). Still, racism remains a divisive issue in this country. The effects of their history continue to limit opportunities and generate stumbling blocks that preclude many African Americans from fully realizing their potential and accessing the advantages this country offers to the privileged. It is small wonder that many African American communities are beset by an array of social ills, and that anger and resentment periodically spill over into the streets. At the present time, roughly 20% of the population of the American South is African American.

Worldview and Health Beliefs

In the process of adapting to their new surroundings, Africans mixed European and Native American traditions with their own cultural backgrounds (Snow, 1993). People of African descent retained many prevention and treatment practices from their original cultures because they considered them to be useful and because of communication barriers (Bloch, 1983) and fear of white physicians. Strong family ties and religious conviction have yielded the family and church as the major sources of strength and support for African Americans (Bloch, 1983; Dressler,1991; Freedman, 1998). The predominant religious sects are Baptist, Pentecostal, and African Methodist Episcopal (AME).

A wide variety of medicinal plants such as *Chenopodium ambrosioides* (Jerusalem oak), *Eupatorium perfoliatum* (boneset), *Aristolochia serpentia* (a snakeroot), and *Podophyllum peltatum* (May apple) traditionally were used extensively. Drugs derived from roots, bark, leaves, fruits, and resins were made into teas, poultices, and powders, or worn in bags around the neck to prevent or cure conditions or diseases such as worms, malaria, croup, pneumonia, colds, teething, and measles. Slave doctors and many other slaves knew how to diagnose and treat illnesses. They made use of preparations such as calomel, blue mass pills, castor oil, ipecac, and tartar emetic and also used tokens, rituals, and ceremonies to restore or maintain health.

Even after one or two centuries in the New World, African American health beliefs and practices still showed similarities to West African and Haitian religion, "voodoo" or "vodoun" (Bloch, 1983). Voodoo medicine consisted of three components—the mystic or supernatural, the psychological, and herbal and folk medicine.

People were thus treated both at the biological and spiritual levels. It survived in the American South because African Americans did not have access to biomedical care. Many of the traditional health practices continue to this day in some areas, particularly among the older population (Bloch, 1983). As African Americans began migrating to northern cities in the mid-1800s, their health beliefs and practices became an amalgam of European folklore, Greek classical medicine, modern biomedicine, vodoun and fundamentalist Christian beliefs, and African folklore. At the same time, some African American beliefs were absorbed into American health practices.

One specific traditional health belief that has persisted among African Americans into contemporary times is the importance of blood, which is the primary health focus among many peoples of African descent. Blood is central to body functioning and physical well-being and is traditionally viewed as constantly responding to internal and external stimuli in a variety of ways (Weidman & Egeland, 1978; Snow, 1993). External factors include the seasons, the ambient temperature, lack of cleanliness, occurrences that trigger strong emotions, and the position of the heavenly bodies. Internal factors may involve the foods one consumes, digestive processes, failure to keep the body clean internally, and illness and its treatment. Age, gender, and body states such as menstruation or pregnancy also have an effect, as can supernatural beings or sorcery. These stimuli can cause a range of changes in the blood: the generation of new blood and disposal of the old; changes in the temperature of the blood, blood volume, consistency, and speed of circulation; shifts in location of the blood, with temporary pooling in various spots; the state of cleanliness of the blood; alterations in the flavor of the blood (bitter, sweet, acidic); or habitation by supernatural creatures. Measures to keep the blood in the right condition require constant attention. Various remedies may be utilized, depending on the particular condition, including blood letting, tonics, roots and herbs, tea, "hot" foods, poultices, salt, poke greens, vinegar, sulphur and molasses, cream of tartar, regular (but not excessive) sexual activity, laxatives, and keeping cool or warm (Snow, 1993). Of particular note are the concepts of "high blood" and "low blood," which refer to high or low blood volume as opposed to the biomedical explanation involving the amount of pressure exerted by the blood on the vessels. "Low blood" also may be characterized as thin blood or anemia. The misunderstandings that may arise because of the differing beliefs about the character of blood disorders could have clinical significance if, for example, the idea of "high blood" results in noncompliance with clinical treatment of hypertension, or if it leads to the use of dangerous or ineffective home remedies for hypertension (Weidman & Egeland, 1978).

African Americans' perception of health typically indicates a high tolerance for discomfort. Minor symptoms are often ignored until they become so severe that normal activities are impaired and the illness becomes obvious to those around them (Bloch, 1983). At that point, health care is sought. Because illness is perceived as a loss of self, isolation from others, and disharmony with one's soul, it is sometimes denied in an effort to maintain harmony. Etiology falls into three categories: environmental hazards, divine punishment, and impaired sociocultural relationships. Illness may be caused by physiological stressors such as inadequate rest, poor nutrition, and germs, or it may be caused by supernatural agents, such as magic, the evil eye, or punishment by God for sins (Bloch, 1983; Snow, 1993).

Because the sick role changes the rights and obligations of the person, African Americans may have difficulty adopting that role behavior. Some relatives and friends may have ambivalent feelings about the sick because they are relieved of normal obligations. However, when illness is recognized, the sick are usually relieved of their duties and receive substantial emotional and physical caring from relatives and friends, particularly adult children (Bloch, 1983; Freedman, 1998). Ill African American elderly receive special attention, generally more formal and informal support than Anglo-American elderly.

The wife, mother, or grandmother typically monitors symptoms and directs intervention for a sick person in the household and cares for elderly parents. In two-parent households, both parents participate in decisions about medical treatment. African Americans are likely to consult with friends and relatives initially rather than go directly to health care professionals, and they usually receive more instrumental and emotional support from these networks than do Anglo Americans. These lay networks employ a variety of home remedies and over-the-counter medicines, including various types of poultices to draw out infection and inflammation, hot lemon water and honey for colds, and hot camphor oil rubs and warm flannel wraps for chest congestion and cough. These home remedies are tried before seeking biomedical treatment and may be continued in conjunction with prescribed medications, usually without the physician's, knowledge (Snow, 1993; Randell-David, 1985).

Indigenous healers known as root workers or root doctors have traditionally been called upon to treat blood irregularities and other illnesses. These practitioners use roots and other herbs in their practices. Rather than going to the woods to dig therapeutic roots, contemporary root workers are more likely to operate herbalism shops in urban areas, selling grocery items and patent medicines as well herbs and roots. Faith healers and practitioners of magic may also be called upon (Hall & Bourne, 1973; Weidman & Egeland, 1978). Traditional treatment costs are relatively low compared with biomedical treatment, making them accessible to lower-income people. These therapies are used in conjunction with standard medical treatments (Hall & Bourne, 1973). Many of the practices are very similar to those of West African folk healers, attempting to treat the person's mind, body, and spirit and return the individual to a state of harmony with nature (Bloch, 1983). In addition to low treatment costs, the benefits these practitioners are believed to offer are allowing patients to remain within their sociocultural environment and exerting some control over the forces that cause health problems that physicians do not. Treatment actions vary according to class, U.S. region, and degree of assimilation into mainstream society. Traditional practices, in general, tend to decrease over time.

Specific Health Problems

Although health and social services usually exist in communities in which African Americans live, transportation difficulties, poverty, and other sociocultural constraints often cause problems in accessing these services (Randell-David, 1985). Racism, lack of education, cultural dissonance with the larger society, and differing definitions of health and illness, lack of trust in Anglo American health care providers, the belief by some African Americans that they do not receive equal quality health care and that providers do not care about them, and the stigma attached to receiving Medicaid may also be factors in accessing services (Griffin, 1994; Bloch, 1983). Many African Americans believe that certain conditions and ailments common in this population tend to be overlooked by Anglo American physicians. There is a preference among many for African American physicians due to the feeling that other physicians may lack the knowledge and understanding of the health problems of African Americans, both from a biological and life situation perspective. Many prefer a physician who is also aware of and appreciative of their spiritual and family lives (Freedman, 1998).

African Americans may deny or not recognize symptoms until a problem is well advanced. Some who suspect they have a terminal illness may delay medical intervention, turning first to the supernatural realm to determine the cause of the illness, and perhaps accepting the illness as God's will. African American women who are sick may have particular difficulty with ambivalent feelings from those around them because they are expected to stay well and take care of their families. Adherence to biomedical treatment protocols may be problematic, perhaps because of the difficulty some may have in understanding what their physicians say to them and their hesitancy to participate actively in discussions with health care providers about their illness and treatment.

African Americans, along with Hispanics and Native Americans, have higher rates of noninsulin dependent diabetes than do Anglo Americans. The rate among African Americans is 1.6 times that of the total U.S. population. This may be related to the high incidence of obesity among African American women. In fact, African American women over the age of 75 are twice as likely to have diabetes than are Anglo American women (Burke & Raia, 1995).

There is also a higher incidence of hypertension and cardiovascular disease in the African American population, and cancer rates have been rising in recent decades.

HIV/AIDS is a critical problem in many African American communities, due mostly to heterosexual transmission and intravenous drug use. Other significant problems that may affect the health of many African Americans include unemployment and underemployment, poverty, violence, a large proportion of single-parent, female-headed households, high rates of homicide among black males, alcoholism, and high rates of depression and suicide among black youth.

Sickle cell anemia, another common disease among African Americans, has received increased attention in recent years, resulting in greater research and counseling efforts. G6-PD enzyme deficiency, a hematological problem affecting 30% of African American males, may result in hemolytic anemia in response to stress, infection, or certain drugs (Bloch, 1983).

Keloid formation, an exaggerated wound-scarring process of the skin, is common in African Americans and may require surgery. Vitiligo, a lack of melanin formation of unknown cause, occurs in any population but is more noticeable in African Americans due to their darker skin tones (Bloch, 1983).

Although the practice has decreased in recent times, pica—the consumption of clay, starch, or flour—was once common, especially among the poor. It may contribute to obesity and result in constipation, fecal impaction, or perforated colon (Burke & Raia, 1995). Lead poisoning, which may lead to retardation or death, is still a hazard for people in older, substandard housing. Children are at particular risk from eating lead paint fragments. African Americans have higher death rates from tuberculosis, influenza, and pneumonia as a result of overcrowding, poor sanitation systems, and poor nutrition (Bloch, 1983).

Diet

African American foodways have origins in Europe and America. Plantation slaves brought new foods with them, including okra, sesame seed (benne), black-eyed peas, peanuts, and other legumes. These were added to items from the American South, such as pumpkin, oysters, corn, cabbage, collard, mustard, dandelion, spinach, pokeweed and turnip greens, onions, peas, sweet potatoes, and squash (Burke & Raia, 1995). Despite the current availability of a wide variety of produce, these vegetables are still preferred by many African Americans. Pork is the traditional favorite source of protein (Schoenberg, 1994). It was thought that fatter pork would give the slaves more energy, so they were usually given the fattier portions of the pig. Organ meats, feet, ears, tongue, tail, and brains were also eaten to reduce waste (Burke & Raia, 1995). Today these items are still commonly consumed by African Americans. A variety of other foods are consumed as well. Vegetables are usually boiled or stewed in water and seasoned with bacon, bacon grease, ham hock, fatback, or lard, and perhaps a little sugar (Schoenberg, 1994; Burke & Raia, 1995). Pressure cooking and frying are also common. Okra, green tomatoes, squash, onion, eggplant, and corn cut from the cob are battered and fried.

Beets, broccoli, string or pole beans, peppers, tomatoes, and rutabagas are popular. Macaroni and cheese, coleslaw, potato salad, chicken cornbread stuffing, and red-eye (ham), sausage, or cream gravies are also commonly consumed. Pickles and relishes, prepared with large amounts of sugar, may accompany meals. Starchy vegetables such as peas and beans, corn and sweet potatoes are staples for many families. Sweet potatoes may be baked, boiled, candied, panfried, or used in pies. Beans or peas combined with a grain, such as Hoppin' John (rice and black-eyed peas), red beans and rice, or beans and cornbread, and succotash (corn and lima beans) are frequent in many homes. Other grains items basic to the diet are grits, cereals, biscuits, and hush puppies. Corn pone (a panfried cake of corn meal and water) and cornbread are sometimes "dunked" in buttermilk or pot liquor (the fatty liquid in which greens are cooked) (Burke & Raia, 1995).

In addition to pork, beef, chicken, and fish are also included in the African American diet, often breaded or battered and fried. Barbecuing is also a favorite cooking method. Oxtail, tripe, tongue, hog maw (pork stomach), pigs' ears and feet, brains, and sousemeat (a mixture of hog

organ meats) are traditional foods that are still consumed today. Crackling (fried pork fat) and chitterlings (hog intestines) are used as well. Game meats are used in some areas. Brunswick stew, a slowly cooked mix of meat, vegetables, and barbecue seasonings is a long-standing favorite. Potted meats and Vienna sausages with crackers or bread are favorites as a snack or light meal, as are bologna and frankfurters (Burke & Raia, 1995).

A variety of fresh, frozen, and canned fruits is utilized. Watermelon, peaches, plums, oranges, apples, honeydew melon, and cantaloupe are particularly popular. Muscadines or scuppernongs, a wild grape, are eaten fresh in season or made into jam or wine. Popular beverages include buttermilk, heavily sweetened iced tea, lemonade, powdered drink mixes, and soft drinks. Desserts are often served daily. Cakes are very popular, such as pound cake, red velvet cake, and caramel, chocolate, or coconut cake. Favored pies are pecan, sweet potato, lemon meringue, coconut cream, mincemeat, chess, and fruit pies, along with fruit cobblers and fried pies (pastries stuffed with stewed dried fruit). Boiled, heavily salted peanuts are a popular snack in the South (Burke & Raia, 1995).

The African American diet is sometimes referred to as "soul food." This term was coined in the 1960s when traditional Southern African American foodways were adopted by African Americans in other areas as a symbol of ethnic solidarity, identity, and recognition of their African heritage (Frank, 1990; Bloch, 1983). The food thus goes beyond merely nourishing the body. It is interwoven with the slave experience, combining foods and preparation methods from Africa with adaptations forced by slavery, and borrowing from food practices of the southern United States (Bloch, 1983; Burke & Raia, 1995). Migration of African Americans and other southerners out of the South has spread these food practices to other parts of the country. Although the components vary from region to region, the core elements remain the same (Burke & Raia, 1995).

The traditional African American diet has a high cholesterol, fat, and sodium content (Schoenberg, 1994; Frank, 1990; Burke & Raia, 1995). In addition, a number of other dietary practices common among African Americans may affect health. Processed and packaged prepared foods now predominate in the African American diet (Baer, Alfonso, Cuenca, Gilbertson, Kealy, & Lehmann, 1997). It is estimated that prepared foods contribute 50% to 75% of the daily sodium intake among African Americans. Fast food restaurant meals are increasingly popular, serving to further increase fat and sodium intake. Traditional southern home cooking has become an occasional practice, used particularly on holidays and special occasions, such as Sunday dinner (Burke & Raia 1995; Baer et al., 1997). Sugar is heavily utilized in food preparation and snacks. Peppermint candies are often consumed to alleviate dry mouth, coughs, and colds and to ward off hunger during long church services. It is commonly thought that it is essential for diabetics to consume the candy in order to prevent hypoglycemia (Burke & Raia, 1995). Many African Americans avoid fresh pork as a way to control hypertension; this practice stems from the folk belief that excess blood goes to the head when large amounts of pork are eaten. This belief is not held about salt-cured pork, which is consumed much more freely and has been implicated in elevated blood pressure (Burke & Raia, 1995). It is also thought that high blood pressure can be controlled through the fat-cutting properties of astringent foods such as vinegar, pickled foods, and garlic (Schoenberg, 1994).

Recommendations to Practitioners

1. Fully explore with patients all treatments and types of healing they have employed to treat their condition (Bloch, 1983). Since little research has been done on folk remedies, some time and effort should be directed toward determining their effectiveness or potential for harm (Randell-David, 1985).
2. Recognize that even though cultural beliefs may not agree with scientific explanations, they have persisted for generations, effectively helping the population. Trying to change deeply held beliefs may fail and will probably alienate the patient in the process. It is important to recognize, understand, and work within the framework of African American health beliefs and practices in order to improve health care delivery and treatment adherence (Bloch, 1983; Randell-David, 1985).
3. Take into consideration socioeconomic status, religious factors, psychological factors, educational and literacy level, differing communication patterns, cooking facilities, physical constraints, and degree of family support when planning health and nutrition education (Bloch, 1983; Freedman, 1998). Negotiate concrete steps toward behavior change.
4. Decreasing the cholesterol, fat, sugar, and sodium content of the diet and controlling weight are of critical importance (Frank, 1990). Traditional foods are important to the culture, so it is helpful to capitalize on their positive aspects and avoid being overly critical in the process of fostering dietary changes. Modifying recipes rather than eliminating foods will likely be more successful (Burke & Raia, 1995; Baer et al., 1997). Encourage dietary substitutions that are compatible with favored food practices (Schoenberg, 1994; Baer et al., 1997). For example, the use of Liquid Smoke gives foods a smokey flavor without the fat and salt. Another approach might be to use smoked turkey as a substitute for pork (Burke & Raia, 1995). Avoid using the term "fresh" as many view fresh foods as undercooked and bland (Schoenberg, 1994). Thorough cooking and seasoning is preferred by most African Americans.
5. Older women have respect from the community and a great deal of responsibility for nutrition and health care (Randall-David, 1985; Snow, 1993). The churches, as well, hold great significance. Employ these resources to effect change. Encourage significant people in the community to deliver health messages (Schoenberg, 1994).
6. Be supportive of the extended family and social network because it is vital to health and survival among African Americans. Since a large proportion of the African American population is involved in health problems, either as patients or caretakers,

community-based education should be implemented (Randall-David, 1985).

7. Work to improve attitudes of health care providers toward Medicaid recipients, and encourage them to treat all African American patients with respect and dignity.

Mexican Americans

Historical Background

Mexican Americans make up the largest segment of the Hispanic population in the United States. Over 2.5 million Mexicans have legally immigrated to this country since 1900, and far more have crossed the border without legal documentation. Mexican immigrants are located primarily in California, Texas, Arizona, Colorado, and New Mexico (Algert & Ellison, 1989). There is tremendous variation in this population, which includes the original Mexican population annexed to the United States after the Mexican-American War, immigrants who have come since the turn of the century, and migrant workers who come for brief periods of time (Schrieber & Homiak, 1981). Mexicans laborers were initially imported to work on the railroads. Migrant Mexican farmworkers are now valued by agribusiness as low-wage workers. More skilled workers may be found in industry and service occupations in urban areas (de Paula, Lagana, & Gonzalez-Ramirez, 1995).

Worldview and Health Beliefs

Although many of the recent immigrants do not speak English, several generations of descendants from earlier immigrants have been born and educated in the United States. There is considerable language diversity among Mexicans, both here and in their own country. Although some Mexican Americans speak only Spanish, most are bilingual or monolingual, speaking only English. There are many indigenous languages in Mexico, so Spanish may be a second language for some Mexicans (de Paula et al., 1995). In addition, word usage varies depending on the region. Educational levels among Mexican Americans vary widely as well, and college education is increasing. Mexican Ameri-

cans whose families have been in this country for generations have been exposed to American cultural values over a long period of time, and some have developed belief systems approaching the typical American ones. Mexican Americans present a full range of beliefs ranging from those of the Native American cultures of Mexico to those of highly westernized upper-income populations (Schrieber & Homiak, 1981; de Paula et al., 1995).

Two important issues for Mexican Americans are family and religion (Schrieber & Homiak, 1981); to understand Mexican Americans is to know their family relationships and their religious beliefs. Both family and religion are dominated by males, whose decisions tend to be the ultimate word in family and social affairs. Mexican life centers around the family and extended family. One of the most important people in the household, in terms of decision making, is the husband's mother. Even if she does not actually live with the family, she will generally live nearby and have a great influence on actions taken in her son's family.

Nonverbal communication is important to note; it is strongly influenced by respeto (respect). Direct eye contact is avoided with authority figures, such as health care providers, or with persons seen to be higher in status, and Mexican Americans may show respect by standing when such a person comes into their presence. Silence may indicate lack of agreement. Exhibiting sympatia (behavior that promotes smooth relationships) does not necessarily mean that acceptance or rapport has been achieved. Touch from strangers is not well accepted, although it is an important part of traditional healing, and a soft handshake is considered polite (de Paula et al., 1995).

Like most Hispanic and Native American groups, Mexican Americans' time orientation is focused on the present and may be relative to the situation. Punctuality in keeping scheduled appointments may not be a priority for some, although the more acculturated Mexican Americans may be more concerned with it (de Paula et al., 1995).

Sensitive personal issues, including health, are usually kept within the Mexican American family (Schrieber & Homiak, 1981). Because of the Catholic bias against contraception and the high value it places on childbearing, women may not disclose the use of contraception even to family members. In general, men tend to be less self-disclosing than do women. Mexican Americans are usually more comfortable discussing personal subjects with individuals of the same gender (de Paula *et al.*, 1995).

The most important aspect of traditional Mexican health beliefs seen in the populations in the United States is the "hot" and "cold" system (Schrieber & Homiak, 1981; Algert & Ellison, 1989). The healthy body is in a state of balance between the contrary qualities of hot and cold. Illness is the outcome of some imbalance between these two qualities through external or internal exposure, or too much heat or too much cold. Hot and cold refer not only to temperature but to more general properties of things, events, and even persons and activities. The nearest approximation to understanding what hot and cold qualities mean in Anglo culture is to think of hot as denoting any strong, invasive, intensely arousing, strongly energetic, or deeply stimulating influence, force, or quality, and cold as denoting any weak, low level, depressing, feeble, delicate, or soft force or quality.

Hot and cold are inherent qualities of medicines, herbs, foods, environments, or objects. Strong emotional experiences are hot, for example. The essence of therapy when someone is ill, therefore, is to try to restore the lost balance between hot and cold in the body of the patient. The belief in this theory seems to be gradually disappearing among Mexican Americans and is being replaced by the modern concept of homeostasis, which retains the concept of balance or internal equilibrium. For instance, loss of blood is believed to impair the internal balance in the body and causing illness. However, hot–cold beliefs are still held in varying degrees by many. This variability within the population makes it difficult to predict the preferred treatment for a given condition. Disease, in general, may be interpreted as the "lack" of something (such as lack of vitamins) or the "excess" of something (such as eating too much salt or too much sugar). Mexican Americans may also relate health to a state of harmonious relations with the social environment and with spiritual forces in the world (Schreiber & Homiak, 1981).

Health is defined as the ability to function adequately, the absence of pain, and the presence of a robust body (Schreiber & Homiak, 1981). The Mexican American conception of appropriate body weight is about 15 pounds heavier than that of the dominant society in this country.

Symptoms of an illness are usually discussed with family members as a first step in treatment (de Paula *et al.*, 1995). The next action may be to consult one of a number of different types of folk healers who are utilized in varying degrees, along with Western health care providers (Schreiber & Homiak, 1981). Traditional healers may be preferred for a number of reasons: they expect a donation for their services, rather than a fixed fee; they prescribe inexpensive herbal remedies; they establish an intimate and warm relationship with the patient and the patient's family; they treat the patient in the presence of the family; and they may allow the family head to take an active role in deciding when treatment should be initiated. These healers, or *curanderos*, can be either male or female and are usually regularly employed persons in the community they serve, practicing healing in addition to their regular employment. They are successful, among other reasons, because they treat their patients within their own cultural frame of reference (Schreiber & Homiak, 1981).

Curanderos are involved in the treatment of four illnesses that are not believed to be treatable by Western health care (Baer & Bustillo, 1998; McVea, 1997; Schreiber & Homiak, 1981). They are believed to attack exclusively people of Mexican descent. These illnesses are:

- *Caida de la mollera* (falling of the fontanelle)
- *Empacho* (akin to gastroenteritis; believed to be caused by an indigestible blockage in the gastrointestinal tract)
- *Mal de ojo* (evil eye or any illness caused by too strong a look given to a child; evil eye refers more to the cause of the disease rather than to the disease itself)
- *Susto* (fright; akin to an emotional disturbance)

In addition, Mexicans may experience *nervios* (a range of mental health conditions, from "stress" through schizophrenia) (Baer, 1996).

Various folk remedies may be used for these and other conditions, including diabetes. Some, like *nopales* (cactus leaves), have been shown to decrease blood glucose. However, some teas and other herbal preparations may interact with other medications. Some folk remedies, such as *vibora de cascabel* (powdered rattlesnake) may be contaminated with potentially deadly Clostridium botulinum (Algert & Ellison, 1989).

In Mexico and other Latin American countries, injectable drugs for self-treatment are readily available without a prescription and are usually administered by laypeople (McVea, 1997). This practice may lead to overuse of antibiotics, use of drugs without any biomedical indication, and transmission of disease as a result of reusing equipment and inadequate sterilization. Obtaining these drugs is easy in border states, and many Mexican Americans bring injection supplies with them and replenish stocks on return trips. Antibiotics, vitamins, hormones for birth control, analgesics, corticosteroids, Valium, and calcium are examples of readily available injectable drugs. Antibiotics are used for conditions such as fevers, colds, sore throats, wounds, toothaches, pain, and insect bites. Vitamins are used for pregnancy, disease prevention, headaches, poor eyesight, fatigue, and inability to gain weight. Injectable drugs are often chosen after consultation with relatives and friends (McVea, 1997).

Specific Health Problems

The general demographic characteristics of Mexican Americans tend to low levels of income and education, poor living conditions, and ethnic segregation. These factors may negatively influence the health status of this ethnic group in the following ways:

- by increasing the risk of contracting infectious diseases as a result of crowded housing and lack of adequate environmental sanitation
- by hampering understanding of preventive efforts in disease control because of literacy problems
- by restricting access to health care because of the lack of money to pay for it
- by creating the grounds for ethnic discrimination in health care delivery (Schreiber & Homiak, 1981)

Those segments of the Mexican American population that work as migrant farmworkers may have additional health problems. Both the undocumented status of many of them and the constant movement required by their work may reduce access to health care.

Mexican Americans are reported to die more frequently than the general American population from cirrhosis of the liver, tuberculosis, diabetes, infectious and parasitic diseases, circulatory diseases, and accidents (Schreiber & Homiak, 1981). Diabetes rates among Mexican Americans are 1.5 to 2.8 times higher than the high rates found among African Americans. Obesity is prevalent among Mexican Americans as well (Algert & Ellison, 1989; Schreiber & Homiak, 1981; de Paula *et al.*, 1995). Underutilization of health care facilities is an important factor in this group's adequate management of their health care needs (Schreiber & Homiak, 1981).

Obstetrical problems may be an important source of health problems in Mexican American communities due to high rates of fertility, although new research seems to show the negative impact of female work outside of home on this indicator. Nutritional problems are seen as largely due to low-income status rather than deficiencies in the traditional food consumption patterns.

The first treatment for most illnesses is at the level of the household, through use of home remedies. Many of these traditional remedies are highly effective, but in some instances they pose health risks. An example is the use of several lead oxides to treat empacho (Trotter, 1985). These substances go by the names of greta, azarcon, and albayalde, and are sold over-the-counter in Mexico. Use of lead-based home remedies must be investigated as a probable cause in all cases of lead poisoning in this population.

Diet

Mexican cooking derives from the blending of Native American, Spanish, and other European food habits and dietary patterns. Historically, the Mexican diet is primarily vegetarian, based on corn, beans, and squash (Algert & Ellison, 1989). The staples of the Mexican diet are beans—of many varieties, the most common being pinto beans; tortillas—a kind of bread made from ground cornmeal (tortillas are also made of wheat flour, but this kind of tortilla has far less calcium and more fat than do corn tortillas); chiles—hot peppers available in 92 known varieties, often made into salsas; chorizos—sausages made from seasoned pork; and tomatoes and onions. Because of regional differences, foods may be known by several names (Alger & Ellison, 1989), but these staples are favorites with all social classes and are found in most daily meals. Tamales, enchiladas, and other more complex dishes, standard fare in Mexican restaurants in this country, are not typical of the food served daily in Mexican American homes. Home cooking is more simple; the complicated dishes are eaten only on special occasions (Algert & Ellison, 1989).

Meal patterns vary according to availability of traditional foods and extent of assimilation into American culture. New foods are added to the diet as a result of the influence of bilingual children and increased levels of education and employment of adult family members. The traditional diet is nutritionally sound, with high levels of complex carbohydrates and frequent use of fruits and vegetables. Processed foods are not often used, and everyday foods are prepared simply and are well-balanced (Algert & Ellison, 1989).

Fresh milk is not widely consumed (high rates of lactose intolerance have been observed in this group), except when mixed with coffee. Children will often drink a *licuado*, which is a blend of milk, banana, and, sometimes, an egg. Cheese is a dietary staple. Vegetables commonly eaten include onions, tomatoes, squash, nopales (cactus), garlic, avocados, and chile. Tomatoes are often the base of vegetable preparations. Fresh salads are rarely eaten, except by the upper classes. Fruits commonly consumed include pineapples, bananas, strawberries, pomegranates, oranges, mangoes, papayas, coconuts, quinces, cherimoyas, apples, and limes. Most fruits are eaten fresh.

Pork and pork products are the favorite meats in Mexican cuisine. Other meats are also eaten, such as goat, beef, and chicken. Fish and seafood are also consumed. Daily use of beans, eaten as a side dish with tortillas, provides an additional source of protein. Beans may be eaten two or three times a day. Corn and beans, eaten in sufficient amounts, provide high-quality, low-fat protein. The use of lime in the preparation of corn tortillas increases niacin and calcium content. Food preparation methods may vary from one area to the other (Algert & Ellison, 1989).

One drawback to the traditional diet is that it may be high in calories and fat. Lard is the most widely used fat in Mexican cooking (Algert & Ellison, 1989). Oils are consumed in small quantities, as well as butter and margarine. Main dishes are often *guisados* (stir-fried), although *caldos* (thick soups that contain less fat) are also acceptable. Sugar is heavily used in cooking dishes such as *churros* (fried pastries), *pan dulce* (sweet bread), and *bunuelos* (fried tortilla dough served with honey). In addition, soft drinks, ice cream, and candy are popular among Mexican Americans (Algert & Ellison, 1989; de Paula *et al.*, 1995).

Recommendations to Practitioners

1. Language will be a problem for some members of this group. The use of bilingual staff or interpreters, or permitting patients to bring family members to serve as interpreters, will be necessary to minimize communication difficulties. However, if family members or others are not knowledgeable about health care it can lead to miscommunication about complex medical terms or sensitive personal issues. A same-gender translator is usually preferred. When speaking in Spanish to a patient, use the formal pronoun *usted*, especially with older people and married women. After rapport has been established over time, the patient or family may indicate that the more familiar forms are appropriate (de Paula *et al.*, 1995).

2. Patients should be questioned about other steps that have been taken up to that point in treating the illness, and specifically what if any home remedies have been tried or are being currently used (Trotter, 1985;

Baer & Bustillo, 1998). Be aware of possible conflicts between folk and biomedical concepts, disease etiology, and labels to decrease possibility of misunderstanding in diagnosis and treatment (Schreiber & Homiak, 1981).

3. For those who must decrease caloric consumption, advise use of caldos versus guisados and corn versus flour tortillas.

4. Patients should not be asked to make on-the-spot medical decisions; it may be necessary to consult other members of the family. In the care of children, the mother of the child may not be the person to make decisions about treatment; consultation with her husband, mother-in-law, and other relatives is expected (Schreiber & Homiak, 1981).

5. Members of this group expect the physician to take a personal interest in their problems. The objective perspective of Western health care professionals will be interpreted as an indicator of coldness and lack of concern (Schreiber & Homiak, 1981).

6. This group also expects that the physician–patient encounter will begin with social amenities, as well as inquiries into the patient's own opinion of his or her condition. "Getting to the point" immediately is interpreted as rudeness (Schreiber & Homiak, 1981).

7. It is better to suggest a course of action than to issue orders (Schreiber & Homiak, 1981).

8. Mexican Americans, being more fatalistic than many other groups, may reject a diagnosis that blames the individual for the illness (Schreiber & Homiak, 1981).

9. There is a general fear of blood loss; reasons for blood tests should be carefully explained and the amount of blood that will be taken clearly indicated (Schreiber & Homiak, 1981).

Mixtecs

It should be noted that it may be difficult to tell if a particular individual is of Mixtec background. Some may be unwilling to identify themselves as such, because they may be undocumented and would prefer to try to blend into the larger Mexican or Mexican American community. Markers of indigenous identity in Latin America are use of indigenous language and clothing. Mixtec women may tend to wear their hair in braids and to carry shawls. Both men and women tend to be shorter and more indigenous in physical appearance than non-Mixtec Mexicans. Men may have a limited command of Spanish; this may not be the case for Mixtec women.

Historical Background

The pre-Columbian inhabitants of the Oaxaca Valley in southern Mexico developed what has been characterized as one of the most complex cultures of their time (Nagengast & Kearney, 1990; Bade 1994). However, the lives of indigenous peoples in Mexico and Central America were permanently transformed by the European conquest of the region several hundred years ago (Nagengast & Kearney, 1990; Zabin, Kearney, Garcia, Runsten, & Nagengast, 1993). Their population declined by 90% during the first 100 years of conquest due to Spanish practices of domination and the devastating diseases they introduced from Europe. Colonial development pushed Mixtec villages from the valley and into the mountains where cultivation was more difficult, in addition to being detrimental to the ecosystem. Hoofed animals introduced by the Spanish also degraded the soil. During this period, deforestation, mining, and plow agriculture caused further deterioration and erosion of arable land in the region, resulting in economic hardship for future generations (Zabin et al., 1993; Bade, 1994). Agricultural technology, Catholicism, and various social and cultural practices were forced upon the Mixtecs.

In spite of this, much of southern Mexico retains indigenous cultural and social forms that are assumed to be survivors from pre-Columbian times. Some of these practices, however, have been covered with a veneer of European influence (Nagengast & Kearney, 1990). It is remarkable that Mixtec culture has been able to survive in light of the cultural differences that exist among their villages and the armed conflict between villages that has been common in the

Mixtec region, and throughout southern Mexico, preventing the formation of solidarity and collective action (Zabin *et al.*, 1993; Bade, 1994). Conflict and boundary disputes between Mixtec communities have largely resulted from population pressure, soil erosion, and land grabs, and hostile efforts are often directed to nearby communities, deflecting attention away from the political and economic powers that are responsible for the harsh conditions (Nagengast & Kearney, 1990; Stephen, 1996; Zabin *et al.*, 1993). In spite of a number of attempts by federal, state, and international programs to address environmental, economic, and social conditions in the region inhabited by the Mixtec, there has been little impact.

In Mexico indigenous people are not held in high regard, even though few Mexicans are without indigenous ancestors; the commonly used epithet *indio* denotes ignorance and stupidity (Nagengast & Kearney, 1990). Mixtecs, one of the largest indigenous minorities in Mexico, have long been exploited and repressed in their own country (Bade, 1994). Driven from their communal villages in Mexico by poor economic conditions, the poorest villagers came to follow the crops along the East and West Coast corridors in the United States harvesting produce such as strawberries, apples, citrus, tomatoes, and grapes in California (Mydans, 1995). Working in over 23 U.S. states, they travel as far north as Oregon, Washington, and Alaska, and can be found working the tomato fields and citrus orchards in Florida, tobacco and sweet potato fields and toy factories in North Carolina, chicken-processing plants and restaurants (as dishwashers) in West Virginia, in restaurants in New York, on poultry farms in Maine, in potato-storage plants in Idaho, and on beet farms in Michigan (Zabin *et al.*, 1993; Runsten & Kearney, 1994). Mixtec Indians from the southern Mexican state of Oaxaca, along with other indigenous groups of menial laborers from Central and South America, are changing the face of the farm labor force in the United States (Mydans, 1995). Farm work in the United States is the primary industry for the Mexican state of Oaxaca, supporting entire villages and providing funding for schools, roads, and water supply (Nagengast & Kearney, 1990; Stephen, 1996). It has been said that the money sent by

migrants to the Mixteca exceeds the total value of agricultural production there (Zabin *et al.*, 1993). When leaving their villages, the migrants leave behind a strong sense of community and shared social responsibility and obligation.

It has been suggested that an increasing proportion of Mixtecs in the migrant labor pool in California has contributed to the decline in migrant living conditions (Zabin *et al.*, 1993; Bade, 1994; Zabin, 1995). Coming from one of the poorest regions of Mexico, they work for less money and receive fewer benefits than do other Mexican migrants (Zabin *et al.*, 1993; Zabin, 1995). Migrant wages, on the whole, have dropped since the 1980s, due at least in part to increased competition in the produce market, particularly between the United States and Mexico. All too often, as a consequence of having little access to cash, families build up large debts to store owners, with interest rates of 20% (Bade, 1994).

Mixtecs tend to be the most migratory of the farmworkers in this country. There is not an accurate count of the magnitude of the farmworker workforce, as many are undocumented workers and are continually on the move (Nagengast & Kearney, 1990; Runsten & Kearney, 1994). Approximately 1 million farmworkers obtained amnesty under a 1986 law, but a significant proportion of more recent arrivals, including Mixtecs, are undocumented (Mydans, 1995). Mixtec ties to their homes are strong. The movement of Mixtecs has been circular in nature, with many workers returning to Mexico at the end of the U.S. growing season (Nagengast & Kearney, 1990; Runsten & Kearney, 1994). Thus Mixtec communities have been characterized as "transnational" (Bade, 1994; Stephen, 1996). Although recent movements have been characterized by stays of increasing length (Greishop, 1997), most workers say they eventually intend to return permanently to Oaxaca. Those involved in circular migration are primarily male; women are much less likely to have returned to Mexico since their arrival in this country. Although the Mixtecs are Mexican citizens and may look like other Mexicans, many of them speak little Spanish and much less English (Nagengast & Kearney, 1990). Mixteco (an unwritten language) is their indigenous language, but there are significant linguistic differences in the language from village to village. There are also differences in clothing styles between Mixtec villages.

The Mixtec community in Mexico, estimated at 400,000 people, is primarily rural, composed of small villages practicing subsistence agriculture and a communal style of government and economic systems (Nagengast & Kearney, 1990; Grieshop, 1997). Wage labor in the villages is virtually nonexistent, although families supplement farm production with the sale of handmade baskets, hats and mats, chairs, pottery, and artwork for meager prices. In recent decades, the villages have become increasingly less populated due to migration to Mexico City, the northern states of Mexico, and the United States (Greishop, 1997). The estimated 50,000 Mixtecs in California represent 15% of the total Mixtec population (Runsten & Kearney, 1994); an additional 25,000 to 40,000 Mixtecs are working in other states (Grieshop, 1997). Mixtec migrants to the United States tend to be less educated and less likely to speak Spanish or English than those who remain in Mexico (Zabin et al., 1993; Zabin, 1995).

Working conditions for Mixtecs and other Indians in Mexico are abysmal (Zabin et al., 1993). In one labor camp, workers were being housed in crowded, windowless, dirt-floored rooms and cooking over open fires. The rooms were typically furnished with packing boxes, boards, and ragged blankets. A central faucet provided water for the entire camp, and toilet facilities consisted of holes dug in the ground enclosed with plastic sheeting (Nagengast & Kearney, 1990). Although living conditions are somewhat less severe in the United States, exploitation at the hands of the mostly Mexican American supervisors on the job has frequently been reported by Mixtec workers. This may take the form of paying them too little and deducting portions of their pay without authorization for such expenses as transportation, housing, and food (Zabin et al., 1993; Zabin, 1995).

Worldview and Health Beliefs

Migratory experiences for the Mixtec are difficult and often degrading and traumatic (Zabin et al., 1993). They have little formal education, limited access to resources, and limited power and choice; the focus of their lives is to serve others. In addition, they are subject to discrimination and pursuit by immigration authorities (Runsten & Kearney, 1994). Despite efforts to maintain transnational ties, significant portions of their communities are lost. Households try to hang on to old ways, but time and the experiences of living in new locations, formal and informal education, and interaction with government services alters them; their lives are changed by the migration experience (Stephen, 1996). They are placed in a position of powerlessness and dependency on the whims of others, which makes them easy targets for exploitation by employers and others (Zabin et al., 1993; Bade, 1994).

To some extent, Mixtecs themselves believe the negative indio stereotype (Zabin et al., 1993). They refer to their language as "poor words." They see themselves as exploited and inferior, and their villages as "sad places" where food and a decent living are hard to obtain and children die of preventable diseases and malnutrition (Kearney & Nagengast, 1989). However, even though this negative view accurately reflects their daily lives in the Mixteca and on both sides of the Mexican–U.S. border, the Mixtecs tend not to accept this impoverished situation as their traditional lot in life. Although Mixtecs have a reputation in the United States for working very hard without complaint and understanding the rules of the migrant worker game, many are involved in movements, centered around a pan-Mixtec ethnic identity, which seek to improve their socioeconomic conditions and power relations, and to address human rights issues (Zabin et al., 1993; Stephen, 1996). In the course of migration, Mixtecs have established migratory patterns and support systems that provide access to jobs and housing for newcomers, and they have begun to organize to protect themselves from exploitation. Organizations in California are focusing on broad issues such as cultural survival, improved living conditions, legal defense, and improved health care and educational opportunities (Nagengast & Kearney, 1990; Zabin et al., 1993). Mixtecs also draw strength from strong religious beliefs. Births, marriage, agricultural seasons, religious celebrations, and healing all involve ritual and prayer to petition the gods, saints, and other supernatural entities. Their lives and culture are characterized by religious meaning and symbolism (Bade, 1994).

Much as the Mixtec migrants can be described as "transnational," their health beliefs and practices can be depicted as "transmedical," by virtue of their exposure to both traditional health practices in Oaxaca and western biomedicine in the United States. Many use local, state, and federal health care programs in the United States as well as indigenous health care practices, depending on the nature, perceived cause, and severity of the complaint; or they may use both the biomedical and traditional systems simultaneously. They often rely on self-treatment or treatment by a traditional healer, utilizing herbs, sweat baths, religious healing ceremonies, and store-bought remedies to treat health conditions. Many of these healers are involved in local, state, national, and international medical organizations devoted to the exchange of healing experiences, concepts, and methods (Bade, 1994).

Presagios, or omens, are commonly reported among Mixtecs in Mexico (Grieshop, 1997). These omens are usually related to animals or dreams, and outcomes may include death, illness, or injury. Although they are not as commonly reported among Mixtecs in the United States, a significant proportion of the population indicates belief in or personal experience with omens. The reverse is true in relation to locus of illness control; migrants are more likely to see the power for illness prevention and control as lying more outside themselves than do Mixtecs who remain in Mexico. This makes sense in light of the daily lives of the migrants; they have little personal control and are subject to powerful external factors. It cannot be assumed that this group is fatalistic and passive, however. They are better described as realistic and compliant, but capable and resilient survivors (Grieshop, 1997).

Spiritual, social, and cosmic factors are believed to have an effect on both the causes and cure of illness. Who the person knows, where he or she has been, and what he or she has done are all considered in determining the cause of illness. Malevolent actions of supernatural, human, or nonhuman agents are central to the eti-ology. Causes of many conditions are attributed to evil spirits, *mal de ojo* (the evil eye), sorcery, the dead, or violation of taboos. There is a strongly held belief that spirits of the dead have an effect on the health of the living. As a result, reverence is shown to the dead through lighting candles on home altars, participating in elaborate ceremonies, and making offerings to keep the spirits content (Bade, 1994).

Mixtecs share a widely held Latin American indigenous belief known as *naugalism* or *tonalism*. A naugal is a person's nonhuman counterpart, usually an animal, that is closely tied to the life of the individual. Naugal sickness, or *cuehe ndacu*, occurs if the person's naugal is hurt; if the naugal dies, the person will die unless preventive measures are performed by a healer. Object intrusion is another form of illness experienced by Mixtecs. In this case, objects such as stones, coins, chiles, needles, and bones are made to enter the body through sorcery. A specialist called *tia tasi* (man who curses, sorcerer) or *tia sa tata* (man of medicine) then sucks the object out through the skin or rubs the affected person with a chicken egg. The illness enters the egg, which can then be destroyed or buried near the house of an enemy, passing the illness on to him or her. Other types of healers include the *chaa tihivi* (man who sucks), *tia jini tuchi* (man who knows how to feel a pulse), and *tia jini naquin in* (man who knows the soil ritual) (Bade, 1994).

Mixtecs also share the belief that illness results from strong emotions, which can cause a person to absorb or transmit illness. Young children are extremely susceptible and must be protected from these emotions. Fright, or *susto* in Spanish and *ni yivi* in Mixtec, results from a shocking experience, causing the soul to separate from the body, perhaps as a result of offending the spirits. It can cause appetite loss, listlessness, diarrhea, and vomiting. The effects may be delayed, often appearing later in life. The cure involves specific rituals and prayers, usually by a healer, and pharmaceuticals or herbs. A Mixtec nursing mother must control her emotions to avoid *cuehe canduu*, or anger sickness in her child. People of all ages, but especially young children, can be victims of mal de ojo, which is caused by jealousy and may be intentional or unintentional. Adults may touch the cheek of a child to break the spell and prevent unintentional evil eye. Again, ritual and prayer involving specific symbolic and religious procedures performed by a healer are key to curing these conditions and sorcery-induced illnesses such as *mal puesto*. Healers must possess divinatory or prophetic skills to determine the cause and appropriate treatment for illness, neutralizing and redirecting malevolent forces. They often use playing cards to divine the cause of illness. Pulsing is a method by which the healer feels the illness through placing his hands on different body parts in order to identify it. This practice also calms and comforts the sick person. Hens and roosters are commonly sacrificed as offerings to the spirits, including God, the Trinity, and numerous saints as well as sacred places, natural phenomena, sacred objects, the dead, and the nagual (Bade, 1994).

The principle of equilibrium is important in Mixtec medical culture. They view the healthy body as maintaining a balance between hot and cold qualities and illness as resulting from destruction of this equilibrium by an excess of either quality. The hot–cold classification system extends to foods and events in the human life cycle and procreation. The principle of equilibrium also applies to social and spiritual relations (e.g., when one asks a favor, the favor is returned; when one is fed, one feeds others, and so on) (Bade, 1994).

The Mixtec see their environment as pervaded by hostile forces, and they hold the idea that powerful desires of others, living and nonliving, can have a negative effect on one's well-being. This fatalistic perception of the motives of others has been attributed to the chronic poverty of the Mixtec indigenous communities, resulting in competition between neighbors over scarce goods (Bade, 1994).

Specific Health Problems

Living conditions for Mixtec migrant workers in Mexico and the United States are harsh. They are subjected to major health hazards from very poor housing conditions and the heavy use of pesticides in agriculture (Nagengast & Kearney, 1990; Stephen, 1996). Life expectancy is lower and morbidity rates are higher in Oaxaca than in the rest of Mexico. Migrants entering the United States may be ill or at risk for serious health conditions (Bade, 1994; Zabin, 1995). A high incidence of upper respiratory illnesses, infectious disease, nutritional problems, and parasitic diseases have been noted among Mixtec migrant workers. High rates of diabetes and anemia occur among women. Dental problems are a major health concern in this population.

Undocumented Mixtec workers are at particularly high risk for labor exploitation and human rights abuses. They are marginalized by virtue of being illegal, poor, Mexican, and *indio* (Nagengast & Kearney, 1990; Zabin *et al.*, 1993). This puts them at even greater risk of health problems than other migrant groups. The seasonal nature of migrant work puts families at risk of malnutrition and other health problems during slack periods (Bade, 1994).

Barriers to biomedical health care for Mixtec migrant populations often include the inability to speak either English or Spanish, lack of transportation, federal aid qualification requirements and paperwork, illiteracy, lack of legal residency documentation, lack of child care, and inappropriate scheduling demands, in addition to poverty. The ailments of uninsured low-income migrants either go untreated, develop into emergency room situations, or are treated through traditional indigenous means. Continuity of care is a challenge because of migratory patterns (Bade, 1994).

Language differences and translation difficulties may interfere with access to appropriate health care. A case in point occurred in central Florida in 1994, when a young pregnant Mixtec woman was unable to communicate her concerns during labor, delivery, and postpartum because she could speak neither Spanish nor English. Hospital staff and social workers did not recognize that she was of Mixtec background. As a result, she was labeled as possibly retarded and rejecting her infant, and she temporarily lost custody of the baby (Hollingsworth, 1994). Mixtecs frequently have difficulty in expressing symptoms to biomedically trained care providers. Differences in concepts of the biological basis of illness and explanations for disease causation greatly affect diagnosis, treatment, and prognosis, as well as the provider–patient interaction. In addition, the often impersonal approach to illness in biomedical systems differs drastically from the physical, emotional, and spiritual support experienced by Mixtecs through their traditional healers and may negatively affect health outcomes.

Diet

Pre-Columbian Mixtec civilization was based on corn, beans, and squash produced by peasant farmers. Those crops continue to be the basis of subsistence agriculture today. Nutritional status in the Mixteca is below national and state averages, with the average daily caloric intake of children being less than two-thirds of the recommended amount. Beans and rice are central to the diet of Mixtecs. *Totopos* (crisp toasted corn tortillas) and *mole de guajolote* (ground chile sauce with turkey) are prepared for celebrations.

Recommendations to Practitioners

1. In planning health education interventions, health care providers will need to develop an understanding and appreciation of the belief systems and the lived experiences of Mixtec migrants if their efforts are to be effective.
2. Personal prevention and treatment strategies should be stressed, with emphasis on the things the individual does have power over and can control both at work and at home.
3. Be alert to the fact that Mixtec migrants, though from a Spanish-speaking country, often speak little or no Spanish. Two interpreters may be required, one to translate from Mixteco to Spanish and the other from Spanish to English. The use of specialized medical terms may cause confusion; simple, familiar terms should be used.
4. Recognize that Mixtecs are culturally, politically, and socially distinct from the mestizo Mexicans who have historically been the predominant migrant labor group in the United States. They present special challenges for health and social service agencies. It is not likely that health care delivery problems will eventually be solved by exposure to biomedicine and assimilation into American culture.
5. Be certain that diagnoses and interventions are understood and that recommendations for health care are realistic for the individual to carry out.
6. Keep in mind that the Western biomedical system is highly institutionalized and technological, very unlike traditional Mixtec health care practices (Bade, 1994).
7. Programs are needed to provide responsive health care and prevent the use of expensive emergency room services for nonurgent health problems. Resolution of Mixtec migrant health problems will require binational and cross-cultural communication, involving governments, Mixtec leaders, Mixtec healers, and the migrants themselves—particularly the mothers, who are the primary health care providers in the family (Bade, 1994).

Guatemalans

It should be noted that it may be difficult to tell if a particular individual is of Guatemalan background. Some may be unwilling to identify themselves as such, because they may be undocumented and would prefer to try to blend into the larger Mexican and Mexican American community. Markers of indigenous identity in Latin America are use of indigenous language and clothing. Guatemalan indigenous women often wear their hair in braids. Both men and women will be shorter and more indigenous in physical appearance than most Mexicans or Mexican-Americans. All will speak an indigenous language (with little or no literacy in this language), and have from minimal (women) to fair (men) command of Spanish.

Historical Background

Although Mayans are the majority population in Guatemala, the society is dominated socially and economically by the Ladino (mestizo) population, with very limited economic mobility and few social or educational services available to the indigenous population (Tedlock, 1992). Many Guatemalan refugees are Mayan

Indians, descendants of a complex Central American civilization now fleeing civil war, poverty, violence, and terrorism in Guatemala (Vlach, 1992; Tedlock, 1992; Burns, 1993). Settlement of Guatemalan refugees began in Indiantown, Florida, in the early 1980s (Miralles, 1989). Indiantown and Los Angeles are the major centers of Mayan immigration (Burns, 1993). Mayans are also found elsewhere in Florida and California, and in Washington, Oregon, Arizona, Texas, New York, Pennsylvania, and Virginia. Often, they escaped death squads or forced relocation through a government hamlet program in their own country. Coming from rural villages in the northwestern highlands, many died as they attempted to cross the border into Mexico. They often arrived in this country as illegal aliens, with little in the way of material resources. It is unlikely that many of the refugees will be able to return to their homeland. Nearly a quarter of a million refugees have fled Guatemala.

Traditionally having practiced subsistence agriculture or worked in small-scale industry in Guatemala, some went to urban areas to find work, while others joined the migrant farmworker streams in the United States. Women may earn additional money by babysitting, doing hand laundry, or cooking for the single men in the migrant community (Miralles, 1989). Scarcity of land, low productivity on available land, and lack of funds for supplies had forced many into supplemental employment before they left their country. Most of the refugees try to leave migrant farm work as soon as they can, preferring safer, less mobile work (Burns, 1993).

Indigenous Guatemalan male refugees often have a good command of spoken Spanish, but few of the women do. Their primary language is usually one of the 26 Mayan dialects found in Guatemala (Burns, 1993).

Worldview and Health Beliefs

Unlike other refugee groups, Guatemalans typically come to the United States in family units—including men and women, who may be widowed or estranged from their spouses (Vlach, 1992)—coming with their children and other family members to establish new lives.

Networks of relatives and friends relocating in the United States encourage neighbors from their original communities to join them, and the newer arrivals count on these networks to help them find housing and work (Vlach, 1992). Baptisms and marriages serve to create *compadrazgo* bonds, forming a structure of social support (Burns, 1993). Parent–child bonds are very strong, extending into adulthood even after the child marries.

The refugees find living arrangements in this country to be very different from those left behind in Guatemala. There the cool, thin mountain air necessitated that houses be closed and dark. Villages were small and widely dispersed, with people meeting when they went to town on market days. In the United States refugees find themselves crowded together as a result of limited housing availability, with two or three families sharing an apartment or house, or families subletting rooms to single people. There tends to be high mobility in refugee communities as people move around in search of better housing (Burns, 1993). Refugees have to learn to negotiate many things that others take for granted, such as post offices, laundromats, an array of products in grocery stores, and enrolling their children in school. Some receive assistance from the Catholic church, refugee service centers, and local people.

The Guatemalan refugee population is relatively young, with the majority being single men and children. Common law marriages are the norm. Most of the adult refugees, particularly the women, have not had any formal schooling. Thus, their written language skills as well as their understanding of scientific or biological concepts may be limited. The majority of children are enrolled in school and are developing fluency in English. Some preschoolers are able to attend day care for migrant families.

Guatemalan refugees are a diverse group, due in part to varying exposure to other cultural groups, particularly Mexicans. The three main religious denominations represented among this group in the United States are Roman Catholic, Seventh Day Adventist, and, to a lesser extent, Evangelical Protestants. The Adventists and Evangelicals are often critical of other groups for heavy drinking and the resulting violence and irresponsible behavior, blaming them for a number of other social ills. A significant number of Guatemalan refugees do not practice any particular religion (Burns, 1993). Catholicism as it is practiced among Mayan people in Guatemala contains many indigenous elements (Tedlock, 1992). The refugees are also a politically diverse group. Early refugees feel they had no choice but to leave their country, whereas more recent arrivals, mostly single males, have come only for jobs and money. Tension and distrust exists among the earlier arrivals as a result of differing experiences with political and military groups in Guatemala.

Guatemalan refugees tend to be wary of other people of color in the United States. Being small in stature and somewhat passive by nature, they are frequently victimized by other groups and have difficulty understanding why this happens to them. Robberies are common because it is widely known that Mayans seldom use banks, but carry their money with them (Burns, 1993).

The refugees have a reputation for being hard workers. In nearly all refugee families, both parents are employed, whereas in Guatemala women seldom do agricultural wage labor. Women retain control over the money they bring in; if only the husband is working, he usually will give his wife money to cover expenses. Relatives often prefer to work together, though women are less likely to work on contract than men (Miralles, 1989). Life for Guatemalans in this country revolves around making a living, and a high premium is placed on good health because it is necessary in order to work hard and earn money. Being ill signifies weakness and inability to carry out responsibilities. Thus, sickness may be denied and treatment delayed.

Social life for the refugees in this country primarily revolves around the family, the church, and recreation. Playing soccer or marimba music, fiestas, and drinking are favored activities (Miralles, 1989). One means of adapting to their new and sometimes frightening way of life is through ceremonies practiced in Guatemala and adapted to life in the United States such as birth celebrations, baptisms, marriages, and funerals. Some associations of Guatemalan Mayans have formed for the purpose of community development and advocacy (Burns, 1993).

Although blue jeans, sneaker and baseball caps are commonly worn, there is still evidence of traditional clothing in refugee communities, especially for special occasions. Many women still wear handwoven and embroidered *huipil* (blouses) and *corte* (skirts), and carry loads in woven blankets. They may wear strands of multicolored necklaces and earrings (Miralles, 1989).

In Guatemala, people maintained health through hard work, attention to religious values, and obtaining biomedical or indigenous health care when needed. In this country, refugees encounter a bewildering array of options for health care; however, most of them are costly, particularly for people with undocumented status. Women, traditionally the experts on food, health, and family security, find this role largely taken from them in this country (Burns, 1993). Uncertainty becomes a way of life for many refugees as they flee their homeland, endure a laborious process to determine eligibility for political refugee status, and face the possibility that they may have to flee again if this effort is not successful. Seldom have Guatemalans been granted political asylum in this country, although many have been granted resident alien status or been given temporary or permanent worker status (Burns, 1993).

Guatemalans, like many other Latin Americans, subscribe to the hot and cold dichotomy of disease causation. It is important to note, however, that the components of this belief system vary from place to place. In Guatemala, the terms *fresco* or *templado* are used in some areas to designate a third category, which is understood as fresh, medium, or neutral (Cosminsky, 1975; Miralles, 1989). The illnesses most commonly attributed by Guatemalans to excessive heat are *diarrea* (diarrhea) and *calentura* (fever). Diarrhea is attributed to hot weather, and is treated by stripping down to diapers or underwear and avoiding the sun or sitting in front of a fan. Drinking cool water or, preferably, Kool Aid or Gatorade are also recommended. It is common to delay treatment for two to three days because it is thought that the condition will resolve without intervention. Although extreme hot and cold can create problems, sudden change from hot to cold or vice versa also creates imbalance and should be avoided. *Mal de estomago* (intestinal pains or upset stomach) may be brought on by either cold or hot conditions, or by something that was eaten that isn't tolerated by the body, such as spicy Mexican food, too much fried meat, and milk. Because many of the herbs used to treat diarrhea and mal de estomago are not available in the United States, the best solution is to refrain from eating or drinking anything for a day or two (Miralles, 1989).

Calentura is diagnosed by feeling the face and neck to see if it is warm. It is caused by extremes of either hot or cold, primarily in reference to the weather. Accompanying symptoms include loss of appetite and irritability. If it is accompanied by diarrhea, it is a sign of something serious that requires medical intervention. Newborn infants are particularly susceptible, and are kept in a closed, warm room. If they must be taken out, they are protected by layers of wrapping and head coverings. Pregnant, lactating, and menstruating women are especially vulnerable to calentura, perhaps because these are hot conditions, or because these are times of weakness, which is considered to be a cold conditions. Tylenol is a commonly used remedy for this malady. *Catarro* (general malaise, head cold) may be a combination of symptoms: fever, cough, sore throat, or sinus pain. The cause is uncertain. Catarro and *gripe* (flu) are generally treated at home with over-the-counter preparations such as Tylenol, aspirin, and cough lozenges or syrups (Miralles, 1989).

More serious diseases that are prevalent among Guatemalan refugees include *dolor de los pulmones* (tuberculosis), *pulmonia* (pneumonia), and intestinal parasites. Pneumonia is considered more dangerous, with more severe symptoms. It is thought to be more of a problem in mountainous areas due to the cold air. Tuberculosis causation, on the other hand, is not clearly identified. It is thought to affect adults primarily (Miralles, 1989). Intestinal parasites, which are very common in Guatemala (Mata, 1995), are believed to grow inside the body and feed off the blood, thereby making a person weak. Adults are usually reluctant to admit they might have intestinal parasites, and delay treatment as a result. Treatment usually involves the entire household, which may be problematic because Guatemalans often do not consider that necessary. In general, they seldom recognize the concept of contagion. There is a belief that intestinal parasites can be picked up from the environment, but the idea of exposure to disease from other individuals is not widely accepted.

In addition to hot–cold imbalance, strength–weakness opposition is viewed as a cause of illness (Cosminsky, 1975). Whether a person is considered strong or weak is not so much due to present circumstances as it is to one's past experiences. For example, a man may be considered strong because he has overcome past hardships, regardless of his present situation. Parents, then, tend to be less concerned about older children who were born in Guatemala and survived the hardships of coming to this country. "Acquired weakness" is a temporary condition that may occur even in a strong person. Strength is related to the good quality and quantity of one's blood (Cosminsky, 1975). As blood is seen as being limited in supply, giving blood samples may cause anxiety, especially for pregnant and postpartum women and their infants. Some believe that it is worth the risk, however, if it aids in diagnosis. A main concern is *bajo* (low) or *debil* (weak) blood. One may be born with the condition, or it may result from excessive blood loss during menstruation or childbirth. The color of the blood is an indicator of quality; women are especially concerned with the color of their menstrual blood. Consuming iron is seen as an effective treatment for blood problems, but there may be confusion as to which foods are good sources (Miralles, 1989).

In general, Guatemalan medicines are considered to be about the same as or better than those available in the United States and remedies, including herbs and injections, are often sent to refugees from home. Injections are considered to be more effective than pills, and refugees may have difficulty understanding why medical doctors in this country prefer expensive pills over injections. Oral medications may be perceived as remaining in the stomach. In spite of reservations about biomedicine, most refugees recognize that they experience fewer kinds of illness and decreased incidence of disease in this country (Miralles, 1989).

Illness may also have supernatural causes, such as *brujeria* (witchcraft) or *Satanas* (diseases caused by Satan). This supernatural belief system has pre-Columbian roots adapted to Catholic beliefs following conquest. It is one of the major explanations of disease causation throughout the Guatemalan highlands. In this country, however, *brujos* (supernatural healers) are not common, although *curanderos* (other indigenous healers) are. The new environment has generated some illnesses among refugees that do not fit traditional health belief models of Guatemala. Among these are fear of poisoning from pesticides and herbicides, urinary tract infections, and vaginitis (Miralles, 1989).

Specific Health Problems

Farmwork becomes dangerous when the workers are not used to using pesticides and agricultural technology (Burns, 1993). In addition, migrants are subjected to crowded housing conditions and poor sanitation. Intestinal parasites are common in this population. Communicable disease rates in Guatemalan migrant communities are high relative to the total population, perhaps a function of not recognizing contagion as a disease etiology. Because people living in the same house may not know each other's names or places of work, it is often difficult to maintain contact over time for adequate health care follow-up.

In crowded housing situations, privacy is lacking and, as a result, tensions between neighbors are common. Stresses also result from the loss of home and family members in Guatemala and from culture shock experienced in their new situation. This may leave Guatemalan refugees vulnerable to illness and subject to posttraumatic stress syndrome. Children in Central America have been heavily affected by political violence and have often been directly involved in combat, which may have implications for their physical and emotional well-being. As a result of past experiences and new stress, anxiety and depression are not uncommon among adolescents (Burns, 1993). Guatemalans frequently must face the triple challenge of being refugees, migrants, and undocumented aliens, and, as such, are not officially recognized by the U.S. government or aid organizations.

Cultural and language differences complicate health assessment and treatment activities and the ability of health care providers to help Guatemalans meet their own needs. Success often requires a degree of flexibility that is difficult to achieve in our rigidly structured health care system.

Guatemalan refugee communities have high rates of alcohol and drug abuse. In some areas, drinking and driving rates are high among Guatemalan refugees. Prostitution is also common in these communities. Weekend violence is a problem, and may lead to fights, accidents, and deaths (Miralles, 1989).

Many of the health care resources used in Guatemala are not available to refugees in migrant farmworker communities, such as *farmacias*, herb vendors, and *curanderos*, or traditional healers. They are accustomed to easy access to a variety of remedies, including injections, which are given by pharmacists without a physician's prescription. Women trained by traditional midwives in Guatemala may be available in some areas to pregnant women. In addition, men who were trained by Catholic missionaries to be *promotores de salud* in Guatemala may be available for first aid and preventive health care, although they are not likely to give injections or medications as they did in Guatemala (Miralles, 1989). Refugees have difficulty finding anyone to administer injections that have been brought from Guatemala. This raises the risk that refugees may ask untrained individuals to administer the injections.

Diet

There is often a sense among Guatemalan refugees that if a food tastes good and does not cause mal de estomago, it must be good for you. A large proportion of the daily calorie intake among the refugees is in the form of candy, soft drinks, potato chips, and other junk food. Sweets are seen to give temporary strength, while a good meal, typically consisting of tortillas and meat, fills the stomach (Miralles, 1989). Overall, Guatemalans historically have consumed a wide variety of foods, including corn tortillas, black beans, squash, green beans, green corn, potatoes, avocados, and greens. Little animal protein and occasional fruit complete the traditional diet (Mata, 1995). Milk products are not commonly used, and because the Mayans are genetically almost 100% Native American, lactose intolerance is common in this population.

The biochemical role of food in good nutrition, disease prevention, and fetal growth is generally not recognized among refugees. Breastfeeding is valued, but it is usually not practical for working mothers, although they may supplement their child's diet with breast milk for two or three years (Miralles, 1989).

Recommendations to Practitioners

1. Be conscious of the chance of misinterpretation of both words and concepts as a result of cultural and language differences and multilevel translation (English to Spanish to Mayan) (Miralles, 1989). Sometimes these language differences may defy translation skills. It is important not to assume that the patient or interpreter understands what is being said—even if they are able to recite what is being told to them, meanings may be misunderstood. Avoid using unfamiliar medical and scientific terms and concepts. Be certain to use appropriate translators for a given condition; for example, although the children may be expert translators, they are not considered appropriate for communicating information concerning reproductive issues and bodily functions (Miralles, 1989). In areas with a high proportion of Guatemalan refugees, developing a program for training community-level health workers may effectively address these issues. In addition to improving communication, these workers can also provide insight into Guatemalan refugee life. Use of gestures may help breach language barriers.
2. Carefully explore to see if traditional remedies are possibly being used prior to initiating pharmacological treatment.
3. Recognize that indigenous disease causation theories determine appropriate intervention and prevention measures, and they must be considered if biomedical treatment is to be effective.
4. Because Guatemalans tend to describe illnesses according to their symptoms, health education efforts may be more successful if the topics focus on specific symptoms of health and illness rather than on diseases and are followed by suggestions for promoting good health (Miralles, 1989). Minimize technological terminology.
5. It is important to emphasize self-reliance and avoid the creating of dependency when providing health and other support services to refugee populations (Miralles, 1989).
6. Those refugees who have entered the migrant stream should know that there is a national migrant health care system and that they can find similar programs as they travel (Miralles, 1989).
7. Use common health problems among Guatemalan refugees as a basis for the development of community health programs (Miralles, 1989). If the issues to be addressed are recognized as a problem by the population being served, health messages are more likely to be accepted.
8. Research needs include study of decision making when facing illness, factors related to emotional and psychological stress, and the process of changing perspectives and medical orientation over time (Miralles, 1989).

Haitians

Historical Background

The history of Haiti has been shaped by foreign powers: Spain, France, and, most recently, the United States (Lassiter, 1998). Following the arrival of Christopher Columbus in 1492, the Spanish proceeded to exploit the resources of the lush island, using and abusing the indigenous people in the process. By 1550, these people had been almost entirely wiped out in violent uprisings or from inhumane treatment and exposure to diseases imported by the Europeans (Civan, 1994). As the indigenous population decreased, the Spaniards turned to West Africa for slaves to replace them (Civan, 1994; Lassiter, 1998). When the economic potential of the area did not materialize, the Spanish gradually lost interest and the French began inching their way into control. Spain relinquished the region to France in 1697, and France proceeded to turn the island into one of its richest colonies through large-scale export of coffee, sugar, cotton, and indigo (Civan, 1994). Slaves continued to be severely mistreated by the French, eventually forming a rebellion that led to freedom from France in 1804, making Haiti the second independent nation in the West and the world's first modern black republic (Civan, 1994; Lassiter, 1998).

Independence brought with it numerous revolts, revolutions, civil wars, and coups over the ensuing decades (Civan, 1994; Bibb & Casimir, 1996; Lassiter, 1998). The United States exerted influence in 1915 when Haitian political instability, American business interests, and growing concern over German interests in Haiti led to invasion and subsequent occupation that lasted 20 years. Conditions improved under American occupation, but the improvements were concentrated around Port-au-Prince, the capital city. Occupation forces were obviously racist and treated Haitians with little regard. All Haitians, mulatto and black, were excluded from real power. As a result, improvements that were made by U.S. occupation were only temporary. When the United States withdrew in 1934, levels of poverty and illiteracy remained unchanged. We left behind a well-trained military force and a strong anti-American feeling (Civan, 1994). The military was the only cohesive institution in Haiti, and the only tool by which government could rule. A series of dictatorships and chaotic social conditions ensued. An opposition movement surfaced, which succeeded in democratically electing a parish priest, Jean-Bertrand Aristede, to the presidency in 1990. He was soon ousted by the military, however. The United States entered the picture once more, applying pressure to the military in the form of trade embargoes, which served largely to make life intolerable for most of Haiti. Threat of invasion finally led to the return of democratic government, and U.S. peacekeeping forces were sent to Haiti to ensure stability (Civan, 1994; Lassiter, 1998).

Since independence in 1804, Haiti has been made up of two distinct societies. Elite mulattos and black generals of the army lived in the towns, controlling the government, the military, and trade. They imitated the French lifestyle and used the French language for public affairs. The black peasants lived in the country, farming small plots of land and having little to do with government or business; in turn, the government paid little attention to improving their conditions. They lived according to African-based traditions and spoke only Haitian Creole, a language that arose from the influence of African, French, Spanish, and English languages. This pattern remains in Haiti to this day. The population of Haiti is 95% black, and about two-thirds lives in rural areas and works in agriculture (Civan, 1994). However, deforestation, land erosion, a declining economy, and the arrival of transnational companies have begun to force peasants to migrate to cities or abroad. A large number work in the Dominican Republic under slave-like conditions. These developments have caused urban problems and social change. Traditionally dependent on the extended family and cooperative labor, urban slum dwelling has weakened these aspects of community life (Sproles, 1990; Civan, 1994).

The first significant Haitian migration to the United States occurred during the 1920s, and a middle class base of professionals and folk healers was established. Since the 1950s, Haitians have migrated to the United States in ever increasing numbers (Civan, 1994). A mass exodus of poor Haitians occurred in the late 1970s through the early 1980s; largely uneducated and with low literacy, they became known as "boat people" (Bibb & Casimir, 1996; Lassiter, 1998). The recent immigrants seek refuge from a country that is distinguished by its poverty and political turmoil. Because the Haitian government is, in name, a democracy, immigrants from that country have not been able to claim political asylum. Consequently, there are large numbers of Haitians living illegally in the United States. Like other newly arrived immigrants, they live in ghettos with poor sanitation, overcrowding, and the intense stresses of poverty, cultural adjustment, and lack of citizenship (Stepick & Portes, 1986).

Haitians have settled mainly in Florida and New York (Sproles, 1990; Lassiter, 1998). Although the immigrants have come from various strata of the Haitian society, they share many of the same cultural standards, the same languages (Creole and French), and the same mix of religions (French Catholicism, American-influenced Protestantism, and voodoo) (Civan, 1994; Bibb & Casimir, 1996).

Haitian communities in the United States form separate ecological niches, most of which have their own community churches, stores, restaurants, social and literary clubs, newspapers, physicians, and folk healers, all of which help the immigrants to maintain their culture. These communities are tightly linked to each other by complex networks of communication and family relationships. Employment migration from one community to another further contributes to the flow of communication (Laguerre, 1981).

Worldview and Health Beliefs

Although 80% of the population is Catholic and 20% is Protestant, voodoo is in fact the national religion of Haiti since most Haitians practice at least some aspects of voodoo or are affected by it in some way (Bibb & Casimir, 1996). A negative stereotype of voodoo has developed as a result of popular misconceptions. Often depicted as a cult of sorcerers practicing "black magic," voodoo is in reality a religion based on generally helpful and protective family spirits (*loas*) that can be called upon for assistance (Lassiter, 1998). The word *voodoo* derives from a West African word meaning *spirit*. Voodoo includes rituals, ceremonies, and altars in which traces of Catholicism and African religious beliefs are evident. The loas are paid, usually in the form of food, drink, or gifts, to bring good fortune or protection or to attack enemies. Belief in voodoo can be so strong that it results in death for a person who is convinced that a hex has been placed on him or her.

The age distribution of Haitian immigrants is biased toward the 10-to-19-year age bracket, with females slightly outnumbering males (Laguerre, 1981). Haitians live in tightly linked social and family networks (Lassiter, 1998). In times of crisis, such as the illness of a family member, friends and relatives are likely to help in diagnosing and curing or advising the patient. However, the way in which Haitians solve their health problems depends on their social and economic backgrounds. Migrants from rural districts were taught to seek help from folk healers, whereas intellectuals educated in France have had little contact with this type of medicine and will probably consult Western physicians (Laguerre, 1981).

Haitians believe in preventive medicine. The most important activities for maintaining good health are eating and resting well and maintaining personal hygiene. Survival in the United States often necessitates long working hours, and very crowded living conditions. In addition the new environment offers many unfamiliar foods, and efforts to eat a balanced meal, in Haitian terms, are often frustrated. Consequently, the factors necessary for healthy living are often absent at a very basic level (Laguerre, 1981).

Upon feeling pain or weakness, the person will consult with the family about the symptom. These family consultations are important, and everyone will try to match the problem with something they have experienced, deciding what caused the illness and how it should be treated. In Haitian culture, illness is considered to have two types of causes (Laguerre, 1981; Lassiter, 1998). If illness (indicated by the presence of pain or weakness) appears very suddenly, it is perceived to be caused by supernatural forces. The problem could be that the individual's spirit protector needs special attention, that the ancestors need propriation, or that sorcery is involved. Consultation with a voodoo priest then becomes necessary for diagnosis and treatment (Laguerre, 1981). On the other hand, illness is seen as having natural causes as well; these illnesses appear slowly, but are of short total duration (Lassiter, 1998). When a problem of this type occurs, there are several treatment options. The preferred first choice is home treatment—home remedies or patent medicines. If the condition persists, a Haitian folk healer may be consulted (Laguerre, 1981). Treatment will include the use of herbs and oils. Use of such healers is a preferred form of treatment among Haitians because it is familiar and non-threatening. Visits with the healer can occur outside of work hours, which prevents losing a day's pay, and the payment can be negotiated. It also has the effect of preserving anonymity within the larger system, a distinct advantage because many Haitians are in the United States illegally. Therefore, when a Haitian appears in a hospital or clinic, it is usually as a last resort (Laguerre, 1981). It should be assumed that the person is feeling very poorly, although due to the Haitian custom of bearing pain stoically, the patient may minimize his or her symptoms.

At the point in which the Western health care is sought, the patient is likely to have a well-developed sense of what the problem is. However, Haitian definitions of causes and symptoms differ greatly from those of biomedicine (Laguerre, 1981). Blood irregularities are perhaps the most significant health concept for Haitians (Lassiter, 1998). Blood can be too thick, thin, hot, cold, weak, dirty, dark, or yellow. Conditions of the blood are related to illness. For example, thick blood can cause hypertension, and is the result of being frightened. Thin blood can be caused by drinking too much alcohol, and will lead to tuberculosis. Physical or mental weakness is the result of weak blood, and necessitates the consumption of red foods and beverages. Thick blood causes itching. To better serve the patient, questions about blood beliefs should be asked, and treatment should include consideration of them. For example, if a diet is being prescribed, red foods could be purposefully included if the patient has included weak blood among his or her symptoms (Laguerre, 1981).

The concept of *gaz* (gas) is also important to Haitians (Laguerre, 1981; Lassiter, 1998). It can be gas as it is normally considered in biomedical terms, or simply air. Air is believed to enter holes in the body, such as the ears and mouth. Gas in the ears can cause headaches, whereas movement of gas through the body may cause pain. For example, back pain may be caused by gas moving from the stomach to the legs (Laguerre, 1981).

Another possible cause of illness is an imbalance of hot and cold factors (Laguerre, 1981). As in Latin American health beliefs, certain foods, medicines, and states of being are classified as hot or cold (Lassiter, 1998). If one is in a hot state, then a cold food or medicine may be necessary. For example, migraines are thought to result from hot blood and may require a cold medicine (Laguerre, 1981).

Specific Health Problems

A major problem for health professionals delivering care to Haitians is the barrier of language (Stepick & Portes, 1986). Most Haitians in the United States are monolingual Creole speakers (Civan, 1994). Most Haitians prefer a member of the family to act as translator.

The widespread poverty in Haiti has affected the health of its people. The infant mortality rates are the highest in the Americas, and the life expectancy of Haitians is the lowest in the Caribbean. Because Haiti has the second-lowest per capita caloric intake in the world, malnutrition is pervasive, particularly among the young and the poor. Medical services are critically lacking in Haiti because of the poor infrastructure in rural areas and the emigration of doctors as a result of political oppression (Civan, 1994).

Chronic conditions reported most often by Haitian families in Miami were serious eye problems, chronic skin problems, nervousness, allergies, arthritis, and rheumatism. Other conditions that health care workers have reported frequently include anemia, parasites, leprosy, malaria, and tuberculosis (Laguerre, 1981). Poor sanitation contributes to many of these illnesses. Skin lesions often thought of as fungus may actually be leprosy; if an antifungal cream is not effective, then leprosy should be considered. Haitians may be at less risk for cardiovascular diseases than the U.S. population in general because most Haitians have retained the island's patterns of extensive physical activity. Many immigrants continue to walk long distances rather than use public or private means of transportation (Laguerre, 1981).

One problem that has mistakenly been associated with the Haitian population is AIDS. The Center for Disease Control has recently removed Haitians from its list of those at risk for AIDS (Civan, 1994; Bibb & Casimir, 1996; Lassiter, 1998). The Haitian community, already under a great deal of stress due to racial discrimination and the inability to gain political asylum in the United States, has been further stigmatized by having been originally, and incorrectly, included on this AIDS list.

Diet

Pork is traditionally the meat most often eaten by Haitians, although the actual preference is for beef, despite its higher price. Chicken, goat, and lamb are also included in the Haitian diet. Meat is often fried. The Haitian diet includes an abundance of fish, usually salted. Turtle, shellfish, and conch are also eaten (Sproles, 1990). Milk is expensive in Haiti, and therefore only the more affluent can afford to consume it, but Haitians seem to be drinking more milk in the United States than they did on the island (Sproles, 1990). A large part of the Haitian diet is made up of beans, primarily red kidney beans as well as black and other types of beans. Haitians eat very little bread; rice is the major staple grain, usually mixed with beans. Sorghum grains (called pitimi) are also a staple (Sproles, 1990). Corn is popular, both boiled and also eaten as a pudding. Haitians eat few green vegetables. They especially like avocados and salads made from hearts of palm sprouts. Preferred fruits include mangoes, bananas, oranges, plantains, coconut, grapefruit, and the star apple. Sugar cane and bamboo shoots are also well liked (Sproles, 1990).

Food is usually fried in oil or lard. Fried pork and fried plantains are among the favorite dishes. Convincing patients to lose weight may be difficult, as there is a cultural bias toward larger body size. It is assumed that thinness reflects poor health and wasting due to emotional and psychological problems (Laguerre, 1981). Lower-income Haitians are the group most likely to show nutritional problems due to low protein intake and heavy consumption of carbohydrate foods. Most Haitians eat large quantities of fatty foods, independent of social class. It may be beneficial to the health of some patients to encourage them to do less frying of foods, or at least use less oil in cooking. Use of lard can be replaced by polyunsaturated vegetable oils. They might also use more fresh greens and leafy vegetables to make up for their low calcium intake when their diet is low in milk (Sproles, 1990).

Recommendations to Practitioners

1. Interpreters should be provided, or a family member permitted to serve in this role.
2. Patients should be asked what they and their families feel the problem is.
3. Prior treatments and other medications being used for the illness should be investigated.

4. Haitian patients have a different view of the importance of location of pain in diagnosing a problem (Laguerre, 1981). The patient will find it meaningless to point out the exact location of the pain; the health care provider should recognize this different perspective.
5. It is believed that any part of the body can be hexed by the use of voodoo. As a result, the patient may be reluctant to give blood or urine samples. Health care workers should reassure the patient that the specimens will be handled carefully.
6. Haitians feel that use of a wheelchair indicates a very serious illness (Laguerre, 1981). If a wheelchair must be used, it should be explained that it is a routine procedure and no cause for alarm.
7. There is an expectation of same-day diagnosis of a problem and a fast-acting treatment (Laguerre, 1981). If this is not to be the case, the situation should be carefully explained to the patient; otherwise it will be assumed that no treatment is being offered.
8. It is believed that new foods may make the patient even more ill; the patient may even fast in a hospital setting rather than eat non-Haitian foods (Laguerre, 1981). If at all possible, patients should be offered familiar foods in these situations.
9. Regardless of the biomedical reality, blaming the patient for his or her condition will have few positive effects.
10. Pregnant and lactating women may be subject to some dietary restrictions (Laguerre, 1981); it may be useful to inquire about these, as well as any foods it is believed these women should preferentially consume.

Conclusion

This overview has stressed the diversity of ideas about and approaches to healthcare seen in rural areas of the American South. Although the discussion was geographically limited, many of the people discussed in this chapter are found in other areas of the country. However, it is critical to avoid stereotyping patients on the basis of their ethnic background. Many beliefs and practices may vary from individual to individual. In addition, health belief systems are mediated by a number of variables, including social class, educational level, length of time in this country, and individual experiences. The best approach is to use the information presented here as a beginning point for exploring whether these beliefs are held by a specific individual rather than a basis for stereotypical assumptions that these beliefs are shared by all members of a particular ethnic group. The generalizations presented in this chapter focus on traditional beliefs and practices that, although held in varying degrees within a population, can still be useful guidelines for understanding underlying attitudes and behaviors.

In addition, the perspective suggested in this chapter may be applied to members of other ethnic groups not covered specifically. The key point is that laypeople, regardless of their ethnic backgrounds, are likely to have perspectives that differ greatly from those of biomedically trained health care workers. Effective care will depend on the ability of the practitioner to learn about the patients' perspectives on their illness and treatment. Issues that must be addressed include these (Kleinman, Eisenberg, & Good, 1978):

- What do you think your problem is?
- What do you think caused your illness?
- Why do you think it started when it did?
- What does your illness do to you?
- How long do you think it will last?
- How have you treated it so far?
- What other kind of treatment would you like to have?
- What are the most important results you would like to get from the treatment?
- What are the main problems your illness has caused you?
- What do you fear most about your illness?

Finally, it is critically important to remember that beliefs of the type discussed in this chapter are extremely difficult to change. Those working in rural health care with patients of different ethnic backgrounds will find that the most successful approach is to adapt biomedical explanations to the worldview of the patient.

References

Algert, S. J., & Ellison, T. H., (1989). *Mexican American food practices, customs, and holidays.* American Dietetic Association and American Diabetes Association.

Bade, B. L. (1994). *Sweatbaths, sacrifice and surgery: The practice of transmedical health care by Mixtec migrant families in California.* Unpublished doctoral dissertation, University of California, Riverside, CA.

Baer, R. D. (1996). Health and Mental Health among Mexican American Immigrants: Implications for Survey Research. *Human Organization, 55*(1), 58–66.

Baer, R. D., Alfonso, M., Cuenca, K. J., Gilbertson, T., Kealy, E., & Lehmann, H. (1997). Dietary change in participants in the St. Joseph's Home Visitor Program: Some suggestions on approaches. (A report to the Home Visitor Program,) Tampa, FL: St. Joseph's Hospital.

Baer, R. D., & Bustillo, M. (1998). Caida de mollera among children of Mexican Migrants: Implications for the study of folk illnesses. *Medical Anthropology Quarterly, 12*(2), 241–249.

Bibb, A., & Casimir, G. J. (1996). Haitian families. In M. McGoldrick, J. Giordano, & J. K. Pearce (Eds.), *Ethnicity and family therapy* (2nd ed.) (pp. 97–111). New York: Guilford Press.

Bloch, B. (1983). Nursing care of black patients. In M. Orgue *et al.* (Eds.), *Ethnic nursing care* (pp. 81–113) St Louis: C.V. Mosby.

Burke, C. B., & Raia, S. P. (1995). *Soul and traditional southern food practices, customs, and holidays.* Diabetes Care and Education, Dietetic Practice Group of the American Dietetic Association.

Burns, A. F. (1993). *Maya in exile: Guatemalans in Florida.* Philadelphia: Temple University Press.

Civan, M. B. (1994). *The Haitians: Their history and culture.* Washington, DC: The Refugee Service Center, Center for Applied Linguistics.

Cobb, J. C. (1984). *Industrialization and Southern society 1877–1984.* Chicago: Dorsey Press.

Cosminsky, S. (1975). Changing food and medical beliefs and practices in a Guatemalan community. *Ecology of Food and Nutrition, 4,* 183–191.

de Paula, T., Lagana, K., & Gonzalez-Ramirez, L. (1995). Mexican Americans. In J. G. Lipson, S. L. Dibble, & P. A. Minarik (Eds.), *Culture and nursing care: A pocket guide.* San Francisco: UCSF Nursing Press.

Dressler, W. W. (1991). *Stress and adaptation in the context of culture: Depression in a Southern black community.* Albany, NY: State University of New York Press.

Flynt, J. W. (1979). *Dixie's forgotten people: The South's poor whites.* Bloomington and London: Indiana University Press.

Frank, M. S. (1990). Southern Black (soul food) food traditions. In L. S. Lieberman & L. B. Bobroff (Eds.), *Cultural food patterns of Florida* (pp. 25–31). Gainesville, FL: Cooperative Extension Service, University of Florida.

Freedman, T. (1998). Why don't they come to Pike Street and ask us: Black American women's health concerns. *Social Science and Medicine, 47*(7), 941–947.

Giordano, J., & McGoldrick, M. (1996). European families: An overview. In M. McGoldrick, J. Giordano, & J. K. Pearce (Eds.), *Ethnicity and family therapy* (2nd ed.) (pp. 427–441). New York: Guilford Press.

Grieshop, J. (1997). Transnational and transformational: Mixtec immigration and health beliefs. *Human organization, 56*(4), 400–407.

Griffin, F. N. U. (1994). Perceptions of African American women regarding health care. *Journal of Cultural Diversity, 1*(2), 32–35.

Hall, A. L., & Bourne, P. G. (1973). Indigenous therapists in a Southern black urban community. *Archives of General Psychiatry, 28,* 137–142.

Hollingsworth, J. (1994, November). I have a right to my baby. *Tampa Tribune,* pp. 1–2.

Kearney, M., & Nagengast, C. (1989). *Anthropological perspectives on transnational communities in rural California* (Working paper no. 3). Davis: California Institute for Rural Studies, Working Group on Farm Labor and Rural Poverty.

Kleinman, A., Eisenberg, L., & Good, B. (1978). Culture, illness, and care: Clinical lessons from anthropological and cross-cultural research. *Annals of Internal Medicine, 88,* 251–258.

Laguerre, M. (1981). Haitian Americans. In A. Harwood (Ed.), *Ethnicity and medical care* (pp. 172–210). Harvard University Press. Cambridge.

Lassiter, S. M. (1998). *Cultures of color in America: A guide to family, religion, and health.* Westport, CT: Greenwood Press.

Mata, L. (1995). The Santa Maria cauque study: Health and survival of Mayan Indians under deprivation, Guatemala. In N. S. Scrimshaw (Ed.), *Community-based longitudinal nutrition and health studies: Classical examples from Guatemala, Haiti, and Mexico* (pp. 29–78). Boston: International Foundation for Developing Countries.

McGill, D., & Pearce, J. (1982). British families. In M. McGoldrick & J. Pearce (Eds.), *Ethnicity and family therapy* (1st ed.) (pp. 457–479). New York: Guilford Press.

McVea, K. L. S. P. (1997). Lay injection practices among migrant farmworkers in the age of AIDS: Evolution of a biomedical folk practice. *Social Science and Medicine, 45*(1), 91–98.

Miralles, M. A. (1989). *A matter of life and death: Health-seeking behavior of Guatemalan refugees in South Florida.* New York: AMS Press.

Mydans, S. (1995, August 24). A new wave of immigrants on farming's lowest rung. *New York Times,* p. A1.

Nagengast, C., & Kearney, M. (1990). Mixtec ethnicity: Social identity, political consciousness, and political activism. *Latin American Research Review, 25*(2), 61–91.

Randell-David, E. W. (1985). *Mama always said: The transmission of health care beliefs among three generations of rural black women.* (Unpublished doctoral dissertation, University of Florida), Gainsville, FL.

Runsten, D., & Kearney, M. (1994). *A survey of Oaxacan village networks in California agriculture.* Davis: California Institute of Rural Studies.

Schoenberg, N. E. (1994). *Dietary adherence among rural African-American elders with hypertension: An ethnographic approach.* Unpublished doctoral dissertation, University of Florida, Gainsville, FL.

Schreiber, J., & Homiak, J. (1981). Mexican Americans. In A. Harwood (Ed.), *Ethnicity and medical care* (pp. 264–336). Cambridge: Harvard University Press.

Scott, A. F. (1970). *The Southern lady: From pedestal to politics 1830–1930.* Chicago: University of Chicago Press.

Snow, L. F. (1993). *Walkin' over medicine.* San Francisco: Westview Press.

Sproles, J. A. (1990). Haitian food traditions. In L. S. Lieberman & L. B. Bobroff (Eds.), *Cultural food patterns of Florida: A handbook* (pp. 86–89). Gainesville: Florida Cooperative Extension Service.

Stans, S. E. (1990). Florida cracker food tradition. In L. S. Lieberman & L. B. Bobroff (Eds.), *Cultural food patterns of Florida: A handbook* (pp. 19–24). Gainesville: Florida Cooperative Extension Service.

Stephen, L. (1996). The creation and re-creation of ethnicity: Lessons from the Zapotec and Mixtec of Oaxaca. *Latin American Perspectives, 23*(2),17–37.

Stepick, A., & Portes, A. (1986). Flight into despair: A profile of recent Haitian refugees in South Florida. *International Migration Review, 20*(2), 329–350.

Tedlock, B. (1982). *Time and the highland Maya.* Albuquerque: NM: University of New Mexico Press.

Trotter, R. (1985). Greta and Azarcon. *Human Organization, 44*(1), 64–72.

Vlach, N. (1992). *The Quetzal in flight: Guatemalan refugee families in the United States.* Westport, CT: Praeger.

Weidman, H. & Egeland, J. (1978). *Miami health ecology project: A statement on ethnicity and health.* Miami: University of Miami Press.

Zabin, C. (1995). Mixtecs and Mestizos in California agriculture: Ethnic displacement and hierarchy among Mexican farm workers. In M. P. Smith (Ed.), *Marginal spaces* (pp. 113–143). New Brunswick, NJ: Transaction Publishers.

Zabin, C., Kearney, M., Garcia, A., Runsten, D., & Nagengast, C. (1993). *A new cycle of poverty: Mixtec migrants in California agriculture.* Davis: California Institute for Rural Studies.

6

The Health of Migrant and Seasonal Farmworkers

BRUCE W. GOLDBERG AND MARIE NAPOLITANO

Introduction

The agricultural industry is among the most vital and strategic industries in the United States. Net farm income in 1998 was estimated at $48 billion and agriculture remains at the economic and cultural foundation of most rural communities (U.S. Department of Agriculture, 1999). It is a critical component of the U.S. economy and helps support and sustain the American lifestyle. Our highly productive system for growing, processing, and distributing agricultural products allows Americans to enjoy a consistent supply of fruits and vegetables that are readily available in our grocery stores and markets. The foundation of the agricultural industry and of many rural communities is the farmworker.

The U.S. agricultural industry employs an estimated 2.5 million farmworkers (U.S. Commission on Agricultural Workers, 1993). The majority of them are either migrant or seasonal. Migrant and seasonal farmworkers perform physically demanding and hazardous work, experience poor living conditions, and have inad-

equate access to medical and social services. Most migrant and seasonal farmworkers are immigrants, and they endure racial discrimination, disruption of cultural traditions and practices, language barriers, and an often unpredictable and stressful lifestyle. Consequently, the frequency and intensity of health problems they experience is greater than the general population.

Estimates of the numbers of migrant and seasonal farmworkers in the United States vary from 1 to 5 million. This disparity is due to differences in definitions, divergent methodologies for estimating the numbers of migrant workers, and whether or not dependents are included. There is no uniform definition of migrant and seasonal farmworkers. The Office of Migrant Health defines migrant farmworkers as those individuals "whose principal employment is in agriculture on a seasonal basis, who has been so employed within the last 24 months, and who establishes for the purpose of such employment a temporary abode" (U.S. Department of Health and Human Services, 1980). Seasonal farmworkers are those who perform seasonal work but do not migrate.

Comprehensive and accurate data on migrant and seasonal farmworkers are lacking. Some data are available on the health, demographics, and socioeconomic status of agricultural workers as a whole. However, it is often difficult to distinguish migrant and seasonal workers from the aggregate. Migrant and seasonal farm-

BRUCE W. GOLDBERG • Department of Family Medicine, Oregon Health Sciences University School of Medicine, Portland, Oregon 97201. MARIE NAPOLITANO • Department of Primary Care, Oregon Health Sciences University School of Nursing, Portland, Oregon 97201.

Handbook of Rural Health, edited by Loue and Quill. Kluwer Academic/Plenum Publishers, New York, 2001.

workers make up two distinct populations, though there are many demographic and occupational similarities among the two groups. Thus, much of the data on these two groups are obtained and reported as an aggregate. When reliable distinctions between groups can be made we will do so, otherwise the term *migrant farmworker* can henceforth be assumed to refer to both migrant and seasonal farmworkers in the aggregate.

The Migrant Farmworker Population

The Office of Migrant Health estimates that there are 3 million migrant and seasonal farmworkers and dependents in the United States (Wilk, 1988). California, with 23%, has the largest share of migrant farmworkers, and Texas is second with 12%. Sixty-eight percent of migrant farmworkers are employed in eight states (in descending order: California, Texas, Florida, Washington, Michigan, Oregon, North Carolina, and Georgia) (Larson & Plascencia, 1993).

The migrant farm labor force in the United States is generally made up of immigrants from Latin American countries (Mines, Gabbard, & Samardick, 1993). Seventy-three percent of all migrant farmworkers are male and 55% were born in Mexico. This is a relatively young population, with a median age of 31 years. Seventy percent of the total migrant workforce is Hispanic. Foreign-born workers make up 60% of the migrant workforce, and this group is almost exclusively (96%) from Latin American countries.

Most foreign-born workers are legally authorized to work in the United States; however, a significant number of migrant farmworkers are unauthorized (Mines, Gabbard, & Boccalandro, 1991). Among all farmworkers, the proportion of unauthorized workers rose considerably between 1988 and 1995, and it is estimated that now as many as 37% of all of them have no work authorization (U.S. Department of Labor, 1997). Legal issues surrounding work status and immigration are extremely sensitive to many migrant workers. Many workers, both authorized and unauthorized, live in fear of immigration and legal authorities. Therefore, the validity of data on numbers of unauthorized workers remains questionable.

Poverty and low education are significant issues among migrant farmworkers. Sixty percent of all farmworker households and more than three-quarters (77%) of undocumented farmworkers live below the poverty threshold (Mines *et al.*, 1993; U.S. Department of Labor, 1997). Yet, despite the high poverty levels, only 20% get need-based social services such as food stamps. Fifty-three percent of migrant workers have less than eight years of formal school-based education. Spanish is the primary language for nearly two-thirds of all migrant farmworkers, and only 40% speak or read English well. Most migrants are married, and 57% reside with their families at their work site.

True migratory farmworkers make up approximately 40% of the farm labor workforce. These migratory workers are primarily employed as harvesters and are usually newer immigrants. About two-thirds of these migratory workers come to the United States from a home base in Mexico, follow crops for a period of time, and then return home. The other one-third remain in the United States, following crops from one location to another (Mines *et al.*, 1993).

Migrant farmworkers historically were thought to confine themselves to three "streams," or geographic areas of employment. The home state was usually south of the eventual work destinations and referred to as "downstream," while the work states were "upstream." The East Coast stream originated from a home base in Florida and extended up the East Coast of the United States to the northern Atlantic states. The midwestern stream originated in Texas and extended throughout the Plains states, midwestern states, and parts of the Rocky Mountain states. The western stream originated in California and Arizona and extended northward to Washington through the agricultural areas west of the Rockies (Meister, 1991). Migrants in the Northwest, Southwest, and Northeast generally work with fruit and nut crops, and those in the Middle West and western Plains states work field crops. The Southeast is predominated by vegetable crops and has the highest percentage of hand-harvesting work in the country. However, as workers increasingly travel throughout the country seeking employment, these "streams" are becoming less distinct.

Recent information points to a more complex and variegated pattern of movement. Three types of migration patterns have been defined: restricted, point to point, and nomadic (Migrant Clinicians Network, 1997). Farmworkers traveling in restricted circuits will travel throughout a season in a relatively small geographic area—for example, chili harvesting in west Texas and southern New Mexico. Those traveling in a point-to-point pattern will travel to the same place or series of places along a route during the course of a season. These people tend to live in home-base areas in southern states, Mexico, or Puerto Rico, and travel for part of the year working in agriculture. Their routes often resemble the previously described streams. Finally, the nomadic farmworkers travel away from home for a period of years, working from farm to farm and crop to crop. Some of these workers may eventually settle in an area, whereas others eventually return to their home base.

There is increasing evidence that over time the immigrant farm labor workforces move away from migratory patterns and tend to settle permanently. This process begins with predominately immigrant workers performing the most difficult and least skilled tasks, such as harvesting. As these unskilled laborers repeatedly work in areas, some eventually become rooted and begin to settle down. Concomitant with this is a tendency for these workers to graduate into more desirable and higher-paying semi-skilled jobs, such as irrigating, pruning, and spraying. Although this pattern is more widespread in the western United States, evidence suggests that it is occurring in increasing numbers in the East (Mines *et al.*, 1993).

Living Conditions

Fifty-six percent of all U.S. male farmworkers live away from their families in housing that they share with unrelated adults. Most occupy labor camps or live jointly with large numbers people in small houses and apartments. Overall, 20% of farmworkers live in housing provided by the employer and about 25% live on the farm where they work (U.S. Department of Labor, 1997).

Among migrant farmworkers, availability of housing is often less than adequate. During migration, they may live in employer-provided housing, private camps, state camps (California), rental apartments, or rental hotel rooms. However, housing is often not available. Data from California, Oregon, and Washington show that private camps, employer-provided housing, and California's state-run camps provide less than 30% of the needed migrant worker housing capacity in those three states (U.S. General Accounting Office, 1992). Employer-provided housing is decreasing as many aging camps are being demolished and not replaced and growers are closing camps rather than pay fines for violations. A survey done by the Community and Shelter Assistance Corporation (CASA) of Oregon in 1990 indicated that the vast majority of farmworkers and their families do not live in labor camps but rather in rental housing under crowded and substandard conditions (Pallack, 1991). Migrant farmworkers face considerable obstacles when attempting to rent housing, such as excessive rent, substantial deposit amounts, long-term leases, lack of credit, discrimination, and a sparse rural rental market (Lopez, 1995). When housing is not available or the obstacles become too great, migrant farmworkers and their families may end up living in their cars.

Inadequate funds are available for construction of sufficient farmworker housing (Lopez, 1995). In a national effort to solve this problem, the Rural Housing and Community Development Service Section 514/516 programs provide loans to growers and loans and grants to nonprofit sponsors of farmworker housing. However, federal funds for farmworker housing have been cut (U.S. General Accounting Office, 1992). Most states and local governments have not addressed this problem. A few exceptions, however, do exist. The state of Oregon grants growers a tax credit to provide housing for farmworkers, and California operates state housing centers. California, Florida, Ohio, Oregon, and Virginia have migrant farmworker housing programs that offer assistance to groups that construct or rehabilitate migrant farmworker housing (U.S. General Accounting Office, 1992). Nonprofit organizations have attempted to fill the void. For example, the Delmarva Rural Program has developed over 30 units of housing in Delaware and Maryland (Lopez, 1995).

In Oregon, the Housing Development Corporation has been building quality migrant farmworker housing for over 13 years in Washington County (approximately 91 units have been contructed to date).

Migrant farmworkers may live in substandard housing such as shacks and barns or in overcrowded bungalows, trailers, dormitories, apartments, or hotel rooms (U.S. General Accounting Office, 1992). They may lack electricity, plumbing, heating or cooling, adequate ventilation, more than one exit, screens over windows, and laundry and recreational facilities. Yet reports state that farmworker housing has improved to some extent (Pallack, 1991; National Advisory Council on Migrant Health, 1995). A survey done by CASA of Oregon in 1990 found that the majority of employer-provided housing was in good physical condition (Pallack, 1991).

The Health of Migrant Farmworkers

The literature suggests that the health of migrant farmworkers is poor and that they have a number of special health concerns. (Goldsmith, 1989; Dever, 1991; National Advisory Council on Migrant Health, 1995; Villarejo & Baron, 1999). However, the available epidemiologic data needed to build a clear picture of their health status are less than adequate. First, as already noted, precise migrant population data are missing and inaccuracies (e.g., the use of different definitions for migrant farmworkers) exist in the data that are available (Rust, 1990). Lack of accurate population data results in inaccurate numbers being used as denominators in morbidity and mortality calculations. Second, comprehensive health data are missing. A national farmworker health data reporting system does not exist nor do population health surveys identify migrant farmworkers in most cases (Slesinger, 1992). And third, the interaction of migration with income, educational level, physical-cultural-social factors, genetic makeup, and past life history and the resultant impact on the health of migrant farmworkers has not been examined. The very nature of the migrant lifestyle contributes to the difficulties in filling in these gaps and results in an uncertain picture of the health status of the population.

The few insights from the literature into the health status of migrant farmworkers come from studies based on migrant health clinic records or convenience samples of small segments of the population. There is uncertainty about just how representative of the entire migrant population these data are. Records from migrant health clinics reveal dermatitis, injuries, respiratory problems, musculoskeletal problems, eye problems, gastrointestinal problems, and diabetes as the most frequently reported health problems (Slesinger, 1992). The majority of clinic encounters tend to be for acute illness rather than chronic illness or preventive care (Wilk, 1986). One larger study by the Migrant Clinicians Network (Dever, 1991) sampled utilization data from four migrant health centers in Texas, Michigan, and Indiana and from community health data collected from two control group counties. This study concluded that migrant farmworkers have more multiple and complex health problems, suffer more frequently from infectious diseases, and they have more clinic visits for otitis media, pregnancy, hypertension, contact dermatitis, eczema, and medical supervision of children. Chronic diseases such as diabetes and hypertension accounted for more visits as age increased.

Occupational and Environmental Health Problems

Farm work exposes the migrant worker to numerous occupational and environmental hazards, many of which have been poorly quantified (Rust, 1990). Occupational and environmental risks are virtually inseparable for the majority of migrant farmworkers. Although hazards may be job-specific (field worker, farm machinery handler, nursery worker, cannery worker), overall this population faces many of the same occupational and environmental risk categories, such as injuries, crowded living conditions, pesticide exposure, lack of field sanitation, and unfavorable climate conditions.

Occupational health risks can and do result in numerous medical problems. A national advisory group organized by the National Institute for Occupational Safety and Health (NIOSH) in 1995 rank-ordered a listing of health problems common to farmworkers (National

TABLE 1. Health Problems Common to Farmworkers.

Common Health Problems	Published Studies
Musculoskeletal	Slesinger & Cautley, 1981; Mines & Kearney, 1982; Wilk, 1986; Estill & Tanaka, 1998; Mobed, 1992.
Pesticide-related	Sharp et al., 1986; Hays & Laws, 1991; Moses et al., 1993; Ciesielski et al., 1994a; Karr et al., 1992; Steenland et al., 1994; Abrams, Hogg & Maibach, 1991.
Traumatic injuries	Ciesielksi, 1991; McDermott & Lee, 1990; Myers, 1997.
Respiratory	Gamsky et al., 1992a; Gamsky, 1992b, Garcia, Dresser, & Zerr, 1996, Schenker, Ferguson. & Gamsky, 1991.
Dermatologic	Schuman & Dobson 1985; O'Malley et al., 1990; Gamsky et al., 1992c; Abrams, et al., 1991.
Infectious disease	Ungar et al., 1986; Kligman et al., 1991; Ciesielski et al., 1992; Ciesielski et al., 1994b; Jacobson et al., 1987; Villarino et al., 1994.
Cancer	Moses, 1989; Zahm & Blair, 1993; Zahm, Ward, & Blair, 1997.
Eye conditions	Myers, 1997; Wilk, 1988.
Mental health	Vega, Warheit, & Palacio, 1985; De Leon Siantz, 1994; De Leon Siantz, 1990; Wiggins & Castanares, 1994.
Disorders of reproduction	De La Torre & Rush, 1989; Whorton et al., 1979; Schwartz & LoGerfo, 1988; Wilk, 1986.
Noise-induced hearing loss	Crutchfield & Sparks, 1991; Bernhardt & Langley, 1993.

Institute for Occupational Safety and Health, 1995). This list in combination with the NIOSH list of leading work-related diseases and injuries (Millar, 1991) for all agricultural workers serves as a worthwhile inventory of the occupational health problems that migrant farmworkers may experience. Although studies exist for migrant farmworkers in each of these categories, they are sporadic and do not present a clear and comprehensive picture of the scope of the health problems encountered by this population in each category. Table 1 presents the list and notes the studies published in each category.

Other health problems secondary to environmental risks include allergic reactions, drowning in ditches, respiratory problems due to exposure to cold and wet weather conditions (National Advisory Council on Migrant Health, 1995), urinary tract infections due to lack of sanitation facilities (Wilk, 1986; Bechtel, Shepherd, & Rogers, 1995), and lower-extremity infections and cellulitis due to inadequate foot protection. Although all occupational and environmental hazards can pose major health threats for the migrant farmworker, the seriousness and presumed prevalence of injuries and pesticide exposures warrant particular attention.

Injuries

Agriculture is consistently rated as one of three most hazardous occupations (Rust, 1990; Schenker, Lopez, & Wintemute, 1995). Injuries are reported as the leading cause of mortality and morbidity among agricultural workers (Wilk, 1986; U.S. Department of Labor, 1988). However, despite their frequency, a comprehensive surveillance system for injuries does not exist and many of the data sources used to compile statistics on agricultural injuries have limitations (Gerberich et al., 1992). For example, workmen's compensation data that are used to compile injury statistics are inconsistent or lacking for agriculture because of exemptions, exclusions, and loopholes in state laws (Mobed, Gold, & Schenker, 1992). Data are also lacking on the nature and consequences of agricultural injuries (Mobed et al., 1992). Therefore, an accurate understanding of the scope and features of injuries for all agricultural workers is currently not possible.

Information on injuries suffered by migrant farmworkers are also limited by reporting inadequacies. For example, federal law exempts farms with fewer than 10 workers from reporting injuries. Yet these account for many of the farms hiring migrant farmworkers. Also, no category exists for migrant farmworkers on farm injury reports; therefore, injury data tend to combine farmers and all types of farmworkers. Still, a broad range of injuries have been identified as significant for migrant farmworkers. These include fractures or sprains from falls from ladders or equipment; sprains or strains from prolonged stooping, heavy lifting, and carrying; amputations, deaths, and crush injuries from tractors, trucks, or other machinery; pesticide poisoning; electrical injuries; carbon monoxide poisoning from running equipment in enclosed areas; and drowning in irrigation ditches (Mines & Kearney, 1982; Ciesielski, Hall, & Sweeney, 1991). The few studies that exist on migrant farmworkers' injuries support this broad range of injury types. One study in California reported injuries from machinery, falling stacks of containers, heavy loads, and falls from ladders (Mines & Kearney, 1982). Another study in North Carolina also reported numerous injuries from machinery (Ciesielski, Hall, & Sweeney, 1991).

Pesticide Exposure

Pesticides are used extensively in agriculture. The Environmental Protection Agency (EPA) estimated that 817 million pounds of pesticides were used for agricultural purposes in 1991 (U.S. Environmental Protection Agency, 1992). Although toxicity data are not complete on all pesticides, many are known to be toxic to humans, causing a wide range of adverse health effects.

The number of migrant farmworkers affected by pesticides and other chemicals, the level of their exposure, and the health consequences are not known. The EPA has estimated that 300,000 migrant farmworkers suffer acute illnesses annually as a result of pesticide exposure (Wilk, 1986). Our poor understanding of this problem is the result of multiple deficiencies. For example, states may lack mandatory reporting; local, state, and federal agencies may not have sufficient resources for identifying violations of required reporting; migrant farmworkers may not seek medical care for known exposures; health professionals may not recognize signs

and symptoms of exposures; and health problems secondary to pesticide exposure may not present for an extended period of time.

The working and living environment of the migrant farmworker offers numerous occasions for pesticide exposure. Mobed *et al.* (1992) categorized them as avoidable (e.g., diluting and mixing pesticides, applying pesticides, being sprayed), unavoidable (drifts, contact with residues), and unknown (use of contaminated water, eating contaminated fruits and vegetables). Pesticides are readily absorbed through the skin and the respiratory and gastrointestinal tracts. The main route for occupational exposures is the skin (Spear, 1991) and there may be greater absorption by migrant farmworkers due to lack of washing facilities (Slesinger & Ofstead, 1990; Zahm & Blair, 1993).

The migrant farmworker's dwelling can be a major source of contamination. Migrant farmworker housing may be located adjacent to fields that have been contaminated with pesticides (Soliman, Derosa, Mielke, & Bota, 1993) and may be exposed to drifts of pesticides during and following their application. Housing may be located where posted signs about pesticide applications cannot be seen by the migrant farmworker and his family. Field-adjacent housing and other housing used by migrant farmworkers may have been sprayed with pesticides to control rodents and roaches. It can also be contaminated by the farmworkers themselves, inadvertently carrying pesticides home from work on their clothes, skin, hair, tools, and vehicles. One study found organophosphate compounds in 62% of household dust samples tested in homes of farmers and migrant farmworker families living within 200 feet of an orchard (Simcox, Fenske, Wolz, Lee, & Kalman, 1995). According to McCauley (1996), pesticides may persist in dwellings longer than in outdoor environments because of the lack of degradative environmental processes such as sun, rain, and microbial activity.

Organophosphate anticholinesterase pesticides are the largest group in current use (Kaloyanova & Batawi, 1991; Lotti, 1992). Acute neurological illness has been shown to be caused by overexposure to these pesticides and other organophosphates and carbamates (Sharp, Eskenazi, Harrison, Callas, & Smith,

1986; Hays & Laws, 1991). Organophosphates and carbamates work by inhibiting the activity of cholinesterase, an enzyme essential for normal neuromuscular functioning. As exposure to these pesticides increases, cholinesterase activity as measured by blood cholinesterase level decreases (McCauley, 1996). Migrant farmworkers and their children who were exposed to pesticides have been found to have lower levels of cholinesterase (Richter, 1992; Ciesielski, Loomis, Mims, & Auer, 1994).

Mild psychological and behavioral deficits such as changes in the speed and precision of answering questions, impaired judgmnt, poor comprehension, and decreased ability to communicate reportedly occur after exposure to anticholinesterase pesticides and can persist for weeks and months (Sidell, 1992). Other acute health manifestations of pesticide exposure include abdominal pain, ataxia, nausea, diarrhea, dizziness, vomiting, headache, malaise, skin rashes, and eye irritation (Wilk, 1986; Moses, 1989). Acute severe pesticide poisoning can result in death (Moses, 1989).

The long-term health effects of acute and low-dose, long-term pesticide exposure are unclear. Because of the exposure risks migrant farmworkers confront, long-term and chronic health problems are a major concern for this population (Sharp et al., 1986; Schenker & McCurdy, 1988; Mobed et al., 1992). However, studying long-term effects in the migrant population poses numerous methodological challenges, such as long-term follow-up and controlling for confounding factors.

Associations have been made between long-term exposure and several types of cancer, neurotoxic effects, and reproductive problems (Sharp et al., 1986; Moses, 1989; Blair & Zahm, 1991). Most epidemiologic studies on carcinogenicity and pesticides have focused on farm owners and farm machinery operators. Studies of farmers consistently have shown increased risk for cancers including leukemia, non-Hodgkin's lymphoma, Hodgkin's disease, multiple myeloma, and cancer of the stomach, prostate, and testis (Zahm & Blair, 1993). The few studies and case reports that exist for migrant farmworkers have similar findings as those for farmers; however, they also have shown excesses for cancers of the buccal cavity, pharynx, lung,

and liver (Moses, 1989; Zahm & Blair, 1993).

Polyneuropathy and neurobehavioral effects are two additional chronic or delayed effects from acute high-dose or chronic low-dose pesticide exposure (Sharp et al., 1986). Findings of the long-term effects from exposure to pesticides on human reproduction are inconsistent except for the relationship between male infertility and dibromochloropropane, which is banned in the United States (Whorton, Milby, Krauss, & Stubbs, 1979; Sharp et al., 1986). Spontaneous abortions, premature births, pregnancy complications, fetal malformation or growth retardation, cancer among offspring, and abnormal development of infants exposed to chemicals through breast milk were cited by Wilk (1986) as potential problems.

Other health problems attributed to chronic pesticide exposure include limb-reduction birth defects (Schwartz & LoGerfo, 1988), and chronic dermatitis, fatigue, headache, sleep disturbances, anxiety, blood disorders, and abnormal liver and kidney function (Wilk, 1986; Moses, 1989).

Other Significant Health Problems Facing the Migrant Population

The number of migrant farmworkers who are HIV-seropositive is higher than in the general population and appears to be increasing (Jones, 1992; Lyons, 1992; Centers for Disease Control, 1992). Included in these numbers are women farmworkers who have been infected through heterosexual contact (Skjerdal, Misha, & Benavides-Vaillo, 1996). The vulnerability of this population stems from a high number of risk factors such as substance abuse (National Migrant Resource Program, 1993; Skjerdal et al., 1996), lack of health education opportunities, and physical and social isolation. Certain cultural factors also contribute to the HIV disease picture for migrant farmworkers. These include the prohibitive use of condoms (Ryan, Foulk, Lafferty, & Robertson, 1988), the multiple-person use of syringes for medications to treat different illnesses ("Be Aware," 1987; Lafferty, 1991), and the use of folk medicine, which can delay diagnosis of AIDS ("Be Aware," 1987). Some of the sexual practices of migrant workers also put them at risk for HIV. A practice known as "becoming milk brothers" has been described in a group of migrant workers and heroin-addicted prostitutes in California (Magana, 1991). This involves several men having sexual intercourse with a single woman in rapid succession. Studies have also found a lack of knowledge about HIV and its transmission among migrant farmworkers (Ryan *et al.*, 1988; Bletzer, 1995; Vasilion, 1992; Skjerdal *et al.*, 1996).

Migrant farmworkers have higher rates of tuberculosis infection than the general population (Centers for Disease Control, 1992). The prevalence of tuberculin reactivity among migrant farmworkers ranges from 23 to 44 % (Wingo et al., 1986; Jacobson, Mercer, Miller, & Simpson, 1987; Ciesielski, Seed, Esposito, & Hunter, 1991). Migratory lifestyle complicates the treatment of active tuberculosis because it requires long-term follow-up, contact screening, and consistent and reliable access to care.

Although diabetes and hypertension are cited as prevalent reasons for clinic encounters, a paucity of information exists on these diagnoses in this population. Predominantly Latino, farmworkers are particularly vulnerable to diabetes and its complications (Council on Scientific Affairs, 1991). Nutritional status, domestic violence, substance abuse, and mental health are also cited as significant health concerns for the migrant farmworker population, yet little information is available. In addition, the health needs of migrant farmworkers from their perspective have not been identified. With regard to perceived health status, Slesinger and Ofstead (1993) reported that one-third (33.6%) of migrant farmworkers surveyed in Wisconsin felt that their health was fair or poor compared with 9.4% of the U.S. population. Only 13.3% of these migrant workers rated their health as excellent, compared with 40.2% of the U.S. population.

Children of Migrant Farmworkers

Children of migrant farmworkers warrant special consideration. They are subject to educational disadvantages and health risks (U.S. General Accounting Office, 1992). The social and emotional impact of migration can bring about unfortunate consequences. Changing schools, especially for short periods of time, and leaving extended family and friends can result in stress and have effects on learning and personality development (De Leon Siantz, 1994; Eshleman & Davidhizar, 1997; Gwyther & Jenkins, 1998). Children who themselves do not migrate are also subject to social disruption. Thirty-eight percent of farmworker parents who have children age 14 and under report that they live apart from them (U.S. Department of Labor, 1997)

The children of farmworkers often live in crowded and unsanitary housing near agricultural fields. They are at risk for pesticide exposure and injury from farm equipment. Poor nutrition, infectious diseases, and lack of up-to-date immunizations are frequently noted among these children (Koch, 1988; Lee, McDermott, & Elliott, 1990; Michael & Salend, 1985). Dental decay, including baby bottle tooth decay, is also a prevalent problem (Koday, Rosenstein, & Lopez, 1990; Woolfolk, Hamard, Bagramian, & Sgan-Cohen, 1984; Call, Entwistle, & Swanson, 1987; Weinstein, Domoto, Wohlers, & Koday, 1992). Lack of dental insurance and the high cost of dental care are mainly responsible for the low incidence of dental care among migrant farmworkers and their children.

Access to Health Care

As previously documented, measures of the health status of migrant farmworkers lag behind those of the rest of the population. Although this can be attributed in part to underlying social and occupational conditions, it is also evident that migrant farmworkers have limited access to medical care. The Migrant Health Act, signed into law in 1962, was established to improve the delivery of primary and supplemental health care services to migrant and seasonal farmworkers in the United States. Funded under Section 329 of the Public Health Service and administered by the Bureau of Primary Health Care, the program currently funds over 100 organizations in 41 states and provides services at more than 400 clinic sites. Yet the program is able to serve less than 20% of the migrant farmworker and dependent population (National Advisory Council on Migrant Health, 1995).

Inability to afford care is among the leading impediments to access to health care. Over half of migrant farmworkers' medical bills are paid by federal migrant health funds, 17% by Medicaid, and approximately 14% by out-of-pocket expenditures (Slesinger & Ofstead, 1993). The Medicaid program was established to assist the poorest Americans gain access to medical care, and indeed most migrant farmworkers fit the profile of the population Medicaid was designed to help. Yet, they appear to have more difficulty accessing Medicaid benefits than any other population in the country (National Advisory Council on Migrant Health, 1995). Although the reasons for this are complex, a great deal is related to a disparity between the organizational structure of the Medicaid program and the farmworker lifestyle.

Although Medicaid is a federal program, it is administered by individual states. Farmworkers must apply within the state in which they reside and there is no transfer of benefits between states. States are allowed up to 45 days to process applications and, depending on the state, eligibility must be revalidated every one to six months. Therefore, migrant farmworkers have often moved on to the next state before eligibility can be established. In addition, the seasonal nature of farm work brings about widely fluctuating monthly incomes, so that during some of the productive months income may actually exclude workers and their families from benefits. Finally, even if farmworkers have Medicaid coverage, they often have difficulty finding providers who will treat them.

Helping people overcome financial barriers to medical care has been a central issue in U.S. health care policy for the past 30 years. However, there is a growing understanding that even if financial access to care is guaranteed, a number of nonfinancial barriers impede access. Unfortunately, few studies have developed models that predict the extent to which these nonfinancial barriers affect access to primary health care (Cary et al., 1995).

Among the most frequently cited nonfinancial barriers to care are language, transportation, culture, mobility, and occupational factors.

Farmworkers often labor far longer than the traditional eight-hour workday, leaving no time to get medical care. In addition, the seasonal nature of agricultural work means that they make every effort to maximize their income whenever work is available. Farmworkers are thus reluctant to take time off to obtain medical care; as any interruption to the workday results in decreased income and, furthermore, may cause employers or crew chiefs to view them as "lazy."

Transportation and geography affect farmworkers' ability to access health care as well. Given the rural locations of work sites, great distances must often be traveled to clinics or hospitals. Transportation is unreliable and expensive, and most migrant farmworkers do not own a vehicle (Mines et al., 1991). Furthermore, because they are so mobile farmworkers have great difficulty in obtaining continuity of care.

Most come from Latin American countries, but they come from a mixture of ethnic and cultural backgrounds. Language and cultural differences may leave farmworkers unaware that the services they need are available. Migrant health centers make every effort to minimize the barriers of language of culture yet often are unable to provide sufficient numbers of bilingual staff. Recent changes in local migrant stream demographics add to these difficulties. For example, over the past 10 years indigenous Guatemalans have become the most rapidly increasing population among the East Coast migrant stream. Of these individuals, roughly 40% speak only a local dialect. In addition, most have never heard about or know how to protect themselves from communicable diseases such as tuberculosis, HIV, and sexually transmitted diseases (East Coast Migrant Health Project, 1996).

Although bilingual and bicultural clinic staff help improve access to care, farmworkers, by the nature of their work and lifestyle, are an extremely hard-to-reach population. Many migrant health clinics have been expanding their community outreach services. Outreach programs take a variety of forms. They may provide home or work site health education, social services, transportation, or "mobile" clinics that provide agricultural field–based or "satellite" medical care. An increasing number of outreach programs employ lay or peer workers recruited from the indigenous cultures of communities that they serve. The lay health worker model is commonly used in developing countries where access to professionals is extremely difficult. In the United States lay health workers have been used increasingly to provide services to poor and medically underserved populations. Lay health worker programs in migrant farmworker communities have been successful in bridging the sociocultural gap and in providing health education and support (Meister, Warrick, Zapien, & Wood, 1992; Warrick, Wood, Meister, & Zapien, 1992).

Legislative and Regulatory Issues

Agricultural employers are exempt from a variety of federal employment and workplace regulations, and federal law treats hired farmworkers differently from employees in other industries (Villarejo & Baron, 1999). For example, the National Labor Relations Act protects the rights of employees to organize and bargain collectively; however, it specifically excludes migrant and seasonal migrant farmworkers. Some states such as California do allow employees this right. The Federal Unemployment Tax Act provides income to workers during periods of unemployment; however, migrant and seasonal migrant farmworkers are again excluded. The Workers' Compensation Law provides assistance to workers injured on the job, but only 27 states provide coverage to migrant farmworkers and only 14 of these provide migrant farmworkers coverage equal to that of other workers (McCauley, 1996).

The General Accounting Office (GAO) analyzed the extent to which selected federal laws, regulations, and programs protect the health and well-being of migrant farmworkers. The report stated that this population is not adequately protected. Therefore, their health and well-being are at risk (U.S. General Accounting Office, 1992). The GAO's five major findings were that there are: (1) inadequate protection from pesticides due to insufficient information and lack of enforcement of regulations; (2) inadequate field sanitation; (3) inadequate protection for children on farms; (4) lack of health care due to inadequate programs; and (5) lack of social se-

curity benefits due to employer underreporting and lack of information on migrant farmworkers.

The Environmental Protection Agency (EPA) regulates pesticides and their uses and maintains specific standards for protecting farmworkers exposed to agricultural pesticides. The EPA modified its standards in 1992 in order to increase protection for migrant farmworkers by preventing exposure to pesticides, mitigating exposures, and providing information to migrant farmworkers about the hazards of the pesticides. Employers must inform workers in writing about the specific pesticides being used and the dangers from exposure. They must also provide training on the prevention of exposure and the treatment of poisoning. Timely warnings must be given to workers who will be in fields treated with pesticides. A lack of enforcement and no reporting mechanism for violations contribute to a large extent to the lack of protection from pesticide exposure for migrant farmworkers. In addition, exemptions from the standards have been granted for such reasons as economic hardship for the employer (National Advisory Council on Migrant Health, 1995).

The responsibility of the Occupational Safety and Health Administration (OSHA) is to adopt and enforce specific standards to help ensure a safe and healthy workplace for all employees. With respect to pesticides at the work site, OSHA has deferred to EPA standards. However, OSHA can approve state plans for worker protection such as pesticide protection that are more stringent than federal regulations. State plans can be more effective; however, states may cite the lack of resources to enforce their plans effectively to protect farmworkers (U.S. General Accounting Office, 1992).

OSHA does require that basic field sanitation be provided to farmworkers. Farms with less than 10 workers are exempted from these regulations except for the states of Washington, Oregon, Arizona, and Alaska, which have more stringent laws. Violations of the law are numerous. A Department of Labor national survey of farmworkers in 1990 revealed that 31% worked in fields without drinking water, handwashing facilities, or toilets (U.S. General Accounting Office, 1992). Other studies have found even less access (Sweeny & Ciesielski, 1990). Limited federal resources prevent effective enforcement of the regulations (U.S. General Accounting Office, 1992).

Toward Improving the Health of Migrant Farmworkers

As this chapter shows, the health of migrant workers is as much related to housing, working conditions, and social factors as to the structure of the health care delivery system. Adequately addressing the health care needs of the migrant worker will require more than simply providing medical services. Also needed are a better understanding of migrant farmworkers' perceptions of their needs and the solutions they envision and desire; a greater scientific understanding of the health problems that affect this population and research into their root causes and potential remedies; and, finally, coordination and integration of the vast array of social, legal, medical, and employment-related services and their delivery in order to minimize barriers and promote accessibility.

Indeed, coordination, integration, and portability are the foundations around which the future health delivery system for migrant workers should be constructed. The lifestyle of migrant workers and the demands of their jobs calls for a system in which they and their families can receive the services they need and interact with the providing agencies and programs in one location. This location should serve as a centralized source of information both for the worker and for the service agencies. Reliable and consistent information would be available and a centralized database would minimize duplicative paperwork, documentation, registration, and other data collection. Funding sources could thus be consolidated and used more efficiently.

In addition to being geographically centralized, services and benefits must be portable. The ability for migrant workers and their families to transfer eligibility for state-administered programs such as Medicaid and cash assistance from one state to another is essential. Such a system would ideally allow migrant workers to receive those benefits for which they qualify seamlessly and without interruption or reapplication, regardless of where they are living or working.

To reduce the barriers to effective service brought about by differences in language, culture, and literacy, all services should be delivered in a culturally and linguistically appropriate manner. Ideally, staff should be multilingual and multicultural. Hours of operation should be designed to meet the needs of the population being served and reliable transportation should be made available.

Within the confines of health delivery system, services will need to be coordinated and consolidated. Mental, dental, and direct medical care should be provided in a centralized location and with a coordinated information and medical record system. The medical record should be accessible to all those providing health care services to migrant workers and their families. To facilitate outreach and work site or camp-based health delivery and education, a complete medical record that can easily be transferred from a health center to another locale is necessary. In addition, such records should be accessible at migrant health delivery sites in other states. The existing technology surrounding computerized medical records is sufficient to allow for such a system. However, the infrastructure and financial support for such a system still need to be established.

References

Abrams, K., Hogan, D., & Maibach, H. (1991). Pesticide related dermatoses in agricultural workers. *Occupational Medicine, 6,* 463–92.

Be aware! Common cultural practices and AIDS. (1987) *Migrant Health Newsline, 4,* 1.

Bechtel, G. A., Shepherd, M. A., & Rogers, P. W. (1995). Family, culture, and health practices among migrant farmworkers. *Journal of Community Health Nursing, 12,* 15–22.

Bernhardt, J., & Langley, L. (1993). Agricultural hazards in North Carolina. *North Carolina Medical Journal, 54,* 512–515.

Blair, A., & Zahm, S. (1991). Cancer among farmers. *Occupational Medicine State of the Art Reviews, 6,* 335–354.

Bletzer, K. V. (1995). Use of ethnography in the evaluation and targeting of HIV/AIDS education among Latino farmworkers. *AIDS Education and Prevention, 7,* 178–191.

Call, R., Entwistle, B., & Swanson, T. (1987). Dental caries in permanent teeth in children of migrant farmworkers. *American Journal of Public Health, 77,* 1002–1003.

Cary, A. H., Goldberg, B. W., Jobe, A. C., McCann, T., Skupien, M. B., Troxel, T. M., & Williams, D. R. (1995). If we fund it, will they come? *Researching nonfinancial barriers to primary health care. Family & Community Health, 18,* 69–74.

Centers for Disease Control. (1992). *Prevention and control of tuberculosis in migrant farmworkers.* (HHS Publication No. [CDC] 92-8017). Washington, DC: U.S. Government Printing Office.

Ciesielski, S. D., Hall, S. P., & Sweeney, M. (1991). Occupational injuries among North Carolina migrant farmworkers. *American Journal of Public Health, 81,* 926–927.

Ciesielski, S. D., Seed, J. R., Esposito, D. H., & Hunter, N. (1991). The epidemiology of Tuberculosis among North Carolina migrant farmworkers. *Journal of the American Medical Association, 265,* 1715–1719.

Ciesielski, S. D., Seed, J. R., Ortiz, J. C., & Metts, J. (1992). Intestinal parasites among North Carolina migrant farmworkers. *American Journal of Public Health, 82,* 1258–1262.

Ciesielski, S., Loomis, D., Mims, S., & Auer, A. (1994a). Pesticide exposure, cholinesterase depression, and symptoms among North Carolina migrant farmworkers. *American Journal of Public Health, 84,* 446–451.

Ciesielski, S., Esposito, D., Protiva, J., & Pielhl, M. (1994b). The incidence of tuberculosis among North Carolina migrant farmworkers, 1991. *American Journal of Public Health, 84,* 1836–1838.

Council on Scientific Affairs. (1991). Hispanic health in the United States. *Journal of the American Medical Association, 265,* 248–252.

Crutchfield, C., & Sparks, S. (1991). Effects of noise and vibration on farmworkers. *Occupational Medicine: State of the Art Reviews , 6,* 355–369.

De La Torre, A., & Rush, L. (1989, January–February). The effects of health care access on maternal and migrant seasonal farmworker women infant health of California. *Migrant Health Newsline, Clinical Supplement, 6*(1).

De Leon Siantz, M. L. (1990). Correlates of maternal depression among Mexican-American migrant farmworker mothers. *Journal of Community Psychology, 3,* 9–13.

De Leon Siantz, M. L. (1994). The Mexican-American migrant family: Mental health Issues. *Nursing Clinics of North America, 29,* 65–72.

Dever, A. (1991). *Profile of a population with complex health problems.* Austin, TX: Migrant Clinicians Network.

East Coast Migrant Health Project. (1996). *Changes in the East Coast migrant stream.* Washington, DC: East Coast Migrant Health Project, Inc.

Eshleman, J., & Davidhizar, R. (1997) Life in migrant camps for children—A hazard to health. *Journal of Cultural Diversity, 4,* 13–17.

Estill, C. F., & Tanaka, S. (1998). Ergonomic considerations of manually harvesting Maine wild strawberries. *Journal of Agri Safety Health, 4,* 43–57.

Gamsky, T. E., McCurdy, S. A., Samuels, S. J., & Shenker, M. B. (1992a). Reduced FVC among California grape workers. *American Review of Respiratory Diseases, 34,* 257–62.

Gamsky, T. E., Schenker, M. B., McCurdy, S. A., & Samuels, S. J. (1992b). Smoking, respiratory systems, and pulmonary function among a population of Hispanic farmworkers. *Chest, 101,* 1361–1368.

Gamsky, T. E., McCurdy, S. A., Wiggins, P., Samuels, S. J., Berman, B., & Shenker, M. B. (1992c). Epidemiology of dermatitis among California farmworkers. *Journal of Occupational Medicine, 34,* 304–310.

Garcia, J., Dresser, K., & Zerr, A. (1996). Respiratory health of Hispanic migrant farmworkers in Indiana. *American Journal of Industrial Medicine, 29,* 23–32.

Gerberich, S., Gibson, R., Gunderson, P., Melton, L., French, L., Renier, C., True, J., & Carr, W. (1992). Surveillance of injuries in agriculture (pp. 161–178). In J. D. Millar (Ed.), *Papers and proceedings of the Surgeon General's Conference on Agricultural Safety and Health.* Cincinnati: National Institute for Occupational Health and Safety.

Goldsmith, M. (1989). As farmworkers help keep America healthy, illness may be their harvest. *Journal of the American Medical Association, 261,* 3207–3213.

Hays, W., & Laws, E. (1991). *Handbook of chemical toxicology.* London: Academic Press.

Jacobson, M. L., Mercer, M. A., Miller, L. K., & Simpson, T. W. (1987). Tuberculosis risk among migrant farmworkers on the Delmarva peninsula. *American Journal of Public Health, 77,* 29–32.

Jones, J. (1992, March–April). HIV-related characteristics of migrant-workers in rural South Carolina. *Migrant Health Newsline, Clinical Supplement,* p. 4.

Kaloyanova, F., & Batawi, M. (1991). *Human toxicology of pesticides.* Boca Raton, FL: CRC Press.

Karr, C., Demers, P., Costa, L. G., Daniell, W. E., Barnhart, S., Miller, M., Gallagher, G. Horstman, S. W., Eaton, D., & Rosenstock, L. (1992). Organophosphate pesticide exposure in a group of Washington State orchard applicators. *Environmental Research, 59,* 229–237.

Kligman, E. W., Peate, W. F., & Cordes, D. H. (1991). Occupational infections in farmworkers. *State Art Review of Occupational Medicine, 6,* 429–446.

Koch, D. (1988). Migrant day care and the health status of migrant preschoolers: A review of the literature. *Public Health Reports, 105,* 317–320.

Koday, M., Rosenstein, D. I., & Lopez, G. M. (1990). Dental decay rates among children of migrant workers in Yakima, WA. *Public Health Reports, 105,* 530–533.

Lafferty, J. (1991). Self-injection and needle sharing among migrant farmworkers. (Letter to the editor). *American Journal of Public Health, 81,* 221.

Larson, A. L., & Plascencia, L. (1993). *Migrant enumeration project 1993.* Rockville, MD: Bureau of Primary Health Care.

Lee, C. V., McDermott S. W., & Elliott C., (1990). The delayed immunization of children of migrant farmworkers in South Carolina. *Public Health Reports, 105,* 317–320.

Lopez, N. C. (1995, Fall). Meeting the challenge: Providing migrant farmworker housing. *Rural Voices,* 3–7 .

Lotti, M. (1992). The pathogenesis of organophosphate polyneuropathy. *Critical Reviews in Toxicology, 21,* 465–487.

Lyons, M. (1992, March-April). Study yields HIV prevalence for New Jersey farmworkers. *Migrant Health Newsline* (Clin. Suppl.), 1–2.

Magana, J. R. (1991). Sex, drugs and HIV: An ethnographic approach. *Social Science and Medicine, 33,* 5–9.

McCauley, L. (1996). Reducing pesticide exposure in minority families. USDHNS-PHS. Grant No. ES-96-005.

McDermott, S., & Lee, C. V. (1990). Injury among male migrant farmworkers in South Carolina. *Journal of Community Health, 15,* 297–305.

Meister, J. L. (1991). The health of migrant farmworkers. *Occupational Medicine: State of the Art Reviews, 6,* 503–510.

Meister, J. S., Warrick, L. H., Zapien, J. G., & Wood, A. H. (1992). Using lay health workers: Case study of a community-based prenatal intervention. *Journal of Community Health, 17,* 37–51.

Michael, R., & Salend, S. (1985). Health problems of migrant children. *Journal of School Health, 55,* 411–412.

Migrant Clinicians Network. (1997). *Redefining migration patterns in the migrant farmworker population.* Austin, TX: Migrant Clinicians Network.

Millar, J. D. (1991). *Papers and proceedings of the Surgeon General's Conference on Agricultural Safety and Health* (pp. 92–105). Cincinnati: National Institute for Occupational Health and Safety.

Mines, R., & Kearney, M. (1982, April). *The health of Tulare County farmworkers: A report of 1981 survey and ethnographic research.* Visalia, CA: Tulare County Department of Health.

Mines, R., Gabbard, S., & Boccalandro, B. (1991). *Findings from the National Agricultural Workers' Survey. (NAWS) 1990: A demographic and employment profile of perishable crop farmworkers.* Washington, DC: U.S. Government Printing Office.

Mines, R., Gabbard, S., & Samadrick, R. (1993). *U.S. farmworkers in the post-IRCA period.* Washington, DC: U.S. Department of Labor.

Mobed, K., Gold, E., & Schenker, M. (1992). Occupational health problems among migrant and seasonal farmworkers. *The Western Journal of Medicine, 157,* 367–373.

Moses, M. (1989). Pesticide-related health problems and farmworkers. *American Association of Occupational Health Nurses Journal, 37,* 115–130.

Moses, M., Johnson, E. S., Anger, W. K., Burse, V. W., Horstman, S. W., Jackson, R. J., Lewis, R. G., Maddy, K. T., McConnell, R., Meggs, W. J. (1993). Environmental equity and pesticide exposure. *Toxicology and Industrial Health, 9,* 913–959.

Myers, J. R. (1997). *Injuries among farmworkers in the United States, 1993.* (Department of Health and Human Services Publication No. 97-115). Cincinnati: OH: National Institute for Occupational Safety and Health.

National Advisory Council on Migrant Health. (1995). *Losing ground: The condition of farmworkers in America.* Bethesda: Department of Health and Human Services / Health Resources and Services Administration, Bureau of Primary Health Care, Migrant Health Branch.

National Migrant Resource Program (1993). *1993 recommendations of the National Advisory Council on Migrant Health.* Austin, TX: National Migrant Resource Program.

National Institute for Occupational Saety and Health, Workgroup on Priorities for Famworker Occupational Health Surveillance and Research. (1995). *New directions in the surveillance of hired farmworker health and occupational safety.* Cincinnati: National Institute of Occupational Health and Safety.

O'Malley, M., Smith, C., Krieger, R., & Margetich, S. (1990). Dermatitis among stone fruit harvesters in Tulare County. *American Journal of Contact Dermatology, 1,* 100–111.

Pallack, K. (1991). *Oregon farm labor housing survey.* Newberg, OR: CASA of Oregon.

Richter, E. (1992). Aerial application and spray draft of anticholinesterases: Protective measures. In B. Ballatyne & T. Aldridge (Eds.), *Clinical and experimental toxicology of organophosphates and carbamates* (pp. 623–631). Oxford: Butterworth-Heinemann.

Rust, G. S. (1990). Health status of migrant farmworkers: A literature review and commentary. *American Journal of Public Health, 80,* 1213–1217.

Ryan, R., Foulk, D., Lafferty, J., & Robertson, A. (1988). *Health knowledge and practices of Georgia's migrant and seasonal workers relative to AIDS: A comparison of two groups.* Stratesboro, GA: Georgia Southern College, Center for Rural Health.

Schenker, M. B., & McCurdy, S. A. (1988). Pesticides, viruses, and sunlight in the etiology of cancer among agricultural workers. In C. Becker (Ed.), *Cancer prevention strategies in the workplace* (pp. 29–37). New York: Hemisphere Publishing.

Schenker, M. B., Ferguson, T., & Gamsky, T. (1991). Respiratory risks associated with agriculture. *Occupational Medicine, 6,* 415–428.

Schenker, M. B., Lopez, R., & Wintemute, G. (1995). Farm-related fatalities among children in California, 1980 to 1989. *American Journal of Public Health, 85,* 89–92.

Schuman, S., & Dobson, R. (1985). An outbreak of contact dermatitis in farmworkers. *Journal of the American Academy of Dermatology, 13,* 220–223.

Schwartz, D. A., & LoGerfo, J. P. (1988). Congenital limb reduction defects in the agricultural setting. *American Journal of Public Health, 78,* 654–657.

Sharp, D. S., Eskenazi, B., Harrison, R., Callas, P., & Smith, A. H. (1986). Delayed health hazards of pesticide exposure. *Annual Review of Public Health, 7,* 441–471.

Sidell, F. (1992). Clinical considerations in nerve agent intoxication. In S. Somani (Ed.), *Chemical warfare agents.* New York: Academic Press.

Simcox, N. J., Fenske, R. A., Wolz, S. A., Lee, I., & Kalman, D. A. (1995). Pesticides in household dust and soil: Exposure pathways for children of agricultural families. *Environmental Health Perspectives, 103,* 1126–1134.

Skjerdal, K., Misha, S., & Benavides-Vaello, S. (1996). A growing HIV/AIDS crisis among migrant and seasonal farmworker families. *Migrant Clinicians Network Streamline, 2,* 1–3.

Slesinger, D. (1992). Health status and needs of migrant farmworkers in the United States: A literature review. *Journal of Rural Health, 8,* 227–234.

Slesinger, D. P. & Cautley, E. (1981). Medical utilization patterns of Hispanic migrant farmworkers in Wisconsin. *Public Health Reports, 96,* 255–263.

Slesinger, D. P. & Ofstead, C. (1990). *Migrant agricultural workers in Wisconsin, 1989: Social, economic, and health characteristics.* Madison: University of Wisconsin, Department of Rural Sociology.

Slesinger, D. P. & Ofstead, C. (1993). Economic and health care needs of Wisconsin migrant farmworkers. *Journal of Rural Health, 9,* 138–148.

Soliman, M. R., Derosa, C. T., Mielke, H. W., & Bota, K. (1993). Hazardous waste, hazardous materials and environmental health equality. (Review). *Toxicology and Industrial Health, 9,* 901–912.

Spear, R. (1991). Recognized and possible exposure to pesticides. In W. J. Hayes and E. Laws (Eds.), *Handbook of pesticide toxicology vol I.: General principles* (pp. 245–274). San Diego: Academic Press.

Steenland, K., Jenkins, B., Ames, R. G., O'Malley, M., Chrislip, D., & Russo, J. (1994). Chronic neurological sequelae to organophosphate pesticide poisoning. *American Journal of Public Health, 84,* 731–736.

Sweeney, M., & Ciesielski, S. (1990, April). *Where work is hazardous to your health.* Raleigh, NC: Farmworkers Legal Services of NC.

Ungar, B. L., Iscoe, E., Cutler, J., & Bartlett, J. G. (1986). Intestinal parasites in a migrant farmworker population. *Archives of Internal Medicine, 146,* 513–515.

U.S. Commission on Agricultural Workers. (1993). *Report of the Commission on Agricultural Workers, November 1992.* Washington, DC: Commission on Agricultural Workers.

U.S. Department of Agriculture. (1999). Agricultural income and finance report. (Report AIS-70). Washington, DC: U.S. Department of Agriculture, Economic Research Service.

U.S. Department of Labor. (1988). Occupational injury and illness incidence rates by industry. *Monthly Labor Review, 111,* 118–119.

U.S. Department of Labor. (1989). *Occupational injury & illnesses, 1989.* Washington, DC: U.S. Department of Labor.

U.S. Department of Labor. (1997). *A profile of U.S. farmworkers: Demographics, Household Composition, Income and Use of Services.* Washington, DC: U.S. Department of Labor.

U.S. Department of Health and Human Services. (1980). *Migrant health program target population estimates.* Rockville, MD: U.S. Department of Health and Human Services.

U.S. Environmental Protection Agency. (1992). *Pesticide industry sales and usage: 1990 and 1991 market estimates.* Washington, DC: U.S. Environmental Protection Agency.

U.S. General Accounting Office. (1992). *Hired farmworkers: Health and well-being at risk.* (Publication No. GAO/HRD-92-46). Washington, DC: U.S. General Accounting Office.

Vasilion, T. M. (1992 March-April). Knowledge of AIDS among female Hispanic migrant farmworkers in Virginia. *Migrant Health Newsline, Clinical Supplements,* 2–4.

Vega, W., Warheit, G., & Palacio, R. (1985). Psychiatric symptomatology among Mexican American farmworkers. *Social Science Medicine, 20,* 39–45.

Villarejo, D., & Baron, S. L. (1999). The occupational health status of hired farmworkers. *Occupational medicine: State of the art reviews, 14,* 613–635.

Villarino, M. E., Geiter, L. J., Schulte, J. M., & Castro, K. G. (1994). Purified protein derivative tuberculin and delayed type hypersensitivity testing in migrant farmworkers at risk for tuberculosis and HIV coinfections. *AIDS, 8,* 477–481.

Warrick, L. H., Wood, A. H., Meister, J. S., & Zapien, J. G. (1992). Evaluation of a peer health worker prenatal outreach and education program for Hispanic farmworker families. *Journal of Community Health, 17,* 13–26.

Weinstein, P., Domoto, P., Wohlers, K., & Koday, M. (1992). Mexican-American parents with children at risk for baby bottle tooth decay: Pilot study at a migrant farmworkers' clinic. *Journal of Dentistry for Children, 59,* 376–383.

Whorton, D., Milby, T., Krauss, R., & Stubbs, H. (1979). Testicular function in DBCP exposed pesticide workers. *Journal of Occupational Medicine, 21,* 161–166.

Wiggins, N., & Castanares, T. (1994). Mental and psychological health issues among migrant and seasonal farmworkers in Oregon: Preliminary research and interventions applications. In H. H. McDuffie, J. A. Dosman, K. M. Semchuk (Eds.), *Agricultural health and safety: Workplace, environment, sustainability.* Boca Raton, FL: CRC Press.

Wilk, V. A. (1986). *Occupational health of migrant and seasonal farmworkers in the United States* (2nd ed.). Washington, DC: Farmworker Justice Fund.

Wilk, V. A. (1988). *Occupational health of migrant and seasonal workers in the U.S.: Progress report.* Washington, DC: farmworker Justice Fund.

Wingo, C., Borgstrom, B., & Miller, G. (1986). Tuberculosis among migrant farmworkers—Virginia. *Journal of the American Medical Association, 256,* 977, 981.

Woolfolk, M., Hamard, M., Bagramian, R., & Sgan-Cohen, H. (1984). Oral health of children of migrant farmworkers in northwest Michigan. *Journal of Public Health Dentistry, 44,* 101–105.

Zham, S. H., & Blair, A. (1993). Cancer among seasonal farmworkers: An epidemiologic review and research agenda. *American Journal of Industrial Medicine, 24,* 753–766.

Zham, S. H., Ward, M. H., & Blair, A. (1997). Pestidicides and cancer. *Occupational Medicine, 12,* 269–89.

7

American Indian and Alaska Native Health Services as a System of Rural Care

EVERETT R. RHOADES

Introduction

With few exceptions (Thornton, Sandefur, & Grasmick, 1982), Indian* life in the Americas has always been rural, a mode that continued with settlement on reservations in the 19th century (Figure 1). Many Native Americans today continue subsistence living—that is, hunting and gathering, and farming—and as will be noted later, many Indian communities are actually frontier in nature. Even with considerable migration to urban areas, especially during and after the Second World War, reservations remained the site of tribal governments. Combined with the strong impulse of Indian people to remain in their local communities, this has resulted basically in a rural setting for Indians, who receive most of their health care from the federal government. The challenges in integrating health programs among small numbers of individuals residing in remote locations are great indeed.

The health care of Indians shares characteristics and concerns with rural health care delivery in general: a relatively small and geographi-

cally dispersed population, small inpatient facilities, a growing need for chronic care but also episodic acute ambulatory care, maintenance of an adequate health care workforce, transportation, and communication. Concerns about the rural nature of Indian health care were reflected in a roundtable discussion by the Indian Health Service (IHS) (1990). However, health care for Indian people differs in a number of important ways from that for the rest of the country, especially in political and administrative arrangements.

American Indians and Alaska Natives

The political characteristics that most distinguish Indians from other American groups are the sovereign nature of Indian tribes and the consequent government-to-government relationship with the United States. The provision of health services to Indian people is the result of agreements, including treaties, executed between two sovereign governments. These agreements may be regarded as binding business arrangements in which the tribes purchased

---

EVERETT R. RHOADES • Native American Prevention Research Center, University of Oklahoma College of Public Health, Oklahoma City, Oklahoma 73104.

Handbook of Rural Health, edited by Loue and Quill. Kluwer Academic/Plenum Publishers, New York, 2001.

*In this chapter, the term Indian will be used interchangeably with other terms that refer to those groups often designated American Indian, Native American, or American Indian and Alaska Native.

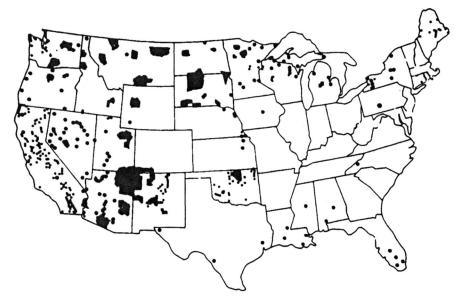

FIGURE 1. Distribution of most federally recognized reservations in the lower 48 states, 1985. (Office of Technology Assessment, 1986).

perhaps the first prepaid health care program in America, paid for through, among other considerations, the cession of lands that became part of the United States. For its part, the federal government assumed certain responsibilities to the tribes, including provision of health services. The concept of sovereignty is so fundamental that it remains the premier preoccupation of tribes and strongly influences all aspects of their relationship with the federal government and, therefore, the federal programs operated on their behalf.

The Indian Health Service

Background

The agency through which the federal government attempts to fulfill its health care obligations to Indians is the Indian Health Service (IHS). Because the IHS is by far the major provider of health services to American Indians and Alaska Natives, it is not possible to discuss these services without discussing the IHS.

It is most helpful to think of the IHS in terms of its 20th-century evolution. A defining event in the development of health services for Indian people was the 1921 Snyder Act, which was the

explicit congressional authorization for federal Indian health services. In it, Congress directed the Commissioner of Indian Affairs to administer funds that "Congress may from time to time appropriate . . . for the relief of distress and the conservation of health . . . of Indians throughout the United States." Thus, more than 75 years ago, a program was defined by language that is now more commonly expressed as *health promotion* and *disease prevention.* The influence of this act on the configuration and operation of the IHS cannot be overemphasized; it defines a program fundamentally different in mission and operation from the rest of the country's health programs. The IHS serves a much larger purpose than simply providing physicians and ancillary medical services. The development of a comprehensive community-oriented primary care program in the IHS may be traced directly to the Snyder Act.

Notwithstanding the forward-looking language of the Snyder Act, health services for Indian people, extremely rudimentary for more than a century, began to take on the attributes of a full-fledged system only after transfer of the IHS from the Department of Interior to the U.S. Public Health Service (USPHS) in 1955. Since then, the IHS has become one of the most complex and successful health programs in existence. With innovations in preventive, curative, rehabilitative, and environmental services, it is an excellent example of *clinical public health*. This evolution was not the result of chance. On the contrary, it was the result of unusual individuals of great foresight and energy who slowly and deliberately, step by step, assembled a modern system.

Following transfer of the IHS to the USPHS, a number of special initiatives began or accelerated. The 1959 Indian Sanitation Facilities Construction Act (P.L. 86-121), provided for construction of safe water and sanitation facilities throughout Indian country; furthermore, it had two important aspects: incorporation of environmental services as an integral component of the overall IHS clinical program and development of true partnerships with tribes. This integration of a variety of environmental and other programs into a national system and the development of partnerships with local communities has seldom, if ever, been duplicated (Indian Health Service, 1985). Other emphases that followed the transfer included maternal and child health, the highest level of professional competence, and institution of a data collection system. In the mid-1970s, legislation strengthened these special programs and added several important features.

The Indian Self-Determination and Education Assistance Act of 1975

Sweeping changes in Indian health care resulted from the 1975 Indian Self-Determination and Education Assistance Act (P.L. 93-638). This act, as the name implies, was intended to strengthen tribal sovereignty—as mentioned earlier, a matter of continuing importance to the tribes. It directed the Bureau of Indian Affairs (in the Department of Interior) and the IHS to turn management of programs over to tribes when they so requested. Only three very narrow grounds for declining were permitted. In 1988, self-determination was further reinforced by amendments to P.L. 93-638, and *self-governance* became an additional mechanism of self-determination (Indian Self-Determination Act Amendments of October 5, 1988, P.L. 100-472). Self-governance provides for even greater control of program design and operation by the

tribes themselves, largely by replacing the unsatisfactory contracting mechanism of P.L. 93-638 with a new instrument, the *compact*. As a result, all tribes now provide at least one or more of their own health programs and some operate their entire health delivery systems.

The Indian Health Care Improvement Act of 1976

The companion legislation to P.L. 93-638 was the 1976 Indian Health Care Improvement Act (P.L. 94-437), also revolutionary in its impact. Innovative provisions included establishment of a manpower development program that provides scholarships for Indian students who wish to pursue a health career, authorization of funds to "close the gap" between the health status of Indians and the general population, specific health planning provisions for each tribe, and more.

Another important element of P.L. 94-437 was promotion of a *resource requirement methodology* (RRM). In the early 1970s, the IHS developed *resource allocation criteria* (RAC), designed to provide objective information for the allocation of resources. RAC used national standards—such as staffing requirements and elements of access, such as driving times—to estimate the comparative resource needs of various programs (Office of Technology Assessment, 1986). During the intervening years, especially with the impetus of P.L. 94-437, the IHS has continued to refine the methodology. It now applies a *resource requirement methodology* to estimate resources needed to bring programs up to acceptable standards. It is particularly useful in preparing an annual budget and establishing priorities that can be used by Congress in making appropriations. A companion methodology, *resource allocation methodology* (RAM), a successor to RAC, is the primary instrument used in allocation of discretionary funds between the many IHS programs.

One of the most dramatic provisions of P.L. 94-437 was the authorization for the Health Care Financing Administration (HCFA) to reimburse the IHS for care rendered to Indians eligible for Medicaid and Medicare services. Funds so generated were to be placed in a special Secretary's fund and used to achieve and maintain accreditation of programs. The result has been universal accreditation of IHS-operated hospitals and clinics, another point of distinction between the IHS and most non-Indian rural facilities.

However, perhaps the most profound provision of P.L. 94-437, often overlooked, was the definition of a specific mission for the IHS. As emphasized in this act and elsewhere, the goal of the IHS is to provide for "the highest possible health status" to Indians, a most salutary complement to the philosophy expressed in the Snyder Act. The importance of this simple vision cannot be overemphasized. It, and the government-to-government relationship, is the basis for all that subsequently distinguishes the IHS from the nonsystem of health care more or less available to non-Indians. It defines a program that goes far beyond simply providing the usual medical services, shifting the focus of health care from the physician and hospital to the community itself. It places primary emphasis on developing programs to address community, rather than individual, problems. The result is a far more proactive, rather than the usual reactive, medical program.

The Organization of Indian Health Services

Several descriptions of the overall IHS program are available (Rhoades, Brenneman, & Santosham, 1993; Rhoades, D'Angelo, & Hurlburt, 1987a; Rhoades, Hammond, Welty, Handeer, & Amler, 1987b; Rhoades, Reyes, & Buzzard, 1987c). The basic IHS organizational element is the Service Unit, a group of ambulatory programs, sometimes with an associated IHS or tribal hospital. Ambulatory programs consist of physician-staffed clinics providing a range of primary medical and dental services, with environmental and community services incorporated into the local program. Many smaller ambulatory facilities (health centers and health stations) are not staffed by full-time physicians but are operated on a day-to-day basis by physician assistants, nurse practitioners, and physicians who visit at intervals. In much of Alaska, the basis of the health care system is specially trained community members, called Alaska Native Community Health Aides (ANCHAs).

In fiscal year 1997, the IHS operated directly 66 Service Units, including 37 hospitals and 113 ambulatory clinics of various sizes. As a result of P.L. 93-638 and its amendments, the tribes operated 84 Service Units with 12 hospitals and 379 ambulatory facilities of various sizes (Indian Health Service, 1997a). Emphasis is on decentralized operations integrated through 12 regions, identified as area offices, and the headquarters located in Rockville, Maryland. Headquarters personnel are concerned with coordination and integration of the many and varied services through formulation of a national budget request, setting of priorities, allocation of resources, and overall program design. In addition to "clinical" professionals, the IHS system includes sanitarians, engineers, injury control experts, health educators, and a variety of other professional providers to a far higher degree than in any other health care system in the United States.

Although specific comparisons have not to this author's knowledge been made, the array of Indian health services, while not always optimal in execution, surely must exceed that available to most rural non-Indians, at least within a single system of care. Services include prenatal and perinatal care, special diabetes programs, mental health services, alcohol and substance abuse services, maternal and child health services, health education, public health nursing, emergency medical services, nutrition, community health representatives, and environmental services. Presently, the IHS provides services to approximately 1.4 million Indians who reside in counties in or near reservations in 35 states from Alaska to Florida and Maine to California (Indian Health Service, 1997a). The fiscal year 2000 budget for the IHS was $2,830,018,000.

Inpatient Care In The IHS

IHS inpatient facilities are on average smaller than non-Indian rural facilities and are often located even more remotely. Of the 49 hospitals operated by the IHS and tribes as of September 3, 1996, 38 (77.6%), contained fewer than 50 beds, compared with 23.1% for U.S. short-stay hospitals. Only 5.4% of U.S. short-stay hospitals have fewer than 25 beds, compared with 38.8% of IHS and tribal hospitals. The IHS and tribes operate no hospitals with more than 200 beds (Indian Health Service, 1997a).

Tertiary care is available at private and public medical centers often located some distance away. Advances in technology, an aging population, and increasingly complex care are placing a severe burden on local Indian communities, quickly exhausting limited budgets. Further, payment for such services has resulted in the IHS becoming a miniature health care financing administration (HCFA).

The Residual Nature of IHS

Under the residual resource rule, the IHS is required to expend funds for the health of Indian people only after all other sources of funding have been exhausted. As a result, IHS encourages Indian people to enroll in appropriate programs for which they are eligible, such as Medicare, Medicaid, and the Children's Health Insurance Program. Collections from Medicaid, Medicare, and private insurance in fiscal year 1999 amounted to $393,886,000 (Department of Health and Human Services, 2000). While this is a substantial contribution to IHS operations, the IHS essentially operates within a "universal cap" as a result of annual congressional appropriations. The IHS, like other payers, seeks to be the payer of last resort. This is important because considerable discrimination continues to be directed to Indians by those who sometimes refer them to the IHS for care, since it is "their" system of care. An important element in IHS operations is that any monies collected from other sources are used to provide additional services. While Indian health services are not an *entitlement,* according to governmental budget terminology, Indian people, notwithstanding their federal programs, cannot be denied any rights, privileges, or services accorded to the general U.S. population. This means that Indian people cannot be denied services elsewhere simply because there is an IHS.

Rationing of Health Care

An important policy that further distinguishes the IHS from other providers is its recognition that rationing of health services is, and has been,

a universal accompaniment of health care, effected through a variety of mechanisms. In the IHS, a distinction exists between the rationing that occurs in programs providing direct services and that involved in payment for care rendered by others. In direct programs, rationing involves two primary mechanisms: allocation of resources between various programs and increased clinic waiting times. Where the IHS is a payer, it generally uses procedures employed by other third-party payers, making decisions about relative priorities for payment of necessary care. Rather than establish a "benefits package" as a specified list of services and procedures, the IHS has defined its payment system as follows: highest priority for payment is for those procedures and/or treatments that, in the judgment of the attending physician, are necessary to prevent loss of life, limb, or one of the senses; or to prevent progression of a medical condition. This definition preserves the judgment of the physician and permits as much flexibility as possible. Thus, the IHS acknowledges the omnipresent rationing of care and attempts to do so based on sound health principles; that is, the effect of programs and resources on the *status of health* of Indian people.

Community and Consumer Involvement

Since the early 1960s, the IHS has formally and informally engaged local communities as partners. It has done this through employment of local health workers, as in the sanitation programs mentioned earlier, and in the establishment of local consumer advisory boards, made up of members of the respective tribes and selected by the tribes themselves. These boards interact with the IHS in varying degrees of collaboration. Although basically advisory, health boards often exercise considerable influence over health programs. Each of the 12 IHS Areas has an area advisory board that functions in much the same way as the Service Unit boards. A national Indian health board provides advice and direction on a range of program and policy matters.

Community relationships are also fostered by the Community Health Representative (CHR) program, in which local indigenous workers coordinate outreach efforts with IHS, tribal, private, and other governmental programs. CHRs are local Indian persons chosen by the tribe who receive training in basic health services and foster health care in the home and the community. Their many activities include blood pressure monitoring, health education, community clean-up campaigns, rabies vaccination of pets, and so on. In addition, they encourage visits to the clinic, often providing an important means of transportation.

Illustrative Rural Programs

Rural Emergency Services for American Indians

The evolution of emergency medical services (EMS) in the IHS offers an excellent case study of challenges faced in implementing rural health services for American Indians and how some have been overcome by local champions. Prior to about 1980, IHS emergency efforts were often primitive, sometimes consisting of no more than a General Services Administration station wagon without radio and often equipped with only a stretcher. Drivers had little or no first aid training and no medical supplies (Rousseau, Jensen, & Decker, 1993). From this modest beginning, a sophisticated EMS program developed through the efforts of energetic tribal and local IHS champions. Contracts to operate EMS were entered into with tribes in the Aberdeen Area in the late 1960s. Modest start-up funds became available through the 1973 Emergency Medical Services Act. In 1976, a Headquarters position was established to provide leadership and soon a national team consisting of a director, research and evaluation consultant, training coordinator, vehicles and communications consultant, and medical director was in place. Program coordinators were appointed in each IHS Area, along with a national EMS advisory group. However, greatest attention to the program remained local, depending on funding by each Area, usually from unobligated year-end funds. Funding was supplemented in 1980 when $1 million appropriated by Congress permitted training of first responders, emergency medical technicians, emergency room nurses and physicians; evaluation of programs; and acquisition of communication equipment. In 1983, funds transferred from the CHR program permitted establishment of well-functioning programs throughout most of Indian country (Rousseau, et al., 1993) (Figure 2). However, the program was not uniformly complete and many communities continued to receive inadequate services.

In 1992, the National Native American EMS Association (NNAEMSA), an education and networking organization, was established. Ad-

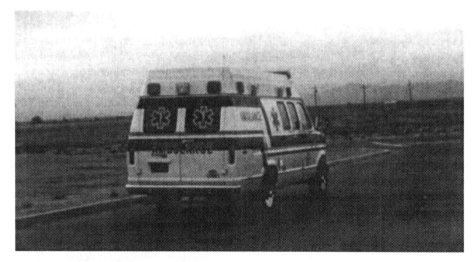

FIGURE 2. Fully equipped prehospitalization units are now available in many Indian communities. Photo courtesy of the Indian Health Service Emergency Medical Services Program, Rockville, MD.

ditional networking outside the IHS has been greatly facilitated through the Mountain Plains Health Consortium (1999), made up of the Veterans Administration, tribes, the IHS, and private organizations. Among other activities, this consortium conducts education programs, many by distance education (Peter Decker, personal communication). There are currently approximately 70 EMS programs, essentially all operated by tribes, in the "lower 48" states, providing the only pre-hospital EMS care to more than 500,000 Native Americans in approximately 20 states (Peter Decker, personal communication). This "bottom-up" approach has characterized many IHS programs. As a result of these individual field efforts, the IHS was able to put into place state-of-the-art EMS for many Indian communities.

However, the efforts to downsize the federal government that began in the 1980s, along with acceleration of individual tribal management of programs, have not been favorable to continuing growth of this important program. A 1993 evaluation by a technical assistance team of the National Highway Traffic Safety Administration, although praising local and individual efforts, was critical of overall IHS support for the program (Indian Health Service, 1993). While recognizing the singular achievements of the IHS field workers, observations by the technical assistance team included these: (1) lack of a comprehensive, coordinated effort; (2) "no clear recognition within IHS that EMS is an integral part of the overall health care system"; (3) an outdated IHS manual; (4) lack of an overall needs assessment; (5) lack of training; and (6) "great disparity between a few model programs and others that do not meet minimum standards" (p. 10). The team also noted, "These efforts have been minimally staffed by some very dedicated individuals with many collateral duties" (p. 7). Sixty-nine recommendations were made covering policy, resource management, training, transportation, facilities, communications, public education and information, medical direction, trauma systems, and evaluation. The report noted that Congress and the IHS should officially recognize EMS as an integral part of the Indian health care program.

Transporting Indian patients under frontier conditions remains a great challenge. A few years ago, an emergency patient in the Havasupai community had to be evacuated by horseback, traversing a seven-mile trail up the side of the Grand Canyon to reach the nearest motorized transportation. It is clear that an EMS operating across the frontier areas of Indian country, frequently with marginal roads, is an expensive undertaking. Considerable effort will be required in order to maintain the system, to say nothing of developing it further. Since injuries remain the leading cause of death of Indians up to age 45 years and approximately half of them are associated with motor vehicle accidents (Indian Health Service, 1997a), the need for sophisticated EMS will continue to increase.

Health Programs for Alaska Natives

Alaska as a Model of Frontier Care

The frontier nature of Alaska Native health care illustrates in sharp detail the various components of rural health care (Alaska Native Health Board, 1991; Alaska Area Native Health Service, 1992; Office of Technology Assessment, 1994). In addition to the extremes of geography, climate, and weather, challenges to health care in Alaska center on the need for primary care providers, transportation, and communication, and also for such basics as sanitation facilities.

The critical determinant of many functions in Alaska is distance. Alaska encompasses an area one-fifth that of the lower 48 states. As illustrated in Figure 3, the challenges of transportation and simple access to clinical care are almost always of paramount concern. As of 1991, the state had approximately 13,000 miles of roads and slightly more than 2,200 miles of ferry transportation, serving only 15% of the approximately 200 Alaska communities (Alaska Area Native Health Service, 1992). Air transportation with its attendant cost, often marginal landing strips, and dependence on weather conditions, remains perhaps the major mode of transportation, although shorter distances may be covered by boat or snowmobile.

The basic community units are the villages. These are characteristically small and remote. One example is Buckland, shown in Figure 4.

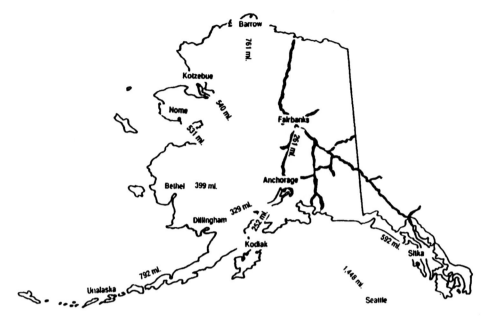

FIGURE 3. Distances between Alaska communities and the Alaska Native Medical Center in Anchorage. The distribution of major roads is also shown. (Adapted from Alaska Area Native Health Board, 1991, p. 11).

This village, located on the Buckland River approximately 75 miles southeast of the nearest tribal hospital in Kotzebue, had a 1999 native population of 363. Basic health care is provided by the Alaska Area Native Community Health Aide (ANCHA) program, which in fiscal year 1998 provided for 3,077 visits. Access to the hospital in Kotzebue depends on air transportation.

Organization of Health Services for Alaska Natives

Perhaps as a result of such impediments, health services for Alaska Natives are remarkably systematized, including three major elements: the Alaska Native Community Health Aides (ANCHAs), regional health care programs, and a medical center in Anchorage. The Alaska Area Native Health Service (AANHS) consists of nine service units (regional health care hubs), which in turn include 26 health centers and 161 village clinics.

The Alaska Native health care program has four tiers: Tier I covers primary diagnostic, assessment, treatment, and referrals under physician orders, well-child clinics, basic laboratory services, and stabilization of emergency patients. Tier I care rests on an infrastructure of

the ANCHAs. These are local individuals, often without high school education, chosen by the local community, who receive training in the diagnosis and management of the most common illnesses, stabilization of the patient, and consultation by radio or telephone with a physician who is often located hundreds of miles away. The village clinic may be no more than a slightly modified residence, often only one or two rooms, equipped with a standing formulary, examination room, and a radio or telephone for consultation. Using standing physician's orders, ANCHAs make an assessment and initiate a plan of treatment. The ANCHAs serve as medics, providing direct health care services, and are not to be confused with the community health representatives (CHRs) who function at a lower level of service. The ANCHA may be the only provider regularly available in many villages, on-call 24 hours a day, often with no local backup.

Tier II care involves 12 regional centers. These provide a broad range of services such as emergency room, inpatient, ambulatory, public health, alcohol abuse treatment, mental health services, and prevention services found in any similar hospital in the United States. As of 1998, Tier I and II centers were staffed by 108 full-

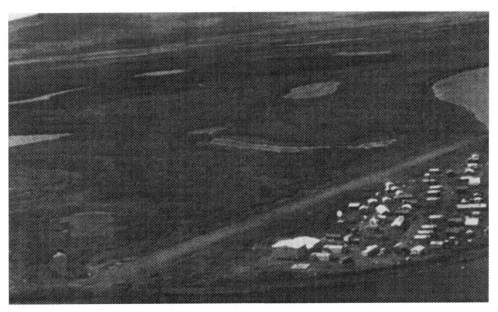

FIGURE 4. The village of Buckland, Alaska. Notable are the absence of roads or automobiles and the prominence of the landing strip. Photo courtesy of the Alaska Area Native Health Service, Anchorage.

and part-time primary care physicians, 74 primary care advanced practice nurses or physician assistants, and 456 ANCHAs (Beck, Saddler, & Ranch, 1998).

Tier III care is provided by the Alaska Native Medical Center (ANMC) in Anchorage, which serves as the central hub for the regional health programs and provides all the services of a typical urban medical center (Alaska Native Health Board, 1991). It also provides telephone consultation services for the many village health centers throughout the state. This system is increasingly linked through a standard and "portable" electronic medical record system and increasing networking through electronic technology (Alaska Native Tribal Health Consortium, 1999). Services requiring a yet higher level of care are available from private and other governmental agencies through the contract health services program.

In addition to basic activities such as transportation, in many villages sanitation and waste disposal are major concerns (Office of Technology Assessment, 1994). A major challenge for sanitation engineers is permafrost; as a result, construction of adequate sanitation facilities is often prohibitively expensive. In a number of villages, this problem has not been solved and

waste is sometimes stored in deteriorating 55-gallon drums.

The AANHS has been extremely resourceful in forming alliances with the private sector, other federal agencies, and especially the state. For example, the public health nursing program is operated by the state. Alaska Natives along with the IHS have developed an integrated, regionalized system of care that has made impressive progress, embracing all the elements required for successful rural programs. The complexity of the overall program is reflected in the fact that all 226 tribal governments operate various programs under self-determination and self-governance.

Changes in Tribal–Federal Administration

Alaska native health care is experiencing fundamental changes in administration. These changes raise questions about the government-to-government relationship, tribal sovereignty, and the ultimate role of the IHS. As a result of self-determination and self-governance, Alaska Native health organizations now control 99% of the IHS funding in Alaska. Transition to this new management system is not yet complete and many problems will undoubtedly be encountered. For example, a recurring question is which entity should operate programs that serve all the tribes and villages. Under the doctrine of tribal sovereignty, entities operating multitribal programs have traditionally required the acquiescence of all the affected tribes. The fiscal year 1998 appropriations act (P.L. 105-83) provided that essentially all of the Alaska area IHS programs at the Area Office (AANHS) and the ANMC would be provided by only two entities. The Southcentral Foundation (SCF) (the nonprofit regional corporation serving Anchorage and the Matanuska–Susitna valley area) was to manage all primary care services provided at or through the ANMC. The newly created Alaska Native Tribal Health Consortium (ANTHC) was to manage all nonprimary care services provided at or through the ANMC, as well as services at the IHS Area Office.

The ANTHC assumed management of the nonprimary care programs of ANMC on January 1, 1999. On this same date, the SCF took over management of all primary care programs, functions, services, and activities of the ANMC. The operating budget of ANMC is allocated approximately two-thirds to the ANTHC (approximately $90 million annually) and one-third to the SCF (approximately $40 million annually). Coordination between the two organizations is through a joint operating board with members named by both organizations. In addition, the two organizations have a revenue-sharing agreement.

In establishing the operating authority in these two organizations, Congress waived the usual requirement for tribal resolutions of support by affected tribes. Further, it prohibited individual tribes from partially or totally leaving an existing tribal organization to manage their own programs. This stay on tribal sovereignty, albeit temporary, may prove to be a precedent that will have future ramifications for the heretofore intensely held concept of tribal sovereignty. It is likely that the rule will ultimately be challenged by a group wishing to remove its shares from the consortium.

The IHS Obstetrics Program as a Model of Organization and Collaboration

Providing obstetrical services in rural locations is a continuing and major concern (Nesbitt, 1996) and many rural areas of the United States are without basic maternity services. Iglesias, Grzybowski, Klien, Gagne, & Lalonde (1998) point out the importance of cooperation between specialists and family physicians and note that decisions about rural maternity care are often between limited or no services. As a result, the concept of low-risk obstetric services in rural communities has been developed to provide safe and accessible maternity care. It is in this context that the IHS may serve as a useful model.

There are approximately 13,000 births each year in IHS, tribal, or contract health facilities (Brenneman, 1999). Although since 1958 Indian maternal mortality rates have fallen by 90%, the three-year average Indian maternal mortality rates since 1986 have been 1.1 to 2.1 times those for American white women (Brenneman, 1999). It should be noted, however, that the small number of Indian births is likely to create artificially high mortality rates. It should also be noted that Indian neonatal mortality rates have consistently been lower than those for the general population. From its inception, a great deal of attention has been devoted to obstetrical services in the IHS. The IHS manual contains a thorough description of procedures considered essential in providing health care to pregnant women and their families, and requires that each facility develop clearly written and understood plans and protocols. The IHS emphasizes standards of care promoted by the American College of Obstetricians and Gynecologists (ACOG), American Academy of Pediatrics, and Joint Commission on Accreditation of Health Care Organizations (JCAHO), including attention to standards for obstetric anesthesia and transportation of patients. In keeping with its own philosophy and tribal sovereignty, the IHS manual recommends that assessment of community needs and desires be taken into account as well as the levels of professional expertise necessary to provide optimal care.

Following common practice, the IHS distinguishes between the capability of programs providing 125 or more deliveries a year and those providing fewer. It recommends that facilities with fewer deliveries seek regional obstetrical care. A few exceptions have been approved in Alaska because of the remoteness of many facilities. The IHS also emphasizes that the local community be fully informed of the state of obstetrical services, the level of care available, and quality of care issues. It further provides for strict credentialing of those providing obstetrical services.

The question of low-risk obstetrics was addressed through a series of lengthy discussions between IHS and JCAHO, sometimes also involving ACOG (Haffner, 1989). The IHS pointed out that its obstetrical services operated within a carefully planned and structured regionalized prenatal and intrapartum care system, with extensive Area and Headquarters support, consultation, and monitoring. The critical issue was the ability of the IHS to demonstrate availability of fully functioning surgical suites with anesthesia services within 30 minutes. A program was established that included close monitoring by JCAHO for low-risk IHS facilities located more than 30 minutes away from regional units. The IHS program includes careful and thorough determination of gestational age dating and prenatal risk assessment. The various elements of the IHS program are reviewed in an annual IHS/ACOG postgraduate course (Haffner, 1989). Also, private physicians serving locum tenens through the auspices of ACOG often provide obstetrical coverage (Zinberg 1996).

The involvement of the ACOG with the IHS began with the establishment of a Committee on Indian Affairs in 1970. Since that time, the association between the two organizations has been intense and ongoing, largely through dedication of the college and its staff, but also because of an IHS senior clinician charged with the responsibility of maintaining the relationship. The relationship fosters a high level of professional competence through evaluations by outside experts and the continuing education program already mentioned (Zinberg, 1996).

According to Brenneman (1999), the ACOG guide *Obstetrical, Neonatal, and Gynecological Care. A Practical Approach for the Indian Health Service* provides excellent recommendations for the program. In addition, the ACOG publishes a series of technical, educational, and practice bulletins for standards of care, available to the general public and to IHS practitioners. These innovations and imaginative approaches are reflected in the fall in Indian maternal mortality rates since 1973 (Figure 5).

Status of Health of American Indians and Alaska Natives

A full discussion of the various parameters of American Indian and Alaska Native health is beyond the scope of this chapter and extensive descriptions are available elsewhere (Indian Health Service, 1997b; Indian Health Service, 1997a). A few examples will serve to illustrate

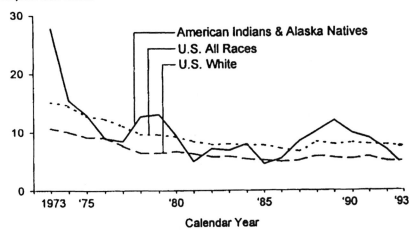

Per 100,000 Live Births

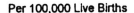

FIGURE 5. Indian maternal mortality rates since 1973. (Indian Health Service, 1997a, p. 43).

the situation. As shown in Figure 6, there has been a steady increase in life expectancy of Indians. Another widely accepted hallmark of the health status of a population is the mortality rates of infants. Few achievements have been as great as the downward trend in infant mortality rates for Indian people; they fell from 22.2 per 1,000 live births in 1972–1974 to 10.9 per 1,000 live births in 1992–1994.

By most indices, improvements in Indian health status have been impressive. However, two important causes of death that have declined among the general population have not done so among Indian people: cardiovascular disease and cancer. In both instances, the present trend for Indian people is static or upward, making it clear that new approaches will have to be taken. In addition, the mortality associated with another important condition, diabetes, is increasing for Indian people at a more rapid rate than for the general population. It remains to be seen if the public health principles that have been so successful in the past will prove to be as effective in dealing with these perhaps more intractable conditions.

Discussion

An extensive literature attests to the challenges of rural health care. Mueller, Ortega, Parker, Patil, & Askenazi (1999) pointed out that existing research does not yet permit any clear understanding of the underlying structures and processes that give rise to racial health disparities and that very little is known about the health of minorities living in some rural areas of the country. Major concerns center on utilization of networks (Moscovice, *et al.*, 1997), partnerships with tertiary level centers (Greene *et al.*, 1999), emergency medical services (Gerard & Stauffer, 1999), use of midlevel practitioners (Knapp *et al.*, 1999), and rural education training tracks for specialists (Landercasper *et al.*, 1997). It is striking that most, if not all, of these concerns have been addressed, sometimes in innovative ways, by the IHS. The examples cited here are but a few of the many approaches taken by the IHS and the tribes.

The IHS approach has embraced certain principles that are perhaps worth reiterating. Paramount among these is a single goal: to elevate the health status of the community. A single goal (or vision) may be the most important basis on which to make very difficult decisions about what services are more urgent than others; that is, decisions about rationing. It is hard to see how the difficult questions of rationing can be approached, at least with some modicum of satisfaction, any other way. This is not to suggest that the IHS system of rationing is necessarily

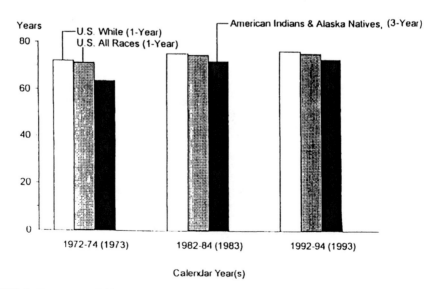

FIGURE 6. Comparison of life expectancy of Indians and that of the general U.S. population. (Indian Health Service, 1997a, p. 134).

the most successful but rather to recommend that rationing be recognized, and dealt with, as the important basis for health policy that it is.

The IHS is presently the only system of health care in the United States that offers a full range of basic services for individuals from antepartum to death. In addition to having a lifetime medical record, the IHS also benefits in having a continuous data monitoring system. The system has a number of flaws, and certain errors are inherent. However, these are recognized and efforts to minimize them are ongoing. The IHS system permits analysis of local, regional, and national databases. This permits comparison of morbidity and mortality rates with those of other populations and also allows examination of various Indian diseases and mortality trends during various time periods. Presently, most analyses compare Indians with the general U.S. population. A more appropriate comparison would be with rural, non-Indian groups.

While maintaining a decentralized system, the vertically integrated IHS organization has a number of important benefits. Vertical integration permits a much greater adherence to standards, as illustrated by the use of the IHS manual described earlier. A degree of authority can be maintained through vertical integration that is not possible with a horizontal organization. For example, the high level of preschool immunizations for Indian children can be traced directly to the management practice whereby Area Directors are evaluated on the basis of the level of childhood immunizations in their respective Areas.

Although it has a vertical organization, the IHS has long engaged in numerous horizontal arrangements, both internally and externally. Achieving proper balance between the two approaches will always be a challenge. Kunitz (1996) has correctly pointed out the possible loss of some of the advantages of vertical integration as tribes take over more and more IHS programs.

The effect on the health of the local populations following assumption of IHS programs by various tribes through self-governance cannot yet be adequately evaluated. There is presently a mix of programs, with some tribes operating their entire programs and others only certain components. Tribes can now generally be divided into two major groups, "self-governance" tribes and those that receive essentially all their services from IHS-operated programs. For many tribes, the flexibility and increased local "ownership" of programs occasioned by self-governance has been quite positive. A number of tribes with considerable income, much of it gained through gaming activities, have supplemented their health programs, with obvious benefit. The same boon is not necessarily seen in some smaller self-governance tribes with less income and smaller staffs. On the other hand, reductions in IHS staff at both the local and area levels as a result of self-governance tribes removing their shares (e.g., funds) and the continued reductions in the federal workforce have had a deleterious effect on tribes electing to receive their services directly from the IHS. The effect has been to force some tribes into self-governance as a way of protecting resources. The ultimate measure of the effect of self-governance will derive from evaluation of medical outcomes, a very difficult area of assessment. Self-governance has resulted in some degree of fragmentation of the IHS information gathering system because some tribes have elected not to participate. This is likely to prove counterproductive. One consequence of these various forces is a noticeably increasing gap between tribes that are well off and tribes that are not. The inherent tendency for the well-off to do better than the less well-off will continue to challenge equitable distribution of resources.

The future of the existing system—with the current public interest in limited government services and possible assumption of management of programs by approximately 500 sovereign entities—is difficult to predict. Certainly, a number of elements that have proved so beneficial to successful programs will be altered, perhaps some of them fatally. However, it is likely that the principles formulated and held to by the IHS over the years will be maintained in some form, perhaps by consortia of tribes or some other configuration. In any event, it is likely that Indian health services will provide opportunities for examining many basic questions of rural health services delivery.

Acknowledgments

The following individuals generously provided great assistance in preparation of this chapter:

George Brenneman of Johns Hopkins School of Hygiene and Public Health, Alan Waxman of the Gallup Indian Medical Center, William Haffner of the Uniformed Services University of Health Sciences, David Schraer of the Alaska Area Native Health Service, Peter Decker of the IHS Emergency Medical Services Program, and Sherry Foster of the Alaska Area Native Health Service.

References

Alaska Area Native Health Service. (1992). *Health care challenges on the last frontier.* Anchorage: Alaska Area Native Health Service.

Alaska Native Health Board. (1991). *Access to care: Crisis for Alaska Natives. Report of task force on patient travel.* Anchorage: Alaska Native Health Board.

Alaska Native Tribal Health Consortium. (1999). *The Alaska Native health care system: A map study of information technology and Native health care in Alaska.* Anchorage: Alaska Native Tribal Health Consortium.

Beck, R. D., Saddler, C., & Ranch, R. 1998. Preliminary experience with an orthopedic teleradiology service at the Alaska Native medical center. *International Journal of Circumpolar Health, 57,* 689–690.

Brenneman, G. (1999). *Revision of the IHS Manual, chapter 13: Maternal and Child Care.* Rockville, MD: Indian Health Service.

Department of Health and Human Services. (2000). *Department of Health and Human Services—Fiscal Year 2001—Indian Health Service. Justification for estimates for appropriations committees.* Rockville, MD: Indian Health Service.

Gerard, W. A., & Stauffer, A. (1999). Rural health care delivery. *Annals of Emergency Medicine, 33,* 725–726.

Greene, P. G. , Smith, D. E., Hullett, S., Kratt, P. P., & Kennard, P. (1999). Cancer prevention in rural primary care. An academic-practice partnership. *American Journal of Preventive Medicine, 16,* 58–62.

Haffner, W. H. J. (1989). IHS low risk maternity units and the JCAHO's anesthesia standard. *IHS Primary Care Provider, 14,* 42–43.

Iglesias, S., Grzybowski, S., Klein, M. C., Gagne, G. P., & Lalonde, A. (1998). Rural obstetrics: Joint position paper on rural maternity care. *Canadian Family Physician, 44,* 831–843.

Indian Health Service. (1985). *The American Indian and Alaska Native: Their environmental health and the environmental health program–A historical perspective, 1955–1985.* Rockville, MD: Environmental Health Program, Indian Health Service.

Indian Health Service (1990). *Tribal Governments as Rural Health Providers.* A roundtable conference on tribal governments as rural health providers—Final report. Rockville, MD: Office of Planning Evaluation and Legislation, Indian Health Service.

Indian Health Service. (1993). *Indian Health Service: An Assessment of Emergency Medical Services.* Report of the Technical Assistance Team, National Highway Transportation Administration. Rockville, MD: Emergency Medical Services Program, Indian Health Service.

Indian Health Service. (1997a). *Trends in Indian Health.* Rockville, MD: Indian Health Service.

Indian Health Service. (1997b). *Regional differences in Indian health.* Rockville, MD: Indian Health Service.

Knapp, K. K., Paavola, F. G., Maine, L. L., Sorofman, B., Politzer, R. M. (1999). Availability of primary care providers and pharmacists in the United States. *Journal of the American Pharmaceutical Association, 39,* 127–135.

Kunitz, S. J. (1996). The history and politics of U.S. health care policy for American Indians and Alaskan Natives. *American Journal of Public Health, 86,* 1464–1473.

Landercasper, J., Bintz, M., Cogbill, T. H., Bierman, S. L., Buan, R. R., Callaghan, J. P., Lottmann, K. J., Martin, W. B., Andrew, M. H., & Lambert, P. J. (1997). Spectrum of general surgery in rural America. *Archives of Surgery, 132,* 494–496.

Moscovice, I., Wellever, A., Christianson, J., Casey, M., Yawn, B., & Hartley, D. (1997). Understanding integrated rural health networks. *Milbank Quarterly, 75,* 563–588.

Mueller, K. J., Ortega, S. T., Parker, K., Patil, K., & Askenazi, A. (1999). Health status and access to care among rural minorities. *Journal of Health Care for the Poor & Underserved, 10,* 230–249.

Mountain Plains Health Consortium. (1999). Ft. Meade, SD: Website at http://www.heds.org.

Nesbitt, T. S. (1996). Rural maternity care: New models of access. *Birth, 23,* 161–165.

Office of Technology Assessment. (1986). *Indian Health Care.* (OTA-H-290). Washington, DC: U.S. Government Printing Office.

Office of Technology Assessment. (1994). An Alaskan challenge: Native village sanitation. (OTA-ENV-591). Washington, DC: U.S. Government Printing Office.

Rhoades, E. R., Brenneman, G., & Santosham, M. (1993). Health on the reservation, 1994 medical and health annual (pp. 96–119). Chicago: Encyclopedia Britannica.

Rhoades, E. R., D'Angelo, A. J., & Hurlburt, W. B. (1987a). The Indian Health Service record of achievement. *Public Health Reports, 102,* 356–360.

Rhoades, E. R., Hammond, J., Welty, T. K., Handler, A. O., & Amler, R. W. (1987b). The Indian burden of illness and future health interventions. *Public Health Reports, 102*, 361–368.

Rhoades, E. R., Reyes, L. ,& Buzzard, G. D. (1987c). The organization of health services for Indian people. *Public Health Reports, 102*, 352–356.

Rousseau, C. J., Jensen, G., & Decker, P. (1993). *National EMS program staff's perspective on emergency medical services in the Indian Health Ser-* vice. Unpublished document. Rockville, MD: Indian Health Service.

Thornton, R., Sandefur, G. D., & Grasmick, H. G. (1982). The urbanization of American Indians—A critical bibliography. Bloomington: Indiana University Press.

Zinberg, S. (1996). ACOG's continuing commitment. Committee on American Indian Affairs 25th anniversary. *ACOG Clinical Review, 1*, 1–14.

8

Rural Women's Health

PATRICIA WINSTEAD-FRY AND ELIZABETH WHEELER

Twenty-five percent of the population of the United States lives in rural areas. Women make up about 52% of these residents (Office of Technology Assessment, 1994). People in rural communities are often poorer than in urban communities; have fewer health resources; have long driving times to health care, and are characterized by familiarity among residents (Bushey, 1998). There are variations within rural communities that need to be considered when generalizing about rural women's health. Before addressing issues in the health of rural women, it is necessary to review issues in women's health generally in order to have a context for discussing rural women's health.

This chapter reviews the scientific assumptions underlying today's health care system as it affects women's health. The authors also discuss literature on selected women's health issues. The literature is confined to that from the United States, as presenting cultural differences as they influence women's health care is beyond the scope of this chapter.

The authors used the American Association of Colleges of Nursing (AACN) definition of women's health in developing the chapter. The definition states, "Women's health refers to wellness and illness issues that are unique to or more prevalent or serious in women, have causes or manifestations specific to women, have outcomes or intervention processes specific to

women, and occur across the lifespan and within the context of women's lives" (American Association of Colleges of Nursing, 1999).

The issue of women's health is often met with questions such as, "Why women's health?" or remarks such as, "Pathophysiology is pathophysiology," or other such comments. The reason for a focus on women's health is there are health care issues, such as reproductive technology, and diseases, such as breast cancer, that are more prevalent or unique in women. Other social issues and diseases, such as depression, obesity, eating disorders, sexual harassment, and child care, while affecting men, have a different manifestation or larger impact on women's lives. To give one example of a condition that has a differential outcome on women's lives, consider incontinence. It is estimated that 50% of nursing home admissions are due to incontinence. Three times as many women as men live in nursing homes (Austin & Jacobson, 1986). If incontinence could be managed to permit more women to live independently in their own homes, their quality of life would be improved and significant economic savings could accrue.

Some justify the lack of focus on women's issues because women outlive men by about seven years. The average life span for people is increasing, but overall men die earlier than women. Although women live longer, they do not necessarily live better. More women suffer chronic diseases; they have higher rates of poverty and experience more days of disability than men. The context of a women's life reflects that more elderly women live alone as widows. Also, more women than men care for a disabled

PATRICIA WINSTEAD-FRY AND ELIZABETH WHEELER • School of Nursing, University of Vermont, Burlington, Vermont 05405.

Handbook of Rural Health, edited by Loue and Quill. Kluwer Academic/Plenum Publishers, New York, 2001.

spouse at home (Johnson & Fee, 1997).

Women also are disadvantaged regarding access to necessary services (time, money, and geography), a critical variable in rural women's health. Nancy Fugate Woods (1992) reported that women earn less than men and therefore have fewer funds for health insurance. More women than men have health insurance, but it is often Medicaid, which limits options for care, as many health care providers will not accept Medicaid patients. For individuals with low incomes, a good proportion of rural dwellers, many do not have adequate coverage from the Medicaid program. In the age group between 45 and 65 years, women are more likely than men to have no health insurance at all. Women workers are more likely to be part-time workers and ineligible for health care as a benefit. They are more likely to drop out of the workforce to care of an ill spouse, aging parent, or grandchild, thus losing benefits they may have had. Thus, a women's marital status becomes a major predictor of her insurance status. Woods (1992) summarizes her review of the status of women stating that we live in a system of "unintended rationing of health care based on gender" (p. 162).

Women have differing life experiences, growing up in quite different social climates, maturing and aging in ways that diverge from men (Benderly, 1997). The biology and physiology of the genders are different. While there have been changes in the expectations of social roles of men and women in the recent past, the two genders still experience differing social status, different roles, and different stresses throughout life. It is not surprising, therefore, that men and women differ in the interaction between genetic endowment and life experience that leads to health or illness.

In order to set a context for women's health, the next section will discuss scientific assumptions operating in the health care system. How these assumptions affect differentials in care for men and women will be presented.

Scientific Assumptions in Health Care

Students and scholars in many fields know the idea of a scientific paradigm. In the field of health care, the prevailing scientific paradigm is the biomedical model. This model is materialistic (positivism), reductionistic, and objective, as is its scientific antecedent in the natural sciences (Harman, 1994). There are debates about the model and some changes are emerging, especially in areas such as consciousness research and alternative therapies. Engel's (1977) biopsychosocial model for medicine has received some attention. Engel posits that in order to understand health or disease, physicians must understand not only biology, but also the psychology and sociology of the patients. The biomedical model, however, is the prevailing paradigm. The idea that medical scientists are separate from what they observe and are objective (not subjective) in their assessment of situations, that mind and matter are two separate provinces of study, that person and environment are separate, are still foundational to modern biomedical thought.

The most basic paradigm in modern medicine is that the "normal" body is the male body. Historically, women were not included in clinical trials (Weisman, 1998). This was not questioned until the 1980s. If there was any reflection on the fact that men and women are different, an argument from "good science" could be made to exclude women from studies that might be less controlled if they were included. For example, most of the psychotropic drugs developed to manage depression did not have women in the clinical trials. To the extent that anyone questioned this fact, a "scientific" logic could be offered that women have menstrual cycles, characterized by mood swings, and these swings could contaminate the research, so excluding them was more scientifically sound. However, when the psychotropic drugs were given in practice, they were prescribed for men and women. The drugs did not work as well to relieve the depressive symptoms in women. Women were told they were "more refractory"—less amenable to treatment than depressed men. This is referred to as "blaming the victim" by women commentators on the phenomenon. It was only during the rise of feminism that this type of "science" was challenged and to some extent modified.

The assumption that the male body is the norm is still dominant. Two of the most flagrant examples of this are a report entitled *Normal Human Aging* (Schok *et al.*, 1984) and the Multiple Risk Factor Intervention Trial (1997). *Normal Human Aging* is an observational study of over 1,000 men. Even though women live longer than men, women were not included in the study. This study conveys the message that the male experience is the normal one. The Multiple Risk Factor Intervention Trial explored the efficacy of cholesterol-lowering drugs. This study enrolled 15,000 men and no women, even though heart disease is the major cause of death for both men and women. Mann (1995) reports the investigators defended the exclusion of women on the grounds their perception was that heart disease is a disease that affects middle-aged men. These studies were expensive and widely reported. Had these findings been accepted as the basis for policy decisions and economic investment, women would have been disadvantaged.

One of the most interesting and least studied questions about women's health is, "Are there cellular differences between men and women that might account for some of the differing outcomes seen in treatment?" This question is important because women are now required to be included in clinical trails by the National Institutes of Health. Suppose a clinical trial of a new drug finds the drug is 90% effective for men and 70% effective for women. How will this finding be interpreted? Will the interpretation be the historical one that women are more refractory to treatment? Will social or developmental cause of the difference be offered, as is frequently the case with differences in achievement and income? Or is it possible that there are cellular differences that account for the difference?

Although science assumes the normalcy of the male body, there are real biologic differences well supported in embryology between men and women that have implications for health care. The XX chromosome configuration gives female fetuses a better chance of correcting genetic diseases (Ramey, 1997). The XY configuration means males have only one chance to correct diseases associated with the X chromosome. The Y chromosome appears only to affect gender. The X chromosome, while affecting gender, also carries, among other things, a

gene for clotting. That is why 85% of hemophiliacs are males. Females, with two X chromosomes, have a backup system that may allow for the correction of some genetically related disease such as learning disabilities, congenital disorders, hemophilia, and inborn errors of metabolism. It is important to note that women do get the genetically caused diseases listed above, so there is more operating here than genetics.

Women have a stronger immune system (Manzi & Ramsey-Goldman, 1999). This is probably related to the presence of two X chromosomes and to estrogen, which stimulates the liver to produce immune globulins. This robust immune system is a two-edged sword. Women manage diseases of bacterial and viral origins well. On the downside, more autoimmune diseases are found in women, such as lupus erythematosus, multiple sclerosis, and rheumatoid arthritis. Again, these are complex relationships as demonstrated by the fact that pregnancy, which reduces immune response, does not affect lupus but often induces a remission in rheumatoid arthritis. Further research could elucidate these complicated phenomena.

Women and Health Research

Aside from the assumptions of modern science, history shows that women have been treated differently in health care. The National Institutes of Health are the largest funders of medical research in the United States, yet it was not until 1986 that NIH developed a policy that required including women in clinical trials. In 1990, the General Accounting office was unable to document any progress in meeting that goal, however (Johnson & Fee, 1997).

Women were not included in the Harvard Physicians Health Study, as an example, the initial research that demonstrated the relationship between taking aspirin and decreased risk of heart disease. The study followed 22,071 men in a randomized clinical trail (Steering Committee of the Physicians Health Research Group, 1989). Women were the subjects in the Nurses' Health Study, which followed 87,000 nurses for six years. This study found that nurses who take one to six aspirin weekly have 25% fewer heart attacks than nurses who don't take aspirin weekly (Manson, Sampler, & Colditz, 1991). The difference between the two studies is significant in that the Harvard physicians study was a randomized clinical trial and the nurses study was a descriptive study with no controls in place. As a result of the outcry over the disparity in the findings between men and women, the same group that conducted the men's study has been funded to follow 41,600 women over 50 years of age for five years.

Until 1990, when the NIH Office for Research on Women's Health was created, research on women was under the National Institute of Child Health and Human Development (NICHD). Most of the research conducted under the auspices of NICHD dealt with pregnancy. Although reproductive health is important, recent statistics on breast cancer, cardiovascular disease in women, and other diseases that disproportionately affect women highlight the need for including women in studies that have historically included only men.

Given the philosophical and historical background of women in health care, it is not surprising that early approaches to women's health focused upon reproduction, the one area where women's biological differences are most apparent. However, recent advances in science make it imperative to explore women's health in a holistic, systematic manner. Gilligan (1982) points out that women are more contextual than men in their thinking, citing ethics as one example. Belenky, Clinchy, Goldberger, and Tarule (1986) in their now classic work *Women's Ways of Knowing* demonstrated significant gender differences in how women develop a sense of self, knowledge, and a voice to express themselves. These differences influence interactions between women and their health care providers.

In the next section, we will explore research available on rural women's health issues and diseases. It should not be surprising that there is a paucity of research on rural women's health. Rural health is not a major focus of funded research, and rural educational and health care institutions often lack qualified researchers, making funded research unlikely. The section will not try to be exhaustive but will present a selection of work that gives readers a sense of where there is substantial knowledge of rural women's health care needs and where there are gaps.

Rural Women's Health: Health and Health Effects

Reproductive Health

A chapter on rural women's health necessarily requires some attention to reproductive issues. However, since historically most research and policy on women's health has dealt with reproductive issues; it will not be a major focus of this work. Family planning and obstetric services will only be presented briefly and emerging areas such as hormone replacement therapy, infertility treatment, and reproductive technology will not be addressed because there is no literature on rural women and the research on urban women is limited. Ethical and policy issues in the area of reproduction, however, emerge every day and reproductive issues continue to be a central component of women's health.

Family Planning

Family planning is becoming a more common concern for rural women, as rural women are getting married at an older age and divorce rates are increasing. They still have more children than their urban counterparts. Federal and state agencies provide most of these services in rural areas so data by state and county is available. Eighty-five percent of U.S. counties have family planning clinics (Frost, 1996). Nationally, Planned Parenthood and health departments are the major providers (30% and 32%, respectively). Family planning clinics are the providers of contraceptive care for poor women and for women under 20 years of age. Sixty percent of these groups attend clinics rather then private physicians. Title X funding is a major source of support for family planning clinics. In nonmetropolitan areas, health departments are the primary providers, followed by community-migrant health centers, independent providers, Planned Parenthood, and hospitals.

While no method of contraception is 100% effective, about one-half of all pregnancies are unplanned and occur with the woman using a contraceptive. Most insurance plans do not cover contraceptives, even when they cover other medications and medical devices. Rural primary care providers are challenged to provide state-of-the art family planning services to their clients, who are often geographically distant from them and may consider discussion of sexual matters inappropriate.

Obstetric Care

The Office of Technology Assessment (1994) estimates that an average of $22,000 is saved for every low birth weight that is prevented. Prenatal care is thought to be a major contributor to delivering a healthy baby. Rural women are more likely to use primary care practitioners or family physicians for obstetric care than urban women (Millman, 1993). However, these practitioners may not deliver babies, so women in labor present themselves at emergency departments. A combination of increased malpractice costs and increased malpractice suits is a major reason why family practice physicians drop obstetrics as part of their practice. Even if a physician is available, there is a tendency to refuse care to high-risk patients. Certified nurse midwives, required by law to treat only low-risk pregnancies, face increased malpractice insurance costs, putting them in a position similar to the physicians. The end result is some rural women with high-risk pregnancies are without a health care provider.

The pregnant woman who has been cared for by a family practice physician or nurse midwife who develops complications is frequently seen in the emergency department of her nearest hospital. This woman is likely to give birth prematurely or to experience more medical complications of pregnancy than her counterpart who is seen by an obstetrician early in pregnancy. One hopeful sign in the area of rural obstetric care is telemedicine. Through this medium, high-risk pregnant women and their family practice physicians can have consultations with obstetric specialists throughout pregnancy, thus decreasing the risk to both mother and infant.

Domestic Violence

Domestic violence is defined as "victimization by an intimate partner" (Surgeon General's Workshop on Violence and Public Health, 1986; Elders & Teuter, 1993). The U.S. Department of Justice (Bachman, 1994) reports that all women are equal candidates for domestic violence and rural and urban differences are not seen. However, Johnson and Elliott (1997) reviewed data on patients seen in primary care settings and found 12% to 28% of patients in these settings report current involvement in a violent relationship. Further analysis found that 28% to 54% of outpatients in primary care settings report some experience with violent partners over their lifetimes. Abused women who visit primary care providers are characterized as seeking help for the stress of the abuse, rather than injuries related to abuse (Koss & Heslet, 1992). These women are also more frequent users of health care resources than nonabused women (Elliott & Johnson, 1995; Saunders, Hamberger, & Hovey, 1993). Health care providers treat the bruises and yet it is estimated that providers identify as few as 1 in 20 abuse cases (Sugg & Inui, 1992).

In one of the few studies that focuses on rural women, Johnson and Elliott (1997) compared women in two rural settings and one small urban clinic. Using a trained interviewer, 127 women were interviewed in the three settings. The rural women were older, had more children, were not employed outside of the home, and did not pursue education after high school (some did not finish high school). Sixty-two of the women (46%) who were interviewed had some experience with violence. Only 22 of the women reported violence in their current relationship, 31 reported violence in past relationships, and 3% reported violence in both relationships. The rural women were more likely to be involved in an ongoing violent relationship, with 25% of them reporting such a relationship compared with 12% of the urban women interviewed.

The women interviewed in the Johnson and Elliott (1997) study experienced abuse once a week. If no abuse occurred within a week, the women were on constant alert for the next abusive incident. Rural abused women, like their urban counterparts, experience social isolation as they withdraw from friends, and families or as the abuser limits their social contacts. Rural women had even greater social isolation because they often did not have cars and lived miles from town. Several women reported that their abusing husbands deliberately disabled their cars. The women were not only physically abused, but were also emotionally and socially abused. Several women reported marital rape at the same rate as urban women: 10% to 14%. One rural woman whose husband held a gun to her head daily did not consider herself abused because her face wasn't bruised like pictures she had seen of abused women on posters.

Assessing abuse in rural women is difficult. Rural women present themselves to health care providers with the same vague symptoms as urban women—migraine headache, neck stiffness, and depression. Further, 92% of women do not discuss physical abuse with their physicians (Johnson & Elliott, 1997). However, if a health care provider directly asks about abuse, many women will acknowledge it if they are in a confidential setting. The familiarity of health care providers in rural communities may present a challenge. On the one hand, providers may be aware that a spouse is quite violent, but on the other hand, providers live in close proximity to the violent individual. Providers could place themselves in danger by aggressively pursuing an abusing spouse or identifying the abuser.

Interventions to decrease domestic violence are increasing. The Family Violence Prevention Fund conducted research on family violence. The 1993 study found that 34% of Americans had witnessed some form of family violence and felt helpless to intervene. The majority of the people interviewed thought family violence was a serious problem. They found a change from 10 years ago when excuses such as "he was drunk" or "she asked for it" were accepted. These same excuses were not accepted in 1993. Based on this study, the Family Violence Prevention Fund concluded that people were ready to do something about the problem, but needed education and guidance in how to approach it. The fund launched a 10-year national project called "There's No Excuse for Domestic Violence" in 1994. In conjunction with the Advertising Council, the fund created newspaper and magazine ads, two radio public service announcements, two television announcements, and bus shelter and billboard ads. In addition, the visual material is multicultural. A national toll-free number exists and action kits are available for communities to learn more about domestic violence. Because of the prevalence and seriousness of abuse, the American Medical Association, the American Nurses Association, and numerous women's groups are also launching initiatives to make assessing and preventing domestic violence a priority.

Mental Health

The mental health of rural women is difficult to determine. It is nonetheless an important aspect of assessing the health of women. The general conclusion from various studies is mental illness is underreported in rural areas (Office of Technology Assessment, 1994). Mental illness is often the result of stress that overrides the coping abilities of the person. Stress is thought to be endemic in agricultural populations due to increasing debt, more work, and selling family farms. It is common for farm families to have the farm to run and an extra job to make ends meet. Often the person with the extra job is the farmer's wife. If the wife has the extra job, the employment may decrease financial stress but add to role stress. Many farm families hold traditional values that include that it is a man's role to provide for his wife who should not work outside of the home. The stress created by altered roles may contribute to mental illness.

Rural populations frequently define health as the ability to do their work; hence, behavior that is not disruptive of performing one's work role may be tolerated even if the behavior is quite bizarre. Families are reluctant to seek mental health services due to the stigma associated with mental illness. Many families will tolerate a level of alcoholism or depression as long as the ill person can maintain some level of functioning that contributes to the family life. Overt psychotic behavior will cause a family to seek care from their family physician with whom they are comfortable. Suggestions that specialized psychiatric service be sought may be resisted.

Thurston-Hicks, Paine, and Hollifield (1998) found psychological distress explained functional impairment more than the severity of a chronic illness in a rural sample. This finding suggests that psychological distress can not only have an impact on the quality of life of a rural person but also affect her ability to function in work roles. It is important for health care providers who work with rural persons to assess satisfaction with their work, since this may be a clue to work performance. Rural persons, who may resist a diagnosis of mental illness based on standard medical criteria, may be more receptive to seeking help if the illness is disrupting their work.

There are often few psychiatrists or other mental health personnel in rural areas to address mental disorders when they are identified. Rural persons, less likely to seek help for emotional distress than their urban counterparts, are treated by primary care physicians when treatment is provided for patients. Primary care physicians are less likely to prescribe adequate amounts of psychotropic drugs or, refer for counseling and lack training in psychiatry (Geller, 1999; Rost, Williams, Wherry, & Smith, 1995). However, some rural women prefer their local primary care physician to other mental health providers, even when professional mental health personnel are available (Hartley, Korsen, Bird, & Agger, 1998).

Assessment of the quality of rural mental health services provided by primary care physicians is complex and requires further elaboration. Geller (1999) conducted a focus group with several rural primary care providers—three physicians, two nurse practitioners, and a physician assistant. Geller found these primary care providers were very aware of their deficiencies in psychiatric care and sought consultation. Geller also found the rate of referral is much higher than the 10% to 30% found in the literature. Part of the confusion arises from the definition of referral. In general medical parlance, a referral means a change of provider. To the rural practitioner in his sample, a referral was seeking out counseling for patients but not turning over the management of the care to the counselor. The Geller study also found that patients and providers reported they were treated badly by psychiatrists. There was little communication from psychiatrists to the referring rural provider. Both patients and providers were concerned about the quality of care rural persons received when referred out of their community. This study highlights the importance of mental health as a significant issue facing rural residents.

Substance Abuse

Substance abuse (alcohol, drugs, and tobacco) in women is a relatively new field of study. Early work focused on men and was generalized to women, often ignoring important biological, immune, and genetic differences between the genders consistent with the prevailing scientific paradigm. Boyd (1998) summarizes the research on women and substance abuse, highlighting that women experience a faster progression of alcohol-related illnesses (e.g., ulcers, cirrhosis, obesity) than men. Women are more likely to present vague complaints to health care providers resulting in delayed treatment or misdiagnosis. Often women have dual disorders that complicate diagnosis as compared with men. For women, depression seems to precede alcoholism—that is, women self-treat depression with alcohol, whereas men become depressed after the development of alcoholism.

Genetic factors undoubtedly contribute to the development of alcoholism. Studies have demonstrated that children of alcoholics raised by abstaining adoptive parents are more likely to develop alcoholism than children with no family history of alcoholism. Low income, unemployment, and an unstable marriage, single status, or divorce is also associated with alcoholism in women. Further, 90% of women in treatment for substance abuse report childhood sexual or physical abuse underscoring the traumas inherent in substance-abusing families. The descriptors of women substance abusers cited here are drawn from research on urban women. Several characteristics are especially common in regard to rural women—notably, low income, unemployment (or underemployment), and depression.

Substance abuse in rural women specifically is rarely studied. Boyd (1998) conducted a significant research study of 34 rural women in West Virginia. Her findings suggest that the profile of rural women alcoholics is similar to their urban counterparts. The majority of the women were white, completed education from seventh grade to one year of college, and worked outside of the home. More were divorced (44%) than married or single, and over 50% lived below 125% of the poverty level as defined by the federal poverty guidelines. Thirty of the 34 women reported some form of childhood victimization.

Twenty-seven women met the National Institute of Mental Health Research Diagnostic Criteria (NIMH, RDC) for depression (Boyd,

1998). Twenty-one met the criteria for generalized anxiety disorder and 19 were scored as concurrently suffering both anxiety and depression. Additionally, each woman reported having several depressed and alcoholic family members.

The majority of the women ($n = 21$) met the National Institute of Mental Health Research Diagnostic Criteria for dual disorder. The drugs most frequently used with alcohol were marijuana, amphetamines, cocaine, and barbiturates (Boyd, 1998). Most of the women had become intoxicated from alcohol by 14 years of age and experienced an alcohol-related health problem by age 21. In this study, the majority of the women began abusing other drugs after the abuse of alcohol, around 18 years of age. Once they began the dual abuse, the length of time to their next health-related problem was two years. The most serious health problems were seizure disorders, cardiac arrest during attempts to detoxify from cocaine, and HIV infection from engaging in unsafe sex. Jail sentences, marital breakup, and loss of jobs were frequent social consequences of their drug use.

Boyd's study, while based on one sample in one geographic location, does suggest that rural practitioners who treat women can be guided by the research on urban women. The lack of mental health facilities that typifies some rural communities and the stigma associated with using them may be barriers to women seeking help. Other barriers to treatment that have been identified are lack of child care, poverty, lack of health insurance, lack of transportation, fear of losing custody of children, job loss, and lack of support from family members (Beckman, 1994; McGrath, Keita, Strickland, & Russo, 1990; Weisner & Schmidt, 1992).

Depression

The incidence of major depressive disorder (MDD) is about 7% of premenopausal women and approaches 50% in low-income urban women (Lyons-Ruth, Connell, Grunebaum, & Botein, 1990). Hauenstein and Boyd (1994) found a 41.5% rate of major depression in rural women living in the Piedmont area of Virginia. The prevalence of depression in other rural areas is also high. Depressed rural women have access barriers to receiving treatment including lack of transportation and child care, poverty, and lack of health insurance (Lewin-Epstein, 1991).

Hauenstein (1996) developed a theoretical basis for nursing practice with depressed rural women. Her model is based on the generic biobehavioral model of stress system disorders developed by Cohen, Kessler, and Gordon. Hauenstein conceptualizes major depression as a special case of stress disorder. In her model, vulnerable individuals who experience stress over time may experience a major depression. If the stressors are modulated by social support and adequate physical resources, depression may be avoided.

Based on her theoretical model, Hauenstein (1996a) developed the Women's Affective Illness Treatment (WAIT) Program for disadvantaged, depressed rural women. The program addresses the needs of women in general and some of the unique environmental and access problems of rural women. An advanced practice nurse implements the program. It can be offered in professional settings or in the patient's home. There are 12 modules that address the etiology and symptoms of depression. The next modules address the personal experience of the depressed woman by identifying stressors, coping methods, and cognitive schema that maintain her depression. The woman then identify behaviors she needs to change. Subsequent modules teach self-care skills such as cognitive restructuring, relaxation methods, and other methods of anxiety control. General areas of health such as adequate sleep, exercise, and good nutrition are taught with the goal of developing a lifestyle that is healthy and stress reducing, thus decreasing the return of depressive symptoms. Appropriate pharmacological treatments are also used.

Outcomes are measured using a series of valid and reliable scales, for example, the Hassles and Uplifts Scale and the Ways of Coping Scale (Hauenstein, 1996b). The program is being evaluated using experimental methods and if it proves successful, it could serve as a model for decreasing other stress-related illnesses in rural women.

Cancer

One of the few illnesses where there is a substantial body of research on rural women is cancer. This research is largely focused on breast cancer and it includes studies on Caucasian, African Americans, Mexican, Latino, and American Indian women. This literature will be reviewed in depth as it illustrates some of the research and intervention issues in rural health care.

Breast cancer is the most frequent cancer in women (Dole & Carney, 1998) and one that is receiving increasing attention. Women have rallied around the issue of breast cancer and have been instrumental in increasing funding for research. Organizations such as the National Association of Breast Cancer Organizations (NABCO) and the National Breast Cancer Coalition (NBCC) have created networks for information exchange and advocacy. Due to the activism of these and other groups, NIH funding for breast cancer diagnosis, treatments, effects of living with cancer, and other outcomes are increasingly being studied.

Research on breast cancer screening (mammography) provides an opportunity to investigate rural samples of women. The location of the researchers in the rural states of Vermont, Louisiana, Kansas, and Arizona suggests their samples are rural in nature. Although the researchers indicate the minority status of the participants, they do not differentiate geographic locations nor do they discuss urban versus rural findings. Although this is a limitation, useful information can be elicited from these studies.

One of the difficult aspects of cancer care is the reluctance of large numbers of women to get mammography. In spite of advances in longevity associated with early diagnosis, many women do not get annual mammograms even when they are offered at no or low cost (Dole & Carney, 1998).

Several studies have focused upon African-American women because in some locations they have less breast cancer than white women but have equal mortality rates due to late diagnosis. More African American women have poorly differentiated cancers and are less likely to have estrogen receptor positive cancers (Moormeier, 1996). Treatment for African-American women tends to be the same as for white women, but the five-year survival rate is 80% in white women compared with 64% in African-American women. Much of the re-

search seeks to understand what barriers exist that prevent African-American women from getting mammograms and what might be done to increase the use of this diagnostic technique to ensure early detection.

Davis, Arnold, Berkel, Nandy, Jackson, and Glass (1996) used a convenience sample of 445 women ages 40 years and older who had not had an annual mammogram. The researchers used a structured interview to assess the women's attitudes toward mammography and their knowledge of it. The researchers also estimated the women's reading ability. Sixty-nine percent of the sample were African-American; 97% had annual incomes of less than $10,000 with a household income of less than $20,000. Seventy-six percent of the women read below the ninth grade level. Fifty-eight percent of the women had not graduated from high school. As the researchers hypothesized, knowledge of mammogram and attitudes toward it were significantly correlated with low literacy. The lower the literacy level, the more likely the woman was to have incorrect knowledge of mammograms, including not knowing what a mammogram is (7%). Additionally, these women had the most negative attitudes toward mammography, characterizing it as harmful, painful, or embarrassing. They also thought that it was difficult to get a mammogram.

The researchers concluded that current attempts to increase mammogram use are effective with women who have some reading skills, but programs are missing the less educated, lower-income women who are the most likely to present with advanced disease. These women are also less likely than more educated women to listen to the doctor's admonition that they get a mammogram. These women listen to friends (51%) and relatives (62%) when it comes to deciding to get health care.

The researchers suggest that more culturally sensitive educational interventions, educating the entire family, and nonprint methods such as videos be used to educate low-income, low-literate women. They point to The Save Our Sister Project as a successful model that might be used with rural African-American women (Eng, 1993).

Lantz, Weigers, and House (1997) in additional research explored how education and income influence rural Wisconsin women's practice of getting a mammogram. The researchers controlled for financial status, knowledge, and attitudinal barriers to seeking health care, as well as other issues affecting access. The random sample consisted of 2,346 rural Wisconsin women over 40 years of age who were interviewed by telephone. The random sample was drawn from eight rural counties that were similar in the number of hospitals, physicians, mammography services, and population. Less than 1% of the women were members of ethnic or racial minorities.

Using logistic regression, several models were developed to explore the predictors of women who used mammography services (Lantz, Weigers, & House, 1997). Regardless of the model, finances were not a major predictor of mammography use. Education was predictive through knowledge and health care access. The best predictors were having a family history of breast cancer, having high scores on the breast cancer knowledge test, available health insurance, having a physician who was seen in the past year, and having a physician who at some point recommended having a mammogram. Not seeing a physician in the past year because of cost, perceiving mammogram results as inaccurate, and perceiving mammogram as inconvenient and uncomfortable were negatively related to having a mammogram.

Friedman, Neff, Webb, and Latham (1998) offer another study that focused on breast cancer knowledge, attitudes, and behaviors as influenced by age. Age increases the risk of breast cancer, yet studies have found that older women tend to think they are at less risk for cancer than younger women (Harris, Fletcher, & Gonzalez, 1991; Mah & Bryant, 1992). The researchers explored breast cancer knowledge, perceived risk, barriers to mammography, recommendations for mammography, health promotion behaviors, intention to obtain a mammography, and mammography use. The majority of the sample was African American and Hispanic (over 70%). Overall, the researchers found no significant differences related to age in their sample that was divided into 30–39, 40–49, and over 50 years. The 30–39 years group was less likely to have a mammogram. More women in the over 40 and 50 age groups reported having

a mammogram or planning to have one. Although the results suggest that women are getting mammograms in an age-appropriate manner, the results were disappointing in that 75% of women over 50 had not had a mammogram in the past two years. This falls below the National Cancer Institute's goal of 80% of women over 50 years of age having an annual mammogram.

There were no age-related differences in barriers to obtaining a mammogram. Younger women said they were "too busy" more often than the older members of the sample. All ages found cost and fear of the results to be barriers. There were also no age-related differences in perceived risk of developing breast cancer. Despite their increased risk, older women may not assess their realistic risk of breast cancer and may not be getting appropriate care and education.

Mexican American and American Indian women are two other groups that have cancer mortality rates that are higher than the national averages. Giuliano, Papenfuss, deZapien, Tilousi, and Nuvayestewa (1998) found that 23% of American Indian women over 50 years of age living on the Arizona Hopi reservation had a mammogram in the past two years. Unfortunately, these low percentages are consistent with other research on Native American women (Agency for Health Care Policy and Research, 1991; Nutting, Calonge, Iverson, & Green, 1994). A similarly low rate of mammography is found in Mexican American women (Samet, Key, Hunt, & Goodwin, 1987). Women who preferred speaking in Spanish had the most anxiety and the poorest communication skills and were least likely to go for screening. Unlike studies on African American women, Lobell and colleagues (1998) found anxiety was inversely related to screening behavior when all other factors were statistically controlled. Knowledge of cancer was positively related to anxiety about cancer and this anxiety decreased their pursuing screening procedures.

The research on mammogram usage among rural women is fragmented and findings vary with ethnic and racial membership of the study group. However, there are strong suggestions that cultural sensitivity, anxiety, negative perceptions, and physician recommendation need to be addressed in any program that seeks to increase mammogram use among rural women. Simply making mammograms affordable will not be sufficient; multifaceted approaches may offer more success.

Cardiovascular Disease

Women have been left out of research on heart disease because the biomedical model assumes it is a male disease. However, cardiovascular disease is the number one killer of women. The National Institutes of Health (1991) and the American Medical Association (1991) have pointed out that women with heart disease are treated less aggressively than men. They are older at diagnosis and have more complications. Fifty percent of women who have a heart attack die within a year, compared with 31% of men. African American women have even worse outcomes.

In spite of the fact that heart disease is the major cause of mortality in women, there is little research on women. The authors found no articles on rural women and cardiac disease. Part of the problem with including women in cardiovascular disease can be traced to the very prestigious Framingham study (Benderly, 1997). This study followed men and women living in Massachusetts who were between the ages of 36 and 68. During the course of the study, three times more men than women died of coronary heart disease. The authors of the study drew the reasonable conclusion that middle-aged men are more likely than women to die of coronary heart disease. However, they then generalized beyond their findings, announcing that women have some sort of protection against heart disease. These findings provided the foundation for subsequent research that excluded women.

There is no evidence that women are protected against heart disease; rather, the disease profile is different in women. They get it later in life, after 75 years of age. Women are more likely than men to die of their first myocardial infarction. Both men and women share the risk of getting coronary heart disease if they smoke, have high blood pressure, and are obese. However, men and women present symptoms differently. Men have myocardial infarcts. Women have angina pectoris and chest pain that may

persist for years without being diagnosed, finally resulting in a fatal heart attack.

Pearson and Lewis (1998) report a study of the epidemiology of rural Otsego County in New York. They found that men and women over 29 years of age had more coronary disease (diagnosed by a physician) as their education level decreased. Persons with less than high school education had more coronary disease, cancer, and diabetes. They found rates of cigarette smoking, obesity, and lack of exercise were related to lower educational attainments. Walking was the most common exercise and most exercisers did not do aerobic exercise. Fully 20% of the county was categorized as obese (defined by body mass index). Fifty percent of men and women under 50 years of age who had not finished high school were smokers. The prevalence of obesity is within the objectives of Healthy People 2000, but the smoking data and exercise data are far below the objectives.

There are no comparative research studies of different rural groups. However, comparing the Otsego data to Vermont Department of Health data demonstrates a more optimistic situation. Twenty-one percent of Vermonters smoke (Vermont Department of Health, 1993). Currently more men than women smoke, but young women are beginning to smoke more than young men. Only 17% of Vermonters exercise three times a week and 20% are obese. As in Otsego County, these figures are related to educational attainment and are below the objectives of Healthy People 2000.

The primary approach to cardiovascular health is prevention. Exercise, smoking cessation (or not starting), and adequate diet are related to most of the chronic diseases that affect the heart. While there is a genetic component, cholesterol can be lowered by diet and exercise. There are also drugs that are effective in lowering cholesterol, if decreasing the intake of fat and cholesterol and losing weight don't successfully manage the problem.

Adequate nutrition, a premise for a healthy cardiovascular system, is a challenge for rural poor (Vermont Department of Health, 1993). Rural persons pay more for fresh vegetables and fruit, mainstays of low fat and low calorie diets, than urban persons (Office of Technology Assessment, 1994). Many rural poor raise fresh vegetables in the summer. However, frequent methods of preparing them are either frying or overcooking.

The use of complex carbohydrates and fiber, except bread, is low. Only 1.9% of Vermonters have five or more servings of vegetable, fruits, and legumes a day. Simple sugars, sodium (salt), and alcohol are used too much. Intake of food high in calcium, iron, and vitamins A, C, and E is also low. Some areas of Vermont don't have fluoride in the water supply. Although the food supply is sufficient, inadequate nutrition results from imbalance in the mix of carbohydrate, fat, and protein or excessive eating.

Chronic Illness

Chronic illnesses persist over time, require ongoing management, and often involve major lifestyle changes and adaptations in one's environment. The illnesses are not reversible, and their manifested effects require special education for the patient to live successfully. These illnesses often require rehabilitation and long periods of observation and care. The overall trajectory of any chronic illness is downhill. The ill woman may experience plateaus when the disease ceases to progress for a while, but over time the illness will worsen. In order to illustrate some of problems attendant to living with chronic illness, three chronic illnesses will be discussed. They are osteoarthritis, diabetes, and osteoporosis.

Osteoarthritis

Osteoarthritis, a disease of the joints, involving the cartilage and surrounding soft tissues, is characterized by pain, joint stiffness and swelling, fatigue, and deformity of the affected area (Primomo, 1995). Osteoarthritis is one of the major causes of days lost from work and of disability in the United States (Fife, 1998). The severity of the disease increases with age and causes increasing dysfunction. In individuals over 65 yeas of age, severe osteoarthritis is reported in 68% of women and 58% of men, yet few studies of gender differences have been conducted (Fife, 1998).

Osteoarthritis develops at a younger age in women and typically involves more weight-bearing joints. Women's hands, knees, ankles, and feet are more affected than men's. The severity of joint damage is also greater in women. Fife (1998) suggests that women are treated less aggressively than men with the disease. Fife points out that men are offered total hip and knee replacements earlier in the course of the disease than women and that women are more functionally impaired when these interventions are offered. Yet, the complication rate and the improvement in functional status after surgery are not gender-related.

Women with osteoarthritis must deal with pain, a loss of mobility, altered body image and self-esteem, and the inability to work and to pursue leisure activities. Although the disease is chronic and not presently curable, women can experience a good quality of life when it is well managed. Women with osteoarthritis need to avoid obesity, balance rest and activity, exercise, protect their joints, manage pain, and eat well (Primomo, 1995). All of the recommendations that lead to well-managed osteoarthritis are more difficult for rural women to implement. Eating well is more expensive for them; obesity is endemic and opportunities for planned exercise may not exist or may be prohibitively expensive. Pain management can be expensive and more potent drugs require physician's prescription. A woman may have difficulty obtaining proper medication if she does not have access to medical care.

Diabetes

Diabetes is another chronic disease that affects women in disproportionate numbers (Primomo, 1995). A deficiency in the amount or efficacy of insulin—a hormone that is necessary to metabolize carbohydrates, fats, and protein—is the major manifestation of the disease. Diabetes is the fifth leading cause of death in women. It is a major contributor to disability and a major cause of kidney failure, blindness, and amputations. Diabetic women experience a more serious course if they suffer stroke, heart disease, or vaginal infections, or become pregnant.

There are three types of diabetes. One is specific to pregnancy and is termed gestational diabetes (Phipps, Long, Woods, & Cassmeyer,

1991). The other types are called Type I and Type II diabetes. Type I diabetics require insulin to manage the disease; Type II diabetics are not insulin-dependent. Regardless of the type of diabetes, treatment of the disease requires persons and families to make major lifestyle changes. Without such changes, treatment will fail and complications will increase.

A woman who is diabetic must become knowledgeable and skillful in understanding the disease and its treatment. Self-care is the best management approach to decrease the complications of the disease. Self-care activities include nutrition planning, focused on sufficient calorie consumption and timing of meals and snacks; self-assessment of blood and urine sugar levels; administration of oral or injected insulin; an exercise regimen; and careful observation of the feet for signs of infection. All of these activities must be planned around the current glucose level, which can vary with stress, a cold, or other "minor" illnesses (Lundman, Asplund, & Norberg, 1990).

Gestational diabetes affects only pregnant women. The treatment for this form of diabetes is dietary management of the pregnant woman. The balance between enough calories to support the woman and the fetus without aggravating the diabetes is a juggling act of great delicacy. Along with dietary management, exercise, which is very helpful in treating diabetes, is controversial in pregnancy. Some studies suggest that exercise induces uterine contractions and may lead to premature labor; other do not support this conjecture (Durak, Jovanovic-Peterson, & Peterson, 1990; Jovanovic-Peterson & Peterson, 1990; Veille, Hohimer, & Burry, 1985).

There is controversial evidence that gestational diabetes affects the intellectual development of the baby. Studies found an inverse relationship between Stanford-Binet IQ scores and maternal diabetes; other research did not confirm this finding (Mulford, Jovanovic-Peterson, & Peterson, 1993; Rizzo, Metzger, & Burns, 1991). Although this type of diabetes often ends with the birth of the child, managing it during pregnancy is a major challenge. For the rural woman who does not have access to high-risk obstetrical care, this highly treatable illness can be a major problem.

Osteoporosis

The last chronic disease to be discussed is osteoporosis, a thinning of the bones that leads to fractures. The loss of bone density occurs with aging in both men and women. Osteoporosis is found in 50% of women and 25% of men over 45 years of age. By 80 years of age, 33% of women will have had a hip fracture. Hip fractures are a potentially terminal illness in the elderly because they can lead to the development of pneumonia (Fogel & Woods, 1995). Hip fractures for elderly rural women can create a situation where they cannot maintain their independence. The ability to drive is an important aspect of rural women's independent living, as they need to drive to shop and to keep medical appointments. If their independence is severely compromised, they may be placed in nursing homes.

Menopause accelerates osteoporosis because of the decline in estrogen that plays a role in calcium metabolism and bone health. The exact relationship between estrogen and osteoporosis is complicated. Studies of women who have undergone surgical menopause find that these women do not have accelerated osteoporosis when compared to women who experience natural menopause (Fogel & Woods, 1995).

While science is exploring causes, osteoporosis prevention should become a goal for women over 35 years of age. Preventive activities can increase or maintain the quality of bone tissue. Even if these activities are begun late in life, such as at 80 years of age, there will be improvement in bone density (Heaney, 1998). Hormone replacement can be used to maintain the level of estrogen in menopausal and postmenopausal women. Calcium interacts with estrogen to increase bone health. Calcium is used more effectively by the body when taken in food; however, supplements can also be helpful. Exercise is critical to bone health as bones adjust their mass based on use. Maintaining an active lifestyle can help maintain bone density (Heaney, 1998).

Osteoporosis is a silent disease, sometimes only detected once a fracture occurs. There are measures of bone mass and bone loss, but presently they are not highly reliable. Current medical opinion is that these measures should be used to guide treatment, not to screen all women (Fogel & Woods, 1995). The best practice for osteoporosis at the present time is a comprehensive assessment of midlife women and intense teaching about the importance of diet and exercise in prevention of illness as one ages. The use of hormone replacement therapy needs to be discussed with women so the best medical plan can be determined with full knowledge of potential side effects. Smoking cessation and decreased alcohol intake are also preventive activities known to be successful for osteoporosis.

The challenge for adequate exercise is especially great in nursing homes where many elderly women spend their last years. If the elderly person was sedentary during their earlier years, designing a program of adequate exercise is difficult. Elders need to be out of doors to experience sun exposure that is essential for the synthesis of vitamin D, necessary for calcium metabolism. Metabolic rates decrease with age, so fewer calories are needed to maintain weight. A sensible diet eaten in a pleasant environment is a major deterrent of obesity in nursing home elders.

In summary, if diet and exercise were improved, chronic diseases that affect women in disproportionate numbers, such as osteoporosis, diabetes, osteoarthritis, and depression could be attenuated to some extent. Because inadequate diet and exercise and smoking have been implicated as causes of osteoporosis, a direct improvement might be achieved from a regular prevention program. Exercise that stimulates the release of natural endorphins can also decrease depression. Hence, an exercise regimen could improve mental health and decrease obesity, a cause of heart disease and a contributor to diabetes, arthritis, osteoporosis, and other chronic illnesses.

Issues and Interventions

Patient Education

Patient education is presented in this chapter because patient participation in health care practices and decisions is critical as medical knowledge increases exponentially. Further, patient education is a foundation of preventive services and a major element of community intervention. The work of Gilligan (1982) and Belenky and her colleagues (1986) demonstrates that women approach problem solving differently from men and may require special educational approaches. Patient participation is essential to managing the chronic illnesses that typify the growing aging population, especially rural women. A well-informed population offers a chance for improved health status.

Understanding illness and how to manage it would presumably be important to rural women who value self-sufficiency and who define health as the ability to do what one has to do (Long & Weinert, 1989, 1998). No research was found on rural women (or men) and patient or health education. When one reads the literature on patient education and physician communication with patients, neither the gender of the physician nor gender of the client is included as a demographic variable or in the data analysis (Calkins, et al, 1997; Levinson & Chaumeton, 1999; Ockene, et al, 1999).

In addition, there are few preventive services and fewer providers so it is a challenge to coordinate health messages. Rural persons with limited education and poor literacy skills may not respond or respond differently to messages that come from radio, television, and print media, for example. Little is known about how rural persons receive health promotion messages. This limitation seriously constrains developing rural health interventions. The core element is health education, but research and demonstration projects specific to rural areas are needed in order to advance geographically specific interventions.

Patient–Provider Communication

At the heart of successful health care is adequate communication between patient and provider. The communication preferences of rural women are poorly studied. We know that most rural women get care from primary care providers. Often there are one or two providers within reasonable travel time. We also know that most providers are either transplanted urbanites or rural persons who went to urban areas for their education. We might assume rural women figure out how to communicate with their primary care provider but we have no studies that address what happens when a rural woman develops a disease that requires referral to an urban health care facility. Can she communicate with her provider in this environment?

Rural living, especially for the poor who may have limited access to health care providers, may be considered a health risk. A major goal for the health of all rural persons is better nutrition and exercise and smoking cessation, yet communicating these health messages is difficult. Rural companies are often small and don't have health promotion programs or health care providers on staff. Further, the context of farm work has changed. Farmers used to balance their caloric intake with hard work and physical exercise, but the mechanization of present-day farm work has decreased the physical activity involved. Developing and delivering appropriate health promotion messages to farm families is a challenge for health care providers. The fact that the health care provider lives in the community can also be a challenge. For example, it would be difficult for a nurse practitioner who smokes to present credible smoking cessation information if her patients see her smoking. On the other hand, if the nurse practitioner announces she is quitting and invites her patients who smoke to join her, she might have a major impact in decreasing the smoking in her community.

Special Populations

Elderly Women

Elderly rural women's health care needs are underresearched. Most research on retirement, resources, and health care for aging persons has focused on men or urban women. In one county in Arizona, one of the most heavily populated with elders, the suicide rate is 32.4 per 100,000, compared with a nationwide rate of 19.4 per 100,000 elders (McIntosh, 1992). As suicide rates denote serious problems for elders, further understanding of how elders fare in rural areas must be explored.

Rural elders have lower average incomes, less health insurance, and higher poverty rates than urban persons (Dimond, 1995). This profile suggests that rural elders are more dependent on Medicare for health services. Historically, many rural physicians kept their costs lower than their urban counterparts. As a result, they are often seriously underpaid by Medicare, leading some of them to refuse Medicare patients (Dimond, 1995). Medicare also does not cover many chronic illnesses. Rural elders who are limited in their activities because of chronic illness may have a very difficult time gaining access to services.

McCulloch (1991) presented the findings of her study on health maintenance practices of older rural women residing in the southeast United States. She compared women who survived and those who did not over a 10-year period (1976 to 1986). She found that her sample of rural elderly women reported arthritis, hypertension, and circulatory problems as their most common health care problems. Aside from these diseases, the women's self-reports of their health status were generally positive. McCulloch suggested these women were a "survivor elite group," characterized by a level of hardiness that is long-standing. These women also did not seem to decline from chronic illness quickly. Their health status over the 10 years of the study was consistently good. Indeed, their arthritis was less troubling after 10 years. McCulloch suggested that improvements in arthritis treatment and self-imposed limitations by the women may have led to this finding.

McCulloch (1991) suggested that health education for rural women needs to take into consideration the unique personalities of these women, who are very proud, fiercely independent, and mistrustful of outsiders, especially when the outsiders represent the government. McCulloch's participants reported a delay in cancer diagnosis, which is attributable in part to their reluctance to make appointments with health care providers, whom they perceived to be outsiders. Thus, culturally sensitive ways to educate rural persons about cancer warning signs need to be developed.

In spite of distrust of the government, over the 10 years of the study, increasing numbers of women used Medicare to pay for health care. They also reported help from family and friends (McCulloch, 1991). As health care costs increase, we can anticipate that families and friends will not be able to help bridge the gap between Medicare dollars and the real cost of service, and thus the quality and quantity of health care may be in jeopardy.

McCulloch's study highlights the need for health care providers and policy makers to be sensitive to the needs of poor rural elderly women. Providers need to find ways to educate patients about circulatory disease, the primary killer of the women in the study. Although McCulloch studied one group of rural women in one section of the country, it is likely that her snapshot is similar to other parts of the country.

Lesbian Rural Women

A group of rural women who are virtually invisible are lesbians. A lesbian who lives in a rural context faces the same issues that heterosexual residents face. Added to these challenges, lesbians frequently encounter stigma associated with their sexual orientation, and isolation from their families of birth is a frequent occurrence. This isolation can exacerbate the endemic loneliness found by Cape (1985) in her study of women and rural life. If the majority of older rural women are, according to Cape "out of sight and out of mind," then rural lesbians are invisible even when in sight.

Rural lesbian women face multiple challenges in constructing the social supports necessary for a safe, productive, satisfying life. Coming out and strategically coping with a larger society that continues to stigmatize lesbians presents constant challenges and choices. The woman may or may not have the support of family members when her sexual identity is either revealed or deduced. Outside the family, when each new social situation is entered, choices about what and how much to relay about one's life is constantly before lesbians (Lindhorst, 1997). Many factors—including age, health, type of employment, single or partnered status, personal constructions of lesbian identity, income level, and the types of daily challenges faced—influence where a woman seeks to build and maintain support networks.

A pivotal variable, however, is the relationship the woman has to her own lesbian identity (Shenk & Fullmer, 1996). The cultural construc-

tion of lesbianism involves the historical and environmental context framed within the meaning of lesbianism in the society. For older women in this culture, the context requires consideration of the understanding of homosexuality prevalent earlier in this century.

Although rural Americans have been determined to be more likely to use informal support networks, they are frequently church-based (Rounds, 1988). Given the current polemics within mainline religions around homosexuality and the attendant condemnation of homosexuals, lesbians may not see this informal support in the same light as their heterosexual rural neighbors and thus be isolated from support networks essential to maintain health.

Health care providers are expected to render equal care to all patients irrespective of sexual orientation, and to be accepting or at least tolerant of diversity in the clients they serve. However, a review of the literature addressing the experiences of lesbians in the health care arena showed that they experienced a mixture of fear, betrayal, and scorn in their health care encounters. The characteristics most frequently reported included unmet needs, negative actions and feelings, heterosexism, and lesbian self-protective strategies.

The analysis of these books and articles also revealed that the primary concern among many lesbians when seeking care was how to balance the need to reveal their lesbianism and the need to conceal it. They spent a great amount of time seeking out a provider who, if not "positive" about lesbians, was at least not negative. They also spent time during the visit to the provider trying to decide how much they should reveal about their lives, whether or not to disclose their sexual orientation, how relevant it was to their health care, and how risky it was to disclose (Flanders, 1992; Hall, 1994a, 1994b; Hitchcock & Wilson, 1992; Robertson, 1992).

Minority Women

Minority women's mortality rate is four to five times that of white women at all ages (Gardner & Hudson, 1996). Yet African American, Latino, and Native American women have one characteristic in common when it comes to health care. That is, the best predictor of their health is their economic status regardless race or ethnicity (Giachello, 1998; Goodwin & Carter, 1998; Wetly, 1998). The minority rural women in the United States are a very diverse group. However, few have high school education, jobs with health care benefits, and other opportunities that are associated with good health. Within-group differences are pronounced due to differences in economics, education, citizenship status and other demographic characteristics (for example, marital status and parenthood) that differentiate all persons. Cancer, heart disease, diabetes, and mental illness are the major health problems of rural minority women (Gardner & Hudson, 1996).

There is little research on rural minority women. The following discussion will draw on the literature on minority women, suggesting that access, cost, literacy, and the other problems that urban women face are multiplied for the rural minority woman. Only African American, Latino, and American Indian women will be included in the discussion, as they are the most frequently studied.

African American Women. African American women experience almost three times the poverty rate of white Americans (31.3% versus 12.3%). While the poverty rate is high, it is even more impressive that the 68.7% of African American who are not poor nonethless have more health problems than their white counterparts (Goodwin & Carter, 1998). Reasons for this are: (1) culturally sensitive health education materials, services, and providers are scarce; (2) high-quality health care is limited in most African American communities; (3) these communities are targeted by the tobacco and alcohol industries for advertising; (4) members of this group often hold jobs that do not include health benefits. Seventy-six percent of poor African American women are single heads of household and have achieved low levels of education. They use emergency departments for health care, resulting in episodic, impersonal care.

Institutional racism causes stress and lowered self-esteem (Goodwin & Carter, 1998). Access to stress management and leisure activities, which are not common in rural areas, are likely more restricted for rural African American women. It is likely that cigarette smoking and alcohol use are substitutes for other forms of stress reduction that do not exist in rural areas. In recent years, persons from the Caribbean, Haiti, and Central and South America have immigrated to the United States and are moving to rural areas. Although many of these people speak English, they have lifeways, cultural patterns, and health beliefs that prevent them from using the health care system, even if they have access. These persons may not understand health interview questions and give answers that result in misdiagnosis. Culturally sensitive information and treatment options need to be developed so appropriate care can be delivered.

Latino Women. The picture is quite similar for Latina rural women (Giachello, 1998). Latina women are among the most diverse women in the country. Some are people of color and experience racism. Some have been here for generations and are citizens; others are new immigrants. The recent immigrants tend to be young and have specific needs for culturally sensitive, bilingual reproductive care.

The Latino culture values family, religion, and traditional self-care practices (Giachello, 1998). A Latina patient is likely to have a Western medical practitioner and a *curandero* or *espiritista* treating the same illness. Some folk healers use herbs that have active ingredients, such as foxglove tea that contains digitalis. If the Western medical practitioner also prescribes digitalis tablets, an overdose may result. In spite of low levels of education and income and nonuse of prenatal services, first-generation Mexicans have few low birth weight babies and a low infant mortality rate (Giachello, 1994). Unfortunately, continued assimilation into the American culture decreases the use of traditional folkways that are beneficial in pregnancy. By the next generation, the incidence of low birth weight and infant mortality, for example, approaches that of other poor women.

Similar to other rural women, Latina women have a distrust of government. They also consider accepting help from someone other than family is charity. Some, as was seen in the section on cancer, either speak only Spanish or prefer Spanish, and are reluctant to approach non-Latino health care providers (Lopez, 1992).

Culturally sensitive health education and health services are not generally available to Latina women and are particularly limited in rural areas.

American Indian Women. The situation of American Indian women is similar to other minority women, with racism, lack of cultural sensitivity, and neglect by the dominant culture contributing to health problems. Until the 1960s, Native Americans often lived in family groups on reservations (Wetly, 1998). They were physically active and used native foods that tend to be low in calories and fat. While health care services on the reservation were minimal, the lifestyle of the people was healthy.

In the 1960s Native Americans began to migrate to cities where stress, processed foods, and sedentary lifestyles were the norm. Alcohol use and cigarette smoking are endemic among Native American women. As would be expected with this lifestyle, heart disease, cancer, injury, diabetes, and stroke are the major causes of mortality (U.S. Department of Health and Human Services, 1994). Genetics also plays a role in the development of diabetes in some American Indian populations. For example, a mutation related to noninsulin dependent diabetes was found almost four times more frequently in a Pima Indian sample (Arizona) than in whites (Walston, Silver, Bogardus, & Knowler, 1995).

In order to plan health services for American Indians, providers need to work with the tribal community (Wetly, 1998). There are vast variations in health; for example, some groups have infant mortality rates and maternal death rates that are lower than the general population. Some generations are more acculturated to the dominant culture than others, creating a situation wherein one generation is quite different than others. For example, Carrese and Rhodes (1995) explored the bioethics around end-of-life issues in a Navajo community. Navajo have a traditional value that avoids death and all discussion of it. Older Navajos in the sample did not want to talk about end of life as it violates their concept of *hozho*.

One service that seems to be needed in American Indian communities is culturally sensitive alcohol counseling (May, 1995). Like other rural women, American Indian women are hampered in their quest for sobriety by lack of child care and sober role models and by poverty and abusive relationships. Preparing educational materials that are relevant for American Indian communities is a challenge because historically the communities were steeped in an oral tradition. Written and visual education imposed on the American Indian in the missionary schools had as a goal the destruction of the native culture. Finding useful means of patient education will require collaboration between health care providers and traditional healers.

Summary

In summary, the authors presented an argument that the biomedical model is unsatisfactory for women's research, making the case that women's health care research needs to be more holistic and environmentally sensitive than the biomedical model allows. The review of rural women's health presented here demonstrates that health care providers have not developed evidence-based practice for rural women, but have relied on evidence of urban women's symptoms and treatment for the management of diseases and subsequent intervention. The burden of a disease is different for rural women because of fewer services, greater geographic distances from essential services, and the lack of social support. Culture-sensitive health education is often lacking and this is an area of great need. Especially sparse is the research on communication between providers and patients, and rural health promotion interventions. Issues of access and aging are major concerns for rural women; especially vulnerable are elderly, lesbian, and minority women. From the research presented here, one can conclude that living in a rural environment is a health risk for some women and exacerbated if a woman is minority status, elderly, poor, or poorly educated.

Policies and research for the future need to test interventions that are sensitive for rural women and model optimal delivery of services suited to rural problems. Policymakers need to be sensitive to the heterogeneity that characterizes rural environments. Immigration increases the diversity of the U.S. population and presents specific challenges in rural areas. Health care providers need to behave in ways that draw out the strengths of health care traditions of persons from nonwhite cultures to assure meaningful and successful health outcomes that will have long-lasting benefits. Specifically, the unique characteristics of rural life and the circumstances of women must be considered in research, design, and delivery of health services and health policy.

References

Agency for Health Care Policy and Research. (1991). *National medical expenditure survey: Access to health care: Findings from the survey of American Indians and Alaska Natives.* Washington, DC: U.S. Government Printing Office (Publication no. DHHS 91-0028).

American Association of Colleges of Nursing. (1999). *Questionnaire on women's issues in baccalaureate curriculum.* Washington, DC: Author.

American Medical Association. (1991). Gender disparities in clinical decision-making. *JAMA, 266,* 559–562.

Austin, L., & Jacobson, B. (1986). Managing incontinence can save dignity and cut costs. *Provider, 12*(7), 44–49.

Bachman, R. (Ed.) (1994). *Violence Against Women: A National Crime Victimization Survey Report.* Washington, DC: U. S. Department of Justice.

Beckman, L. J. (1994). Treatment needs of women with alcohol problems. *Alcohol Health & Research World, 18*(3), 206–211.

Belenky, M. F., Clinchy, B. M., Goldberger, N. R., & Tarule, J. M. (1986). *Women's ways of knowing: The development of self, voice, and mind.* New York: Basic Books.

Benderly, B. L. (1997). *In her own right.* Washington, DC National Academy Press.

Boyd, M. R. (1998). Substance abuse in rural women. *Nursing Connections, 11*(2), 33–45.

Bushey, A. (1998). Health issues of women in rural environments: An overview. *JAMA, 53*(2), 53–56.

Cape, E. (1985). Out of sight, out of mind: Aging women in rural society. *Women and Environments, 7*(3), 4–6.

Carrese, J., & Rhodes, L. (1995) Western bioethics on the Navajo reservation: Benefit or harm? *JAMA, 274,* 826–829.

Davis, T. C., Arnold, C., Berkel, H., Nandy, I., Jackson, R. H., & Glass, J. (1996). Knowledge and attitude on screening mammography among low-literate, low-income women requires study. *Cancer, 79*(9), 1912–1920.

Dimond, J. (1995). Determinants of quality of life for rural elders. *Journal of Rural Health, 11*(2), 146–154.

Dole, G. R., & Carney, P. A. (1998). Characteristics of underserved women who did and those who did not use a free/low-cost voucher as a part of a mammography screening program. *Journal of Cancer Education, 13*(2), 102–107.

Durak, E. P., Jovanovic-Peterson, L., & Peterson, C. M. (1990). Comparative evaluation of uterine response to exercise on five aerobic machines. *American Journal of Obstetrics and Gynecology, 162,* 754–756.

Elders, J. M., & Teuter, J. M. (1993). Public health. In B. A. Elliott, S. J. Price (Eds.), *Visions 2010: Families and health care* (pp. 2–3). Minneapolis, MN: National Council of Family Relations.

Elliott, B. A., & Johnson, M. M. (1995). Domestic violence in a primary care setting: Patterns and prevalence. *Archives of Family Medicine, 4,* 113–119.

Eng, E. (1993). The Save our Sister project: A social network strategy for reaching rural black women. *Cancer, 72*(3), 1071–1077.

Engel, G. I. (1977). The need for a new medical model: A challenge for biomedicine. *Science, 196,* 129–136.

Fife, R. S. (1998). Osteoarthritis in elderly women. In L. A. Wallis (Ed.), *Textbook of women's health.* (pp. 439–444). Philadelphia: Lippincott-Raven.

Flanders, L. (1992). Nowhere to hide: AIDS, an equal opportunity killer, invades the lesbian community. *New Directions for Women, 25,* 6–7.

Fogel, C. I., & Woods, N. R. (1995). Midlife women's health. In C. I. Fogel & N. F. Woods. (Eds.), *Women's health care,* (pp. 79–100). Thousand Oaks, CA: Sage.

Friedman, L. C., Neff, N. E., Webb, J. A., & Latham, C. K. (1998). Age-related differences in mammography use and in breast cancer knowledge, attitudes and behaviors. *Journal of Cancer Education, 13,* 26–30.

Frost, J. (1996). Family planning clinic services in the United States, 1994. *Family Planning Perspectives, 28*(3), 92–100.

Gardner, P., & Hudson, B. L. (1996). Advance report of final mortality statistics 1993. *Monthly Vital Statistics Report, 44*(7). National Center for Health Statistics.

Geller, J. M. (1999). Rural primary care providers' perceptions of their roles in the provision of mental health services: Voices for the plains. *Journal of Rural Health, 15*(3), 326–334.

Giachello, A. L. (1994). Maternal/perinatal health issues. In C. W. Molina, M. Aguirre-Molina (Eds.), *Latino health in the U.S.: A growing challenge* (pp. 48–59). Washington DC: American Public Health Association.

Giachello, A. L. (1998). Hispanic/Latino women's health. In L. A. Wallis (Ed.), *Textbook of women's health.* (pp. 69–76). Philadelphia: Lippincott-Raven.

Gilligan, C. (1982). *In a different voice: Psychological theory and women's development.* Cambridge, MA: Harvard University Press.

Giuliano, A., Papenfuss, M., deZapien, J., Tilousi, S., & Nuvayestewa, L. (1998). Breast cancer screening among southwest American Indian women living on reservations. *Preventive Medicine, 27,* 135–143.

Goodwin, M. J., & Carter, A. B. (1998). African-American women. In L. A. Wallis (Ed.), *Textbook of women's health* (pp. 63–67). Philadelphia: Lippincott-Raven.

Hall, J. M. (1994a). Lesbians recovering from alcohol problems: An ethnographic study of health care experiences. *Nursing Research, 43*(4), 238–244.

Hall, J. M. (1994b). How lesbians recognize and respond to alcohol problems: A theoretical model of problematization. *Advances in Nursing Science, 16*(3), 46–63.

Harman, W. (1994). A re-examination of the metaphysical foundations of modern science: Why is it necessary? In W. Harman & J. Clark (Eds.), *New metaphysical foundations of modern science* (pp. 1–14) Sausalito, CA: Institute of Noetic Sciences.

Harris, R. P., Fletcher, S. W., & Gonzalez, J. J. (1991). Mammography and age: Are we targeting the wrong women? A community survey of women and physicians. *Cancer, 67,* 2010–2014.

Hartley, D., Korsen, N., Bird, D., & Agger, M. (1998). Management of patients with depression by rural primary care practitioners. *Archives of Family Medicine, 7,* 139–145.

Hauenstein, E. (1996a). Testing innovative nursing care: Home intervention with depressed rural women. *Issues in Mental Health Nursing, 17,* 33–50.

Hauenstein, E. (1996a). A nursing practice paradigm for depressed rural women: Theoretical basis. *Archives of Psychiatric Nursing, 10*(5), 283-292.

Hauenstein, E., & Boyd, M. (1994). Depressive symptoms in young women of the Piedmont: Prevalence in rural women. *Women & Health, 21*(2/3), 105–123.

Heaney, R. P. (1998). Osteoporosis. In L. A. Wallis (Ed.), *Textbook of women's health* (pp. 445–454). Philadelphia: Lippincott-Raven.

Hitchcock, J. M., & Wilson, H. S. (1992). Personal risking: Lesbian self-disclosure of sexual orientation to professional health care providers. *Nursing Research, 41*(3), 178–183.

Johnson, M., & Elliott, B. A. (1997). Domestic violence among family practice patients in midsized and rural communities. *Journal of Family Practice, 44*(4), 391–400.

Johnson, T. L., & Fee, E. (1997). Women's health research: An introduction. In F. P. Haseltine & B. G. Jacobson (Eds.), *Women's health research* (pp. 3–26). Washington, DC: Health Press International.

Jovanovic-Peterson, L., & Peterson, C. M. (1990). Fuel metabolism in pregnancy - clinical aspects. In R. A. Mittelmark, R. A. Wiswell, & B. L. Drinkwater (Eds.), *Exercise in pregnancy* (pp. 45–60). Baltimore, MD: Williams and Wilkins.

Koss, M. P., & Heslet, L. (1992). Somatic consequences of violence against women. *Archives of Family Medicine, 1,* 53–59.

Kuhn, T. (1970). *The structure of scientific revolutions* (2nd ed.). Chicago: University of Chicago Press.

Lantz, P. M., Weigers, M. E., & House, J. S. (1997). Education and income differentials in breast and cervical cancer screening. *Medical Care, 35*(3), 219–236.

Lewin-Epstein, N. (1991). Determinants of regular source of health care in black, Mexican, Puerto Rican, and non-Hispanic white populations. *Medical Care, 29,* 543–557.

Lindhorst, T. (1997). Lesbians and ginned men in the country: Practice implications for rural social workers. *Journal of Gay and Lesbian Social Services, 7*(3), 1–11.

Long, K. A., & Weinert, C. (1989). Rural nursing: Developing the theory base. *Scholarly Inquiry for Nursing Practice: An International Journal, 3,* 113–127.

Long, K. A., & Weinert, C. (1998). Rural nursing: Developing the theory base. In Helen J. Lee (Ed.), *Conceptual basis for rural nursing* (pp. 3–18) New York: Springer.

Lopez, C. (1992). *Reaching and serving Hispanic elderly: A guide for non-Hispanic organizations.* Washington, DC: National Council of LaRaza Office of Institutional Development.

Lundman, B., Asplund, K., & Norberg, A. (1990). Living with diabetes: Perceptions of well-being. *Research in Nursing and Health, 13,* 255–262.

Lyons-Ruth, K., Connell, D., Grunebaum, H., & Botein, S. (1990). Infants at social risk: Maternal depression and family support services as mediators of infant development and security of attachment. *Child Development, 61,* 85–98.

Mah, Z., & Bryant, H. (1992). Age as a factor in breast cancer knowledge, attitudes and screening behaviour. *Canadian Medical Association Journal, 146,* 2167–2174.

Mann, C. (1995). Women's health research blossoms. *Science, 269,* 766–770.

Manson, J. E., Sampler, M.D., & Colditz, G. A. (1991). A prospective study of aspirin use and primary prevention of cardiovascular disease in women. *JAMA 266,* 521–527.

Manzi, S., & Ramsey-Goldman, R. (1999). Autoimmune diseases. In R. B. Ness & L. H. Kuller (Eds). *Health and disease among women: Biological and environmental influences* (pp. 342–372). New York: Oxford University Press.

May, P. A. (1995). The epidemiology of alcohol abuse among American Indians: The mythical and real properties. *The HIS provider, 20,* 41–50.

McIntosh, K. (1992). Epidemiology of suicide in the

elderly. *Suicide & Life-Threatening Behavior, 22*(1), 15–35.

McCulloch, J. (1991). Health and health maintenance profiles of older rural women, 1976–1986. In A. Bushey (Ed.), *Rural nursing* (Vol. 1; pp. 281–296). Thousand Oaks, CA: Sage.

McGrath, E., Keita, G., Strickland, B., & Russo, N. (1990). *Women and depression: Risk factors and treatment issues* (Final report of the American Psychological Association National Task Force on Women and Depression). Washington, DC: American Psychological Association.

Millman, M. (1993). *Access to health care in America.* Washington, DC: National Academy Press.

Moormeier, J. (1996). Breast cancer in Black women. *Annals of Internal Medicine, 124*(10), 897–905.

Mulford, M. I., Jovanovic-Peterson, L., & Peterson, C. M. (1993). Alternative therapies for the management of gestational diabetes. *Clinical Perinatology, 20*, 619–634.

Multiple Risk Factor Intervention Trial Group. (1997). Statistical design considerations in the NHLI Multiple Risk Factor Intervention (MRFIT). *Journal of Chronic Diseases, 30*, 261–275.

National Institutes of Health. (1991). *Opportunities for research on women's health.* Washington, DC: Author.

Nutting, P., Calonge, N., Iverson, D., & Green, L. (1994). The danger of applying uniform clinical policies across populations. The care of breast cancer among American Indians. *American Journal of Public health, 84*, 1631–1636.

Office of Technology Assessment. (1994). *Health care reform: Current trends in health care costs and health insurance coverage.* Washington, DC: U.S. Government Printing Office.

Pearson, T., & Lewis, C. (1998). Rural epidemiology: Insights fro m arural population laboratory. *American Journal of Epidemiology, 148*(10), 949–957.

Phipps, W., Long, B., Woods, N. F., & Cassmeyer, V. (1991). *Medical-surgical nursing* (4th ed.). St. Louis, MO: C. V. Mosby.

Powers, M. (1986). *Oglala women: Myth, ritual, and reality.* Chicago: University of Chicago Press.

Primomo, J. (1995). Chronic illnesses and women. In C. I. Fogel & N. F. Woods (Eds.), *Women's health care* (pp. 651–669). Thousand Oaks, CA: Sage.

Ramey, E. (1997). How female and male biology differ. In F. P. Haseltine & B. G. Jacobson (Eds.), *Women's health research: A medical and policy primer* (pp. 47–62). Washington, DC: Health Press International.

Rizzo, T., Metzger, B. E., & Burns, W. J. (1991). Correlations between antepartum maternal metabolism and intelligence of offspring. *New England Journal of Medicine, 325*, 911–916.

Robertson, M. M. (1992). Lesbians as an invisible minority in the health services arena. *Health Care for Women International, 13*(2), 155–163.

Rost, K. Williams, C., Wherry, J., & Smith, G. R. (1995). The process and outcomes of care for major depression in rural family practice settings. *Journal of Rural Health, 11*,114–120.

Rounds, K. (1988). Responding to AIDS: Rural community strategies. *Social Casework, 69*(6), 360–364.

Samet, J., Kay, C., Hunt, W., & Goodwin, J. (1987). Survival of American Indian and Hispanic cancer patients in New Mexico and Arizona. *Journal of National Cancer Institute, 79*, 457–463.

Saunders, D. G., Hamberger, L. K., & Hovey, M. (1993). Indicators of woman abuse based on a chart review at a family practice center. *Archives of Family Medicine, 2*, 537–543.

Schock, N. W., Greulich, R. C., Andres, R., Arenberg, D., Costa, .T., Lakatta, E. G., & Tobin, J. D. (1984). *Normal human aging: The Baltimore longitudinal study of aging.* Washington, DC: US Government Printing Office.

Shenk, S., & Fuller, E. (1996). Significant relationships among old women: Cultural and personal constructions of lesbianism. *Journal of Women and Aging, 8*(3), 75-89.

Steering Committee of the Physicians Health Study Research Group. (1989). Final report on the aspirin component of the ongoing physicians health study. *New England Journal of Medicine, 321*, 129–135.

Sugg, N. K., & Inui, T. (1992). Primary care physicians' response to domestic violence: Opening Pandora's box. *JAMA, 276*, 3157-3160.

Surgeon General's Workshop on Violence and Public Health. (1986). *Surgeon General's workshop on violence and public health: Report.* Washington, DC: U. S. Department of Health and Human Services, Public Health Service.

Thurston-Hicks, A., Paine, S., & Hollifield, M. (1998). Functional impairment associated with psychological distress and medical severity in rural primary care patients. *Psychiatric Services, 49*(7), 951–955.

U.S. Department of Health and Human Services. (1994). *Trends in Indian health 1989 and 1994. Washington, DC:* Public health Service, Indian Health Service, Office of Planning Evaluation and Legislation, Division of Program Statistics.

Veille, J. C., Hohimer, R. A., Burry, K. (1985). The effect of exercise on uterine activity in the last eight weeks of pregnancy. *American journal of Obstetrics and Gynecology, 151*, 727–730.

Vermont Department of Health (1993). *Healthy Vermonters 2000.* Montpelier, VT: Author.

Walston, J., Silver, K., Bogardus, C., Knowler, W. C. (1995). Time of onset of non-insulin-dependent diabetes and genetic variation in the beta 3 adrenergic receptor gene. *New England Journal of Medicine, 333*, 343–347.

Weisman, C. S. (1998). *Women's health care.* Baltimore, MD: Johns Hopkins Press.

Weisner, C., & Schmidt, L. (1992). Gender disparities in treatment for alcohol problems. *JAMA, 268,* 1872–1876.

Wetly, E. R. (1998). American Indian/Alaska Native women. In L. A. Wallis (Ed.). *Textbook of Women's Health* (pp. 77–83). Philadelphia: Lippincott-Raven.

Woods, N. F. (1992). Status of women's health care. *Institute of Medicine 1992 Annual Meeting.* Washington, DC: National Academy Press.

9

Pediatric and Adolescent Health

NEVA ABBOTT AND KAREN OLNESS

Children and adolescents who live in rural areas anywhere in the world will experience different cultures, health risks, and health care delivery systems than will those who live in metropolitan or urban areas. Throughout the world there are geographic barriers to child health services and this is reflected in health-related statistics. The intention of this chapter is to review information about the health of children and adolescents who live in rural areas of the United States, compare the health status of these children with those who live in urban areas, and make recommendations for improvement of health care of rural children.

Demography and History

Rural children in the United States make up a much more heterogeneous group than they did in past generations when they were more comparable to rural children in less developed countries. There, children are a significant part of the rural economy that, in turn, is almost entirely dominated by agriculture. It is important to have many children to do the manual labor of agriculture, to assure there will still be enough children if some die (which is considered in-

evitable in many cultures), and to care for parents and grandparents in their older years.

Today in the United States, as a result of ever-increasing technology and mobility, less than 2% of the nation's population lives on farms (Simon, 1999). With the 1997 Census of Agriculture calculating the average age of farm operators to be 54 years, it may be that the percentage of children living on farms is less than the percentage of children in the total population. It is impossible to say for sure because the Census of Agriculture is so geared to economic issues that it counts livestock but ignores children. Farm operators, in addition to increasing in average age over the years, are also decreasing in numbers (as farms become larger), and are more likely to be female, to be of a race other than white, and to have a principal occupation other than farming. The number and nature of children on the farm are also influenced by the presence of migrants who are hired to work on farms, usually performing tedious hand labor. These workers may have children or be adolescents themselves.

The Census Bureau estimates the present nonmetropolitan population to be about 20% of the entire population of the United States. The last time that the bureau compared urban to rural population was in the 1990 census when it was considered to be 75% urban and 25% rural (U.S. Bureau of the Census, 1997). How the present nonmetropolitan population may be divided into urban and rural is not clear. The actual numbers are about 270 million for the entire population of the country, 54 million of whom live outside metropolitan areas. Of the

NEVA ABBOTT • Monroe, North Carolina 28110. KAREN OLNESS • Department of Pediatrics, Case Western Reserve University, and Rainbow Center for International Child Health (RCIC), Rainbow Babies and Children's Hospital, Cleveland, Ohio 44106-6003.

Handbook of Rural Health, edited by Loue and Quill. Kluwer Academic/Plenum Publishers, New York, 2001.

latter about 14 million (26%) are under the age of 18.

Accuracy in enumerating persons becomes very important to individual states and counties because the amount of Medicaid and other federal funds received are directly linked to population (Goodman, 1999). Union County in North Carolina is a rural county that is experiencing tremendous growth in its Hispanic population. The Census Bureau now estimates that it missed 38% or about 30,000 people in this county in 1990 through undercounting in African American and Hispanic neighborhoods. Recent immigrants can also create a need for health expenditures. For example, much of the Hispanic population in Union County has come directly from regions of Mexico that do not immunize their children. This has resulted in the need for the Health Department to pay significant sums of money to control outbreaks of rubella among young Hispanic adults.

There is no one demographic factor relating to health—other than distance to medical care—that distinguishes the entire rural population from the urban population in the United States. Even distance to care varies enormously among rural communities. Consider California and Montana: California's population is 93% urban while Montana's is 52% urban according to the 1990 census, but California has three and a half times as many farms as Montana. The farms are so much larger and the population so much more scattered in Montana that it is generally more difficult for rural people to access medical care there than it is in California.

Aggregate statistics from the entire nation's nonmetropolitan population do not adequately define individual rural communities. Health care services and delivery systems must be tailored to the particular demographic, social, political, historical, and environmental realities of each rural service area.

Access to Health Care

Children and adolescents living in rural areas usually have limited access to care for certain medical conditions because of the lack of specialized personnel and facilities in rural clinics and hospitals. During the past 25 years there have been great advances in development of regional services to make specialized medical services more easily available for adults and children. Children are often transported to regional centers to receive neonatal or intensive care for injuries. Such transport is associated with expense, inconvenience, and additional stress for families. There is excess morbidity associated with interhospital transport (Kanter, Boeing, Hannan, & Kanter, 1992).

A recent study in Washington State (Melzer, Grossman, Hart, & Rosenblatt, 1997) examined the delivery of hospital services for rural children younger than 18 years via a retrospective review of statewide hospital discharge data. This review found that, of 69,690 pediatric hospital discharges during the study period, 16% were rural residents and 10% were from rural hospitals. Rural hospitals cared for 59% of hospitalized rural children. The urban hospitals in Washington had two-thirds of discharges for diseases requiring chemotherapy, psychiatric disorders, and neonates with multiple severe problems. The rural hospitals had the majority of discharges for gastrointestinal diagnoses, respiratory conditions, or minor neonatal problems. Rural hospitals with staff pediatricians had higher annual pediatric discharges, total charges, lengths of stay, and sick newborns compared with hospitals without pediatricians. However, there was no evidence that the hospitals with pediatricians served as local referral centers, although the average rural pediatrician cared for five times as many inpatients as a rural family practitioner. Intrarural transfer of hospitalized children was uncommon and patients in the catchment areas of hospitals without pediatricians were either being treated locally in those hospitals or referred to urban centers. The authors noted that the low transfer rate may reflect a failure of family practitioners to recognize a difference in competency between themselves and rural pediatricians, an unwillingness on the part of rural pediatricians to accept transfers from outside their catchment areas, or financial or medicolegal concerns related to the types of patients received in transport. They concluded that family practitioners contemplating rural practice should receive training in general inpatient pediatrics and that pediatricians in rural practice must be prepared for a high volume of inpatient care. Clinical and educational links between urban regional centers and rural providers is important.

Of children living in rural areas, those who are in families of migrant workers are among the most deprived with respect to access to health care services. Their utilization of medical services is often episodic and their frequent movement to new work sites makes it unlikely that they will have a medical home. Although these children may be legal immigrants, if they entered the United States after 1996 they are eligible for Medicaid only after five years. Both legal and illegal immigrants not eligible for Medicaid are covered for emergency services but not for preventive services such as well child care. The children of migrant children may not have access to immunizations. They are likely to have more nutritional problems, dental problems, and infectious diseases than rural children who live in a more stable environment. A recent study suggested innovative nursing strategies to improve access to health care for migrant children. These included the training of lay community outreach workers and the development of information tracking systems (Gwyther & Jenkins, 1998).

A study of barriers to child health services in rural northern New England between 1980 and 1989 found that travel times to physicians decreased only slightly during the decade. Of 363,443 children living in 936 nonmetropolitan areas, 15.5% were more than 30 minutes from pediatricians in 1989 and travel to emergency rooms was more than 30 minutes for 10% of the children. In contrast, only 1.8% of children faced excessive travel times to family practitioners (Goodman, Barff, & Fisher, 1992).

A number of studies have documented that emergency room resources and use for children and adolescents vary depending on whether they come from rural or urban areas (Svenson, Nypaver, & Calhoun, 1996; Smith, Thompson, Shields, Manley, & Haley, 1997). In rural areas of Kentucky it was noted that trauma accounted for nearly half of all emergency room runs, and ambulance time was prolonged. Advanced life support procedures were performed infrequently, especially in younger patients. There is evidence that emergency care personnel in rural areas are not sufficiently experienced in management of acutely ill and injured children. A study of death rates from trauma among children in Kentucky found them to be much higher in rural settings (Svenson, Spurlock, & Nypaver, 1996a).

Economic Issues

A study of adolescent health care from 1990 found that nonmetropolitan adolescents made fewer physician visits and were more apt to delay seeking physician care than were metropolitan adolescents. Adolescents in rural areas were 39% more likely to be hospitalized and 30% had no form of health insurance. Although the adolescents in rural areas came from families with higher rates of poverty, they were 20% less likely to be publicly insured (McManus, Newacheck, & Weader, 1990).

The health care utilization and costs of previously uninsured rural children were examined by Tilford, Robbins, Shema, & Farmer (1999) through four years of claims data from a school-based health insurance program located in the Mississippi Delta. All children who were not Medicaid-eligible, or were uninsured, were eligible for limited benefits under the program. The 1987 National Medical Expenditure Survey (NMES) was used to compare utilization of services. The study represents a natural experiment in the provision of insurance benefits to a previously uninsured population. Premiums for the claims cost were set with little or no information on expected use of services. Claims from the insurer were used to determine the response to insurance for several categories of health services. The use of services increased over time and approached the level of utilization in the NMES. Actuarial estimates of claims cost greatly exceeded actual claims cost. The provision of a limited medical, dental, and optical benefit package cost approximately $20 to $24 per member per month in claims paid. The study's authors concluded that an important uncertainty in providing health insurance to previously uninsured populations is whether a pent-up demand exists for health services. Evidence of a pent-up demand for medical services was not supported in this study of rural school-age children. States considering partnerships with private insurers to implement the state-based Children's Health Insurance Program could lower premium costs by assembling basic data on previously uninsured children.

Special Hazards

There are few studies documenting the unique hazards for children who live in rural areas and those that have been done may not be applicable to all rural areas throughout the entire nation.

Environmental Hazards

The Environmental Protection Agency (EPA, 1996) states that children are particularly at risk from environmental hazards in three ways:

- Because children's systems are developing—including rapid changes in growth, immature body organs and tissues, and weaker immune systems in infancy—they are more susceptible to environmental threats.
- Because children eat proportionately more food, drink more fluids, and breathe more air per pound of body weight than adults, and because they play outside more, they are more exposed to environmental threats.
- Because children are least able to protect themselves, their behavior—such as crawling on the ground or the floor—exposes them to different environmental hazards.

Although all children are at risk for damage from environmental hazards, children who live on farms are at even greater risk. Many agricultural activities generate dust (from soil, hay, or grain) and children may inhale allergens or microbial agents such as coccidioidomycosis and blastomycosis. Children on farms are exposed to many animals, including cats and dogs as well as cattle, pigs, and sheep. These animals may spread allergens or infectious diseases such as camplyobacter jejuni diarrhea, rabies, brucellosis, cyptosporidiosis, Escherichia coli 0157:H7 diarrhea, leptospirosis, and cat scratch disease (Bartonella henselae bacteria). Recent studies of feedlots have found that more than 80% of cattle have been infected with Escherichia coli 0157:H7. Children in farming environments are more likely to be exposed to clostridium species (gas gangrene) and to tetanus spores than are urban children. They are at a greater risk of being exposed to Lyme disease, Borrelia (relapsing fever), and Rocky Mountain Spotted Fever. They are at risk of being exposed to toxic gases in silos or near manure pits. And children living on farms are more likely to be exposed to herbicides, insecticides, and allergens.

A 1989 survey of 50 migrant farm-working youths under 18 years found that 11% had mixed or applied pesticides, despite child labor laws that prohibit work with hazardous chemicals (Pollack, Landrigan, & Mallino, 1990). More than 15% of these adolescents had symptoms consistent with organophosphate poisoning but few had sought medical care. Forty percent had been sprayed with pesticides directly by crop-dusting planes or indirectly by drifting chemicals from planes or tractors. Forty percent had worked in fields wet with pesticide for which there was a field reentry time. It is likely that these children did not know about restrictions on reentry or about the risk of pesticides.

One recent study compared the prevalence of Helicobacter pylori (HP) in children from urban and rural areas of West Virginia (Elitsur, Short, & Neace, 1998). Blood samples were collected from 1,164 children. Overall, 40% of samples were positive for HP. HP acquisition was associated with increasing age, crowding, and rural location but not with gender, water source, or socioeconomic status. The reason for the increased likelihood of HP infection in children from rural areas was not clear.

Lead poisoning can cause learning disabilities, behavior problems, and neurological damage in children. According to a newspaper article, some states are lax in insisting that doctors test children on Medicaid for lead poisoning (Pear, 1999). Many doctors do not see lead exposure as a problem for their patients or are unaware of the federal requirements. Also, many poor children do not see a doctor until they are sick, and most children with high levels of lead in the blood display no obvious symptoms at first. About 890,000 children ages 1 through 6 are thought to be poisoned by lead and about 535,000 of these children are enrolled in Medicaid, but fewer than 20%—1.2 million of the 6.3 million recipients—are ever tested. However, in Alaska, universal lead screening for Medicaid-enrolled children is not an effective use of public health resources because the prevalence of lead exposure was very low, although the average blood level of lead in the blood was higher in rural children than in urban children (Robin, Beller, & Middaugh, 1997). The findings provide an example of the importance of considering local and regional differences when formulating screening recommendations and regulations, and continually reevaluating the usefulness of federal regulations.

Physical Injuries

Children and adolescents who live on farms are at special risk from machinery accidents used both for work and recreation. In spite of major publicity efforts to make parents aware of these risks, many children under age 16 continue to operate farm vehicles. They play and work in the same place that their parents work and like to emulate them.

A recent descriptive study of factors influencing exposure of children to major hazards on family farms found that parents were usually knowledgeable about high-risk activities and yet allowed their children to be active participants in hazardous work (Lee, Jenkins, & Westaby, 1997). A sample of 1,255 Wisconsin dairy farm fathers provided data regarding decisions to expose children younger than 14 years to risks of injuries. Fathers' attitudes were the strongest predictors of behavioral intentions, and grandparents and mothers exerted limited influence. Groups such as health care providers, 4-H clubs, Future Farmers of America, and insurers exerted only a modest influence on fathers' feelings of social pressure. The study did not find specific demographic characteristics of the family or farm that were predictive of fathers' intentions to expose children to hazards.

A survey of 169 farm families in Iowa (Hawk, Gay, & Donham, 1991) reinforces this important issue of the disparity between knowledge and behavior. Analysis of these data indicated several issues to target for intervention efforts. One is lack of supervision—more than 40% of children who operate equipment do so unsupervised. Approximately 30% of children over 3 years old play alone in work areas, and 80% of

these children play near machinery in operation. Another issue is operation of farm machinery by very young children—respondents' children began operating equipment at an average age of 12 years. Yet the parents believe their children are not capable of operating equipment until age 15.

A study from Kentucky (Svenson, Spurlock, & Nypaver, 1996b) found that children from rural areas were at increased risk for firearm-related mortality even after controlling for availability of a hospital with 24-hour emergency services, 911 services, and pre-hospital advanced life support. The reason for this is not clear. One can speculate that rural children may be less closely supervised than their urban counterparts and may have observed more firearm use by older family members.

Svenson et al. (1996a) also examined medical and demographic factors associated with traumatic deaths among children in Kentucky. All 1,024 pediatric trauma deaths that occurred from 1988 to 1992 were analyzed. Death rates were calculated for each type of trauma for each county in the state. Motor vehicle accidents accounted for most of the pediatric deaths, but this finding was markedly age-dependent. Death rates were higher in rural Kentucky for all forms of trauma and were highest in the Appalachian region. Rural setting was associated with higher traumatic death rates, whereas the availability of a hospital with 24-hour emergency services in the county and the presence of advanced life support prehospital care were associated with lower death rates. Children in Appalachia were at an increased risk compared with other Kentucky children, even when controlling for the rural nature of Appalachia. The authors' conclusion is that demographic and medical system factors are associated with traumatic death rates in Kentucky children. Both access to care and advanced prehospital support were significantly associated with lower pediatric death rates. Increased access to quality care and training of prehospital providers in advanced life support should be priorities in the planning of trauma systems for this state.

Vane and Shackford (1995) studied the epidemiology of traumatic death in pediatric patients in Vermont. They reviewed all deaths caused by injury in victims under 19 years old between 1985 and 1990. They hypothesized that mortality would be higher than equivalent populations in urban areas. During the study period, 5,322 children were hospitalized for trauma (14% of total admissions for children in the state) and 36 died (0.67%). For this subgroup, head injury was the most common cause of death (72%). When compared with data from the National Pediatric Trauma Registry from urban centers, the mortality rate for hospitalized children in this rural state was lower (0.67% versus 2.7%, $p < 0.001$). On review of the population-based statistics for the entire state, they found that these numbers were deceptively low. In all, 731 children died during the study period; of these, 283 were determined by autopsy or coroner's report to have died of trauma (38.7%). Eighty-seven percent of the children who died never reached the hospital. Mortality (age-adjusted) was highest in the 15- to 18-year-olds (68.5 of 100,000), than in those under one year old (26.8 of 100,000), 1- to 5-year-olds (15.6 of 100,000), and 5- to 14-year-olds (11.8 of 100,000), which significantly exceeds the predicted national averages for these age groups.

Rausch, Sanddal, Sanddal, & Esposito (1998) measured pediatric injury deaths per 100,000 population in the state of Montana from October 1989 to September 1992 with regard to intentionality of injury, mechanism of injury, and use of protective devices. They compared these with previous data about childhood injuries (1980 to 1985) collected by Baker & Waller (1989). Of 121 patients reviewed, 56% were male and 44% were female. Mean age was 7.0 years (median, 8.0). Eighty-one percent of patients were Caucasian and 16% were Native American. The leading cause of injury was motor vehicle crashes, which was followed by drowning, unintentional firearm injuries, deaths related to house fires, homicides, and suicides. Overall, 87% of injuries were unintentional and 13% were intentional, with 62% of these suicides and 38% homicides. When considered independently of intent, firearm-related injuries ranked second. Earlier data showed motor vehicle crashes ranking second, unintentional firearm injuries seventh, and homicides fourth. Comparison of death rates per 100,000 people for the two time periods showed increases in suicide deaths (3.2 versus 0.8) and unintentional firearm injury deaths (2.3 versus 0.6). The authors concluded that the epidemiology of rural pediatric injury-related deaths has changed. Deaths related to suicide and firearms have increased. Violent deaths related to injuries caused by firearms are at a magnitude approaching all other causes. These findings have implications for public health education and injury control strategies in rural areas.

Dunn, Cline, Grant, Masius, Teleki, Snow, Katz, & Carroll (1993) described preventable pediatric injuries and the proportion receiving documented injury prevention instruction by emergency department personnel by reviewing charts retrospectively at a rural Level I trauma center. All injured children aged birth through 15 years presenting to the hospital from January 1, 1987, through December 31, 1987 were included. During the study period, 1,449 injuries presented to the trauma center. Motor vehicle crashes caused the largest number of preventable injuries (71), although the proportion of preventable injuries was higher among poisonings, burns, and pedestrian–automobile collisions. Among the 1,313 patients available to emergency department (ED) personnel at discharge, injury prevention instruction was indicated in 27% of cases but documented in the medical record in only 3%. ED personnel were more likely to document instruction for preventing poisoning than other causes of injury. Most preventable pediatric injuries treated and released by ED personnel do not receive documented injury prevention instruction.

Residential Fires

A study of fatal and nonfatal residential fires in predominantly rural areas of North Carolina found that most fatal fires were due to smoking. People living in mobile homes were at greater risk for death if a fire occurred. The presence of an alcohol-impaired person was also a strong risk factor for death in case of a fire (Runyan, Bangdiwala, Linzer, Sacks, & Butts, 1992). A study of the relationship between social conditions and fire mortality among children in New Mexico found that mobile homes, homes without plumbing, and negligence of adults were associated with death (Parker, Sklar, Tandberg, Hauswald, & Zumwalt, 1993). Of 57 children, 82% died at the scene; only 11% reached a burn center.

Drug Use Among Rural Students

Recent studies have examined the differences in the prevalence of drug use among adolescents who live in rural and in suburban areas. Cronk & Sarvela (1997) concluded there were few differences in drug use practices between rural and urban adolescents. A study of 464 12th-grade students in west central Ohio were a subset of the larger Dayton Area Drug Survey (DADS) of 1,898 students (Falck, Seigal, Wang, & Carlson, 1999). Schools located in towns with less than 4,000 people and at least 25 miles from Dayton were designated as rural. Of concern was the overall high number of students who indicated lifetime use of selected drugs as well as the percentage of students reporting five or more alcoholic drinks in a row in the preceding two-week period. The study found that 45% of suburban boys compared to 21.5% of rural boys had five or more alcoholic drinks in a row during the preceding two weeks and that 26% of suburban girls compared to 17.6 % of rural girls reported five or more alcoholic drinks. Only 21% of suburban boys and 36% of rural boys reported they had never been drunk compared with 30.5% of suburban girls and 30.2% of rural girls. Significantly more suburban boys (62.3%) than rural boys (38.5%) had used marijuana, whereas 53% of suburban girls and 46.5% of rural girls had used marijuana. Overall, there were no statistically significant differences between girls. Across all drug classes, larger percentages of suburban boys reported use than did rural boys. The authors noted that significantly fewer rural boys held jobs away from home or school when compared with rural girls and suburban peers. They speculated that rural boys were more likely to be under the watchful eye of a parent or teacher. Such surveillance could put them under the tutelage of people who guided them away from drug involvement. The authors also noted that, since rural youths are better known by neighbors and people in the community, behaviors like drug misuse are more difficult to conceal than in more densely populated areas. The relationship between employment and drug use needs further study. Employ-

ment may increase or decrease drug use, depending on the role-modeling of employers and co-employees.

A recent study of parents in Alaska who had children in Head Start programs found that use of smokeless tobacco, marijuana, and tobacco was much higher than in the 1995 National Household Survey estimates (Stillner, Kraus, Leukefeld, & Hardenbergh, 1999). For example, tobacco use in the previous month was 56% compared to 34.7% in the National Household Survey. For parents between 26 and 34 years, previous-month alcohol use was 63% compared to 38% in the National Household Survey. Families in this study lived in villages with populations under 700 people. School officials complained that children and adolescents in these villages roamed about all night because the parents were drinking. Yet 86% of parents reported that it was wrong to take drugs, to drink a lot, or for someone to force another person to drink, and one-third of parents reported problems related to their drinking such as memory loss and passing out. The authors noted the importance of taking into account the traditional governance of Eskimos before planning programs to reduce drug use among parents of young children.

A study of crack cocaine use among 771 rural migrant workers in South Florida found that they used crack an average of 14 of the previous 30 days (Weatherby, McCoy, Metsch, Beltzer, McCoy, & Da la Rosa, 1999). Among women, however, living with children was negatively related to crack use. Living with children had no significant association with crack use among men. Authors noted that recent participation in drug user treatment seemed to result in more and not less drug use and that social support can be either supportive or destructive. The issue of impact on the children was not addressed in this paper. A limitation in this and similar studies is a failure to do detailed learning assessments among parents. Interventions probably need to take into account specific learning disabilities that may affect both parents and children.

HIV Disease and Rural Children

HIV infection occurs in rural areas. From 1991 to 1992 the increased percentage of cases was higher in nonmetropolitan areas than in any other areas of residence. Unfortunately, good epidemiological studies of HIV in rural areas are lacking, and children of HIV-infected parents are at risk. In general it is believed that those at greatest risk are migrant and seasonal farmworkers, people who abuse alcohol, prostitutes, black women, and users of intravenous drugs and crack cocaine (Berry, 1993). HIV infection is associated with drug use. Because of high rates of drug use among migrant farmworkers, the National Institute on Drug Abuse funded the Migrant Health Study to examine HIV risk behaviors among drug-using farmworkers and their sexual partners. A recent study described the behaviors of 151 migrant farm workers in South Florida. Of them, 6% were HIV-positive (Inciardi, Surratt, Colon, Chitwood, & Rivers, 1999). Another study in South Carolina assessed 265 workers ages 16 and older in 15 migrant camps; 13% were HIV-infected and 16% had tests that were reactive for syphilis. Of the 166 who responded to the question on condoms, 46% said they never use them (Jones, Rion, Hollis, Longshore, Leverette, & Ziff, 1991). Although treatment with AZT in pregnancy can reduce transmission to infants to as low as 6%, this is unlikely to occur in migrant families. They are less likely to receive regular prenatal care and to have testing for HIV status. Therefore, there is also an increased likelihood that infants will be born with HIV infection and that this may not be recognized for some time. A recent study of women with HIV disease living in rural communities found that almost half of the women felt stigmatized due to having HIV (Sowel, Lowenstein, Moneyham, Demi, Mizuno, & Seals, 1997). Yet most had disclosed their HIV status to health care workers, sexual partners, and family members.

Rural Children and Disasters

Disasters involve the destruction of property, cause injury and loss of life, and affect large populations. They may be natural such as floods, technological such as radioactive or chemical releases, or complex humanitarian disasters that evolve from civil conflict, economic collapse, and population displacement (Mandalakas, Toresen & Olness, 1999).

Children living in rural areas are at risk of disasters, as are urban children. However, in general, they have less immediate access to treatment for both medical and psychological effects of disasters. Disasters in rural areas can include tornadoes, blizzards, forest fires, floods, hurricanes, earthquakes, avalanches, and chemical disasters such as those related to train derailments or grain bin explosions. Children in the rural areas of the United States were exposed to the disasters of drought and grasshopper invasions in the 1930s. All disasters have psychological and economic effects and most are likely to have lifelong effects on families.

Gaps in a country's infrastructure are most easily exposed during disasters. In rural areas, deficiencies in the ability to handle medical emergencies become evident (Hayes & Baginski, 1993; Koehler & Van Ness, 1993; Danbom, 1993).

Most vulnerable in any disaster are infants, preschool children, pregnant and lactating women, the elderly, and the handicapped. Disasters may be evaluated in three distinct stages: the early or acute emergency phase, the late or recovery phase (1 to 6 months following the disaster) and the rehabilitation phase (more than 6 months after the disaster). During the acute phase the most urgent survival needs of the most vulnerable must be met. These include food, water, shelter, and clothing. Children have unique requirements that make them more vulnerable than adults. They lack the reserves required to endure acute stress. Due to their small size and higher rate of metabolism, they develop dehydration, malnutrition, and fatigue more quickly. They have immature immune systems and are more likely to contract infectious diseases than adults. Hence, the delivery of basic needs is different for children in disaster situations.

If mothers are breast-feeding in disaster situations, it is important to provide them with adequate fluids, food, and as stress-free an environment as possible. A high priority is to facilitate provision of regular breast-feeding for infants. Toddlers on solid foods require smaller, more frequent portions of food. Food distribution plans must take this into account. Giving young children their total caloric requirement for 24 hours in one feeding leads to malnutrition because these children cannot eat so much at one time and because older children or adults may steal food from them.

Shelter and protection from the elements for children must take into account protection from exploitation, abuse, and negative influences of some adults. Children are also the easiest targets for corrupt adults who may be present in disaster situations. In some disaster situations, especially if children have been separated from parents, it may be important to create separate facilities for children.

With respect to sanitation, younger children present a special challenge because, if not toilet-trained, they may contribute to transmission of infectious diseases. Adults who are organizing facilities after a disaster must be aware of this and make special arrangements for very young children who may be without adults and not yet toilet-trained.

With respect to children without family (unaccompanied minors), it is important to identify them in disaster situations and then to find foster care families as soon as possible. If foster care is likely to take time, then it is helpful to find volunteer adult women who will stay with a few unaccompanied minors both day and night. The failure to provide caretakers for children who are displaced from their families may lead to tragic physical and psychological problems.

Children always suffer some psychological consequences from disasters. The event leading to the disaster—tornado or flood or hurricane, for example—may have been intrinsically frightening. Displacement from one's home, familiar objects, and predictable daily life is very frightening. Children may show symptoms of emotional trauma that vary, depending on their age, and may not be obvious to adults (Table 1). They may regress developmentally. Children who were toilet-trained may no longer have bladder and bowel control. They may be more hyperactive and inattentive. Some children become more aggressive and others more withdrawn.

Ideally, child health specialists should be present in disaster situations to provide early intervention for prevention of severe posttraumatic stress symptoms. However, monitoring

Table 9.1. Developmental Responses to Trauma

Toddlers

- Similar reaction to that of parents
- Regression in behaviors
  (e.g., may forget toilet-training)
- Decreased appetite
- Nightmares
- Muteness
- Clinging
- Irritability
- Exaggerated startle response

School-Age Children

- Marked reactions of fear and anxiety
- Increased hostility with siblings
- Somatic complaints (e.g., stomachaches)
- Sleep disorders
- School problems
- Decreased interest in peers, hobbies, school
- Social withdrawal
- Apathy
- Reenactment via play
- Posttraumatic stress disorder

Preadolescents

- Increased hostility with siblings
- Somatic complaints
- Eating disorders
- Sleep disorders
- Decreased interest in peers, hobbies, school
- Rebellion
- Refusal to do chores or to help
- Interpersonal difficulties
- Posttraumatic stress disorder

Adolescents

- Decreased interest in social activities
- Decreased interest in peers, hobbies, school
- Anhedonia
- Decline in responsible behaviors
- Rebellion, behavior problems
- Somatic complaints
- Sleep disorders
- Eating disorders
- Change in physical activity (both increase and decrease)
- Confusion
- Lack of concentration
- Risk-taking behaviors
- Posttraumatic stress disorder

Note: These typical responses to disasters may vary according to the culture and prior living situations.

can be done via family members, teachers, food servers, and all adults who are around children in a disaster. One approach is to talk with parents and caretakers about their children. What behavioral changes do they note? Do young children cry constantly, or are they mute? Do they manifest head-banging and rocking or other self-stimulatory behaviors? Are they unresponsive to physical contact? Do they show developmental regression? Does their play seem normal? Are they acting out the recent events of disasters? Some principles related to prevention involve simple interventions as follows:

1. Develop predictable schedules as soon as possible. These relate to meals, bathing, and daily activities.
2. Initiate school programs as soon as possible. Although some aspects of the school must be jerry-built, it is therapeutic for school-age children to attend school.
3. Initiate organized games, religious services, music, and recreation programs for children and get the older children involved in their planning.
4. Attempt to provide food, sleep rituals, clothing, and toys that are familiar to young children.
5. Support parents as much as possible, depression in parents will contribute to symptoms in their children.

Fortunately, in the United States, most disasters are relatively short and children return to their neighborhoods and homes. This does not mean that they will be spared posttraumatic stress disorder (PTSD). The diagnosis of PTSD is made when the following symptoms persist for more than one month:

- Reexperiencing the event through play, nightmares, or flashbacks; distress with events that resemble or symbolize the trauma
- Routine avoidance of reminders of the event or a general lack of interest in life
- Increased sleep disturbances, irritability, poor concentration, startle reaction, and regression
- Mutism, refusal to speak

Such symptoms require therapeutic intervention. An example is a women in her 90s who had been a child in a farmhouse struck by lightening when she was 7 years old. The farmhouse burned and the family escaped. However, she continued to regress to acute anxiety whenever dark clouds appeared on the horizon. She did this throughout her life, aware on a cognitive level about the origins of her severe anxiety but unable to change it on her own. Early psychological intervention could have prevented her symptoms.

Health Benefits for Children Who Live in Rural Areas

Although our literature search for this chapter did not provide data on specific health benefits from living in rural areas, it is likely that there are several benefits. We strongly encourage research in this area. The statements in the next paragraph reflect personal experience in growing up in a rural area, providing health care for rural children, and, more recently, observing grandchildren in a rural environment.

Children living in small towns and on farms are much more likely to be known to many adults and to be observed more frequently by adults whom they know. This can be an advantage with respect to avoiding health-risk factors. Although managed care gyrations have forced rural families to change health care providers more frequently, in general rural families are more likely to be followed over many years by the same health care provider who can evaluate problems in the broad family sense. Children living in small towns and on farms probably have more opportunities to get exercise and to be part of sports teams than do children in urban areas. It would be interesting to compare weights of grade-school children in urban and in rural environments. Children in small towns and on farms probably see grandparents and relatives more often than do their urban counterparts. They have more awareness of the occupations and activities of their adult mentors than do urban children. Children who participate in rural organizations such as 4-H have opportunities for responsibilities that are rarely accorded their urban counterparts. They also have more organized activities available during summers. Consider the children who learn to care for and then exhibit animals at local fairs (Figure 1), demonstrate their skills in cooking or baking, or raise grain or vegetables. As they learn these skills, they receive recognition from adults and increase confidence in their personal ability to succeed. The work they participate in is real work, necessary, and provides them with purpose, in contrast to some of the contrived or superficial activities of their urban counterparts. They observe the cycle of life at an early age. They are likely to be involved in religious activities. The observing and caring adult community around them is more likely to intervene if they do things that are dishonest or unethical. They will experience adolescent upheavals but they also are likely to have a broad support base during those periods.

Interventions to Improve Health

There are relatively few reported recent intervention studies reported that relate to children and adolescents who live in rural areas. One model study evaluated a community-based program to improve infant immunization rates in rural Minnesota (Hellerstedt, Olson, Oswald, & Pirie, 1999). Communities Caring for Children (CCC) is a collaborative effort of 10 community health service agencies that provide public health services in 13 rural counties, the Northwest District Office of the Minnesota Department of Health, and local organizations and businesses. When the CCC was established in 1991, the 13-county area had an infant mortality rate 50% higher than in the rest of Minnesota, and the immunization rate for 2-year-olds was 58%. Goals of the CCC were to increase the number of infants and children who received age-appropriate well-child examinations and to increase the number who received timely immunizations. The program involved educational campaigns through public media, outreach to health providers, and active enrollment of new mothers in the CCC program. Enrollees in the program received a newsletter two weeks before every well-child exam and immunization deadline. The newsletter contained information specific to the age of the infant or child and a "refrigerator memo" with child and family care telephone numbers.

Evaluation of the program included surveys of all mothers who had delivered singleton liveborns between May 1 and December 31, 1995. Of the total women who gave birth during that period, 776 women or 65.7% were enrolled in the CCC and 421 of them completed the telephone survey. Compared with CCC enrollees, nonenrollees were older, better educated, more likely to be white, and of higher parity. There

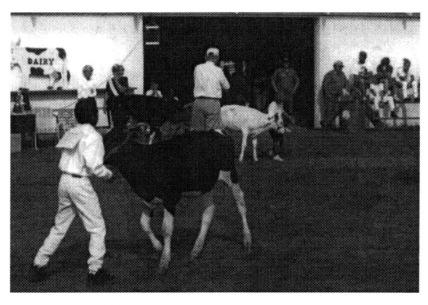

FIGURE 1. Farm boy with calf at county fair.

were few differences in concern about side effects from infant immunizations, or in beliefs that immunizations are effective. Fifty-seven percent of CCC enrollees and nonenrollees said they were "somewhat worried" or "very worried" about side effects from infant immunizations. Twenty-eight percent of CCC and 32% of non-CCC enrollees agreed that polio vaccines could be dangerous. Survey subjects were asked whether certain infant illnesses would cause them to delay an immunization visit. There were no differences, by CCC enrollment, but more than one-third reported they would cancel a visit if the infant had a cold, a mild ear infection, or a mild fever. Most of the mothers interviewed recognized that diseases such as pertussis, measles, diphtheria, meningitis, and hepatitis may be serious. Ninety-eight percent of the subjects reported that their infants had at least one well baby health visit, and there were no differences according to CCC enrollment. With respect to age-appropriate immunizations, women enrolled in CCC were 1.7 times more likely than nonenrollees to have an immunization card. For infants younger than eight months and older than eight months, infants of CCC enrollees had higher levels of immunization compliance. However, in all groups more than 70% were compliant with all recommended immunizations. The authors noted that all those surveyed, regardless of CCC enrollment, represented a more health-conscious group than those who could not be reached by telephone. In the 1997 Minnesota legislature session, a proposal for a statewide childhood immunization registry was defeated, primarily because of data privacy concerns.

Smith, Thompson, Shields, Manley, & Haley (1997) evaluated the effectiveness of a rural emergency medical and trauma services project in increasing the knowledge and confidence of emergency care personnel in the management of acutely ill and injured children. This prospective, quasi-experimental study used an untreated control group design with pretest and posttest of prehospital and hospital-based emergency care personnel in two rural counties in central Ohio. Project evaluation compared 50 emergency care providers from the intervention county with 43 emergency care providers from the control county. Changes in knowledge and confidence of these personnel in the assessment and management of pediatric emergencies were compared. Providers in the intervention county demonstrated a significantly greater increase in test scores regarding knowledge of pediatric emergencies than did providers in the control county ($p = .001$). Significantly greater improvement was also seen when comparisons of test scores were made for field ($p = .02$) and hospital ($p = .03$) emergency care personnel separately. Self-reports on a visual analog scale indicated that providers in the project intervention county had a significantly greater decrease in anxiety than did control subjects when presented a scenario of a child experiencing a respiratory arrest ($p = .01$). On the basis of scores from a five-point Likert scale, emergency personnel in the intervention county had a greater increase in confidence regarding management of the pediatric airway ($p = .0003$). They also had a greater increase in the belief that they had adequate pediatric training ($p = .000001$) after participating in the project than emergency personnel in the control county. The rural pediatric emergency medical and trauma services project was effective in increasing the knowledge and confidence of emergency care personnel in the management of acutely ill and injured children. This project offers a model that can be replicated in other rural areas nationally.

Public Health Recommendations

The population of each local rural area must be assessed with special emphasis on identifying groups of children whose access to health care is compromised by distance, financial disadvantage, or cultural factors. The means should be developed to ensure that these groups, as well as all other children of the area, receive appropriate care. Appropriate care begins with the basics: health education, immunizations, and well-child visits. It also includes good primary care and effective emergency service in the rural community. Finally, secondary and tertiary care must be available to all children and adolescents of the community when needed.

County health departments usually have a special mandate to seek out and serve infants and young children who are unable to access the private care system. There are several other reasons local health departments can help communities achieve appropriate care for their children. The state health department provides them with a strong infrastructure, they are the first recipients of reports of communicable disease in the community, they serve as a connecting link between statewide organizations and local agencies, and they can do the basics of child health care economically and efficiently.

Slifkin, Clark, Strandhoy, and Konrad used county-level immunization data generated by state public health agencies to explore the rural–urban variation in the delivery of childhood immunizations in the public sector (1997). Public health department–documented immunization coverage rates for 1995 were obtained from 882 counties in 11 states east of the Mississippi River. In all states except West Virginia, nonmetropolitan counties averaged higher completion rates than metropolitan counties. Consistent with the descriptive statistics, in the regression analysis nonmetropolitan counties had average immunization rates 2.47 percentage points higher than metropolitan counties, even when controlling for county socioeconomic characteristics. For the 11 states in the analysis, rural children immunized in the public sector had higher completion rates compared with urban children. These data reflect the dependence of rural families on the public health system and the potential for successful health care delivery through public clinics. The investigators believe that, as new health care systems are brought into rural areas, the success of this existing avenue for care must not be overlooked.

The Basics

Health Education

Health education should involve the community as much as possible. Ideally, groups and individuals within the community should help identify health education goals and assist in the teaching necessary to achieve them. Realistically, however, this may be difficult to accomplish (Lee, Jenkins & Westaby, 1997). Accurately or not, rural people are known to be "set in their ways" and slow to adapt to new ideas. Health education issues, particularly with regard

to safety, may vary somewhat according to the local situation but should include the following subjects: sexual abuse, safety, violence, guns, discipline, TV, protection against infectious diseases, substance abuse, protection from environmental toxins, and dental hygiene.

Health education appropriate to the age and lifestyle of the child should be a part of almost every visit to a primary care provider. Physicians generally enjoy a high degree of respect in rural communities and their advice is sometimes heeded when other educators fail. The present system of reimbursement for physicians' services is not conducive to physicians spending a great deal of time on this activity, however; educational videotapes in the waiting area, brochures, and advice from other members of the office staff may have to suffice. Public health nurses can be extremely knowledgeable and committed in the area of health education. Although they may not command the same respect accorded to physicians, they are often able to relate in a way that makes mothers feel more relaxed and thus more receptive to extensive teaching.

Immunizations

Children require 15 to 19 doses of vaccine by the age of 18 months to be protected against 10 childhood diseases, including diphtheria, tetanus, whooping cough, bacterial meningitis, polio, hepatitis B, chicken pox, measles, mumps, and rubella. Community providers need to be alert to the special immunization needs of groups such as immigrants.

Well-Child Visits

Well-child visits should include a general physical assessment, developmental testing, identifying behavioral problems, screening for lead poisoning in areas where this occurs, screening for sickle cell disease in nonwhite populations, bringing immunizations up to date, and health education. In some areas it may be appropriate for public health nurses to apply fluoride varnish to young children's teeth. Tuberculosis screening is appropriate for children of recent immigrants from countries that have a high rate of tuberculosis.

Primary Care in Rural Areas

Primary care providers in rural areas—be they nurse practitioners, physician assistants, family practitioners, or pediatricians—must be able to deal skillfully with two special types of situations. These are identification and management of children whose airway is severely threatened, and conditions that will not be deemed by parents to necessitate specialized care, such as dermatological conditions. Skin conditions are common among children and adolescents. Parents are grateful when their child's rash can be diagnosed and treated by the primary caregiver; almost all adolescents suffer to some extent from acne, which can significantly affect them both socially and pyschologically.

Emergency Care

Serious emergency cases will usually be transported to hospitals where specialists will provide definitive care; in the meantime and during the transport, the child or adolescent needs not only to be kept alive but in such a condition that long-term function and appearance will be optimal. Rural trauma teams are at a disadvantage in that they do not care for large numbers of patients and therefore do not have the opportunity to practice their skills as do their urban counterparts. Training programs focusing on pediatric patients are a must.

Availability of Specialist Care

Telemedicine has proven useful for many kinds of care, ranging from pediatric cardiology (Murdison, 1997) to psychotherapy for children and adolescents (Ermer, 1999), and may be of great value to rural children who live long distances from specialist care. Even where available, however, telemedicine cannot always substitute for actual contact between the specialist and the child. It is valuable to identify all possible sources of transportation before the need arises. One mode that may be more feasible for small children than for recumbent adults is the light airplane. Even small towns often have airports and sometimes farmers own airplanes that are kept on their farms, using a field as a runway.

Summary

There are 14 million children and adolescents who live in areas defined as rural in the United States. They do not have access to health care that is equivalent to that of their urban peers. Although they are often transported to regional centers for serious problems such as neonatal disease or injuries, there is excess morbidity associated with such interhospital transport. Children involved in disasters such as tornadoes, hurricanes, or forest fires are less likely to receive rapid acute care or excellent treatment for posttraumatic stress than children living in urban areas. Of children who live in rural areas, those in families of migrant workers are most deprived with respect to access to all health services, including preventive services. Children and adolescents who live in rural areas are subject to some specific hazards that are less likely in urban areas. These include infectious diseases such as campylobacter diarrhea, leptospirosis, or Lyme disease, accidents involving machinery, exposure to pesticides, and exposure to allergens. Advantages for children in rural areas include closer observation of their activities by adults in small communities, more opportunities to be involved in community activities, and a greater likelihood of regular exercise. They do not get involved with drugs as early or as extensively as do their urban counterparts.

There are model public health programs that focus on the special needs of rural children to provide thorough preventive care, including anticipatory guidance related to specific rural risks to good health. Several of these programs include home visits to rural children. As telemedicine becomes more sophisticated and available this is likely to increase the availability of specialized medical diagnostic and treatment services to children in all rural areas. In the meantime, there is a need for ongoing health services research related to the special situation of rural children and the interventions that are most appropriate, efficient, and acceptable.

References

Baker, S. P., & Waller, A. E. (1989). *Childhood injury: State by state mortality facts*. Baltimore: Johns

Hopkins Injury Prevention Center.

Berry, D. E. (1993). The emerging epidemiology of rural AIDS. *Journal of Rural Health, 9*(4), 293–304.

Cronk, C. E., & Sarvela, P. D. (1997). Alcohol, tobacco, and other drug use among rural/small town and urban youth: a secondary analysis of the monitoring the future data set. *American Journal of Public Health, 87,* 760–764.

Danbom, R. A. (1993). Small and isolated. The solution is community. *Caring, 12,* 62, 64–66.

Dunn, K. A., Cline, D. M., Grant T., Masius, B., Teleki, J. K., Snow C., Katz, E., & Carroll, E. (1993). Injury prevention instruction in the emergency department. *Annals of Emergency Medicine, 8,* 1280–1285.

Elitsur, Y., Short, J. P., & Neace, C. (1998). Prevalence of Helicobacter pylori infection in children from urban and rural West Virginia. *Digestive Disease Science, 43,* 773–778.

Environmental Protection Agency (1996). Environmental health threats to children. EPA-F-96-001 (November 14, 1997); http://www.epa.gov/epadocs/child.htm

Ermer, D. J. (1999). Experience with a rural telepsychiatry clinic for children and adolescents. *Psychiatric Services, 50*(2), 260–261.

Falck, R. S., Siegal, H. A., Wang, J., & Carlson, R. G. (1999). Differences in drug use among rural and suburban high school students in Ohio. *Substance Use and Misuse, 34,* 567–577.

Goodman, D. C., Barff, R. A., & Fisher E. S. (1992). Geographic barriers to child health services in rural northern New England: 1980 to 1989. *Journal of Rural Health, 8,* 106–113.

Goodman, W. (July 28, 1999). Stand up and be counted. *The Charlotte Observer,* p. U6.

Gwyther, M. E., & Jenkins, M. (1998). Migrant farmworker children: Health status, barriers to care, and nursing innovations in health care delivery. *Journal of Pediatric Health Care, 12,* 60–66.

Hawk, C., Gay, J., & Donham, K. J. (1991). Rural Youth Disability Prevention Project Survey: Results from 169 Iowa farm families. *Journal of Rural Health, 7*(2), 170–179.

Hayes, K., & Baginski, Y. (1993). Earthquake! *Caring, 12,* 38–41.

Hellerstedt, W. L., Olson, S. M., Oswald, J. W., & Pirie, P. L. (1999). Evaluation of a community-based program to improve infant immunization rates in rural Minnesota. *American Journal of Preventive Medicine, 16,* 50–57.

Inciardi, J. A., Surratt, H. L., Colon, H. M., Chitwood, D. D., & Rivers, J. E. (1999). Drug use and HIV risks among migrant workers on the DelMarVa Peninsula. *Substance Use and Misuse, 34,* 653–666.

Jones, J. L., Rion, P., Hollis, S., Longshore, S., Leverette, W. B., & Ziff, L. (1991). HIV-related characteristics of migrant workers in rural South Carolina. *Southern Medical Journal, 84,* 1088–1090.

Kanter, R. K., Boeing, N. M., Hannan, W. P., & Kanter, D. L. (1992). Excess morbidity associated with interhospital transport. *Pediatrics, 90,* 893–898.

Koehler, G. A., & Van Ness, C. (1993). The emergency medical response to the Cantara hazardous materials incident. *Prehospital Disaster Medicine, 8,* 359–365.

Lee, B. C., Jenkins, L. S., & Westaby, J. D. (1997). Factors influencing exposure of children to major hazards on family farms. *Journal of Rural Health, 13,* 206–215.

Mandalakas, A., Torjesen, K., & Olness, K. (1999). *Helping the children: A practical handbook for complex humanitarian emergencies.* Kenyon, MN: Health Frontiers.

McManus, M. A., Newacheck, P. W., & Weader, R. A. (1990). Metropolitan and nonmetropolitan adolescents: Differences in demographic and health characteristics. *Journal of Rural Health, 6,* 39–51.

Melzer, S. M., Grossman, D. C., Hart, L. G., & Rosenblatt, R. A. (1997). Hospital services for rural children in Washington State. *Pediatrics, 99,* 196–203.

Murdison, K. A. (1997). Telemedicine: A useful tool for the pediatric cardiologist. *Telemedicine Journal, 3*(2), 179–184.

Parker, D. J., Sklar, D. P., Tandberg, D., Hauswald, M., & Zumwalt R. E. (1993). Fire fatalities among New Mexico children. *Annals of Emergency Medicine, 22,* 517–522.

Pear, R. (1999, August 22). States lax in testing for lead in poor kids. *Charlotte Observer,* p. 4A.

Pollack, S. H., Landrigan, P. J., & Mallino, D. L. (1990). Child labor in 1990: Prevalence and health hazards. *Annual Review of Public Health, 11,* 359–375.

Rausch, T. K., Sanddal, N. D., Sanddal, T. L., & Esposito, T. J. (1998). Changing epidemiology of injury-related pediatric mortality in a rural state: implications for injury control. *Pediatric Emergency Care, 14*(6), 388–392.

Robin, L. F., Beller, M., & Middaugh, J. P. (1997). Statewide assessment of lead poisoning and exposure risk among children receiving Medicaid services in Alaska. *Pediatrics, 99*(4), E9.

Runyan, C. W., Bangdiwala, S. I., Linzer, M. A., Sacks, J. J., & Butts J. (1992). Risk factors for fatal residential fires [see comments]. *New England Journal of Medicine, 327,* 859–863.

Simon, S. (1999, July 26). As crop supplies soar, prices plunge. *Charlotte Observer,* p A1.

Slifkin, R. T., Clark, S. J., Strandhoy, S. E., & Konrad, T. R. (1997). Public-sector immunization coverage in 11 states: The status of rural areas. *Journal of Rural Health, 13*(4), 334–341.

Smith, G. A., Thompson, J. D., Shields, B. J., Manley, L. K., & Haley, K. J. (1997). Evaluation of a model for improving emergency medical and trauma services for children in rural areas. *Annals of Emergency Medicine, 29*(4), 504–510.

Sowell, R. L., Lowenstein, A., Moneyham, L., Demi, A., Mizuno, Y., & Seals, B. F. (1997). Resources, stigma, and patterns of disclosure in rural women with HIV infection. *Public Health Nurse, 14,* 302–312.

Stillner, V., Kraus, R. F., Leukefeld, C. G., & Hardenbergh, D. (1999). Drug use in very rural Alaska villages. *Substance Use and Misuse, 34,* 579–593.

Svenson, J. E., Nypaver, M., & Calhoun, R. (1996). Pediatric prehospital care: epidemiology of use in a predominantly rural state. *Pediatric Emergency Care, 12*(3), 173–179.

Svenson, J. E., Spurlock, C., & Nypaver, M. (1996a). Factors associated with the higher traumatic death rate among rural children. *Annals of Emergency Medicine, 27*(5), 625–632.

Svenson, J. E., Spurlock, C., & Nypaver, M. (1996b). Pediatric firearm-related fatalities. Not just an urban problem. *Archives of Pediatric and Adolescent Medicine, 150, 6,* 583–587.

Tilford, J. M., Robbins, J. M., Shema, S. J., & Farmer, F. L. (1999). Response to health insurance by previously uninsured rural children. *Health Services Research, 34*(3), 761–775.

U.S. Bureau of the Census (1997). *Statistical Abstract of the United States.* Washington, DC: U.S. Government Printing Office.

Vane, D. W., & Shackford, S. R. (1995). Epidemiology of rural traumatic death in children: A population-based study. *Journal of Trauma, 38*(6), 867–870.

Weatherby, N. L., McCoy, H. V., Metsch, L. R., Bletzer, K. V., McCoy, C. B., & de la Rosa, M. R. (1999). Crack cocaine use in rural migrant populations: Living arrangements and social support. *Substance Use and Misuse, 34,* 685–706.

10

Infectious Diseases

KEITH B. ARMITAGE AND GARY I. SINCLAIR

Rural Americans may experience a variety of infections that are rare or unusual in urban or suburban dwellers. Rural dwellers are more likely to have occupations (e.g., agriculture) or avocations (e.g., hunting, trapping) that expose them to microbes carried by animals and insects (Donham & Mutel, 1982). They are more likely to be exposed to untreated or contaminated water due to poverty or underdeveloped water and sanitation systems. Most physicians and other health care professionals train in urban or suburban setting, and may have little or no experience with infectious diseases occurring in rural dwellers. Both classic infectious diseases rarely seen in the modern era (e.g., plague, anthrax) and new and emerging diseases (e.g., *Hantavirus sp.*) are most often encountered in rural settings.

In this chapter we discuss infections that are uniquely encountered or have an increased incidence in rural dwellers. We have subdivided these by the type of exposure (animal, water) and route of transmission. This is followed by a brief discussion of selected infections that have an increased incidence in specific populations. As is the case with all infections, treatments may evolve rapidly with time, and practitioners should consult a more recent reference for some specific therapeutic recommendations.

KEITH B. ARMITAGE • Division of Infectious Diseases, Case Western Reserve University, Cleveland, Ohio 44106-4984. **GARY I. SINCLAIR** • School of Medicine, Case Western Reserve University, Cleveland, Ohio 44106-4984.

Handbook of Rural Health, edited by Loue and Quill. Kluwer Academic/Plenum Publishers, New York, 2001.

General Approach

The evaluation of rural dwelling patients presenting with signs and symptoms of infection should include a careful history of exposure to animals, insects, and water. Many of the infections discussed here have dermatological manifestations, and the physical exam should include a careful exam of the skin. Lab testing (specifically serologies) should be guided by knowledge of the local incidence of particular infections.

Zoonoses

The term *zoonosis* refers to infections normally found in the nonhuman animal world or having a primary animal reservoir, with incidental human infection. Zoonoses include viruses, bacteria, and protozoa. The mode of transmission of zoonotic pathogens from the animal reservoir to humans is variable and includes direct contact, ingestion, inhalation, insect vectors, and animal bites. Clinically, zoonotic infections can be asymptomatic or life-threatening. Outdoor recreation and occupations and exposure to wild animals are the most important risk factors for zoonosis in the United States (Weber & Rutala, 1999). Approximately 10,000 zoonotic infections are reported to the CDC per year; the majority (6,000 to 8,000) are Lyme disease. The risk of zoonosis varies by geography, changes in the population of the animal host or insect vector, alterations in ecosystems, and modifications in human activity. Zoonotic in-

Table 10.1. Zoonotic Infections Likely to be Encountered by Rural Americans

Infection	Route of Transmission or Vector	Reservoir
Anthrax	Direct contact, inhalation	Mammals
Arboviral encephalitis	Insect bites	Birds, mammals
Cryptosporidiosis	Ingestion (water)	Cattle
Babesiosis	Tick bites	Rodents
Borrelia sp. (Lyme disease)	Ticks	Deer, mice
Brucellosis	Ingestion	Goats, sheep, swine, dogs
Echinococcosis	Ingestion	Dogs, sheep, goats
Ehrlichiosis	Ticks	Mammals
Giardiasis	Ingestion (water)	Wild and domestic animals
Hantavirus	Inhalation	Mice
Leptospirosis	Ingestion of urine	Wild and domestic animals
Psittacosis	Inhalation	Domestic birds
Plague	Insects	Rodents
Q fever	Inhalation	Cattle, sheep, goats
Rabies	Animal bites	Bats, mammals
Rickettsia sp.	Ticks	Mammals
Toxocariasis	Ingestion	Dogs
Tularemia	Direct contact, insect bites	Mammals, birds
Vesiculovirus	Direct contact	Wild and domestic animals

fections likely to be encountered by rural Americans are listed in Table 1. Rural dwelling patients presenting for clinical evaluation should be asked about outdoor activity and exposure to domestic or wild animals to determine risks for zoonotic infections.

Zoonoses Contracted via Direct Contact, Bites or Inhalation

Hantavirus

In the spring of 1993 a cluster of cases of severe respiratory distress syndrome was seen in the Four Corners area of the southwest United States. Investigation led to the discovery of a newly identified virus of the Hantavirus genus (subsequently called the *Sin Nombre* virus) and the description of a severe clinical syndrome that results from infection (the Hantavirus pulmonary syndrome). Hantavirus infection around the world previously was associated with renal diseases. Mice carry the virus, and human infection occurs most often via inhalation of desiccated, aerosolized mice feces. Infection has been seen most often in individuals living in poor housing conditions and in rural areas where field mice seek shelter in human dwellings.

The initial symptoms of Hantavirus pulmonary syndrome may be indistinguishable from common viral upper respiratory illnesses. However, as the illness progresses severe respiratory compromise develops with dsypnea, rales, fever, pleuritic chest pain, and hemoptysis. Laboratory findings include thrombocytopenia, neutrophilia and an increased hematocrit due to hemoconcentration. There is rapid development of diffuse pulmonary infiltrates and severe respiratory failure, often resulting in death within 48 hours. The case fatality rate is 60%. Hanatvirus pulmonary syndrome should be suspected in the patient who presents severe URI symptoms with the associated hematologic abnormalities. Early treatment with the antiviral agent ribavirin may be beneficial. Otherwise, treatment consists of supportive care.

Rabies

Rabies is now rare in the United States with an average of five cases per year, most of which are imported. In the United States, rabies is found in dogs, raccoons, skunks, foxes, and bats. Any bite from a potentially infected animal must be treated with rabies immune globulin and vaccination. Many experts recommend postexposure treatment after handling a living or dead bat, skunk, or raccoon. The risk of acquiring rabies from this type of exposure is very low, but even a very small risk of acquiring this untreatable, usually fatal illness should prompt consideration for treatment. One well-documented case of rabies acquired in the United States in the past decade occurred in a child who did not report any animal bites but was living in a suburban house where a bat was found. Many authorities now recommend postexposure prophylaxis for individuals who find a bat in their dwelling, even if no bite is reported. Postexposure prophylaxis consists of administration of rabies immune globulin and the rabies vaccine, and is expensive (average cost over $1,000). Rabies vaccination should be considered in individuals in occupations with exposure to potentially infected animals. Administration of the vaccine should also be considered for individuals likely to have frequent exposure to bats.

Rabies virus causes a fatal meningoencephalitis. The incubation period averages 20 to 90 days but can range from 4 days to years. Vague symptoms of fever and malaise may precede the onset of encephalitis, which in acute cases is followed by the rapid onset of paralysis and death. There is no specific therapy and the mortality rate approaches 100%. Reports of supposed cures have been open to question as to the diagnosis. The diagnosis can be made by demonstration of the virus in pathologic specimens or serologically.

Tularemia

Francisella tularensis is a small bacillus acquired by direct contact with rabbits, other small mammals, and birds, or from bites of insects (particularly ticks and biting flies) infected by feeding on small mammals. Aerosolized transmission from inhalation of infected animal products, which can occur during the dressing and cleaning of game, has been reported. Infected patients present most often with fever and swollen lymph glands, usually with an ulcer at the site of inoculation. Infection can also produce a severe febrile illness with associated headache, chills, and abdominal pain. Without treatment fever can persist for several weeks. An oculoglandular form results from inoculation of the conjunctiva; patients present with conjunctivitis lid edema and regional adenopathy. Patients may present with pneumonia due to inhalation or hematogenous spread.

In the United States, infection is associated with the hunting and skinning of rabbits and hares, and with tick bites. People in occupations associated with tularemia include farmers, veterinarians, sheep workers, hunters and trappers, and meat handlers. The annual incidence is 0.05 to 0.15 cases per 100,000 population, with most cases occurring during the summer in the Southeast and Midwest. The diagnosis is most often made serologically. Suspected cases should be treated on the basis of clinical suspicion without waiting for serologies. Antibiotic therapy with streptomycin, gentamicin or one of the tetracyclines for 10 to 14 days is the usual treatment. The mortality rate is 1 to 3%.

Toxocariasis

Toxocara canis is a parasite of dogs. Human infection occurs after the ingestion of eggs found in dog feces. Infection is associated with contact with puppies and dogs, and with eating soil (pica). Infection takes one of two forms: systemic and ocular. In the systemic form (known as visceral larva migrans) the toxocara larva migrates in the viscera, producing hepatosplenomegaly, pulmonary disease, and eosinophilia. Systemic toxocariasis is usually self-limited, and the parasite is unable to survive for more than a few weeks. Antihelminthic therapy may have a role in very symptomatic cases. Ocular toxocariasis produces ocular inflammation, visual symptoms, and in severe cases can lead to visual impairment Consultation with an opthamolgist to confirm the diagnosis should be done when possible. Seroepidemiologic studies have demonstrated an association between rural residence and an increased risk of toxocariasis in children (Herrmann, Glickman, Schantz, Weston, & Domanski, 1985).

Tick-Borne Diseases

Many rural Americans have outdoor occupations or avocations that place them at risk for several tick-borne illnesses, such as tularemia (discussed above), ehrlichiosis, Lyme, Rocky Mountain spotted fever (RMSF), other rickettsioses, babesiosis, and relapsing fever (Walker, 1998; Varde, Beckley, & Schwartz, 1998). Each of these infections is discussed below. With only one exception (babesiosis), all are susceptible to the antibiotic doxycycline. Some of these infections can be rapidly fatal (e.g., RMSF) and empiric therapy with doxycycline should be considered for individuals with outdoor exposure who present with nonspecific febrile syndromes during summer and fall (Goodman, 1999).

Rocky Mountain Spotted Fever

Rickettsia sp. are maintained in nature through a cycle involving reservoirs in animals and insect vectors, with humans incidentally infected. *Rickettsia rickettsii* is the cause of Rocky Mountain Spotted Fever and is the most important *rickettsia* species in the United States. Infection usually occurs in the spring and summer and is associated with peak tick activity. The prevalence of RMSF is highest in the south Atlantic states (0.83 per 100,000 inhabitants) and the south central states (0.53 per 100,000 inhabitants) and is comparatively rare in the Rocky Mountain states (Thorner, Walker & Petri, 1998). Rural counties in the south Atlantic states have the highest local prevalence (as high as 14.59 per 100,000). Infection is associated with outdoor recreational and occupational activity.

The classic manifestations after an incubation period of 2 to 14 days are headache, fever, and rash, including a rash on the wrist and palms. "Spotless" RMSF occurs, particularly in older patients and in African Americans, and the absence of a rash should not dissuade clinicians from considering the diagnosis. Other symptoms may be protean and include myalgia, nausea, vomiting, and stupor. Untreated RMSF can lead to death or severe illness with permanent neurologic sequelae. Therapy with tetracyclines or chloramphenicol usually leads to rapid improvement. Even in the antibiotic era the mortality of RMSF is 3 to 4%. The diagnosis can be suspected on the basis of clinical and epidemiological features and confirmed by serologic tests or isolation of the organism from blood or tissue samples in specialized labs.

Other *Rickettsia* species (e.g., *R. prowazekii*) occur in the United States. They may present with a mild to severe febrile illness without rash. Most cases have been seen in individuals with outdoor occupations or avocations (McDade & Sheppard, 1980).

Ehrlichiosis

The genus *Ehrlichia* contains several rickettsia-like species that are spread by ticks and produce a febrile illness in humans. *Ehrlichia sp.* had been recognized in animals for several decades, but it was not until 1986 were they recognized as human pathogens. The first case was a 56-year-old man bitten by ticks in rural Arkansas. The vast majority of cases occur in a rural setting and have been associated with outdoor recreational, peridomestic, occupational, and military activities (Comer, Nicholson, Olson, & Childs, 1999; Fritz & Glaser, 1998). In some series 11% of patients suspected of having RMSF had ehrlichiosis (Fritz & Glaser, 1998). Most cases have been seen in the southeast states and Texas, Arkansas and Oklahoma, but cases have been reported in the Northwest, Midwest, and California (Bakken *et al.*, 1998; Fritz *et al.*, 1997; "Human Ehrlichiosis," 1996). The two species that infect humans are *E. cannis* and *E. chaffeensis*. *E. cannis* is acquired from ticks that feed on the canine reservoirs (dogs, coyote, fox, and jackal). The animal reservoir for *E. chaffeensis* is not clearly established but is also thought to be dogs.

Illness due to *Ehrlichia sp.* may be mild and indistinguishable from a mild febrile viral illness or may be severe and characterized by fever, hypotension, confusion, renal failure, pancytopenia, and coagulopathy. The mortality rate is 2%. Therapy with tetracycline or doxycycline usually leads to rapid recovery.

Arboviral Encephalitis

In the United States, several viruses have in common an animal reservoir (primarily avian), transmission to humans via mosquito bites, and a resulting encephalitis in humans. These include Eastern equine encephalitis (EEE), Western equine encephalitis (WEE), St. Louis encephalitis (SLE), and California group encephalitis (CE) (Powell & Kappus, 1978). Fully symptomatic infection is characterized by fever, headache, nausea, and vomiting, followed by mental confusion and coma.

EEE virus infection is rare (less than 15 cases per year) but has a high mortality rate (50 to 70%). EEE is a summertime disease and is most often seen along the Eastern seaboard and Gulf states, but has been reported in other parts of the country. The risk is highest during peak mosquito activity. The primary animal reservoir is an avian species, with spread to humans and horses by mosquitoes.

WEE is a disease of humans and horses seen in states west of the Mississippi. Risk factors for infection include rural living and agricultural employment. The number of cases per year varies from none to 200 cases. The case fatality rate is lower than EEE (3 to 4%), and asymptomatic infection is common in adults; cases are more often symptomatic in young children.

SLE occurs throughout the United States; clinically it produces an illness similar to WEE but symptomatic infection is more common in the elderly than children (Reisen & Chiles, 1997). In the past decade SLE has been the most frequently documented arboviral encephalitis; one outbreak in 1975 affected 1,815 people.

The diagnosis of a specific arboviral encephalitis can be made by acute and convalescent serologies. There is no specific therapy for arboviral encephalitis. Prevention efforts are directed at control of the mosquito vector and avoidance of mosquito bites.

CE group virus and related *bunyaviruses sp.* rank second in incidence to SLE, with 60 to 130 cases reported per year (McJunkin, Khan, & Tsai, 1998; Reisen, Chiles, Lothrup, Presser, & Hardy, 1996). These viruses infect a variety of mammals and are transmitted to humans by mosquito bites. Infection occurs in the fall and summer in individuals living near or entering forests. Patients present with fever, seizures, and altered mental status. Illness tends to be more severe in children. Infection with this class of encephalitis-producing viruses has been seen in all regions of the country with significant mosquito populations, including Alaska (Walters, Tirrell, & Shope, 1999). Each specific virus has a particular ecological niche; detailed discussions of these are beyond the scope of this chapter. The diagnosis of a specific virus can be established serologically.

Babesiosis

Babesia sp. are malaria-like parasites long known as a disease of cattle and wild animals. In the last 30 years it has been shown that humans can also be infected with *Babesia*. In healthy humans *Babesia* produces a mild, self-limited illness, but it can inflict a severe illness characterized by hemolysis in the immunocompromised or asplenic patient (White, Talarico, Chang, Birkhead, Heimberger, & Morse, 1998). Most cases have been seen in the northeast coast, as well as in Wisconsin and Washington State (Herwaldt *et al.*, 1996; Herwaldt *et al.*, 1995; Meldrum, Birkhead, White, Benach, & Morse, 1992). Over 100 cases have been documented, but the incidence is thought to be much higher as mild or asymptomatic cases usually go undiagnosed. The parasite is found in rodents and is transmitted to humans by the same tick species responsible for transmission of Lyme disease. Co-infection with the bacterium responsible for Lyme disease is common. Transfusion-related cases have been reported. Babesiosis is diagnosed by examination of blood smears or by serologies. Minimally symptomatic cases require no therapy; more severely infected patients can be treated with clindamycin and quinine. Profoundly ill patients have been treated with exchange transfusion.

Lyme

Lyme disease is the most common vector-borne disease in the United States, with over 50,000 cases reported from 1982 to 1995 (Centers for Disease Control, 1996). Lyme disease is caused by the spirochete *Borrelia burgdorferi* and spread by ticks of the *Ixodes* genus. The animal reservoir for *B. burgdorferi* includes mice, deer and several other animals. Deer in particular seem to be important to the life cycle and spread of Lyme disease. Lyme disease is primarily an illness of suburban dwellers who live in close proximity to protected deer populations in the Northeast, Atlantic seaboard, Wisconsin, Minnesota, Northern California, and Oregon. Rural dwellers in these areas are also at risk.

An expanding annular rash at the site of the

tick bite is characteristic of primary Lyme disease. Muscle aches, headaches, fever, chills, arthralgias, and other symptoms may also occur. Untreated, the Lyme spirochete disseminates, and later stages of Lyme disease involve joints, the central nervous system, and the cardiac conduction system. Many of the manifestations of late Lyme disease respond to therapy, but permanent neurologic impairment can occur. Cases of early Lyme disease can be diagnosed clinically and are treated with doxycycline or amoxicillin. The diagnosis of later stages of Lyme disease is usually based on the clinical presentation and serologies, and may require parenteral antibiotics.

Plague

Plague, a disease of antiquity thought responsible for killing one-fourth of Europe's population in the Middle Ages, exists today in several areas of the world, including the southwestern states (Butler, 1983; Crook & Tempest, 1992). Plague results from infection with a bacterium, *Yersinia pestis*. Modern plague is primarily a zoonosis, transmitted from animals to animals and animals to humans by fleabites, and rarely by ingestion (orally or by inhalation) of infected material. Human-to-human respiratory spread is rare in the modern era, and is seen only in the setting of large outbreaks in developing countries. In the United States the primary reservoirs for *Yersinia pestis* are ground squirrels, rock squirrels, and prairie dogs. Humans are accidental hosts bitten by infected rodent fleas. Most cases occur during the months of May to October, when people are more likely to come into contact with rodents. In the United States the highest incidence is in young American Indians living in the Southwest (1.4 cases per 100,000 population). In addition to animal contact, risk factors also include the availability of stored food that attracts rodents and possibly failure to control fleas on pets.

There are several clinical syndromes. Bubonic plague results from inoculation of the skin by a fleabite, followed two to eight days later by tender adenopathy in the region of the bite, and fever, chills, weakness, and headache. The lymph node swelling progresses to a bubo, an intensely tender, oval fluctuant mass. Examination of the skin may reveal the fleabite, an ulcer, vesicles, or pustules. Other infection can provoke tender regional adenopathy (e.g., tularemia), but the rapid development of the bubo is unique to plague. Untreated, bubonic plague can progress to sepsis and death within two to four days. Septicemic plague occurs when infection produces severe sepsis without a clinically apparent bubo. In New Mexico in the 1980s, septicemic plague accounted for 25% of all cases and had a mortality of 33%. Pneumonic plague occurs from hematogenous spread to the lung or by primary respiratory infection. Plague can also present as meningitis, pharyngitis, or gastroenteritis.

The diagnosis of plague should be considered in the patient with a compatible clinical syndrome who has a history of contact with prairie dogs or squirrels. The diagnosis can be made by stain and culture of a bubo aspirate or by blood cultures. Serologic tests can also be used. Without treatment, plague has 50% mortality. Streptomycin is the drug of choice. Tetracyclines can be used when oral therapy is desired, or when the patient is allergic to streptomycin. A vaccine is available for individuals who handle or are likely to have frequent contact with rodents. Other preventive measures include improvement in housing and food storage, and use of protective clothing to minimize fleabites. The Plague Branch of the Centers for Disease Control, located in Fort Collins, Colorado, investigates each case.

Infections Related to Agricultural Exposure

Rural dwellers are more likely to be employed in agricultural occupations than city dwellers, and as a result are more prone to a variety of animal and plants related diseases. With the mechanization and reduction of the agricultural labor force over the past half-century, most of these diseases have drifted into obscurity. Yet on occasion the rural provider will encounter one of these illnesses. Recognition and treatment remains crucial, as many of these illnesses carry a high fatality rate in the untreated form but have a high cure rate with simple therapies such as doxycycline. A complete list of agriculturally associated illnesses would be beyond the scope of this discussion (see Mandell, Bennet, & Dolin, 1995). Examples of some relatively common agricultural illnesses follow.

Brucellosis

Brucella sp. is a small gram-negative coccobacillus, which can be mistaken for a more common pathogen (*Moraxella catarrhalis*) on gram stain. Multiple species of *Brucella* chronically infect a wide range of animals, including cattle, goats, sheep, swine, and dogs. The organism is particularly abundant in the reproductive tracts of animals and large numbers of organisms are spread through milk, urine, and placenta. In humans, the organism is virtually always acquired from infected animals, especially through unpasteurized dairy products. The incidence in the United States is less than 1 case in 200,000, with most cases confined to Texas, California, Virginia, and Florida (Centers for Disease Control, 1994).

Infection is via contact with nonintact skin, mucous membrane exposure, inhalation, and ingestion. An incubation period of two to eight weeks is followed by a flulike illness with fevers, chills, sweats, myalgia, headache, and stiff neck. Lymphadenopathy and splenomegaly may also occur. All organ systems can and usually are involved (Young, 1995). Untreated, the illness becomes chronic with a waxing and waning course and a mortality of about 2% (Eyre, 1908).

Diagnosis is made based on a combination of clinical history, cultures, and serologic tests. The organism can be isolated from blood in 15 to 70% of cases. Of note, standard Bactec collection systems are capable of identifying the organism, but should be held for delayed growth (>30 days) (Young, 1995).

A six-week course of oral doxycycline generates an initial response, but relapse rates are estimated between 5 and 40%. Thus, doxycycline is usually combined with either rifampin or streptomycin and continued for 45 days for uncomplicated cases (Young, 1995). Quinolones and TMP/SMX are used as additional agents for complicated cases such as endocarditis and CNS infection.

Histoplasmosis

Histoplasma capsulatum is a fungus found in high concentrations in soil in the central river valleys of the United States. Previous minimally symptomatic infection is ubiquitous in adults in these areas. The droppings from chickens as well as other birds enrich soil and improve its ability to support *histoplasma*, but the birds themselves are not carriers of the organism. Bats can be infected with *histoplasma* and excrete the fungus in their droppings, thus creating the association between spelunking and histoplasmosis (Bullock, 1995).

Humans inhale the organism from aerosolized soil particles. In 90% of cases, a self-limiting, asymptomatic pneumonic process ensues, leaving behind calcified pulmonary granulomas that mimic resolved primary tuberculosis. During the acute phase, patients may complain of flulike symptoms. In the minority of immunocompetent patients and in many immunocompromised patients, the disease is not self-limiting and can progress to a chronic pulmonary syndrome with upper lobe disease resembling tuberculosis. Rarely histoplasmosis infection produces an exuberant inflammatory reaction in the mediastinum leading to mediastinal fibrosis. A progressive disseminated histoplasmosis syndrome can occur, particularly in the immunocompromised, and affect virtually every organ system in the body (Bullock, 1995).

Diagnosis is based on clinical presentation, culture of the fungus, and serology. In the disseminated form of the disease, particularly in immunocompromised patients, assaying the urine for *histoplasma* antigen is a particularly sensitive and specific test (Bullock, 1995; Wheat, 1994).

For severe cases, the disease is treated with amphotericin B or itraconazole (Bradsher, 1996). Mild, self-limited cases of primary histoplasmosis in otherwise healthy subjects do not need to be treated.

Blastomycosis

Blastomyces dermatitis is a fungus that causes an illness very similar to histoplasmosis. Blastomycosis, however, is much less common, having only been reported in small clusters and in sporadic cases, and thus its epidemiology, natural reservoir, and overall pathogenesis are less well understood. Efforts to better understand the epidemiology of blastomycosis have been hampered by the lack of an available skin-testing reagent (which is available for histoplasmosis). Some evidence suggests that the disease is most prevalent in middle-aged men with outdoor occupations and soil exposure. Environmental studies suggest that the organism lives best in warm moist soils of wooded areas with abundant decaying vegetation. In the United States, cases are most common in the Mississippi and Ohio River basins, the Midwest in general, and the southeastern and south central states (Chapman, 1995).

Similar to *histoplasma sp.*, *blastomyces sp.* enters via the lungs. Asymptomatic pulmonary infection probably does occur, but the exact incidence is unknown. The infection can be self-limiting, or it can be progressive and infect virtually every organ system in the body. Pulmonary disease mimics both histoplasmosis and tuberculosis. Skin infection is common and mimics a wide range of other processes (Chapman, 1995).

Diagnosis is made best by smears, histopathology, and culture of affected organs. Serologies do exist, but their predictive value is somewhat low (Chapman, 1995; Bradsher & Pappas, 1995).

Amphotericin B and itraconazole are efficacious in disseminated or severe cases. Mildly symptomatic cases of primary pulmonary disease do not require treatment (Bradsher, 1996).

Psittacosis

Psittacosis refers to human infection with the organism *Chlamydia psittaci*, normally a pathogen of avian species. All birds are susceptible, and many tend to shed the organism when sick. Turkey-associated psittacosis has the highest attack rate in psittacosis epidemics (Schlossberg, 1995), and poultry farmers are at significant risk.

The most common presentation is an atypical pneumonia beginning 7 to 14 days after exposure (Grayston, 1990). However, the disease can disseminate and affect virtually any organ system.

Diagnosis is difficult, as no good serologic markers exist and culture is both difficult and dangerous to laboratory personnel (Mesmer, Skelton, & Moroney, 1997). The CDC views a clinical history plus a complement fixation titer of 1:32 or greater as a confirmed case (Wong, Skelton, & Daugharty, 1994). Treatment with tetracycline or doxycycline usually results in a dramatic clinical improvement. Erythromycin is a second-line treatment (Schlossberg, 1995).

Leptospirosis

Leptospirosis is a spirochetal disease contracted via exposure to wild and domestic animals. In the United States, the most important vectors are dogs, livestock, rodents, wild mammals, and cats. Most cases occur in young adult men involved in agricultural activities during summer or early fall (Farrar, 1995).

Leptospires can persist in the urine of many mammalian hosts for long periods of time without causing disease. Humans are exposed by direct contact with water and soil contaminated with urine (Farr, 1995).

Leptospires penetrate mucous membranes or nonintact skin. The infection is usually subclinical with 15% of abattoir workers and veterinarians having serologic evidence of infection without a history of compatible disease (Farrar, 1995). In those individuals experiencing clinical leptospirosis, two phases have been identified. The first phase begins one to two weeks after exposure and presents as a nonspecific flulike illness that resolves spontaneously. The patient appears well for one to two days when the second or "immune mediated" phase begins. Aseptic meningitis, uveitis, rash, and fever characterize this phase. Weils's syndrome is a severe form of leptospirosis involving jaundice, hemorrhage, renal failure, and myocarditis (Farr, 1995).

Diagnosis is based on a combination of clinical suspicion, identification of organisms by darkfield microscopy, special media cultures, and titers (Farr, 1995). Treatment is traditionally with ampicillin or tetracycline, though mild disease is usually self-limiting and controlled studies have been difficult to do in more severe disease (Farr, 1995).

Q Fever

Q fever is caused by the rickettsia-like intracellular pathogen, *Coxiella burnetti*. It is a zoonosis with the most common reservoir in cattle, sheep, and goats, though many animals and some arthropods can harbor the organism. The organism resists desiccation and is found in particularly high concentrations in animal urine, feces, milk, and birth products. Humans are infected by inhalation of contaminated aerosols, and after an incubation period of two to six weeks, develop fevers, chills, myalgias, and headache. The disease is usually self-limited, lasting one to two weeks, but can be complicated by atypical pneumonia, culture negative endocarditis, hepatitis, osteomyelitis, and encephalitis (Marrie, 1995).

Diagnosis is often made in a person with the appropriate exposure (particularly to parturient cows), a compatible clinical illness, and negative cultures when more common pathogens have been excluded. Cultures are not done routinely in clinical labs, and serologic testing, though helpful, is complicated by the fact that the organism exists in two morphologically similar phases with different surface antigens (Raoult & Marrie, 1995).

Treatment of the more severe manifestations of Q fever is usually accomplished with doxycycline, though other antibiotics also have activity and are sometimes used in combinations (Marrie, 1995).

Echinococcosis

Echinococcosis is a disease of carnivorous dogs and ungulates (primarily sheep) that is transmitted to humans by contact with eggs in dog feces. Infection in humans produces two distinct syndromes based on the species of *Echinococcus* producing the infection.

E. granulosus and *E. vogeli* cause hydatid or unilocular cyst disease. Domestic dogs in livestock breeding areas are the usual primary hosts, and sheep, goats, camels, and sometimes humans serve as the intermediate hosts. In North America, the syndrome is seen (rarely) in the southwestern United States. It is acquired via ingestion of parasite eggs from dog feces. The organism lives as a tapeworm form in the alimentary canals of dogs, wolves, and foxes, and eggs are excreted in the stool. Eggs are highly resistant to desiccation, and can be ingested by livestock, or by humans under conditions of poor sanitation. After ingestion, the eggs hatch to form immature cysts (oncospheres), which penetrate the gut mucosa and are disseminated via the circulation. The immature cysts most commonly grow to mature hydatid cysts in the liver (50 to 70%) or lung (20 to 30%) but can occur anywhere in the body. They grow to a size of 5–10 cm within the first year but can remain silent for decades unless symptoms related to their mass effect appear (Schantz & Okelo, 1990).

The most common way to diagnose hydatid cysts is by the classic radiographic appearance on CT, ultrasound, or MRI. Diagnosis can be confirmed via IgG or IgE serologies available through the CDC, which are 80 to 100% sensitive and 88 to 96% specific for patients with liver cysts but less than 50% sensitive when other organs are involved (Aziz, 1998). Hydatid cyst diseases should be considered in the differential of more common diagnoses such as pyogenic liver abscess when the appropriate exposure history is elicited.

Optimal treatment involves surgical or CT-guided drainage with concomitant antihelminthic therapy (albendazole or mebendazole). Complications include anaphylaxis and dissemination of daughter cysts. Expert surgical and infectious diseases consultation should be sought (King, 1995).

E. multilocularis causes a similar syndrome, but tends to be more aggressive than *E. granulosus*. *E. multilocularis* cysts reproduce by asexual budding and tend to form tumorlike masses. Biopsy often gives the first clue to an infectious process, and serologies can be helpful in establishing the diagnosis. In the United States, this disease is seen (rarely) in the northern forest regions. Treatment is by combined surgical resection of the cysts and surrounding tissues with concomitant administration of antihelminthic agents (King, 1995).

Sporotrichosis

Sporotrichosis is a fungal infection caused by the fungus *Sporothrix schencki*. Exposure generally occurs during farming or gardening when individuals come into contact with thorned plants, timber, sphagnum moss, armadillos, or soil (Rex, 1995).

Cutaneous sporotrichosis is the most common form in immunocompetent individuals. A cellulitic or nodular lesion arises at the site of inoculation and spreads lymphangitically, usually as subcutaneous nodules. Cooler portions of the body are preferred.

On rare occasions the organism can be inhaled and cause a granulomatous pneumonitis. Even rarer, the organism can disseminate hematogenously and cause multifocal disease, often with multiple cutaneous sites.

Diagnosis is made by culture of a suspicious lesion. Confirmatory immunoblot assays for *Sporothrix sp.* IgG are available, and have excellent sensitivity and specificity (Scott & Muchmore, 1989). Treatment of cutaneous disease can be accomplished by use of saturated potassium iodide solution taken orally (Rex, 1995). Itraconazole may be an effective alternative.

Disseminated disease is difficult to treat, requiring amphotericin B with subsequent itraconazole (Rex, 1995).

Anthrax

Anthrax, due to infection with *Bacillus anthracis*, remains rare in the United States, but is seen in agricultural workers with exposure to animal hides and hair. Cutaneous anthrax presents initially as a painless, itchy papule that becomes vesicular and then forms a black eschar. Untreated lesions can disseminate and lead to sepsis or meningitis. The organism can usually be cultured from the lesion; and the lesions can be infectious. Cutaneous anthrax responds to penicillin, erythromycin, or chloramphenicol. Anthrax also produces inhalation/pulmonary or gastrointestinal syndromes, due to inhalation or ingestion of the spores, respectively. Both pulmonary and gastrointestinal forms of anthrax usually proceed rapidly to sepsis and have high fatality rates. Anthrax has recently gained prominence as a vehicle of bioterorism.

Vesiculovirus

Vesiculoviruses are pathogens of wild and domestic animals. One particular subtype, VSV-

New Jersey, is endemic in the southeastern United States. It causes a stomatitis in horses and cattle, and the disease can also be seen in swine. Humans contract the virus by direct contact with oral secretions from these animals. An incubation period of 24 to 48 hours is followed by a self-limiting flulike illness of four to seven days in duration. The disease is almost invariably self-limiting and treatment is rarely required (Fine, 2000).

Infections Related to Sanitation and Water

Giardiasis

Rural dwellers who rely on wells or untreated surface water for their drinking water are at risk for infection with *Giardia lamblia*, a protozoan parasite acquired by ingestion of the cysts in contaminated water. Person-to-person transmission occurs, particularly among children in day care centers. Infection results in watery diarrhea that is usually self-limited but can be severe in immunosuppressed patients. Chronic infection can occur, particularly in individuals with IgA deficiency. In the United States contaminated surface water has been seen most often in the mountainous regions of the Northeast, the Northwest, and the Rocky Mountain states. Natural infection occurs in sheep, cattle, beavers, deer, dogs, and cats. Several outbreaks have been associated with contamination of surface water by wild mammals. *Giardia* is most commonly treated with metronidazole (Flagyl).

Cryptosporidium

Cryptosporidium parvum is a protozoan parasite that causes gastroenteritis. Crytosporidium is acquired from water contaminated with animal feces, usually cattle. Infection produces a self-limited watery diarrhea in healthy individuals but can produce severe long-lasting infection in immunocompromised patients. In the United States cattle are the primary reservoir. Infection has been documented in dairy farmers and other persons who have contact with cattle (Lengerich, Addiss, Marx, Ungar, & Juranek, 1993). Treatment consists primarily of supportive care; a variety of therapies have been tried in severely affected immunocompromised patients without success.

Hepatitis A

Hepatitis A is a viral infection of the liver spread by the fecal oral route. Infection in small children usually produces a mild, nonspecific illness. In adults infection can produce marked jaundice but mortality is rare (< .3%) and long-term sequelae do not occur. Infection occurs via contaminated water and by direct contact. In the United States the seroprevalence is 40% and is associated with lower socioeconomic status (Alter & Mast, 1994). Hepatitis A is diagnosed by serologies. Therapy consists of supportive care. A vaccine is available, and is indicated for travelers, military personnel, and sanitation workers. In epidemics of Hepatitis A, intramuscular immunoglobulin is effective in preventing infection in household contacts of known cases or other high-risk individuals.

Strongyloidiasis

In many developing tropical countries, rural living and poor sanitation are associated with intestinal parasites such as hookworm, *Strongyloides*, *ascaris,* and whipworm. These helminths are acquired by direct contact with soil contaminated with human feces. With improvements in sanitation, acquisition of these parasites is very uncommon in the United States (Mahmoud, 1995). *Strongyloides stercoralis* is an important exception, and has been found in rural dwellers particularly in the South and Appalachia. The unique life cycle of *S. stercoralis* (the organism can complete its life cycle without passage outside the body, unlike other helminths) produces autoinfection, resulting in persistent infection that can span decades. Transmission of *Strongyloides* is now uncommon, but infection is seen in older adults who live or grew up in rural poverty or acquired the infection abroad. Patients may present with symptoms of infection years after acquiring the parasite. Autoinfection can produce mild symptoms of peri-rectal itching and eosinophilia years after exposure, and immune-deficient patients can present with severe disease. Immunosupression due to medications

such as corticosteroids or underlying disease including HIV infection can lead to the hyperinfection syndrome with dissemination of the parasite into many organs, including the lungs. Polymicrobial bacteremia and meningitis with adult respiratory distress syndrome can also occur. The diagnosis can be made by identification of *Strongyloides* larva in the sputum or stool. Supportive care and therapy with thiabendazole or ivermectin are indicated, but the syndrome has a high mortality. Care should be taken in giving immunosuppressive therapy to subjects who may harbor *Strongyloides stercoralis*, and screening examinations of the stool should be undertaken before such therapy is undertaken (Mahmoud, 1995).

Special Issues

HIV/AIDS in Rural Populations

The HIV epidemic that became apparent in the early 1980s was largely centered in urban centers. Though most states have mandatory reporting of positive HIV tests and diagnoses of AIDS, testing is not mandatory and the epidemiology of the epidemic is not fully understood. Nevertheless, most experts agree that the epidemic has decentralized with many of the infected returning to their birthplaces for terminal care and for other reasons. Cases of HIV and AIDS have been reported in all 50 states (Centers for Disease Control, 1999). Furthermore, some HIV providers who have established outreach clinics in rural communities report as many as 25 regular HIV patients in places where local physicians had previously reported no HIV within their service area (personal communication with Anderson Clinical Research, April, 1999).

In addition, of the 900,000 presumed HIV-infected individuals in the United States only 300,000 are thought to be receiving care specifically for their illness (Bozzette, 1999). Thus, rural providers are likely to encounter "occult" HIV patients in their practices, albeit in low numbers.

With the advent of potent antiretroviral therapy in 1996, the prognosis for HIV infection has dramatically improved. Former residents of AIDS hospices have regained their health and returned to work, and nationally, HIV-related deaths have fallen dramatically. However, the decline in death rates appeared to have leveled off at a small but nontrivial number in 1997 (Palella, Delaney, Moorman, Loveless, Fuhrer, Aschman, & Holmberg, 1998), and some reports suggest a slight upturn in HIV-related deaths in 1999 (Chowdhry, Valdez, Assad, Wooley, Davis, Davidson, & Lederman, 2000).

Many studies have shown that the success of HIV therapy strongly correlates with the experience of the provider. For this reason, the Human Resources Service Administration (HRSA) has developed a system of AIDS Education and Training Centers (AETC) to service rural providers who are likely to encounter low number of HIV-infected individuals in their practices. Though prescription of antiretroviral medications is an exceedingly complicated and rapidly changing field best left to experts, rural providers should be educated on recognition of HIV in previously undiagnosed patients, the importance of strict adherence to HIV medications, and antiretroviral related side effects and emergencies. For additional information, we recommend contacting the local AETC or the AIDS center at the nearest tertiary care center.

Infectious Diseases in Migrant Workers

Migrant farmworkers present a unique challenge for rural health care providers, as they present with infections acquired in their home country that are rare in the United States or are uncommon in the rural setting. For example, in the United State tuberculosis is primarily a disease of urban poor, alcoholics, homeless, and drug users, but it also has a relatively high incidence among migrant farmworkers (Haas & Des Prez, 1995). Diseases that have a long incubation or a delayed presentation are of particular concern because the illness may become clinically apparent only after the patient has left his native county. For example, transmission of malaria is exceedingly rare in the United States but can have a prolonged or delayed course and is seen in migrant workers from Central and South America. Chronic carriage of intestinal helminths is very common among the poor in tropical countries. The majority of patients with intestinal worms are asymptomatic, but patients may present with anemia, malabsorption, or abdominal pain.

Neurocystercicosis

Neurocystercicosis is the term for CNS infection with tapeworm cysts, and it results from the ingestion of tapeworm eggs. Neurocytercicosis is common in Mexico and Central and South America (Del Brutto & Sotelo, 1988). When tapeworm eggs are ingested they may migrate to any part of the body, but cysts outside of the CNS tend to be asymptomatic. In CNS disease, symptoms occur years after infection. After the cysts locate in the CNS they may slowly expand for years, producing few or no symptoms. Eventually the cyst will die, producing inflammation and frequently leading to seizures, and less commonly intracranial hemorrhage and other neurologic syndromes. The diagnosis should be suspected in immigrants from endemic areas who have new seizures or other neurologic syndromes. The diagnosis can be made on the basis of characteristic CT or MRI findings and by serologies. Treatment with the antiparasitic drug albendazole or praziquantel and supportive care is successful in most patients.

Amebiasis

Amebiasis is very common in Mexico and Central and South America. *Entamoeba histolytic*, the causative agent of amebiasis, is a protozoan parasite acquired by ingestion of contaminated food or water. The most common clinical syndrome of *E. histolytica* infection is amebic dysentery, which occurs within a few days of ingestion. Of more concern to the rural health provider in the United States is amebic liver abscess, which can present months after the initial *E. histolytica* infection and may be asymptomatic. Patients with amebic liver abscess present with right upper quadrant pain and fever. Ultrasound or CT scans reveal a space-occupying lesion in the liver. The diagnosis can be confirmed by serology. Drainage is not needed; amebic liver abscess responds well to therapy with oral metronidazole.

Chagas Disease

Chagas disease is endemic in Mexico and Central and South America, and it is estimated that there are more than 50,000 infected immigrants in the United States (Kirchhoff & Neva, 1985; Winkler, Brashear, Schur, Lee, & Hall, 1992). Chagas disease results from infection with the protozoan parasite *Trypanosma cruzi*, transmitted to humans by the bite of the bloodsucking reduvid bugs. *T. cruzi* has a natural reservoir in a variety of mammalian species. Human infection occurs most often where the insect vector lives in substandard human dwelling built near forests and comes into contact the residents. Transmission also occurs via blood transfusion. Acute Chagas disease is usually mild. Patients may present with swelling at the site of the insect bite, and fever and malaise. The infection may also involve the CNS or heart. Health care practitioners in the United States are more likely to encounter patients with chronic Chagas disease, which occurs years or even decades after initial infection. The heart is the organ most frequently involved and patients present with arrhythmia and congestive heart failure. Gastronintestinal manifestations also occur and include megaesophagus and megacolon. Patients present with difficulty swallowing or chronic constipation. Antiparasitic therapy is not helpful in chronic Chagas disease, and therapy is aimed at management of symptoms.

References

Alter, M. J., & Mast, E. E (1994). The epidemiology of viral hepatitis in the United States. *Gastrointestinal Clinics of North America, 23,* 437–453.

Aziz, D. C. (1998). Echinococcus spp. In J. B. Peter (Ed.), *Use and interpretation of laboratory tests in infectious disease* (5th ed., pp. 72–73). Santa Monica, CA: Specialty Laboratories.

Bakken, J. S., Goellen, P., Van Etten, M., Boyle, D. Z., Swonger, O. L., Mattson, S., Krueth, J., Tilden, R. L., Asanovich, K., Walls, J., & Dumler, J. S. (1998). Seroprevalence of human granulocytic ehrlichiosis among residents of northwestern Wisconsin. *Clinical Infectious Diseases, 27,* 1491–1496.

Bozzette, S. (1999, January 31–February 4). Presentation at the sixth Conference on Retroviruses and Opportunistic Infections, Chicago.

Bradsher, R. W. (1996). Histoplasmosis and blastomycosis. *Clinical Infectious Diseases, 22*(2), S102–111.

Bradsher, R. W., & Pappas, P. G. (1995). Detection of specific antibodies in human blastomycosis by enzyme immunoassay. *Southern Medical Journal, 88,* 1256–1259.

Bullock, W. E. (1995). Histoplasma capsulatum. In G. L. Mandell, J. E. Bennett, & R. Dolin (Eds.), *Mandell, Douglas, and Bennett's principles and practice of infectious diseases* (4th ed.; pp. 2340–2352). New York: Churchill Livingstone.

Butler, T. (1983). *Plague and other Yersinia infections.* New York: Plenum.

Centers for Disease Control and Prevention. (1994). Brucellosis outbreak at a pork processing plant—North Carolina, 1992. *Morbidity and Mortality Weekly Report, 43,* 113–116.

Centers for Disease Control and Prevention. (1996). Lyme disease—United States, 1995. *Morbidity and Mortality Weekly Report, 45,* 481–484.

Centers for Disease Control and Prevention. (1999). HIV testing—United States. *Morbidity and Mortality Weekly Report, 48,* 52–55.

Chowdhry, T., Valdez, H., Assad, R., Wooley, I., Davis, T., Davidson, R., & Lederman, M. M. (2000, January 31–February 3). *The changing spectrum of HIV mortality: An analysis of 249 deaths between 1995–1999.* Paper presented at Conference on Retroviruses and Opportunistic Infections,, San Francisco.

Chapman, S. C. (1995). Blastomyces dermatitidis. In G. L. Mandell, J. E. Bennett, & R. Dolin (Eds.), *Mandell, Douglas, and Bennett's principles and practice of infectious diseases* (4th ed.; pp. 2353–2365). New York: Churchill Livingstone.

Comer, J. A., Nicholson, W. L., Olson, J. G., & Childs, J. E. (1999). Serologic testing for human granulocytic ehrlichiosis at a national referral center. *Journal of Clinical Microbiology, 37,* 558–564.

Crook, L. D., & Tempest, B. (1992) Plague: A clinical review of 27 cases. *Archives of Internal Medicine, 152,* 1253–1256.

Del Brutto, O. H., & Sotelo, J. (1988). Neurocysticercosis: An update. *Review of Infectious Diseases, 10,* 1078–1087.

Donham, K. J., & Mutel, C. F. (1982). Agricultural medicine: The missing component of the rural health movement. *The Journal of Family Practice, 14,* 511–520.

Eyre, J. H. (1908). Melitensis septicemia (Malta or Mediterranean fever). *Lancet, 1,* 1747–1752.

Farr, R. W. (1995). Leptospirosis. *Clinical Infectious Diseases, 21,* 1–8.

Farrar, W. E. (1995). Leptospira species (Leptospirosis). In G. L. Mandell, J. E. Bennett, & R. Dolin (Eds.), *Mandell, Douglas, and Bennett's principles and practice of infectious diseases fourth edition* (pp. 2137-2141). New York: Churchill Livingstone.

Fine, M. S. (2000). Vesicular stomatitis and related viruses. In G. L. Mandell, J. E. Bennett, & R. Dolin (Eds.), *Mandell, Douglas, and Bennett's principles and practice of infectious diseases* (5th ed., pp. 1809–1811). Philadelphia: Churchill Livingstone.

Fritz, C. L., & Glaser, C. A. (1998). Ehrlichiosis. *Infectious Disease Clinics of North America, 12,* 123–136.

Fritz, C. L., Kjemtrup, A. M., Conrad, P. A., Flores, G. R., Campbell, G. L., Schriefer, M. E., Gallo, D. & Vugia, D. J. (1997). Seroepidemiology of emerging tickborne infectious diseases in a Northern California community. *Journal of Infectious Diseases, 175,* 1432–1439.

Goodman, J. L. (1999). Ehrlichiosis—ticks, dogs, and doxycycline. *New England Journal of Medicine, 341,* 195–197.

Grayston, J. T. (1990). Chlamydia. In K. S. Warren & A. A. F. Mahmoud (Eds.), *Tropical and geographical medicine* (2nd ed.; pp. 644–660). New York: McGraw-Hill.

Haas, D. W. & Des Prez, R. M. (1995). Mycobacterium tuberculosis. In G. L. Mandell, J. E. Bennett, & R. Dolin (Eds.), *Mandell, Douglas, and Bennett's principles and practice of infectious diseases* (4th ed.; pp. 2215–2216). New York: Churchill Livingstone.

Herrmann, N., Glickman, L. T., Schantz, P. M., Weston, M. G., & Domanski, L. M. (1985). Seroprevalence of zoonotic toxocariasis in the United States 1971–1973. *American Journal of Epidemiology, 122,* 890–896.

Herwaldt, B. L., Springs, F. E., Roberts, P. P., Eberhard, M. L., Case, K., Persing, D. H., & Agger, W. A. (1995). Babesiosis in Wisconsin: a potentially fatal disease. *American Journal of Tropical Medicine and Hygiene, 53,* 146–151.

Herwaldt, B, Persing, D. H., Precigout, E. A., Goff, W. L., Mathiesen, D. A., Taylor, P. W., Eberhard, M. L., & Gorenflot, A. F. (1996). A fatal case of babesiosis in Missouri: identification of another piroplasm that infects humans. *Annals of Internal Medicine, 124,* 643–650.

Human ehrlichiosis–Maryland, 1994. (1996). *Morbidity and Mortality Weekly Report, 45,* 798–802.

King, C. H. (1995). Cestodes (Tapeworms). In G. L. Mandell, J. E. Bennett, & R. Dolin (Eds.), *Mandell, Douglas, and Bennett's principles and practice of infectious diseases* (4th ed.; pp. 2544–2553). New York: Churchill Livingstone.

Kirchhoff, L. V., & Neva, F. A. (1985). Chagas' disease in Latin American immigrants. *Journal of the American Medical Association, 254,* 3058–3060.

Lengerich, Ej, Addiss, D. G., Marx, J. J., Ungar, B. L., & Juranek, D. D. (1993). Increased exposure to cryptosporidia among dairy workers in Wisconsin. *Journal of Infectious Diseases, 67,* 1252–1255

Mahmoud, A. A. F. (1995). Intestinal Nematodes. In G. L. Mandell, J. E. Bennett, & R. Dolin (Eds.), *Mandell, Douglas, and Bennett's principles and practice of infectious diseases* (4th ed.; pp. 2530–2533). New York: Churchill Livingstone.

Mandell, G. L., Bennett, J. E., & Dolin, R. (Eds.). (1995). *Mandell, Douglas, and Bennett's principles and practice of infectious diseases* (4th ed.). New York: Churchill Livingstone.

Marrie, T. J. (1995). Coxiella burnetii (Q Fever). In G. L. Mandell, J. E. Bennett, & R. Dolin (Eds.), *Mandell, Douglas, and Bennett's principles and practice of infectious diseases* (4th ed.; pp. 1727–1735). New York: Churchill Livingstone.

McDade, J. E., & Sheppard, C. C. (1980). Evidence of Rickettsia prowazekii infections in the United States. *American Journal of Tropical Medicine and Hygiene, 29,* 277–284.

McJunkin, J. E., Khan, R. R., & Tsai, T. F. (1998). California—La Crosse encephalitis. *Infectious Disease Clinics of North America, 12,* 83–93.

Meldrum, S. C., Birkhead, G. S., White, D. J., Benach, J. L., & Morse, D. L. (1992). Human babesiosis in New York State: an epidemiological description of 136 cases. *Clinical Infectious Diseases, 15,* 1019-1023.

Mesmer, T. O., Skelton, S. K., & Moroney, J. F. (1997). Application of a nested, multiplex PCR to psittacosis outbreaks. *Journal of Clinical Microbiology, 35,* 2043–2046.

Palella, F. J., Delaney, K .M., Moorman, A. C., Loveless, M .O., Fuhrer, J., Aschman, D. J., & Holmberg, S. D. (1998). Declining morbidity and mortality among patients with advanced human immunodeficiency virus infection. *New England Journal of Medicine, 338,* 853–860.

Powell, K. E., & Kappus, K. D. (1978). Epidemiology of St. Louis encephalitis and other acute encephalitides. *Advances in Neurology, 19,* 197–213.

Raoult, D., & Marrie, T. (1995). Q fever. *Clinical Infectious Diseases, 20,* 489–496.

Reisen, W. K., & Chiles, R. E. (1997). Prevalence of antibodies to Western equine encephalomyelitis and St. Louis encephalitis in residents of California exposed to sporadic and consistent enzootic transmission. *American Journal of Tropical Medicine and Hygiene, 57,* 526–529.

Reisen, W. K., Chiles, R. E., Lothrup, H. D., Presser, S. B., & Hardy, J. L. (1996). Prevalence of antibodies to mosquito-borne encephalitis viruses in residents of the Coachella Valley, California. *American Journal of Tropical Medicine and Hygiene, 55,* 667–671.

Rex, J. H. (1995). Sporothrix schenckii. In G. L. Mandell, J. E. Bennett, & R. Dolin (Eds.), *Mandell, Douglas, and Bennett's principles and practice of infectious diseases* (4th ed.; pp. 2321–2324). New York: Churchill Livingstone.

Schantz, P. M., & Okelo, G. B. A. (1990). Echinococcosis (Hydatidosis). In K. S. Warren & A. A. F. Mahmoud (Eds.), *Tropical and geographical medicine* (2nd ed.; pp. 505–518). New York: McGraw-Hill.

Schlossberg, D. (1995). Chlamydia psittaci (Psitacosis). In G. L. Mandell, J. E. Bennett, & R. Dolin (Eds.), *Mandell, Douglas, and Bennett's principles and practice of infectious diseases* (4th ed.; pp. 1693–1695). New York: Churchill Livingstone.

Scott, E. N., & Muchmore, H. G. (1989). Immunoblot analysis of antibody responses to *Sporothrix Schenckii*. *Journal of Clinical Microbiology, 27,* 300–304.

Thorner, A. R., Walker, D. H., & Petri, W. A. (1998). Rocky Mountain spotted fever. *Clinical Infectious Diseases, 27,* 1353–1359.

Varde, S., Beckley, J., & Schwartz, I. (1998). Prevalence of tick-borne pathogens in Ixodes scapularis in a rural New Jersey county. *Emerging Infections, 4,* 97–99.

Walker, D. H. (1998). Tick-transmitted infectious diseases in the United States. *Annual Review of Public Health, 19,* 237–269.

Walters, L. L., Tirrell, S. J., & Shope, R. E. (1999). Seroepidemiology of California and Bunamwera serogroup (Bunyaviridae) virus infections in native populations of Alaska. *American Journal of Tropical Medicine and Hygiene,* 60, 806–821.

Weber, D. J., & Rutala, W. A. (1999). Zoonotic Infections. *Occupational Medicine, 14,* 247–284.

Wheat, L. J. (1994). Histoplasmosis: Recognition and treatment. *Clinical Infectious Diseases, 19,* S19–27.

White, D. J., Talarico, J., Change, H. G., Birkhead, G. S., Heimberger, T., & Morse, D. L. (1998). Human babesiosis in New York State: Review of 139 hospitalized cases and analysis of prognostic factors. *Archives of Internal Medicine, 158,* 2149–2154.

Winkler, M. A., Brashear, R. J., Schur, J. D., Lee, H., & Hall, H. J. (1992). Prevalence of seropositive antibodies to Ditrypansoma cruzi in Hispanic and non-Hispanic blood donors in the United States. (Abstract). *Journal of Parasitology, 78*(Supplement), 73.

Wong, K. H., Skelton, S. K., & Daugharty, H. (1994). Utility of complement fixation and microimmunofluorescence assays for detecting serologic responses in patients with clinically diagnosed psittacosis. *Journal of Clinical Micorobiology, 32,* 2417–2421.

Young, E .J. (1995). An overview of human brucellosis. *Clinical Infectious Diseases, 21,* 283–289.

11

Chronic Disease in Rural Health

LESLIE K. DENNIS AND STACIE L. PALLOTTA

Chronic Diseases

As a large proportion of the American population grows into old age, it is important to understand how long-term illnesses are affecting us. Chronic disease refers to a health-related state, lasting a long time, often defined as three months or longer (Timmreck, 1988). Risk factors for chronic diseases are genetic, environmental, behavioral, and social. For the purposes of this chapter, we will refer to behavioral and social risk factors as lifestyle factors in comparison to genetic or environmental factors. Some environmental factors may be related to lifestyle factors such as occupation; however, we will address these as environmental factors. Over the past decade there has been an increase in stress, sedentary lifestyles, high-density-population living, poor diet, crime, drugs, gangs, poverty, and pollution, many of which lead to chronic diseases (Timmreck, 1988). Rural health has been examined by looking at farmers, nonmetropolitan health centers, populations not adjacent to a metro area, and populations with less than 20,000 residents.

Only a limited number of studies have examined chronic diseases in rural areas. Differences in chronic disease rates among urban and rural

LESLIE K. DENNIS • Department of Epidemiology, College of Public Health, University of Iowa, Iowa City, Iowa 52242-1008. STACIE L. PALLOTTA • Department of Epidemiology and Biostatistics, School of Medicine, Case Western Reserve University, Cleveland, Ohio 44106.

Handbook of Rural Health, edited by Loue and Quill. Kluwer Academic/Plenum Publishers, New York, 2001.

communities may stem from a variety of factors. The morbidity associated with chronic disease is affected by unique aspects of rural America (Schwartz, 1999). Rural health risks may arise from agricultural exposures including organic and inorganic airborne dusts and gases, microbes, fertilizers, insecticides, herbicides, fungicides, and diesel exhaust fumes, along with physical and mechanical hazards, stress, and behavioral factors (Zejda, McDuffee, & Dosman, 1993). In addition, access to care in rural communities varies from urban areas in that there are often long distances to health care services, fewer individuals with health insurance, and few specialty clinics. Among agricultural communities, the major perceived problems include respiratory disorders, cancer, neurologic problems, injuries, skin diseases, hearing loss, and stress (Zejda, McDuffee, & Dosman, 1993).

Many rural populations reported higher rates of chronic disease at the end of the 20th century than their urban counterparts. In North Carolina, six of nine major chronic diseases had higher rates in rural areas, including stroke, coronary heart disease, diabetes, cervical cancer, colorectal cancer, and cirrhosis (Stoodt & Lengerich, 1993). In Oklahoma, medical diagnoses at admission were compared between metropolitan and nonmetropolitan adult day centers. Admissions to metropolitan centers were more likely to be diagnosed with Alzheimer's disease whereas admissions to nonmetropolitan centers were more likely to be diagnosed with musculoskeletal, respiratory, cardiovascular, or endocrine conditions and have

189

cancer (Travis & McAuley, 1999). Rates of heart disease, cancer, and diabetes mellitus in rural New York were found to exceed the average U.S. rates for urban areas (Pearson & Lewis, 1998). A study of chronic illness among a rural population in India found that 20% were suffering from chronic diseases, accounting for 59% of ill persons (Garg, Mishra, Bhatnagar, Singh, Srivastava, & Garg, 1986). However, the prevalence of chronic diseases decreased with increase in educational level, suggesting that in India the urban–rural differences in chronic diseases may be related to factors affected by education levels (Garg *et al.*, 1986). Similarly, in West Africa a gradient of lifestyle factors from rural to poor urban to urban workers saw changes associated with urbanization for hypertension and body mass index (Kaufman, Owoaje, James, Rotimi, & Cooper, 1996). Similar changes in China have been seen with rural–urban migration for serum lipid levels that appear to be related to lifestyle and diet changes (He *et al.*, 1996). Overall, these studies at the end of the 20th century suggest higher rates for many chronic diseases in rural populations that may be related to lifestyle factors.

Rural populations have often been considered to have healthy lifestyles, with some advantages over crowded urban areas (Pearson & Lewis, 1998). However, in the late part of the 20th century the predominance of cardiovascular disease switched from urban to rural areas. This may reflect what Pearson & Lewis call "slow adopter" behavior often associated with rural populations; that is, they were slower than urban populations to adopt unhealthy lifestyles and then slow to adopt healthy behaviors. In the 1990s urban areas seemed to be benefiting from reduced unhealthy behaviors, and adoption of healthy behaviors whereas rural areas were seeing the effects of adopting unhealthy "urban" behaviors. In addition, rural areas tend to show less usage of preventive services (Pearson & Lewis, 1998). The lack of health care providers and large distance to the nearest provider may present important barriers to preventive health services for chronic disease in rural communities. Rural health care providers too may be "late adopters" due to heavy patient load, travel time, and lack of accessible continuing medical education. Thus, the more recent higher rates of chronic disease in rural areas may reflect a lack of access to health care in addition to behavioral changes (Pearson & Lewis, 1998). The inadequate access to health care among rural Americans may require novel intervention strategies to reduce chronic disease among them (Schwartz, 1999).

The literature on the burden of chronic diseases in rural health is limited. After review of what is available, we have grouped the risk factors for disease into five categories:

1. Genetic factors—genetic predisposition to a specific disease
2. Environmental factors—natural or man-made, but vary in frequency by geographic area
3. Lifestyle factors—such as smoking, diet, and exercise—which are modifiable factors that affect the general population but may be differentially distributed in some rural areas
4. Social factors—social norms of communities that affect behavior
5. Access to health care—may affect long-term disability and mortality

Access to care will be discussed within specific diseases and lifestyle factors. While grouping risk factors may be somewhat arbitrary, these five categories do affect how chronic disease issues in rural health may resemble or vary from the same issues in urban areas.

In general, lifestyle factors tend to affect urban and rural areas in similar ways. However, as stated previously, some of these risk factors (both positive and negative) may translate to rural areas more slowly. Lifestyle factors are also important in understanding rural health because knowledge about their relation to chronic disease in urban studies will often translate directly to rural health. However, knowledge from urban studies may not translate to rural settings for social norms and beliefs or for issues related to access to care.

In this context, we reviewed chronic disease and lifestyle risk factors in relation to rural health. Because studies on chronic disease in rural areas were scarce, we also examined the distribution of chronic disease in the Medicare data for 1993 by urban and rural counties in the United States. In the following sections, major chronic disease categories and how they relate to rural health are reviewed.

Cardiovascular Disease

Cardiovascular disease (CVD) includes a variety of heart and blood vessel diseases, such as coronary heart disease, cerebrovascular disease, hypertension, stroke, and rheumatic heart disease. Cardiovascular disease is believed to develop slowly from deposits of fat, cholesterol, and other substances on the artery walls (Smith & Pratt, 1993). It usually manifests in middle age. Potentially modifiable risk factors include high blood pressure, high cholesterol, cigarette smoking, physical inactivity, diabetes, and obesity (Labarthe, Eissa, & Varas, 1991). Some studies have examined high blood pressure, hypertension, and elevated blood cholesterol as precursors or markers of cardiovascular disease and thus have examined behavioral factors associated with these precursor conditions.

An excess of coronary disease emerged in rural areas in the 1970s and 1980s (Schneider & Greenberg, 1992; Ingram & Gillum, 1989). This may reflect lower socioeconomic levels as income in farming communities decreased or more high-fat and high-calorie diets. There does not appear to be evidence of specific environmental exposures in rural areas related to cardiovascular disease. Variations in cardiovascular disease between urban and rural areas are more likely to reflect variation in modifiable lifestyle risk factors. This idea was supported by the increase seen over time in rural Crete of coronary heart disease and cardiovascular diseases that was related to dietary and lifestyle changes (Voukiklaris, Kafatos, & Dontas, 1996). Interventions for coronary heart disease in rural areas need to address individual factors related to smoking, diet, and obesity, along with community issues related to access to health care.

Cancers

Cancer includes a variety of diseases with varying risk factors. Cancers are classified according to their histologic features and according to the organ they affect (Brownson, Reif, Alavanja, & Bal, 1993). Agricultural communities are commonly exposed to herbicides, insecticides, and fungicides that possess some level of carcinogenic activity in animals (Zejda et al., 1993; Kay, 1974; International Agency for Research on Cancer, 1980). However, it is unclear what percent of the excess cancer cases in rural America are related to carcinogenic chemicals or to differences in behavioral factors.

Several studies have reported higher rates of specific cancers in rural areas that appear to be related to environmental exposure to pesticides and other carcinogenic chemicals. In rural areas heavy pesticide use was associated with an overall increase in cancer rates and specifically lung cancer and female hormone–related cancers (Wesseling, Antich, Hogstedt, Rodriquez, & Ahlbom, 1999). In rural Iowa, cancers of concern include non-Hodgkin's lymphoma, leukemia, and prostate, stomach, and brain cancers, which may be related to environmental effects of pesticides, chemical solvents, and excessive sunlight (Barrett, 1999). Non-Hodgkin's lymphomas have been observed in populations exposed to herbicides, insecticides, and organic solvents (Masala et al., 1996).

Other studies have reported unexplained variations in cancer rates in rural areas. In Minnesota, both increased and decreased standardized cancer mortality rate ratios were seen for varying cancers when comparing forest and urban areas to corn and soybean agricultural regions, potato/wheat/sugar beets regions, or wheat/corn/soybean regions (Schreinemachers, Creason, & Garry, 1999). In Texas, rural counties had similar or lower rates than urban areas for most cancers; the only increase seen was for melanoma among females. Among white males, rural rates were lower for buccal cavity, colorectal, larynx incidence, lung mortality, prostate incidence, bladder, and incidence of non-Hodgkin's, but similar patterns were not seen among Hispanic or African American males (Risser, 1996). This lack of consistent findings suggests random variation or variation in modifiable risk factors rather than a common rural environmental exposure. In Norway, a slight urban dominance was seen in prostate cancer incidence (Harvei, Tretli, & Langmark, 1996). Small or no rural variation was seen for breast cancer in New Zealand (Armstrong &

Borman, 1996). In Costa Rica, rural areas reported increased rates of gastric, cervical, penile, and skin cancers whereas urban areas saw increased rates of lung, colorectal, breast, uterus, ovary, prostate, testis, kidney, and bladder cancers (Wesseling *et al.*, 1999). Various rural areas have reported an increase in cervical cancers (Thistle & Chirenje, 1997; Biswas, Manna, Maiti, Sengupta, 1997). These unexplained cancer rates may reflect differences in lifestyle factors within rural communities. Variation in cancer mortality rates may reflect poor access to care or differences in diagnosis and reporting patterns.

Based on the work of Doll and Peto (1981) and Miller (1992), cancer deaths that can be attributed to occupational factors range from 4% to 9% of cancer deaths, whereas 29% to 30% are attributed to tobacco and 20% to 35% to dietary factors. Although, environmental and occupational exposure to pesticides, herbicides, insecticides, and fungicides needs to be addressed in farming and other rural communities, smoking and dietary patterns are important lifestyle factors that also relate to cancer risk.

Treatment patterns for various cancers are different in rural areas than in urban regions. In Australia and the United States, breast conserving surgery is less common in rural areas (Farrow, Hunt, & Samet, 1992; Byrne *et al.*, 1997). While little data are available on prostate specific antigen (PSA) screening rates in urban and rural areas, reduced PSA use in some rural areas may account for lower rates of localized prostate cancer. The well-documented increased risks among farmers may account for the increase in prostate cancer seen in other rural areas (Keller-Byrne, Khuder, & Schuub, 1997). More research on possible variations in treatment and the reasons for such variations may help us to understand better how these variations may affect mortality rates.

Cancer intervention programs specific to rural communities have been limited in number. A video intervention study among rural elders showed a decrease in cancer fatalism (Powe & Weinrich, 1999). Although low socioeconomic status and poor health care access have been related to increases in some cancer rates in rural areas (Biswas *et al.*, 1997), removal of eco-

nomic barriers among rural Wisconsin women did not lead to increased cervical or breast cancer screening and therefore had little effect on mortality (Lantz, Weigers, & House, 1997). Some cancer interventions validated in urban settings should apply to rural communities; however, special attention will need to be directed to issues related to access to care that are specific to rural communities. As seen in the Wisconsin intervention study, simple removal of economic barriers may not be enough to effect change. More research into interventions in rural areas is needed. A better understanding of economic barriers specific to rural health and ways to change them is needed. In addition, further research into the cost-effective approach of video interventions in waiting areas of community health centers could be translated to various other chronic health issues in rural communities (Powe & Weinrich, 1999).

Chronic Lung Diseases and Respiratory Diseases

An excess of respiratory problems among farmers has been found in various populations (Yesalis, Lemke, Wallace, Kohout, & Morris, 1985; Morgan, Smith, Lister, Pethybridge, Gilsob, Callaghan, & Thomas, 1975; Dosman, Graham, Hall, VanLoon, Bhasin, & Froh, 1987; Warren, Holford-Strevens, & Manfreda, 1987; do Pico, 1996). Studies of respiratory diseases among farmers have included chronic bronchitis, asthma, chronic obstructive pulmonary disease, hypersensitivity, pneumonitis, organic-dust toxic syndrome, and lung function changes (Zejda *et al.*, 1993; do Pico, 1996). The prevalence of chronic bronchitis ranges from 5.6% to 21.0% among farmers and 17.0% to 49.0% among grain workers—almost twice as high as among nonfarming control subjects (Morgan *et al.*, 1975; Dosman *et al.*, 1987; Vohlonen, Tupi, Terho, & Husman, 1987; Iverson, Dahl, Korsgaard, Hallas, & Jensen, 1988; Chan-Yeung, Shutzer, MacLean, Dorken, & Grzybowski, 1980; Cockroft, McDermott, Edwards, & McCarthy, 1983; Cotton, Graham, Li, Froh, Barnett, & Dosman, 1983; do Pico, Raddan, Tsiatis, Peters, & Rankin, 1984; Yach, Myers, Bradshaw, & Benatar, 1985). Respiratory symptoms including wheezing and shortness of breath were found in three times the number of retired Iowa farmers compared to retired nonfarmers (Yesalis *et al.,* 1985). Wheezing was also present in 12% to 30% of swine farmers (Donham, Haglind, Peterson, Rylander, & Belin, 1989; Bongers, Houthuijs, Reemijn, Brouwer, & Biersteker, 1987). Unlike many other chronic diseases, respiratory diseases are thought to be more highly attributable to environmental factors than to lifestyle factors (Goldring, James, & Anderson, 1993).

Organic dusts are important rural environmental factors known to cause asthma and other lung diseases (Schwartz, 1999; Barrett, 1999). Common allergens, animal proteins, and irritants in rural communities also contribute to the development of airway disease (Schwartz, 1999). Dairy farmers in Sweden have developed more respiratory symptoms over time thought to be related to storage mites as allergens (Kronqvist, Johansson, Pershagen, Johansson, van Hage-Hamsten, 1999). Some researchers have suggested decreased chronic lung diseases in rural settings related to decreased pollution; however, there is little concrete evidence of this.. Measurement of population pollution exposure while controlling for individual exposure to smoking and other lifestyle factors is next to impossible.

Prevalence rates of asthma tend to be bimodal, describing both childhood and adult onset of asthma; however, diagnostic criteria for asthma are not standardized, causing great variation in reported prevalence rates. Asthma may be classified into allergic (atopic) or nonallergic (nonatopic) categories (Goldring *et al.,* 1993). Differences in diagnostic criteria make it difficult to compare rates between studies; therefore, examining differences within studies is more productive. There is little evidence of urban–rural differences in asthma prevalence rates, but this mostly reflects a lack of research in this area. No differences were seen in a study between asthma rates in rural and urban England (Devereux, Ayatollahi, Ward, Bromly, Bourke, Stenton, & Hendricle, 1996). However, a nonsignificant slight increase in asthma was seen in nonmetropolitan areas of Great Britain (Kaur, Anderson, Austin, Burr, Harkins, Strachan, & Warner, 1998). To better identify risks of asthma, childhood asthma is often examined. There are

multiple barriers that adversely affect the health of children with asthma in rural America, including poverty, geographic barriers to health care, less health insurance, and poorer access to health care providers (Schwartz, 1999). Lack of close access to care may have a negative affect on controlling asthma (Jones & Bentham, 1997). Mortality related to asthma in low-density populations with large distances to health care services has been higher than in urban areas (Garrett, 1997; Jones & Bentham, 1997; Schwartz, 1999). Several studies have shown lower prevalence rates of allergic diseases in rural populations than urban populations (Braback & Kalvesten, 1991; Bjorksten, 1994; Popp, Zwick, Streyrer, Rauscher, & Wanke, 1989). One study conducted in a rural community found that factors related to parental occupation of farming decreased the risk of children becoming atopic and developing symptoms of allergic rhinitis (Braun-Fahrlander *et al.,* 1999). Another study found lower asthma, allergies, and bronchial problems in children living in homes that used coal or wood as an indoor heating source (von Mutius, Illi, Nocolai, & Martinez, 1996). These findings may represent an immune resistance built up by early exposure.

Overall, chronic lung diseases and respiratory diseases are important in rural health. While research on these diseases in rural areas is limited, the environmental factors associated with respiratory diseases clearly put many rural residents at higher risk. However, there are few differences in reported prevalence rates of asthma between urban and rural populations. It is unclear if this accurately reflects rural asthma or if it reflects differences in diagnostic criteria and treatment. Research on both the preventative measures and the medical management of respiratory diseases in rural communities is needed.

Musculoskeletal Diseases

Musculoskeletal diseases are the most common causes of physical disabilities in the United States (Kelsey & Hochberg, 1988). The literature on musculoskeletal disease and rural health is scarce, with most of it focusing on arthritis. One study indicates arthritis is reported more often among residents of rural areas (Kaplan,

Alcaraz, Anderson, & Weisman, 1996). Another study found urban residents more likely to have been diagnosed with osteoarthritis but rural residents more likely to be diagnosed with rheumatoid arthritis (Saag, Doeebbeling, Rohrer, Kolluri, Mitchell, & Wallace, 1998). Another finding is that rural residents tend to experience more arthritis and disability than urban dwellers. However, rural patients with either osteoarthritis or rheumatoid arthritis are more mobile than urban patients despite similar degrees of functional disability (Jordan, Linder, Renner, & Fryer, 1995). These studies do not provide a clear picture of arthritis in rural areas. Understanding the effect of arthritis in rural communities is dependent on understanding the lifestyle factors related to arthritis and how such factors are distributed in rural populations.

There are more than 100 musculoskeletal disease, most of them are uncommon with unknown causes, allowing little opportunity for prevention (Scott & Hochberg, 1993; Hochberg, 1992). However, osteoarthritis and osteoporosis account for the majority of disability due to musculoskeletal disease. Risk factors for osteoarthritis include injuries, obesity, and repetitive usage, whereas osteoporosis is related to immobility, thin body build, heavy alcohol use, long-term corticosteroid use, lack of estrogen replacement, smoking, physical inactivity, and low calcium intake (Scott & Hochberg, 1993). These risk factors are lifestyle factors. Differences in musculoskeletal disease seen between urban and rural areas most likely reflect differences in these lifestyle factors.

Neurologic Disorders

Many diseases fit the definition of chronic neurologic disorders, including Alzheimer's disease, Parkinson's disease, multiple sclerosis, amyotrophic lateral sclerosis (ALS), Guillain-Barre syndrome, epilepsy, and migraine headache. Research has evaluated potential agricultural factors frequently found in rural populations and their role in neurologic disease. Agricultural workers are thought to suffer from neurologic effects of the toxicologic properties of pesticides, solvents, and other chemicals used by farmers (Zejda et al., 1993). Several neurologic disorders including Parkinson's disease,

Alzheimer's disease, and chronic encephalopathy have been associated with rural residence based on exposure to agricultural chemicals, while other neurologic diseases are associated with genetics or lifestyle factors (Franklin & Nelson, 1993).

Rural residence has been evaluated as a potential risk factor for both Alzheimer's disease and Parkinson's disease in several recent studies. It has been associated with a higher risk of Alzheimer's disease than urban residence (OR = 2.49) (Hall et al., 1998). This may reflect exposure to organic solvents, since other risk factors for Alzheimer's disease, including Down's syndrome, head injury, and maternal age, appear to have little association with rural residence (Franklin & Nelson, 1993). Studies of Parkinson's disease suggest a similar relationship. Factors associated with rural living, such as pesticide exposure and occupational farming, appear to increase the risk for Parkinson's disease (Gorell, Johnson, Rybicji, Peterson, & Richardson, 1998). Herbicide and insecticide exposure increases the risk of Parkinson's disease with an OR = 4.10 and OR = 3.55, respectively (Gorell et al., 1998). Pesticide use has also been reported as a risk factor for Parkinson's disease elsewhere (Hubble, Cao, Hassanein, Newberger, & Koller, 1993). Exposure to chemical agents in general also increases risk for Parkinson's, as reflected by an OR = 5.87 (Werneck & Alvarenga, 1999).

Amyotrophic lateral sclerosis (ALS), or Lou Gehrig's disease, is known to be associated with athletes and vigorous physical activities. There also appears to be a genetic component with an autosomal dominant inheritance. Other risk factors for amyotrophic lateral sclerosis include agricultural work along with work in leather, manufacturing plastics, or exposure to heavy metals, organic solvents, and electrical shock (Franklin & Nelson, 1993). Further research examining amyotrophic lateral sclerosis in agricultural workers related to organic solvents while controlling for physical activity could expand our understanding of the independent association with solvents.

Multiple sclerosis (MS) has been widely studied in rural health. Some studies about multiple sclerosis report a more frequent occurrence of the disease in rural regions (Swank, Lerstad,

Strom, & Backer, 1952; Rinne, Panelius, Kivalo, Hokkanen, & Palo, 1966; Wilkstrom, 1975; Shepherd & Downie, 1980). Others suggest a higher risk in urban communities (Dassel, 1960; Beebe, Kurtze, Korland, Auth, & Nagler, 1967; Verdes, Petrescu, & Cernescu, 1978; Lensky, 1979). Still other studies report no difference between rural and urban environments (Neutel, 1980; Poskanzer, Sheridan, Prenney, & Walker, 1980). Most of the studies of multiple sclerosis examined prevalence or mortality rates at current residence. It has been suggested that current residence is not suitable for the etiological considerations of multiple sclerosis since childhood and adolescence appear to be the most relevant time periods of exposure. This may explain some differences in findings. Data collected from patients who grew up in rural environments may lead to more dependable results about how rural residence may be related to development to multiple sclerosis (Lauer & Firnhaber, 1985). However, it should be noted that the most widely supported risk factors for multiple sclerosis are genetic susceptibility and a possible interaction between genetic susceptibility and a childhood virus. Furthermore, whites are more susceptible than other races, with prevalence rates increasing with increasing distance from the equator (Franklin & Nelson, 1993). Most risk factors for multiple sclerosis do not appear to be related to factors specific to rural health.

Guillain-Barre syndrome is generally associated with a viral infection. However, one study suggests that up to 90% of patients with Guillain-Barre syndrome with acute motor axonal neuropathy reside in areas without running water; many such areas are rural (Paradiso, Tripoli, Galicchio, & Fejerman, 1999). It is unclear what the lack of running water or rural residence may contribute to this neurologic disease. Other neurologic disorders including epilepsy and migraine headache do not appear to be more prevalent in rural areas than in urban areas. Risk factors for these neurologic disorders appear to be related to lifestyle factors, infections, and some other disease occurrences (Franklin & Nelson, 1993). While these disorders are not seen disproportionately in rural areas, treatment in rural areas may be inadequate. One study reported that 70% of those with epilepsy in rural

areas were receiving no or inadequate treatment (Sridharan & Murthy, 1999). Treatment from specialists such as neurologists may require traveling long distances.

In addition to specific neurologic disorders, general neurologic effects of residing in a rural environment are important. Most commonly, research has focused on neurologic effects of toxicologic properties of pesticides, solvents, and other chemicals used by farmers. The possible neurotoxicity of such chemicals is a major public health concern. The neurologic effects of long-term exposure to agricultural chemicals has been limited by nonspecific and subtle symptoms (Zejda et al., 1993). Adding to researchers' concern is the recently emerging information about delayed nervous system effects of various pesticides and agricultural chemicals (Mushak & Piver, 1992). As already noted, current evidence suggests increased risks of Parkinson's disease and amyotrophic lateral sclerosis in rural communities, with insufficient research on other neurologic disorders there. As research continues, work associated with a rural residence, specifically farming, may prove to be the primary link between rural health and chronic neurologic diseases.

Psychiatric Illnesses

Population-based data on psychiatric problems and stress in rural areas are limited (Zejda et al., 1993). Most studies of chronic mental illness have included samples collected from large urban areas (Department of Health and Human Services, 1993). Studies have provided limited information specifically in regard to diagnosis and symptomatology among rural clients (Dottl & Greenley, 1997). Overall, reliable data of the prevalence of mental disorders in rural residencies are scarce (Office of Technology Assessment, 1990). Measurement of psychiatric illnesses presents many challenges. Many studies focus on the prevalence and symptom intensity of specific mental disorders. The inclusion criteria for certain psychiatric illness have changed over time; therefore, early studies that measured a specific mental illness may not correlate with a recent study of the same condition. Some studies may rely on self-report while others rely on medical records. Often psychiatric illnesses do not have clear-cut diagnostic definitions. This can make comparisons of studies or populations difficult, particularly when examining psychiatric illness in rural populations.

Schizophrenia has shown prevalence rates in rural U.S. areas equal to half that found in urban areas (Cooper, Goodhead, Craig, Harris, Howat, & Korer, 1987; Link & Dohrenwen, 1980; Wing, 1978). Similarly, one study found rural clients less likely to be diagnosed with schizophrenia when compared to urban counterparts (Sommers, 1989). Yet another study reported no rural–urban differences in rates of schizophrenia (Blazer *et al.*, 1985). Bipolar disorder has been reported with equal frequency in both rural and urban settings, but findings on unipolar depression often conflict among researchers (Sommers, 1989; Davies, Bromet, Schulz, Dunn, & Morgenstern, 1989; DeLeon, Wakefield, Schultz, Willaims, & Vanden Bos, 1989; Crowell, George, Blazer, & Landerman, 1986; Commerce Clearing House, 1990). Other specific mental disorders that have been examined include anxiety disorders, which were more prevalent among urban residents, and antisocial personality, which showed no difference between rural and urban residents (Sommers, 1989). Overall, psychiatric disorders seem to be less frequently diagnosed in rural settings. It is unclear if this represents a true decrease among rural residents or differences in diagnosis. Diagnosis of psychiatric diseases in rural communities may be affected by the lack of physician time to address such issues and social stigmas about seeing a doctor for psychiatric symptoms.

An important aspect of mental health in rural settings is the availability, utilization, and accessibility of services. In an attempt to care for their mentally ill, many rural areas rely on emergency mental health services such as crisis services. Because many rural communities lack other mental health treatment options, crisis services are especially important (Sommers, 1989). Such services face various problems in a rural environment. Rural crisis services reportedly use fewer techniques for need assessments, provide less public education about the service, and provide more limited training of crisis workers than urban crisis services (Miller, 1982). While general acute care community hospitals are the most common providers of inpatient mental health services in rural areas, rural acute care community hospitals have fewer short-term psychiatric inpatient beds than urban hospitals, with an average of 1.5 versus 5.9 beds per hospital respectively (Office of Technology Assessment, 1990). This may suggest that, in addition to the greater number of specialty clinics for mental health in urban areas, urban general community hospitals are also better equipped than rural hospitals to deal with the mentally ill. Or this may reflect a reduced need for such centers in rural areas. Rural communities are also often at a disadvantage when it comes to appropriate mental health care because of the barriers of cost and long distances to care centers (Miller, 1982). Unfortunately, recent information on mental health service delivery in rural areas is minimal (Office of Technology Assessment, 1990). The data that are available suggest rural patients with mental illness do not receive adequate outpatient care (Fortney, Lancaster, Owen, & Zhang, 1998). Rural patients are also less likely to visit specialty care clinics, and according to one other study, they have three times the odds of urban patients of being admitted through the emergency room for mental health problems (Rost, Zhany, Fortney, Smith, & Smith, 1998). Use of antidepressant drugs in rural populations is also below national trends, suggesting an underutilization of this form of treatment, a reduction in the number of cases that are diagnosed, or a reduced risk of depression (Ganguli *et al.*, 1997). However, this finding may also suggest overutilization of antidepresent drugs elsewhere.

Overall, the prevalence of psychiatric illness in rural settings is thought to equal that in urban settings. However, this is not substantiated by data, with higher prevalence rates often reported in urban areas. Mental health treatment services are more difficult to utilize in many rural communities and the need for them is unclear. More research in the area of psychiatric illness and rural environments needs to be undertaken in order to substantiate prior studies which lack appropriate control groups, have inconsistent disease definitions, or report speculative results. An understanding of other rural health issues along with the social stigmas related to psychiatric treatment in rural settings is vital.

Other Chronic Diseases

Rates of hypertension, diabetes, and high cholesterol in rural areas may be increased due to a higher percentage of obese residents (Willems, Saunders, Hunt, & Schorling, 1997). National data suggest that nonmetropolitan residents had higher age-adjusted rates for arthritis, cataracts, hearing impairment, orthopedic impairments, ulcers, diabetes, kidney trouble, bladder disorders, hypertension, and emphysema than metropolitan residents (National Center for Health Statistics, 1994). The rural excess for many chronic diseases may be related to differential environmental exposures, lower socioeconomic status, and reduced access to quality medical and rehabilitative care (Wallace & Wallace, 1998). Residents of rural communities also have higher rates of activity limitations due to chronic conditions, and a lower percentage of rural residents than urban residents perceive their health to be excellent (Hicks, 1992). Excess chronic disease in rural populations may also reflect variations in lifestyle factors, including obesity, diet, exercise, tobacco smoking, and so on, that are related to various chronic diseases.

Medicare Prevalence Rates

Methods

We examined all U.S. Medicare claims for 1993 among patients age 65 and older across counties. A county was defined as urban if it had a population of 2,500 or more and rural if it was completely rural or had a population of less than 2,500 (Butler & Beale, 1994). Patients were considered prevalent cases for a given chronic disease if they had a diagnosis for that disease on any admission in 1993.

Poisson regression was used to examine the relationship between urban and rural counties for prevalent cases in 1993 of all residents age 65 or older, controlling for race and sex as well as age. Since admissions for 1993 only were examined, there may be underestimation of prevalent cases. The prevalence rates were adjusted to the 1993 urban population (for race, sex, and age). It should be noted that due to the large number of claims available in the Medi-

care database, the power of these analyses is high, so statistical significance may not represent clinical significance. Another limitation of these analyses is that the data come from discharge data, where there may be preferential coding of some conditions based on reimbursement issues.

Results

Table 1 reports the prevalence rates for each major chronic disease category for both urban counties and rural counties. The rural percent increase represents the ratio of the rural prevalence rate to the urban prevalence rate. For most chronic diseases reported, rural populations had a higher prevalence than the urban populations. However, higher rates were seen in urban areas for alcohol-related illnesses, liver disorders, and neurological disorders. No differences were seen for hypertension, all cancers combined, lung cancer, colorectal cancer, breast cancer, or lymphoma. The highest rural percent increases over the urban prevalence rates were seen for cervical cancer, osteoarthritis, and chronic lung diseases. In general, these findings are consistent with the preceding literature review of these chronic diseases in rural health. Differences in most of these chronic disease categories may reflect differences in urban and rural lifestyle factors. Therefore urban–rural differences in lifestyle factors are also reviewed in the following section.

Lifestyle Risk Factors

Various national surveys continue to examine risk factors in populations. However, they seldom break out lifestyle factors separately by urban and rural areas. In addition, how such factors vary may change over time. Since chronic diseases are characterized by long latency periods, a lag time in the distribution of risk factors in relation to the development of chronic disease must be considered. Similarly, residence at diagnosis of a disease is of less interest than residence 10 to 30 years prior to diagnosis. Many studies that have compared chronic disease in urban and rural areas may not have adjusted for possible migration, this could explain some of

TABLE 1. U. S. Prevalence Rates per 100,000 Population for Chronic Diseases in Medicare Population Age 65+, 1993[a]

Disease (ICD-9 Code)	Urban	Rural	Rural Percent Increase	P-value
Coronary heart disease (410-414; 429.2)	5075.00	5275.15	3.9	<0.001
Cerebrovascular disease (430-438)	2128.27	2229.65	4.8	<0.001
High blood pressure/hypertension (401-405)	5631.21	5627.94	-0.1	0.90
Elevated blood cholesterol (272.0-272.4)	596.03	649.29	8.9	<0.001
Cancers (140-208)	2372.27	2373.74	0.1	0.93
Lung cancer (162)	377.98	372.96	-1.3	0.42
Colorectal cancer (153-154)	278.38	270.19	-2.9	0.12
Breast cancer (174)	210.91	211.47	0.3	0.91
Cervical cancer (180)	11.57	16.47	42.4	<0.001
Prostate cancer (185)	375.3	416.36	10.9	<0.001
Lymphoma (200-202)	113.84	108.77	-4.5	0.14
Leukemia (204-208)	106.37	116.31	9.3	0.002
Chronic lung diseases[b]	3642.03	4143.10	13.8	<0.001
Asthma (493)	434.53	469.60	8.1	<0.001
Chronic obstructive pulmonary disease (490-492;496)	3074.64	3525.22	14.7	<0.001
Occupational lung disease (493; 500-504; 506;507.8; 515-517)	662.57	767.56	15.8	<0.001
Diabetes (250)	3080.19	3339.49	8.4	<0.001
Chronic liver diseases (571)	158.33	127.04	-19.8	<0.001
Alcohol-related diseases[c]	248.07	209.16	-15.7	<0.001
Musculoskeletal diseases (274; 710-739)	3162.23	3629.42	14.8	<0.001
Osteoarthritis (715)	1289.83	1628.52	26.3	<0.001
Rheumatoid arthritis (714)	208.15	224.97	8.1	<0.001
Gout (274)	167.96	183.64	9.3	<0.001
Osteoporosis (733.0-733.09)	284.25	308.00	8.4	<0.001
Neurologic disorders[d]	1731.67	1698.19	-1.9	0.013

[a]Causes of death were coded according to International Classification of Disease, Ninth Revision (referred to as ICD-9) (World Health Organization, 1977).
[b](490-496; 500-504; 506; 507.8; 515-517)
[c](291; 303; 305; 357.5; 425.5; 572-571.39; 535.3; 790.3; E8600; E8601)
[d](290.4; 331.0; 332.0; 335.2; 340; 345.0-345.9; 346.0-346.9; 354.0; 357.0; 358.0; 722.1-722.2; 722.52; 722.6; 724.02; 724.2-724.6; 800-801; 803-804 (except .0 & .5); 806.0-806.9; 847.2; 850-854; 952.0; 952.9)

the conflicting findings for certain chronic diseases.

The distribution of many lifestyle factors varies between urban populations and rural populations. Studies have related rural life stresses to increased poor health behaviors, including alcohol and drug abuse, along with increases in child and spouse abuse (Pothier, 1991; Summer, 1991). Education level, which has been found to differ between rural and urban populations, may act as a risk factor for poor health behaviors, including alcohol abuse (Booth, Ross, & Rost, 1999). Examination of current trends in lifestyle factors, such as obesity and smoking, may assist rural communities in planning for their health care needs in the future. Available information on how lifestyle factors may affect rural communities are reviewed below.

Obesity and Diet

As previously stated, studies have reported higher rates of obesity in rural communities, which may affect rates of hypertension, diabetes, and cholesterol among other chronic conditions (Willems et al., 1997). Studies have suggested a possible association between obesity and colorectal cancer (Brownson et al., 1993). Coronary heart disease has been shown to be weakly associated (relative risk of less than 2) with obesity, as was breast cancer with post-menopausal obesity (Smith & Pratt, 1993; Brownson et al., 1993). A moderate association (relative risk of 2 to 4) was reported between osteoarthritis and obesity, carpal tunnel syndrome and obesity, and a thin body build and osteoporosis (Scott & Hochberg, 1993; Franklin & Nelson, 1993). A strong association (relative risk greater than 4) has been seen between obesity and diabetes (Bishop, Roesler, Zimmerman, & Ballard, 1993). Diet also effects chronic disease in varying ways. In general, high-fat and high-salt diets are associated with an increase in a several chronic diseases. A protective effect was seen among rural children who consumed fewer foods containing fat and more fruits and vegetables than their urban counterparts (Proctor, Moore, Singer, Hood, Nguyen, & Ellison, 1996). Overall obesity and some dietary factors are associated with chronic disease; however, few studies have examined specific effects on rural health. Although it is commonly assumed that obesity is a problem in rural areas, the evidence to support this is unclear. Research on diets in rural areas is also scarce.

Smoking

Smoking has been suggested as a possible risk factor for diabetes (Bishop et al., 1993) and Parkinson's disease (Scott & Hochberg, 1993). Weak associations have been seen for cervical cancer (Brownson et al., 1993) and osteoporosis (Scott & Hochberg, 1993). Environmental tobacco smoke was weakly associated with childhood asthma (Goldring et al., 1993). Moderate associations with smoking have been seen for coronary heart disease and stroke, and a strong association is commonly known to exist between lung cancer and tobacco smoking (Smith & Pratt, 1993). As stated previously, 29% to 30% of cancers are suggested to be attributable to tobacco smoking (Doll & Peto, 1981; Miller, 1992). While tobacco smoking is a clear risk factor for many chronic diseases, the prevalence of tobacco smoking in rural areas is unclear. The few studies that have compared urban and rural smoking rates have had conflicting results. If rural communities are "slow adopters," as suggested by Pearson & Lewis (1998), then a better understanding of current smoking habits in rural populations will help these communities plan future health care needs.

Substance Abuse

One of the most common types of substance abuse is alcohol use. Alcohol abuse is reported to be as serious and prevalent in rural areas as in urban settings. Likewise, other substance abuse has proven to be as much of a problem in rural settings as in urban locations (U.S. General Accounting Office, 1990; Hilton, 1991). However, generalizations between rural and urban substance abuse may not always be appropriate. Numerous researchers assume that factors affecting urban substance abuse affect rural substance abuse in the same way, and they generalize findings to rural settings based solely on results from urban study samples (Weisner, 1993; Room, 1989; Hingson, Scotch, Day, & Culbert, 1980; Hingson, Mangione, Meyers, & Scotch, 1982; Beckman & Kocel, 1982; Bannenberg, Ratt, & Plomp 1992; Jordon & Oei, 1989; Weisner & Schmidt, 1992; Schmidt, 1992). By implementing such generalizations, characteristics unique to rural substance abuse are likely being overlooked.

It has been suggested that utilization of alcohol abuse services probably differs between rural and urban settings, although little research supporting this speculation has been reported (Booth et al., 1999; Metsch & McCoy, 1999). Researchers have questioned if treatment for problem drinkers differs between urban and rural settings and if this would interfere with attainment of accurate prevalence rates. One recent study found rural problem drinkers use fewer alcohol treatment services than their urban counterparts (Booth et al., 1999). Whether treatment differences are due to availability of resources, access to resources, or social and cultural norms may be an important factor in rural alcohol research and the issue warrants further investigation. For example, rural populations may be less likely to utilize substance abuse treatment centers because of local cultural norms. Religious beliefs and the role of the church or fear of lack of privacy may discourage rural alcohol abusers from seeking treatment (Metsch & McCoy, 1999). Similarly, the rural work ethic has been suggested to play an important role in rural alcoholism; the importance of independence, self-sufficiency, and being able to work and function in productive roles can deter people from seeking help for an alcohol-related disorder (Donham & Mutel, 1982; Soweel & Christensen, 1996; Weinert & Long, 1990). Another possible explanation for the lack of alcohol treatment utilization in rural settings is that reliance on extended family for help—a tradition in many rural communities—causes people to avoid social services assistance (Weinert & Long, 1990).

Alcohol abuse in rural settings cannot simply be measured by prevalence rates of treatment, and risk factors should not be automatically deemed comparable to those associated with abuse in urban locations. The existing research is scarce, and the unique components of rural alcohol abuse, including treatment utilization and risk factors, have rarely been considered. Researchers do agree, however, that rural alcohol abuse needs to be separated from urban abuse in order to be appropriately evaluated, and future research is expected to follow this suggestion (Booth *et al.*, 1999; Metsch & McCoy, 1999).

Nonalcohol Substance Abuse

The current literature on prevalence rates of other substance abuse in rural areas is conflicting (Logan, Schenck. Leukefeld, Meyers, & Allen, 1999; Yawn, Yawn, & Uden, 1992; Whitehead, Chillag, & Elliott, 1992). Examined less frequently than alcohol abuse, nonalcohol substance abuse studies are difficult to locate. Nonetheless, substance abuse rates in rural communities are expected to be comparable to those in urban settings. Specifically, like alcohol, other substance abuse is considered as important a problem in rural settings as in urban locations (U.S. General Accounting Office, 1990; Hilton, 1991). Because attitudes about substance use influence rates of abuse, various studies have examined rural attitudes toward substance use and abuse. One study, which examined rural beliefs about drug abuse, reported half the sample disapproved of all drug use behaviors including cigarette smoking (Logan *et al.*, 1999). Marijuana use is reported to be lower in rural areas than the national estimates, with a sug-

gestion that peer perception influenced the lower marijuana use rate (Substance Abuse and Mental Health Services Administration, 1996; Pruitt, Kingery, Mirzaec, Heuberger, & Hurley, 1991). Contrary to this, another study reported that marijuana was the easiest drug to obtain by rural residents and that it was considered the least risky substance to take among those who did not oppose all drug use behaviors (Logan *et al.*, 1999). Attitudes and beliefs are thought to affect more than marijuana abuse in rural locations. Cocaine, opiate, and amphetamine use is uncommon in the rural pregnant population and this may be due to strict social norms (Yawn *et al.*, 1992). Conversely, anabolic steroid and cigarette use occurs at equal rates in urban and rural settings (Whitehead *et al.*, 1992). This coincides with the attitudes among rural residents that neither steroid abuse nor cigarette smoking is a significant concern (Whitehead *et al.*, 1992). A better understanding of the prevalence rates of drug use and what may affect these rates in rural settings is needed.

Lack of rehabilitation services, reduced availability of services, reduced access to treatment centers, lack of utilization of treatment, and the inability to afford services are all thought to affect the rural substance abuser more than his urban counterpart (Robertson & Donnermeyer, 1997). Acceptability of services is also suggested as a barrier (McBride, Mutch, Kilcher, Inciardi, McCoy, & Pottieger, 1996). Even when treatment is available, rural residents may be reluctant to take advantage of it. Recruitment and retainment of substance abuse professionals is also traditionally difficult in rural areas (Howland, 1995; Murray & Keller, 1991; Mintzer, Culp, & Puskin, 1992; Robertson & Donnermeyer, 1997; Soweel & Christianson, 1996). Although little empirical rural research has focused on substance abuse treatment programs, researchers suggest that rural treatment seekers for nonalcohol-related substance abuse face more barriers than urban abusers (Robertson & Donnermeyer, 1997; McBride *et al.*, 1996; Soweel & Christianson, 1996).

Physical Activity and Inactivity

Possible associations with physical inactivity have been reported for stroke (Smith & Pratt,

1993) and breast cancer (Brownson *et al.,* 1993). Weak associations with physical inactivity have been reported for a variety of chronic diseases, including coronary heart disease (Smith & Pratt, 1993), colorectal cancer and breast cancer (Brownson *et al.,* 1993), diabetes (Bishop, Roesler, Zimmerman, & Ballard, 1993), and osteoporosis (Scott & Hochberg, 1993). At the other extreme, vigorous physical activity is associated with amyotrophic lateral sclerosis (Scott & Hochberg, 1993). While physical activity or inactivity has been associated with various chronic diseases, it is unclear how physical activity among rural residents may differ from their urban counterparts. One study reported that physical activity among rural children was more than twice that of urban children, with most of the physical activity for rural children being work-related (Proctor *et al.,* 1996). This level of physical fitness may act as a protective factor among rural children for many chronic diseases. Research on physical activity levels in rural populations is sparse, however, and there are many opportunities to explore how physical activity in rural residents, especially farmers, may affect their health.

Adolescent Health Concerns and Risk Behaviors

Youth risk behavior trends have become of increasing interest over the last several years (Kann *et al.,* 1996). Tobacco use, drug use, birth control pill use, and involvement in physical activity, however, have significantly worsened among high school students (Kann, Warren, Harris, Collins, Williams, Ross, & Kolbe, 1996). Still other behaviors considered risky have stayed the same or demonstrated inconsistent patterns of change from 1991 to 1997 in U.S. youth; these behaviors include suicide attempts, lifetime cigarette use, current sexual activity, and enrollment in physical education (Kann *et al.,* 1996). Risk behavior is closely related to perceptions of health (Vingilis, Wade, & Adlaf, 1991). Perceptions of health, in turn, are dependent on several factors. Economic, social, psychological, behavioral, and school competency factors have all shown to influence adolescents' perception of health (Vingilis *et al.,* 1991; Weston, Bell Brown, & Stewart, 1989). Rural

adolescents, facing recent depressions in agricultural economy and increases in life stresses, may be at an especially high risk of poor health perception (Puskar, Tusaie-Mumfdord, Sereika, & Lamb, 1999). These poor health perceptions influence decision making and involvement in risk-taking behaviors.

Rural students are reported to be more accepting of alcohol abuse (Larson, 1978; Chimonides & Frank, 1998), more likely to suggest violence as an appropriate intervention, and less accepting of depression (Chimonides & Frank, 1998) than urban students. Hence, rural adolescents may be a unique subset of adolescents in terms of at-risk behaviors. However, many studies show no significant difference in health concerns and risk behavior between rural and urban youth. In one study, major health concerns of rural adolescents were fatique, frequent headaches, weight problems, and depression. The most frequent risk behaviors reported were alcohol and tobacco use and minimal concern about venereal disease and AIDS (Puskar *et al.,* 1999). Such findings are consistent with national statistics, largely representing urban adolescents, compiled from the Youth Risk Behavior Survey (Kann *et al.,* 1996) and the Add Health Project (National Longitudinal Study of Adolescent Health, 1989). Overall, health concerns and risk behaviors of adolescents may differ slightly between rural and urban students, but the most common concerns and behaviors seem universal across geographic locations.

Conclusions

Some chronic diseases appear to be more prevalent in rural communities than in urban communities. Consistently higher prevalence rates in rural areas have been seen for chronic lung diseases (respiratory diseases) and neurologic disorders, specifically Parkinson's disease and amyotrophic lateral sclerosis. Some higher prevalence rates may reflect increased exposure to farming-related chemicals. Urban populations have higher prevalence rates of psychiatric disorders, including schizophrenia and anxiety disorders. It is unclear if the higher urban psychiatric prevalence rate is a true difference or if it reflects differences in diagnosis and referrals to urban areas for psychiatric patients. Most of the variation in chronic diseases between urban and rural populations appears to reflect variation in lifestyle factors. Lifestyle factors comprise the majority of risk factors for cardiovascular disease, most cancers, and musculoskeletal disorders. Variation or lack of variation in lifestyle factors between urban and rural populations may be highly correlated with the relative rates of most chronic diseases in these populations. Many lifestyle factors are modifiable. Therefore, behaviorial interventions for rural communities may be developed based on urban models that also consider rural social norms and issues of access to care specific to rural communities.

The greatest difference between the two populations is a reduction in access to good quality health care in many rural areas. Access to care is an important factor in interventions because it may affect the diagnosis and treatment of some chronic conditions and therefore the duration, morbidity, and mortality of chronic diseases. More research into how barriers to access to health care in rural areas differ from those in urban areas is needed, along with an understanding of how these barriers can be effectively modified.

Physicians are also an important component of chronic disease prevention because 80% of the U.S. population sees a doctor each year (Stoodt & Lengerich, 1993). Research into how to work effectively with rural primary care providers without increasing their burden is needed.

Overall, reduction of chronic disease in rural areas needs to focus on lifestyle changes and on barriers to lifestyle changes that are specific to rural settings. Lifestyle changes needed in rural populations are similar to those needed in urban areas. Barriers to change in rural areas include prohibitive costs, long distances to treatment, social stigmas about both diagnosis and treatment, heavy patient load among physicians, lack of accessible continuing medical education for physicians, and community knowledge and attitudes about risk factors, prevention, and treatment. The limited available research on chronic disease in rural communities provides opportunities for researchers willing to focus on rural health.

References

Armstrong, W., & Borman B. (1996). Breast cancer in New Zealand: Trends, patterns, and data quality. *New Zealand Medical Journal, 109,* 221–224.

Bannenberg, A. F. I., Ratt, H., & Plomp, H. N. (1992). Demand for alcohol treatment by problem drinkers. *Journal of Substance Abuse Treatment, 9*(1), 59–62.

Barrett, J. (1999). A focus on farming health in Iowa. *Environmental Health Perspectives, 107,* A142–143.

Beckman, L. J., & Kocel, K. M. (1982). The treatment-delivery system and alcohol abuse in women: Social policy implications. *Journal of Social Issues, 38*(2), 139–151.

Beebe, G. W., Kurtzke, J. F., Kurland, L. T., Auth, T. L., & Nagler, B. (1967). Studies on the natural history of multiple sclerosis—3. Epidemiologic analysis of the army experience in World War II. *Neurology, 17,* 1–17.

Bishop, D. B., Roesler, J. S., Zimmerman, B. R., & Ballard, D. J. (1993). Diabetes. In R. C. Brownson, P. L. Remington, & J. R. Davis (Eds.), *Chronic disease epidemiology and control* (pp. 221–240). Washington, DC: American Public Health Association.

Biswas, L. N., Manna, B., Maiti, P. K., & Sengupta, S. (1997). Sexual risk factors for cervical cancer among rural Indian women: A case-control study. *International Journal of Epidemiology, 26*(3), 491–495.

Bjorksten, B. (1994). Risk factors in early childhood for the development of atopic diseases. *Allergy, 49,* 400–407.

Blazer, D., George, L. K., Landerman, R., Pennybacker, M., Melville, M. L., Woodbury, M., Manton, K. G., Jordan, K., & Locke, B. (1985). Psychiatric disorders: A rural/urban comparison. *Archives of General Psychiatry, 43*(12), 1142.

Bongers, P., Houthuijs, D., Remijn, B., Brouwer, R., & Biersteker, K. (1987). Lung function and respiratory symptoms in pig farmers. *British Journal of Industrial Medicine, 44,* 819–823.

Booth, B. M., Ross, R. L., & Rost, K. (1999). Rural and urban problem drinkers in six southern states. *Substance Use & Misuse, 34*(4&5), 471–493.

Braback, L., & Kalvesten, L. (1991). Urban living as a risk factor for atopic sensitization in Swedish schoolchildren. *Pediatric Allergy & Immunology, 2,* 14–19.

Braun-Fahrlander, C. H., Gassner, M., Grize, L., Neu, U., Sennhausers, F. H., Varonier, H. S., Vuille, J. C., Wuthrich. B. (1999). Prevalence of hay fever and allergic sensation in farmer's children and their peers living in the same rural community. *Clinical & Experimental Allergy, 29,* 28–34.

Brownson, R. C., Reif, J. S., Alavanja, M. C. R., & Bal, D. G. (1993). Cancer. In R. C. Brownson, P. L. Remington, & J. R. Davis (Eds.), *Chronic disease epidemiology and control* (pp. 137–168). Washington, DC: American Public Health Association.

Butler, M. A., & Beale, C. L. (1994). *Rural-urban continuum codes for metro and nonmetro counties, 1993.* (Staff report no. 9425.) Washington, DC: Agricultural and Rural Economy Division, Economic Research Service, U.S. Washington, D.C.: Department of Agriculture.

Byrne, M. J., Jamrozik, K., Parsons, R. W., Fitzgerald, C. J., Dewar, J. M., Harvey, J. M., Sterrett, G. F., Ingram, D. M., Sheiner, H. J., Cameron, F. G. (1993). Breast cancer in Western Australia in 1989. II. Diagnosis and primary management. *Australian & New Zealand Journal of Surgery, 63,* 624–629.

Chan-Yeung, M., Schulzer, M., MacLean, L., Dorken, E., & Grzybowski, S. (1980). Epidemiologic health survey of grain elevator workers in British Columbia. *American Review of Respiratory Disease, 121,* 329–338.

Chimonides, K. M., & Frank, D. I. (1998). Rural and urban adolescents' perceptions of mental health. *Adolescence, 33*(132), 823–832.

Cockroft, A. E., McDermott, M., Edwards, J. H., McCarthy, P. (1983). Grain exposure—Symptoms and lung function. *European Journal of Respiratory Diseases, 64,* 189–196.

Commerce Clearing House. (1990). *Medicare and Medicaid guide.* Chicago: Commerce Clearing House, Inc.

Cooper, J. E., Goodhead, D., Craig, T., Harris, M., Howat, J., & Korer. J. (1987). The incidence of schizophrenia in Nottingham. *British Journal of Psychiatry, 151,* 619–626.

Cotton, D. J., Graham, B. L., Li, K. Y. R., Froh, F., Barnett, G. D., Dosman, J. A. (1983). Effects of grain dust exposure and smoking on respiratory symptoms and lung function. *Journal of Occupational Medicine, 25,* 131–141.

Crowell, B. A., Jr., George, L. K., Blazer, D., & Landerman, R (1986). Psychosocial risk factors and urban/rural differences in the prevalence of major depression. *British Journal of Psychiatry, 149,* 307–314.

Dassel, H. (1960). A survey of multiple sclerosis in a northern part of Scotland. *Acta Neurologica Scandinavica, 35* (suppl. 147), 64–72.

Davies, M. A., Bromet, E. J., Schulz, C., Dunn, L. O., & Morgensterm, M. (1989). Community Adjustment of chronic schizophrenic patients in urban and rural settings. *Hospital and Community Psychiatry, 40*(8), 824–830.

DeLeon, P. H., Wakefield, M., Schultz, A. J., Williams, J., & VandenBos, G. R. (1989). Rural America, Unique opportunities for health care delivery and health services research. *American Psychologist, 44*(10), 1298–1306.

Department of Health and Human Services. (1993). *Taking rural into account: Report on the National Public Forum.* Lincoln, NE: Department of Health and Human Services.

Devereux, G., Ayatollahi, T., Ward, R., Bromly, C., Bourke, S. J., Stenton, S. C., & Hendrick, D. J. (1996). Asthma, airways responsiveness and air pollution in two contrasting districts of northern England. *Thorax, 51,* 169–174.

Doll, R., & Peto, R. (1981). *The causes of cancer: Quantitative estimates of avoidable risks of cancer in the United States today.* New York: Oxford University Press.

Donham, K. J., & Mutel, C. F. (1982). Agricultural medicine: The missing component of the rural health movement. *Journal of Family Practice, 14,* 511.

Donham, K., Haglind, P., Peterson, Y., Rylander, R., & Belin L. (1989). Environmental and health studies of farm workers in Swedish swine confinement buildings. *British Journal of Industrial Medicine, 46,* 31–37.

do Pico, G. A. (1996). Lung (agricultural/rural). *Otolaryngol Head and Neck Surgery, 114*(2), 212–216.

do Pico, G. A., Raddan, W., Tsiatis, A., Peters, M. E., & Rankin, J. (1984). Epidemiologic study of clinical and physiologic parameters in grain handlers of northern United States. *American Review of Respiratory Diseases, 130,* 759–765.

Dosmon, J. A., Graham, B. L., Hall, D., VanLoon, P., Bhasin, P., & Froh, F. (1987). Respiratory symptoms and pulmonary function in farmers. *Journal of Occupational Medicine, 29,* 38–43.

Dottl, S. L., & Greenley, J. R. (1997). Rural-urban differences in psychiatric status and functioning among clients with severe mental illness. *Community Mental Health Journal, 33*(4), 311–332.

Farrow, D. C., Hunt, W. C., & Samet, J. M. (1992). Geographic variation in the treatment of localized breast cancer. *New England Journal of Medicine, 326,* 1097–1101.

Fortney, J. C., Lancaster, A. E., Owen, R. R., & Zhang, M. (1998). Geographic market areas for psychiatric and medical outpatient treatment. *Journal of Behavioral Health Services and Research, 25*(1), 108–116.

Franklin, G. M., & Nelson, L. M. (1993). Chronic neurologic disorders. In R. C. Brownson, P. L. Remington, & J. R. Davis (Eds.), *Chronic disease epidemiology and control* (pp. 307–336). Washington, DC: American Public Health Association.

Furnival, C. M. (1997). Breast cancer in rural Australia. *Medical Journal of Australia, 166*(1), 25–26.

Ganguli, M., Mulsant, B., Richards, S., Stoehr, G., & Mendelsohn, A. (1997). Antidepressant use over time in a rural older adult population: The MoVIES project. *Journal of the American Geriatrics Society, 45*(12), 1501–1503.

Garg, S. K., Mishra, V. N., Bhatnagar, M., Singh, R. B., Srivastava, R. B., & Garg, A. (1986). Chronic illness among rural population. *Indian Journal of Medical Sciences, 42*(3), 60–62.

Garrett, J. E. (1997). Health service accessibility and deaths from asthma. *Thorax, 52*(3), 205–206.

Goldring, J. M., James, D. S., & Anderson, H. A. (1993). Chronic lung diseases. In R. C. Brownson, P. L. Remington, & J. R. Davis (Eds.), *Chronic disease epidemiology and control* (pp. 169–198). Washington, DC: American Public Health Association.

Gorell, J. M., Johnson, C. C., Rybicki, B. A., Peterson, E. L., & Richardson, R. J. (1998). The risk of Parkinson's disease with exposure to pesticides, farming, well water, and rural living. *Neurology, 50*(5), 1346–1350.

Hall, K., Gureje, O., Gao, S., Ogunniyi, A., Hui, S. L., Baiyewu, O., Unverzagt, F. W., Oluwole, S., & Hendrie, H. C. (1998). Risk factors and Alzheimer's disease: A comparative study of two communities. *Australian & New Zealand Journal of Psychiatry, 32*(5), 698–706.

Harvei, S., Tretli, S., Langmark, F. (1996). Cancer of the prostate in Norway, 1957–1991: A descriptive study. *European Journal of Cancer, 32A*(1), 111–117.

He, J., Klag, M. J., Wu, Z., Qian, M. C., Chen, J. Y., Mo, P. S., He, Q. O., & Whelton, P. K. (1996) Effect of migration and related environmental changes on serum lipid levels in southwestern Chinese men. *American Journal of Epidemiology, 144*(9), 839–848.

Hicks, L. L. (1992). Access and utilization; special populations-special needs. In L. A. Straub & N. Walzer (Eds.), *Rural health care: Innovations in a changing environment* (pp. 20–25). London: Praeger.

Hilton, M. E. (1991). The demographic distribution of drinking patterns in 1984. In W. B. Clark & M. E. Hilton (Eds.), *Alcohol in America: Drinking practices and problems* (pp. 75–86). Albany, NY: State University of New York Press.

Hingson, R., Scotch, N., Day, N., & Culbert, A. (1980). Recognizing and seeking help for drinking problems: A study in the Boston metropolitan area. *Journal of Studies on Alcohol, 41*, 1102–1117.

Hingson, R., Mangione, T., Meyers, A., & Scotch, N. (1982). Recognizing and seeking help for drinking problems: A study in the Boston metropolitan area. *Journal of Studies on Alcohol, 43*(3), 273–288.

Hochberg, M. C. (1992) Arthritis and connective tissue diseases. In J. Thoene (Ed.), *Physician's guide to rare diseases* (pp. 907–959). Montvale, NJ: Dowden.

Howland, R. H. (1995). The treatment of persons with dual diagnoses in a rural community. *Psychiatry Quarterly, 66*(1), 33–49.

Hubble, J. P., Cao, T., Hassanein, R. E., Neuberger, J. S., & Koller, W. C. (1993). Risk factors for Parkinson's disease. *Neurology, 43*(9), 1693–1697.

Ingram, D. O., Gillum, R. F. (1989). Regional and urbanization differentials in coronary heart disease mortality in the United States, 1968–1985. *Journal of Clinical Epidemiology, 42*, 857–868.

International Agency for Research on Cancer (IARC). (1980). An evaluation of chemicals and industrial processes associated with cancer in humans based on human and animal data. *Cancer Research, 40*, 1–12.

Iverson, M., Dahl, R., Korsgaard, J., Hallas, T., & Jensen, E. J. (1988). Respiratory symptoms in Danish farmers: An epidemiological study of risk factors. *Thorax, 43*, 872–877.

Jones, A. P., Bentham, G. (1997). Health service accessibility and deaths from asthma in 401 local authority districts in England and Whales, 1988–1992. *Thorax, 52*, 218–222.

Jordon, C. M., Oei, T. P. S. (1989). Help-seeking behavior in problem drinkers: A review. *British Journal of Addiction, 84*, 979–988.

Jordan, J. M., Linder, G. F., Renner, J. B., & Fryer, J. G. (1995). The impact of arthritis in rural populations. *Arthritis Care & Research, 8*(4), 242–250.

Kann, L., Warren, C. W., Harris, W. A., Collins, J. L., Williams, B. I., Ross, J. G., & Kolbe, L. J. (1996). Youth risk behavior surveillance—United States, 1995. *Journal of School Health, 66*(10), 365–377.

Kaplan, R. M., Alcaraz, J. E., Anderson, J. P., & Weisman, M. (1996). Quality-adjusted life years lost to arthritis, effects of gender, race, and social class. *Arthritis Care Research, 9*(6), 473–482.

Kaufman, J. S., Owoaje, E. E., James, S. A., Rotimi, C. N., & Cooper, R. S. (1996). Determinants of hypertension in West Africa: Contribution of anthropometric and dietary factors to urban–rural and socioeconomic gradients. *American Journal of Epidemiology, 143*(12), 1203–1218.

Kaur, B., Anderson, H. R., Austin, J., Burr, M., Harkins, L. S., Strachan, D. P., & Warner, J. O. (1998). Prevalence of asthma symptoms, diagnosis, and treatment in 12–14 year old children across Great Britain. *British Medical Journal, 316*, 118–124.

Kay, K. (1974). Occupational cancer risks for pesticide workers. *Environmental Research, 7*, 243–271.

Keller-Byrne, J. E., Khuder, S. A., & Schaub, E. A. (1997). Meta-analyses of prostate cancer and farming. *American Journal of Industrial Medicine, 31*(5), 580–586.

Kelsey, J. L, & Hochberg, M. C. (1988). Epidemiology of chronic musculoskeletal disorders. *Annual Review of Public Health, 9*, 379–401.

Kronqvist, M., Johansson, E., Pershagen, G., Johansson, S. G., & van Hage-Hamsten M. (1999). Increasing prevalence of asthma over 12 years among dairy farmers on Gotland, Sweden: Storage mites remain dominant allergens. *Clinical & Experimental Allergy, 29*(1), 35–41.

Labarthe, D. R., Eissa, M., & Varas, C. (1991). Childhood precursors of high blood pressure and elevated cholesterol. *Annual Review of Public Health, 12,* 519–541.

Lantz, P. M., Weigers, M. E., & House, J. S. (1997). Education and income differentials in breast and cervical cancer screening. Policy implications for rural women. *Medical Care, 35*(3), 219–236.

Larson, O. F. (1978). Values and beliefs of rural people. In T. R. Ford (Ed.), *Rural USA: Persistence and change* (pp. 33–35). Ames: Iowa State University Press.

Lauer, K., & Firnhaber, W. (1985). Epidemiological investigations into multiple sclerosis in Southern Hesse: The influence of urban and rural environment on disease risk. *Acta Neurologica Scandinavica, 72,* 403–406.

Lensky, P. (1979). Geographical disproportions of multiple sclerosis in Czechoslovakia. *Geographia Medica, 9,* 1–7.

Link, B., & Dohrenwend, B. P. (1980). Formulation of hypotheses about the ratio of untreated to treated cases in the true prevalence studies of functional psychiatric disorders in adults in the United States. In B. D. Dohrenwend & B. S. Dohrenwend (Eds.), *Mental illness in the United States: Epidemiological estimates* (pp. 1–161). New York: Praeger Special Studies.

Logan, T. K., Schenck, J. E., Leukefeld, C. G., Meyers, J., & Allen, S. (1999). Rural attitudes, opinions, and drug use. *Substance Use & Misuse, 34*(4&5), 545–565.

Masala, G., Di Lollo, S., Picoco, C., Crosignani, P., Demicheli, V., Fontana, A., Funto, I., Miligi, L., Nanni, O., Papucci, A., Ramazzotti, V., Rodella, S., Stagnaro, E., Tumino, R., Vigano, C., Seniori Costantini, A., & Vineis, P. (1996). Incidence rates of leukemias, lymphomas, and myelomas in Italy: Geographic distribution and NHL histotypes. *International Journal of Cancer, 68*(2), 156–159.

McBride, D. C., Mutch, P. B., Kilcher, C., Inciardi, J. A., McCoy, H. V., & Pottieger, A. E. (1996). Barriers to treatment among crack-dependent and other drug-abusing inner city women. In D. D. Chitwood, J. E. Rivers & J. A. Inciardi (Eds.), *The American Pipe Dream, Crack, Cocaine, and the Inner City* (pp. 7–10). Ft. Worth, TX: Harcourt Brace.

Metsch, L. R., & McCoy, C. B. (1999). Drug treatment experiences: Rural and urban comparisons. *Substance Use & Misuse, 34*(4&5), 763–784.

Miller, F. T. (1982). Emergency crisis services in rural mental health centers. In P. A. Keller & J. D. Murray (Eds), *Handbook of rural community mental health* (pp. 1–230). New York: Human Science Press.

Miller, A. B. (1992). Planning cancer control strategies. In Health and Welfare (Eds.), *Chronic diseases in Canada.* Vol. 13, No. 1. Toronto, Ontario: Health and Welfare.

Mintzer, C. L., Culp, J., & Puskin, D. S. (1992). *Health care reform: What it means for rural America.* Rockville, MD: National Advisory Committee on Rural Health, Office of Rural Health Policy.

Morgan, D. C., Smyth, J. T., Lister, R. W., Pethybridge, R. J., Gilson, J. C. Callaghan, P., & Thomas, G. O. (1975). Chest symptoms in farming communities with special reference to farmer's lung. *British Journal of Industrial Medicine, 32,* 228–234.

Murray, J. D., & Keller, P. A. (1991). Psychology and rural America. *American Psychologist, 46*(3), 220–231.

Mushak, E. W., & Piver, W. T. (1992). Agricultural chemical utilization and human health. *Environmental Health Prospectives, 97,* 269–274.

National Center for Health Statistics. (1994). Current estimates from the National Health Interview Survey, 1992. *Vital & Health Statistics Series 10: Data from the National Health Survey, 10,* 189.

National Longitudinal Study of Adolescent Health. (1989). *MMWR, 38*(9), 147–149.

Neutel, C. I. (1980). Multiple sclerosis and the Canadian climate. *Journal of Chronic Diseases, 33,* 47–56.

Office of Technology Assessment. (1990). Health care in rural America (OTA-H-434). Washington, DC: U. S. Government Printing Office.

Paradiso, G., Tripoli, J., Galicchio, S., & Fejerman, N. (1999). Epidemiological, clinical, and electrodiagnostic findings in childhood Guillain-Barre syndrome: A reappraisal. *Annals of Neurology, 46*(5), 701–707.

Pearson, T. A., & Lewis, C. (1998). Rural epidemiology: Insights from a rural population laboratory. *American Journal of Epidemiology, 148*(10), 949–957.

Popp, W., Zwick, H., Steyrer, K., Rauscher, H., & Wanke, T. (1989). Sensitization to aeroallergens depends on environmental factors. *Allergy, 44,* 572–575.

Poskanzer, D. C., Sheridan, J. L., Prenney, L. B., & Walker, A. M. (1980). Multiple sclerosis in the Orkney and Shetland Islands. II. The search for an exogenous aetiology. *Journal of Epidemiology & Community Health, 34,* 240–252.

Pothier, P. (1991). Demythologizing rural mental health. *Archives of Psychiatric Nursing, 5*(3), 119–120.

Powe, B. D., & Weinrich, S. (1999). An intervention to decrease cancer fatalism among rural elders. *Oncology Nursing Forum, 26*(3), 583–588.

Proctor, M. H., Moore, L. L., Singer, M. R., Hood, M. Y., Nguyen, U. S., & Ellison, R. C. (1996). Risk profiles for noncommunicable diseases in rural and urban schoolchildren in the Republic of Cameroon. *Ethnicity & Disease, 6*(3-4), 235–243.

Pruitt, B. E., Kingery, P. M., Mirzaee, E., Heuberger, G., & Hurley, R. S. (1991). Peer influence and drug use among adolescents in rural areas. *Journal of Drug Education, 21*(1), 1–11.

Puskar, K. R., Tusaie-Mumford, K., Sereika, S., & Lamb, J. (1999). Health concerns and risk behaviors of rural adolescents. *Journal of Community Health Nursing, 16*(2), 109–119.

Rinne, U. K., Panelius, M., Kivalo, E., Hokkanen, E., & Palo, J. (1966). Distribution of multiple sclerosis in Finland with special reference to some geological factors. *Acta Neurologica Scandinavica, 42*, 385–399.

Risser, D. R. (1996). Cancer incidence and mortality in urban versus rural areas of Texas: 1980–1985. *Texas Medicine, 92*(1), 58–61.

Robertson, E. B., & Donnermeyer, J. F. (1997). Illegal drug use among rural adults, mental health consequences and treatment utilization. *American Journal of Drug & Alcohol Abuse, 23*(3), 467–484.

Room, R. (1989). The U.S. general population's experiences of responding to alcohol problems. *British Journal of Addiction, 84*(11), 1291–1304.

Rost, K., Zhang, M., Fortney, J., Smith, J., & Smith, G. R. (1998). Rural-urban differences in depression treatment and suicidality. *Medical Care, 36*(7), 1098–1107.

Saag, K. G, Doebbeling, B. N., Rohrer, J. E., Kolluri, S., Mitchell, T. A., & Wallace, R. B. (1998). Arthritis health service utilization among the elderly: The role of urban–rural residence and other utilization factors. *Arthritis Care & Research, 11*(3), 177–185.

Schmidt, L. (1992). A profile of problem drinkers in public mental health services. *Hospital and Community Psychiatry, 43*, 245–250.

Schneider, D., & Greenberg, M. R. (1992). Death rates in rural America, 1939–1981. Convergence and poverty. In W. M. Gesler & T. C. Ricketts (Eds.), *Health in rural North America. The geography of health care services and delivery* (pp. 55–85). New Brunswick, NJ: Rutgers University Press.

Schreinemachers, D. M., Creason, J. P., & Garry, V. F. (1999). Cancer mortality in agricultural regions of Minnesota. *Environmental Health Perspectives, 107*(3), 205–211.

Schwartz, D. A. (1999). Etiology and pathogenesis of airway disease in children and adults from rural communities. *Environmental Health Perspectives, 107*(3), 393–401.

Scott, J. C., & Hochberg, M. C. (1993). Arthritis and other musculoskeletal diseases. In R. C. Brownson, P. L. Remington, & J. R. Davis (Eds.), *Chronic disease epidemiology and control* (pp. 285–306). Washington, DC: American Public Health Association.

Shepherd, D. I., & Downie, A. W. (1980). A further prevalence study of multiple sclerosis in northeast Scotland. *Journal of Neurology Neurosurgery & Psychiatry, 43*, 310–315.

Smith, C. A., & Pratt, M. (1993). Cardiovascular disease. In R. C. Brownson, P. L. Remington, & J. R.

Davis (Eds.), *Chronic disease epidemiology and control* (pp. 83–108). Washington, DC: American Public Health Association.

Sommers, I. (1989). Geographic location and mental health services utilization among the chronically mentally ill. *Community Mental Health Journal, 25*(2), 132–144.

Soweel, R. L., & Christensen, P. (1996). HIV infection in rural communities. *Nursing Clinics of North America, 31*(1), 107–123.

Sridharan, R., & Murthy, B. N. (1999). Prevalence and pattern of epilepsy in India. *Epilepsia, 40*(5), 631–636.

Stoodt, G., & Lengerich, E. J. (1993). Reducing the burden of chronic disease in rural North Carolina. *North Carolina Medical Journal, 54*(10), 532–535.

Substance Abuse and Mental Health Services Administration. (1996). *National Household Survey on Drug Abuse, 1995.* Washington, DC: U.S. Department of Health and Human Services.

Summer, L. (1991). *Limited access: Health care for the rural poor.* Washington, DC: Center on Budget and Policy Priorities.

Swank, R., Lerstad, O., Strom, A., & Backer, J. (1952). Multiple sclerosis in rural Norway—Its geographic and occupational incidence in relation to nutrition. *New England Journal of Medicine, 246*, 721–728.

Thistle, P. J., & Chirenje, Z. M. (1997). Cervical cancer screening in rural populations of Zimbabwe. *Central African Journal of Medicine, 43*(9), 246–251.

Timmreck, T. C. (1988). *An introduction to epidemiology* (2nd ed.). Sudbury, MA: Jones and Bartlett.

Travis, S. S., & McAuley, W. J. (1999). Preexisting medical conditions in adult day services: An examination of nonmetropolitan and metropolitan admissions. *Journal of Gerontology, 54*A(5), M262–266.

U.S. General Accounting Office. (1990). *Rural drug abuse—Prevalence, relation to crime, and programs.* Washington, DC: U.S. General Accounting Office.

Verdes, F., Petrescu, A., & Cernescu, C. (1978). Epidemiologic survey of multiple sclerosis in the Bucharest city and suburban area. *Acta Neurologica Scandinavica, 58*(2), 109–120.

Vingilis, E., Wade, T., & Adlaf, E. (1991). What factors predict student self-rated physical health? *Journal of Adolescent Psychiatry, 21*(1), 83–97.

Vohlonen, I., Tupi, K., Terho, E. O., & Husman, K. (1987). Prevalence and incidence of chronic bronchitis and farmer's lung with respect to the geographical location of the farm and to the work of farmers. *European Journal of Respiratory Diseases, 152* (suppl.), 37–46.

von Mutius, E., Illi, S., Nicolai, T., & Martinez, F. D. (1996). Relation of indoor heating with asthma, allergic sensitization, and bronchial responsiveness, survey of children in south Bavaria. *British Medical Journal, 312*, 1448–1450.

Voukiklaris, G. E., Kafatos, A., & Dontas, A. S. (1996). Changing prevalence of coronary heart disease risk factors and cardiovascular diseases in men of a rural area of Crete: 1960 to 1991. *Angiology, 47*(1), 43–49.

Wallace, R. E., & Wallace, R. B. (1998). Rural-urban contrasts in elder health status: Methodologic issues and findings. In R. T. Coward & J. A. Krout (Eds.), *Aging in rural settings: Life circumstances and distinctive features* (pp. 67–840). New York: Springer.

Warren, C. P. W., Holford-Strevens, V., & Manfreda, J. (1987). Respiratory disorders among Canadian farmers. *European Journal of Respiratory Diseases, 154* (suppl.), 10–14.

Weinert, C, & Long, K. A. (1990). Rural families and health care: Refining the knowledge base. *Marriage & Family Review, 15,* 57.

Weisner, C. (1993). Toward an alcohol treatment entry model: A comparison of problem drinkers in the general population and in treatment. *Alcoholism Clinical & Experimental Research, 17*(4), 746–752.

Weisner, C., & Schmidt, L. (1992). Gender disparities in treatment for alcohol problems. *Journal of the American Medical Association, 268*(14), 1872–1876.

Werneck, A. L., & Alvarenga, H. (1999). Genetics, drugs and environmental factors in Parkinson's disease. A case-control study. *Arquivos de Neuro-Psiquiatria, 57*(2B), 347–355.

Wesseling, C, Antich, D., Hogstedt, C., Rodriguez, A. C., & Ahlbom, A. (1999). Geographical differences of cancer incidence in Costa Rica in relation to environmental and occupational pesticide exposure. *International Journal of Epidemiology, 28*(3), 365–374.

Weston, W. W., Bell Brown, J., & Stewart, M. A. (1989). Patient-centered interviewing. Part I. Understanding patients' experiences. *Canadian Family Physician, 35,* 147–151.

Whitehead, R., Chillag, S., & Elliott, D. (1992). Anabolic steroid use among adolescents in a rural state. *Journal of Family Practice, 34*(4), 401–405.

Wilkstrom, J. (1975). Studies on the clustering of multiple sclerosis in Finland. II. Microepidemiology in one high-risk county with special reference to familial cases. *Acta Neurologica Scandinavica, 51,* 173–183.

Willems, J. P., Saunders, J. T., Hunt, D. E., & Schorling, J. B. (1997). Prevalence of coronary heart disease risk factors among rural blacks: A community-based study. *Southern Medical Journal, 90*(8), 814–820.

Wing, J. K. (1978). *Schizophrenia: Towards a new synthesis.* London: Academic Press.

World Health Organization (WHO). (1977). *ICD-9: International Classification of Disease, Ninth Revision.* Geneva, Switzerland: World Health Organization.

Yach, D., Myers, J., Bradshaw, D., & Benatar, S. R. (1985). A respiratory epidemiologic survey of grain mill workers in Cape Town, South Africa. *American Review of Respiratory Disease, 131,* 505–510.

Yawn, B. P., Yawn, R. A., & Uden, D. L. (1992). Substance use in rural midwestern pregnant women. *Archives of Family Medicine, 1*(1), 83–88.

Yesalis, C. E. III, Lemke, J. H., Wallace, R. B., Kohout, F. J., & Morris, M. C. (1985). Health status of the rural elderly according to farm work history: The Iowa 65+ rural health study. *Archives of Environmental Health, 40,* 245–253.

Zejda, J. E., McDuffie, H. H., & Dosman, J. A. (1993). Epidemiology of health and safety risks in agriculture and related industries: Practical applications for rural physicians. *Western Journal of Medicine, 158*(1), 56–63.

12

Rural Occupational Health and Safety

LORANN STALLONES

Approximately 20% of the U.S. population, or 53 million Americans, reside in rural areas, but as with many issues in rural health, there is little published information in occupational safety and health specifically for rural residents. In Colorado, between 1982 and 1987, 16% of the total workforce was employed in rural counties (Colorado Department of Health, 1990). The majority of rural residents who do not commute to urban areas are likely to work in the production of goods and they are often self-employed. Because small businesses are primary employers in rural areas, information is not readily available from the Bureau of Labor Statistics, which focuses largely on businesses that employ 11 or more workers who are 14 years of age or older (Pratt, 1990). The most extensive work on occupational safety and health in rural areas has been done among agricultural workers (Donham et al., 1997), including migrant and seasonal workers, yet this group makes up only about 2% to 5% of the total population and a small percentage of all rural workers.

No single handbook, manual, or other source contains essential information on the hazards that exist specific to occupation. A wide array of hazards are included in workplace settings, including acute trauma; physical hazards such as ionizing and non-ionizing radiation; chemical hazards that can have immediate or delayed effects; biological hazards; and ergonomic and social hazards (Key et al., 1977). Extensive information has been compiled on chemical hazards, including reproductive effects of occupational exposures (Paul, 1993). The International Labour Organization (ILO) has proceeded with the development of international safety datasheets on occupations. The catalogue being developed will include job profiles, including definitions and descriptions, tasks performed, related occupations, primary equipment used, industries that have the occupation in common, and hazards (Donagi & Aladjem, 1998). Hazards are grouped much as noted earlier in this paragraph: acute traumatic events, physical hazards such as ionizing and nonionizing radiation, chemical hazards related to nonaccidental exposures, and biological, ergonomic, and social hazards.

The U.S. Department of Labor was created by Congress in 1913 to promote the welfare of working people, to improve working conditions, and to enhance opportunities for profitable employment (U.S. Department of Labor, 2000). The department originally consisted of four bureaus: the Bureau of Labor Statistics, the Bureau of Immigration, the Bureau of Naturalization, and the Children's Bureau. A service was added to mediate labor disputes, and in 1915

LORANN STALLONES • Colorado Injury Control Research Center, Department of Environmental Health, Colorado State University, Fort Collins, Colorado 80523-1676.

Handbook of Rural Health, edited by Loue and Quill. Kluwer Academic/Plenum Publishers, New York, 2001.

a small employment service was added. Issues that were of concern then and that are still the focus of department activities include workers' wages and hours, working conditions and employment opportunities, employment discrimination, cooperative labor–management relations, and labor's role in national industrial productivity. Landmark laws were developed to protect wage earners, and the department became a principal regulatory and enforcement agency. During the 1920s the department promoted vocational training for youth and helped migrant workers find jobs in labor-short areas. Immigration laws were changed from a free-immigration policy to a quota system through laws enacted in 1921 and 1924. During this decade, the Women's Bureau was founded to promote employment opportunities for women. Frances Perkins was appointed as Secretary of Labor by President Franklin Roosevelt in 1933, the first woman appointed to a cabinet post, and she served longer than any other person in that position (1933 to 1945). During her tenure standards were developed—including minimum wage, overtime, and child labor—that are contained in the Fair Labor Standards Act (FLSA). Currently, both the FLSA and workers' compensation are located under the Employment Standards Administration (ESA) within the Department of Labor. Health and safety enforcement began in 1958 when standards were passed to protect dock and harbor workers from many hazards. This role expanded with the 1970 passage of the Occupational Health and Safety Act and then again in 1978 when responsibility for mine safety and health was transferred to the Department of Labor. Currently, the principal regulatory agencies involved with occupational safety and health regulation in the United States are the Occupational Safety and Health Administration (OSHA) and the Mine Safety and Health Administration (MSHA). OSHA governs employees in the private sector and MSHA governs miners. The agencies are charged with adopting legally enforceable standards based on the best scientific evidence to ensure that no worker will suffer illness if exposed to his or her work throughout a lifetime. The second criterion for regulation is that the standards be technically feasible. Standards that are covered include limits on the concentration and duration of exposure to hazardous substances, work practices, medical surveillance, personal protective devices, responsibility of the employer to inform workers about hazards through warning labels, education, and training. Most standards, however, are related to permissible exposure limits (PELs). Most of the safety standards that are adopted are based on safety codes developed by professional organizations or by consensus standards organizations. A list of these includes: the American National Standards Institute (ANSI), the National Fire Protection Association; the National Electrical Code, the American Society for Testing Materials, the American Welding Society, and the American Society of Mechanical Engineers. ANSI standards relevant to occupational safety and health include respiratory protection devices, industrial ventilation, lasers, and quality standards for compressed gas. Standards set by OSHA and MSHA cover about 600 of the 60,000 chemicals used in industrial countries (Weeks, Levy, & Wagner, 1991).

Two notable additional regulatory agencies also have occupational health and safety responsibility. The Environmental Protection Agency (EPA) regulates users of pesticides and has the authority to issue licenses to those who apply restricted-use pesticides (Weeks et al., 1991). Authority for registration and use of pesticides comes to EPA through the Federal Insecticide, Fungicide, and Rodenticide Act (FIFRA). The act requires that EPA protect against any unreasonable adverse effects to humans and the environment and includes a requirement to balance the costs and benefits of use of all pesticides (National Research Council, 1998). EPA worker protection standards were developed in 1992 and implemented in 1996 and apply to all employees who handle agricultural pesticides and who cultivate and harvest plants on farms or in greenhouses, nurseries, or forests. The regulations are intended to eliminate or reduce exposure to pesticides, mitigate exposures that occur, and inform employees about pesticide hazards. The regulations include provisions regarding use of personal protective equipment, setting reentry times for workers entering treated fields, notification of workers about areas that have been treated, and training of employees in basic pesticide-safety measures (National Research Council, 1998). Under the Toxic Substances Control Act (TSCA), an inventory of over 70,000 existing chemicals is maintained (Stellman, 1998). Prior to manufacture or importation, chemicals that are not on the list must have a premanufacture notice submitted to EPA, and EPA may impose testing or other requirements based on a review of the notice. The Nuclear Regulatory Commission (NRC) regulates users of radioactive materials and also has the authority to issue licenses (Weeks et al., 1991).

The National Highway Safety Administration, the Federal Aviation Administration, the Federal Railroad Administration, and the U.S. Coast Guard are all located in the Department of Transportation. When work-related deaths and injuries involve transportation safety, these organizations become involved. They govern such things as vehicular and aircraft integrity, limitations on the hours of work allowed, and licensure of airline pilots and water transportation captains (Weeks et al., 1991).

As in urban settings, these agencies become involved in rural occupational safety and health as their various mandates require. Regulations that apply in urban settings are the same as those that apply in rural settings. There are variations across states in how the regulatory agencies operate; some of the variations are provided below.

Occupational Safety and Health Administration (OSHA)

Established in 1971 as a unit of the Department of Labor, OSHA's mandate is to set health and safety standards and to enforce compliance with these standards by inspecting workplaces and issuing citations for noncompliance. OSHA has jurisdiction over employers in the private sector excluding railroads, merchant marine, and dock employees, mines, and highway traffic. States can implement their own OSHA programs instead of the federal program, but they must be determined to be as effective as the federal program. Federal employees are supposed to be covered by plans implemented by the employing agencies.

Employers with 10 or more employees are required to keep records of workers' job-related injuries and illnesses and, if requested, make the information available to OSHA inspectors, workers and worker representatives (Weeks et al., 1991). In addition, employers are responsible for being familiar with all standards that apply to their workplace, to control hazards, to inform and train workers about the hazards, and to ensure that workers have and use protective equipment. Employers are also required to report workplace fatalities and serious injuries to OSHA.

OSHA employs approximately 650 inspectors nationwide to cover more than 5 million workplaces. Priorities for conducting inspections are: (1) imminent dangers; (2) fatalities or catastrophes; (3) employee requests; and (4) general schedule or random selection. Imminent dangers are conditions under which death or serious harm will occur immediately or before the danger can be eliminated through normal enforcement procedures. Workers have limited legal protection to refuse to work under such conditions, and inspectors may seek a temporary restraining order to shut down a workplace for up to five days. Reporting of work-related death is mandatory. Annually, OSHA investigates only about 1,500 fatalities of the estimated 8,000 that occur. Employees may request an inspection and these requests may be anonymous, but requests must be in writing and the inspection is likely to include only those items listed in the complaint. Each field office determines which criteria to use to select certain industries or workplaces for general schedule or random inspections (Weeks et al., 1991).

A mandatory standard called the Hazard Communication Standard (HCA) was developed as to ensure that all chemicals produced in or imported to the United States are evaluated. Hazard information related to chemicals must be transmitted to employers and workers through a program that includes labeling, other forms of warnings, chemical safety data sheets, and training (Stellman, 1998).

MINE SAFETY AND HEALTH ADMINISTRATION (MSHA)

MSHA was established as a unit of the Department of the Interior in 1969 with jurisdiction limited to coal mines. The statute was amended in 1977 and responsibility moved to the Department of Labor, with jurisdiction extending to all underground and surface mines and attached facilities in the United States. The enforcement powers of MSHA are significantly greater than OSHA's. MSHA is required to inspect each underground mine four times each year and each surface mine twice each year. Citations and penalties for noncompliance are mandatory. MSHA inspectors can shut down all or part of mines they consider to present imminent dangers. In contrast, OSHA cannot shut down an operation without a court order.

Special Populations in Rural Occupational Safety and Health

In rural communities, several groups require specific attention. The first group is migrant and seasonal farmworkers, and they have been discussed elsewhere and so will not be presented here. The second group includes farm owners and operators and farmworkers who are not seasonal or migrant workers. The third group is made up of the youth who work in rural communities, primarily on farms. The second two groups will be discussed below.

Agricultural Workers

Four basic facts related to production agriculture differentiate it from industrial settings: (1) a lack of uniformity and control of workplaces and work activities; (2) the overlap of residence and workplace; (3) a majority of family-operated farms without age restrictions for workers; and (4) relatively little government regulation of work hazards (Murphy, 1992). As a result of these unique circumstances the prevention and control strategies employed for the reduction of illnesses and injuries have been different in agriculture than in other industries. In addition, there are more government agencies that serve agriculture and a wider array of

nongovernmental agencies involved in all aspects of agriculture, from lobbying groups to nonprofit organizations with specific goals. Farms are also exempted from many health and safety standards under the Occupational Safety and Health Act. Congressional riders are included in annual appropriations bills that prohibit the OSHA from spending money to prescribe, issue, administer, or enforce any standard, regulation, or order in farms that do not have temporary labor camps and that have 10 or fewer employees (National Research Council, 1998).

During the past 40 years, farms have become larger, and the number of farm workers has declined by more than 70% since the 1950s (Myers, Herrick, Olenchock, Myers, Parker, Hard, & Wilson, 1992). Increased availability of machinery, chemicals, water, and improved seed and livestock has resulted in a substitution of capital for labor. The incidence of workplace illnesses and injuries among workers on farms with 10 or more employees is exceeded only by construction and mining. The working population in the United States consists of approximately 2.7 million farm operators, 2.2 million hired farmworkers, and 2.9 million unpaid farmworkers. In addition, there are approximately 1.2 million children under 14 years of age who reside with farm operators and are likely to help with farm chores, and an additional 800,000 children of hired farmworkers who may work with parents. Further, most farm operators are white (97%), a majority are male (77%), and the median age is 47 years (Myers et al., 1992). Relevant to safety and health issues, almost half do nonfarm work during the year, averaging 213 days of paid work off the farm. The average number of days operating a farm is 235 per year, with about 58% working 250 days or more.

In 1991, the Surgeon General convened a conference on agricultural safety and health, as mandated by Congress (Myers et al., 1992). Leading causes of illnesses and injuries among the agricultural workers that were identified and discussed included occupational lung diseases (e.g., farmers' lung disease, asthma, hog lung, silo fillers' disease, organic dust toxic syndrome); musculoskeletal injuries (e.g., milkers' knee, tractor drivers' syndrome, tendinitis, repetitive motion trauma); occupational cancers (e.g., skin, bladder, brain, leukemia); traumatic injuries (machine-related fatalities, electrocutions, suffocation, suicide, amputations, eye injuries); occupational cardiovascular disease (heat stroke); reproductive disorders (infertility, miscarriages); neurological disorders (dementia, neurologic dysfunction); noise-induced hearing loss; dermatological disorders (dermatitis); psychological disorders (stress-related conditions, depression); and infectious diseases (zoonoses, tuberculosis) (Myers *et al.*, 1992). Despite the traditional perspective that agricultural workers other than migrants are a healthy group, there is increasing evidence that they are not. The exposures they receive in the workplace are similar in nature to those of many industrial workers; the differences are in the amount and duration of exposure over a working year. Farmers work on a schedule that is dictated more by weather conditions than any other working population. As a result, they work extremely long hours for short periods during a year. In doing so, they resemble shift workers and new employees to a great extent, and this is reflected in high rates of traumatic injury. Although a farmer may become very familiar with the equipment in use during one season, the equipment is put away and brought out again months later, so there is a period of becoming accustomed to the machinery each time it is used during a working lifetime. In addition, there may be no one around to retrain a farmer about proper use and safety requirements. In the event that a farmer is injured, it can be hours before someone realizes there is a problem. Increasingly, spouses are working off the farm to augment income and provide access to lower-cost medical insurance. This further delays discovery of an injured farmer and increases the likelihood of worsening the outcome of the injury. Another consequence of this is that the spouses are less and less familiar with the operation of the farm and the equipment, making them less likely to be able to locate someone who has been injured and less likely to know how to extricate the injured person from entrapment. As the complexity of the machinery increases, so does the importance of having familiarity with how it works in order to shut it off. With fewer people involved in farming, the population density in those ar-

eas of intense agriculture is further reduced, exacerbating problems of discovering an injury has occurred, of rapid response to medical emergencies, and of availability of medical care.

Children and Adolescent Labor Issues

The hours of work and types of jobs that children and adolescents may perform are governed by state and federal regulations (National Research Council, 1998). The primary law governing the protection of children at work is the Fair Labor Standards Act (FLSA). Those who are under 16 years of age are to confine their employment to hours and types of work that will not interfere with their schooling, health, and well-being. Those who are 16 to 17 years of age are not covered, but the Secretary of Labor may prohibit them from working at hazardous jobs. FLSA applies only to those businesses engaged in interstate commerce with annual gross income in excess of $500,000. No data are available on how many of the 6.5 million workplaces with 110 million employees are children or adolescents. Children who work in agriculture are subject to different regulations from those not employed in agriculture. Specific differences include the age at which hazardous jobs can be performed: 18 years in nonagricultural work and 16 years in agricultural work. In addition, hours and hazardous orders, even for the same hazard, vary for youth involved in agriculture. Youth under the age of 16 who work on a farm owned and operated by their parents are allowed to work during school hours, unlike any other employed youth under 16 years of age. In fact, youth working on their parents' farms are exempted from coverage under FLSA, regardless of age, hazards related to the job, or hours worked, unlike all other children who are prohibited from hazardous jobs even if working with parents. Regulations prohibit certain types of work by age, but ignore conditions of work in permissible jobs (National Research Council, 1998). Hazardous jobs that are prohibited, except for youth employed in agriculture, include the following: manufacturing or storing explosives; driving a motor vehicle and being an outside helper on a motor vehicle; coal mining; logging and sawmilling; using power-driven wood-working machines; being exposed to radioactive substances and ionizing radiation; using power-driven hoisting apparatus and power driven-metal forming, punching, and sheating machines; mining other than coal mining; slaughtering, meat packing, processing, or rendering; using power-driven bakery machines and power-driven paper products machines; manufacturing brick, tile, and related products; using power-driven circular saws, band saws, and guillotine shears; and carrying out wrecking, demolition, and ship-breaking operations, roofing operations, and excavation operations. Eleven hazardous farm jobs are not allowed for youth below the age of 16, but children and adolescents who work for their parents are exempt from the prohibitions. These jobs are: (1) operating a tractor of over 20 power-take-off horsepower and connecting or disconnecting an implement or any part of an implement to a tractor as described above; (2) operating or assisting to operate the following machines: corn picker, cotton picker, grain combine, hay mower, crop dryer, forage blower, auger conveyor, forage harvester, hay baler, potato digger, mobile pea viner, feed grinder, crop dryer, unloading mechanism of a nongravity type self-unloading wagon or trailer, power post-hole digger, power post driver, or nonwalking type rotary tiller; (3) operating or assisting to operate trencher or earth moving equipment, forklift, potato combine, and power driven circular, band or chain saws; (4) working on a farm in a yard, pen, or stall occupied by a bull, boar, or stud horse maintained for breeding purposes and sow with suckling pigs or cow with newborn calf (with umbilical cord still present); (5) felling, buckling, skidding, loading, or unloading timber with a butt diameter of more than 6 inches; (6) working from a ladder or scaffold at a height of over 20 feet; (7) driving a bus, truck, or car while transporting passengers, or riding as a passenger or helper on a tractor; (8) working inside a fruit, forage or grain storage unit designed to retain an oxygen deficient or toxic atmosphere or in an upright silo within two weeks after silage has been added or when a top loading device is in operation position or in a manure pit or in a horizontal silo while operating a tractor for packing purposes; (9) handling or applying pesticides and other agricultural chemicals classified as Category I or II of toxicity by the Fed-

eral Insecticide, Fungicide, Rodenticide Act (FIFRA); (10) handling or using a blasting agent including black powder, sensitized ammonium nitrate, blasting caps, and primer cords; and (11) transporting, transferring, or applying anhydrous ammonia. For several of these restrictions exceptions are made for student learners (1,2,3,4,5,6) and for participants in 4-H training programs or vocational agricultural training programs (1,2).

Conclusion

Limited information is currently available on occupational illnesses and injuries among rural workers other than those involved in agriculture. Researchers need to delineate the magnitude of the problem among rural residents in order to determine differential patterns of employment and risk. The absence of emergency medical care and hospitals, and the distance from major medical care centers, argue for more emphasis on prevention programs in rural areas, but the programs cannot be appropriately developed without baseline information to target the areas to be addressed. Child and adolescent labor issues also need further attention. As the population in rural areas declines, the propensity to hire any available worker to fill a job may place rural youth at higher risk of exposure to occupational injuries and illnesses than urban and suburban youth.

References

Colorado Department of Health. (1990). *Occupational injury deaths in Colorado, 1982–1987.* Denver: Health Statistics and Vital Records.

Donagi, A., & Aladjem, A. (1998). Systematization of occupational hazards by occupation. J. M. Stellman (Ed.), *Encylopaedia of occupational health and safety,* (4th ed., Vol. 4.). Geneva, Switzerland: International Labour Office.

Donham, K. J., Rautiainen, R., Schuman, S. H., & Lay, J. A. (1997) *Agricultural health and safety: Recent advances.* New York: Haworth Medical Press.

Key, M. M. , Henschel, A. F., Butler, J., Ligo, R. N., & Tabershaw, I. R. (1977). *Occupational diseases: A guide to their recognition.* Washington, DC: U.S. Government Printing Office.

Murphy, D. J. (1992). *Safety and health for production agriculture.* St. Joseph, MI: American Society of Agricultural Engineers.

Myers, M. L., Herrick, R. F., Olenchock, S. A., Myers, J. R., Parker, J. E., Hard, D. L., & Wilson, K. (1992). *Papers and proceedings of the Surgeon General's Conference on Agricultural Safety and Health* (DHHS (NIOSH) publication no. 92-105). Washington DC: U.S. Government Printing Office.

National Research Council. (1998). *Protecting youth at work: Health, safety, and development of working children and adolescents in the United States.* Washington, DC: National Academy of Sciences.

Paul, M. (1993). *Occupational and environmental re-productive hazards: A guide for clinicians.* Baltimore, MD: Williams & Wilkins.

Pratt, D. S. (1990). Occupational health and the rural worker: Agriculture, mining, and logging. *Journal of Rural Health, 6,* 399–417.

Stellman, J. M. (1998). *Encylopaedia of occupational health and safety* (4th ed., vol. 3). Geneva, Switzerland: International Labour Office.

U.S. Department of Labor. (2000). DOL historical information (May 3, 2000); http://www.dol.gov/dol/asp/public/programs/history/main.htm

Weeks, J. L., Levy, B. S., & Wagner, G. R. (1991). *Preventing occupational disease and injury.* Washington, DC: American Public Health Association.

13

Oral Health

ROBERT ISMAN

Why include a chapter on oral health in a rural health textbook? Is dentistry so unique among the health professions that it warrants a separate discussion from a more generic discourse on health services? The answer is yes . . . and no. On one hand, there are a number of unique features about oral health and oral health services that set them apart from other health services. On the other hand, just as the mouth is part of the body, oral health is an essential and integral component of overall health and should not be isolated from any analysis of health services.

Unfortunately, oral health represents a much overlooked component of health and health care. This chapter will examine why oral health services are so often undervalued, and will provide a brief description of the epidemiology of major oral diseases and conditions, access to and financing of oral health services, the prevention of oral disease, oral health care delivery system issues, and dental workforce issues. In addition, some suggestions for dealing with the oral health problems of rural communities will be offered.

Oral Health: An Integral Component of Primary Health Care

While it may seem intuitively obvious that oral health care is an integral and essential com-

ROBERT ISMAN • California Department of Health Services, Office of Medi-Cal Dental Services, Rancho Cordova, California 95670, and University of California at San Francisco, San Francisco, California 94143.

Handbook of Rural Health, edited by Loue and Quill. Kluwer Academic/Plenum Publishers, New York, 2001.

ponent of primary health care, the "obvious" has often escaped the unsympathetic ears of physicians and policymakers. Reasons include these: (1) a tendency toward professional isolationism within the dental profession; (2) a misperception of dentistry as a specialty of medicine that has often caused nondental professionals to be undereducated about oral health; (3) relatively little interaction between dentists and other health care providers, external regulatory bodies, and community agencies, resulting in limited involvement in matters related to major health policy issues; (4) lack of experience of better educated health professionals with the kinds of dental problems faced by less affluent individuals, leading to an underestimation of the significance of oral health problems compared with other health problems; and (5) major oral diseases—dental caries (tooth decay) and periodontal disease (gum disease)—are so pervasive as to be considered an inevitable part of life (Isman, 1993).

Why should oral health services be considered a part of primary care? One of the most important reasons is that the effects of oral health problems are not limited to the mouth; often, they also profoundly affect general health. For example, while there is rightly much national attention and funding support for research on cervical cancer, it is largely unknown that oral cancer kills more Americans than cervical cancer (American Cancer Society, 1999). Although it occurs in the mouth, oral cancer is a threat to *health*, not just to oral health. Similarly, the first indication of HIV infection often occurs in the mouth and is detected by dental professionals.

The early interventions afforded by early detection of symptoms allow HIV-infected persons to lead longer, higher-quality, and more productive lives. The oral manifestations of HIV, although they occur in the mouth, are threats to *health*, not just to oral health.

In recent years, the evidence linking oral and systemic disease has become even stronger. Periodontal disease now is clearly associated with preterm low birth weight (Offenbacher, Katz, Fertik, Collins, Boyd, Maynor, McKaig, & Beck, 1996), cardiovascular disease (Grau *et al.*, 1997), diabetes (Grossi & Genco, 1998), and respiratory disease (Scannapieco, Papandonatos, & Dunford, 1998).

Epidemiology of Oral Diseases

Dental Caries

Dental caries is one of the most prevalent of human diseases, and the most prevalent chronic disease of children, occurring approximately five to eight times more frequently than asthma (Edelstein, 1998). By the time they graduate from high school, almost 80% of all children in the United States have experienced tooth decay (Kaste, Selwitz, Oldakowski, Brunelle, Winn, & Brown, 1996a). By middle age, United States adults have more than half their teeth affected

by decay (National Institute of Dental Research, 1987).

Almost 55% of 5 to 17-year-olds have experienced no caries in their permanent teeth, and 62% of 2 to 9-year-olds have experienced no caries in their primary teeth. However, the proportion of children who are caries-free declines dramatically with age, so that although 74% of 5 to 11-year-olds have never had a decayed permanent tooth, only one-third of 12 to 17-year-olds have had no decay in the permanent dentition (Figure 1). Girls have a slightly higher prevalence of caries in the permanent dentition than do boys of similar ages, but there is little difference in caries experience between girls and boys in the primary dentition.

Caries is not uniformly distributed among all children. Rather, 25% of the children with at least one permanent tooth have 80% of the caries (Kaste *et al.*, 1996a). There are no recent national data comparing caries prevalence in urban and rural areas. Earlier studies indicated that children from rural areas have a higher percentage of decayed and missing teeth than urban children (Public Health Service, 1991). Most of the disease is concentrated among those with low income and low educational attainment and among minorities, although there are some exceptions.

Family income and education have a pronounced relationship to caries prevalence. Fig-

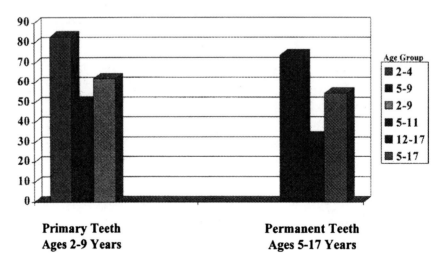

FIGURE 1. Percentage of children with no tooth decay, by age group, 1988–1994. From National Center for Health Statistics, 1999.

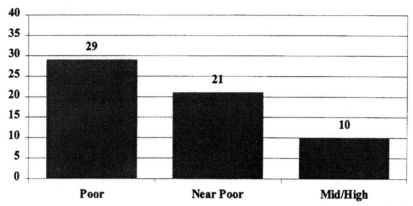

FIGURE 2. Percentage of children ages two to four years who have ever had tooth decay, by family income, 1988–1994. From National Center for Health Statistics, 1999.

ure 2 shows that among 2 to 4-year-old children, about three times as many children from poor families have experienced caries as children from middle- and high-income families. Similarly, twice as many 15-year-olds from families with less than a high school education had untreated caries as from families with more than a high school education (Figure 3) (National Center for Health Statistics, 1999).

Among adults, for every population subgroup, the prevalence of enamel caries (caries on the crowns of teeth—above the gums) increased with age (Winn, Brunelle, Selwitz, Kaste, Oldakowski, Kingman, & Brown, 1996). Males had lower overall caries experience than females, and non-Hispanic whites had more than non-Hispanic blacks, who in turn had more than Mexican Americans. The prevalence of root

caries increased with age in almost every demographic group. Overall, one out of every four adults who still had teeth had root caries. More men than women had root caries, and differences between racial/ethnic groups were small.

Periodontal Diseases

Periodontal diseases refer to diseases of the tissues that support the teeth in the jaws. Gingivitis (inflamed and bleeding gums), loss of the bone supporting the teeth in the jaws, receding gums, accumulation of bacterial plaque, calculus (tartar), poor oral hygiene, and tooth loss have all been used in epidemiologic studies as surrogates for "periodontal disease." Periodontal disease is often stated to be the leading cause of tooth loss among adults in the United States,

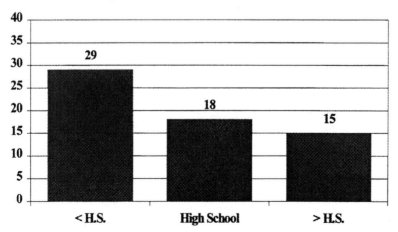

FIGURE 3. Percentage of children age 15 with untreated tooth decay, by education level of parents, 1988–1994. H. S. Education = high school education, head of household. From National Center for Health Statistics, 1999.

although some more recent studies have found dental caries to result in more tooth loss.

More than 90% of persons 13 years of age or older have experienced some clinically evident loss of periodontal attachment, but only 15% exhibited more severe periodontal destruction (loss of tissue attachment of 5 mm or more) (Brown, Brunelle, & Kingman, 1996). Overall, females exhibited better periodontal health than males, and non-Hispanic whites exhibited better periodontal health than either non-Hispanic blacks or Mexican Americans. No data on urban–rural differences were reported.

Tooth Loss and Edentulism

The overall prevalence of tooth loss and edentulism (loss of all natural teeth) have been declining in the United States over the past several decades, but important differences still exist between different subpopulations. During 1988–1991, about 10% of United States adults were edentulous, with no differences by gender. Among racial/ethnic categories, Mexican Americans were the most likely and white non-Hispanics the least likely to have at least one tooth. Age was inversely associated with every indicator of tooth retention and directly associated with every indicator of tooth loss (Marcus, Drury, Brown, & Zion, 1996).

Oral Cancer

The term "oral cancer" includes a diverse group of tumors arising from the oral cavity. Usually included are cancers of the lip, tongue, pharynx, and oral cavity. The annual incidence of oral cancer in the United States is about 11/100,000 population, with rates in males more than twice as high as those in females (Ries, Miller, Hankey, Kosary, Harras, & Edwards, 1994; American Cancer Society, 1999). Oral cancer is responsible for 2% of all cancer deaths in the United States and is projected to account for more than 29,800 new cases and about 8,100 deaths in 1999. Overall five-year survival is 53% (American Cancer Society, 1999).

The natural history of each type of cancer can be quite different. Cancer of the lip accounts for 11% of new cases of oral cancer but only 1% of deaths, while cancer of the pharynx accounts for 31% of new cases of oral cancer but 50% of deaths. Ninety-five percent of oral cancer occurs in persons over age 40, and about half of all oropharyngeal cancers and the majority of deaths from this disease occur in persons over age 65 (Ries et al., 1994).

Use of tobacco in all forms and, to a lesser extent, alcohol abuse are the major risk factors for the development of oral cancer (Vokes, Weichselbaum, Lippman, & Hong, 1993) and account for 90% of oral cancer in the United States (Silverman, 1990). The risk of oral cancer is increased 6 to 28 times in current smokers (Centers for Disease Control and Prevention, 1993). Even with recent advances in prosthetic replacements of oral-facial structures, surgery to remove and repair the effects of oral cancer can still be significantly debilitating and have long-lasting psychosocial effects.

Table 1 presents incidence, mortality, and five-year survival rates for oral cancer in comparison to other malignancies. Surprising to many is the fact that oral cancer occurs more frequently than many cancers, including cancer of the cervix, kidney, liver, ovary, pancreas, stomach, leukemias, and melanoma (National Cancer Institute, 1999). Black males have the highest incidence, followed in decreasing frequency by white males, black females, and white females. The mortality rate for black males is double that of white males, and females of both races are considerably less likely to die from the disease.

Cleft Lip/Cleft Palate

Approximately 7% of children in the United States are born with craniofacial deformities. The most common of these is cleft lip and/or cleft palate. The overall incidence of cleft lip and/or palate is one in 700 births, making this deformity the fourth most common birth defect in the United States (American Society of Plastic Surgeons, 1999). Children with clefts may experience speech, masticatory, and esthetic complications as a result of their condition. They may also be alienated or otherwise mistreated by their peers (Caplan & Weintraub, 1993). New advances in surgery, however, continue to reduce the previously devastating effects of these conditions.

TABLE 1. Incidence, Mortality, and Five-year Survival Rates for Selected Cancers[a]

Type	Incidence 1992–1996	Mortality 1992–1996	Survival Rate 1989-1995
Breast (females)	110.6	25.4	84.7
Cervix	4.1	1.5	69.7
Colon	31.9	–	61.6
Kidney	9.3	3.5	60.3
Leukemias	10.3	6.3	43.1
Liver	3.1	2.8	5.7
Lung/bronchus	57.0	49.5	13.8
Melanoma	13.0	2.2	87.7
Non-Hodgkin's lymphoma	15.8	6.8	51.0
Oral cavity/pharynx	10.3	2.7	53.3
Ovary	7.9	4.3	50.0
Pancreas	8.9	8.4	4.1
Prostate (males)	156.5	25.6	91.9
Stomach	7.0	4.2	21.1
Urinary bladder	16.8	3.2	80.7

[a]Incidence and mortality rates are per 100,000 and are age-adjusted to the 1970 United States standard population. Survival rates are expressed as percents.
Note: From SEER Cancer Statistics Review, 1973–1996, by the National Cancer Institute, 1999.

More than a quarter of a million people living in the United States have one or more cleft abnormalities. About 50% have both cleft lip and cleft palate, while 30% have only cleft palate and 20% have only cleft lip. Native Americans appear to have the highest prevalence of cleft lip or palate of any racial group, followed by Japanese and Chinese. Whites and blacks are affected even less. Males have a higher incidence of cleft lip, with or without cleft palate. Females have a higher occurrence of cleft palate alone (University of Medicine and Dentistry of New Jersey, 1996).

Oral Injuries

Although oral injuries include injuries to the teeth as well as to the jaws, face, lips, tongue, gums, and other oral soft tissues, most studies of oral injuries have only addressed the teeth. Traumatic injuries to the teeth are among the most serious of dental conditions because of critical sensory, communicative, gustatory, and psychosocial functions of the teeth and mouth (Kaste, Gift, Bhst, & Swango, 1996b).

Seventy-five percent of oral injuries have been reported to occur in children under 15 years of age (Bhat & Li, 1990). The most recent national survey found that more than 38 million persons

6 to 50 years of age in the United States—about one-quarter of this age group—were estimated to have evidence of trauma to at least one of their incisors (front teeth). Males had more incisal trauma than females, with a ratio of 1.5:1. The prevalence of incisal trauma in all racial or ethnic categories was very similar and appeared to be positively associated with age (Kaste *et al.*, 1996b).

Access to Oral Health Services

Access is used as a shorthand term for a broad set of concerns that center on the degree to which individuals and groups are able to obtain needed services from the health care system. The Institute of Medicine (IOM) defined it as *the timely use of personal health services to achieve the best possible health outcomes* (Institute of Medicine, 1993).

Many measures have been used to define access, but health services utilization rate is probably the most common. However, although utilization rates are important and useful indicators of access, they fail to reveal its many dimensions. In particular, they do not reveal whether people receive the services they need. For this reason, looking at health care outcomes is a complementary approach to measuring access, although access is only one of a number of factors that stand between the use of health care services and desired health outcomes. Perhaps the most important access consideration is whether people have the opportunity for a good outcome—especially in those instances in which health care can make a difference. When those opportunities are systematically denied to groups in society because they face barriers to care, there is an access problem that needs to be addressed.

The issues and difficulties in defining and measuring access to *oral health* care are no different than those applying to access to health services in the United States today. The most common indicators of oral health services utilization are the proportion of the population with a dental visit in the past year, and the number of visits per person in the past year.

Utilization of Dental Services in the United States

Overall, if measured using these traditional indicators, access to dental care in the United States increased for every age group, both sexes, all income levels, all levels of education, and the major racial-ethnic groups between 1983 and the most current national surveys in 1988–1994. In some cases, these increases have been dramatic, as with for persons ages 75 years and over (Isman & Isman, 1997).

Use of dental services by some racial-ethnic and income groups—for example, gains among blacks relative to whites—suggests that differences in access attributable to race and income are becoming less important and that we are moving toward a more equitable distribution of services. As encouraging as these trends appear, they are no cause for complacency, as overall trends tend to mask more subtle, but important, differences between populations that continue to exist. These differences illustrate why just looking at overall utilization rates gives an incomplete, and in many ways inadequate, picture of access.

Lave and colleagues (Lave, Keane, Lin, Ricci, Amersbach, & LaVallee, 1998a) found that the largest amount of unmet need or delayed care reported for children newly enrolled in a health insurance program was for dental care; the longer children remain without insurance, the more likely they are to have unmet health care needs. Children with dental coverage also were more likely than uninsured children to have a regular dentist and to make use of preventive dental services (Lave, Keane, Lin, Ricci, Amersbach, & LaVallee, 1998b).

A persistent racial difference is in the use of preventive services and in particular the use of dental sealants to prevent tooth decay. For example, among 5 to 17-year-olds, the percentage of white children who have had one or more sealants applied to their permanent teeth is three times that of black and Mexican American children (Selwitz, Winn, Kingman, & Zion, 1996).

One of the lowest rates of dental service use in the past year is among the edentulous population ages 65 years and over; only 10% to 11% of this group had a dental visit in the past year, which is less than one-fourth that of the entire population in this age group (Gift, 1995). However, because rates of edentulism are continuing to decline, the steady increase in use of dental services by the elderly population is predicted.

Utilization of Dental Services in Rural Areas

A number of studies have demonstrated lower patterns of dental utilization in rural areas and have consistently found that urban residents use dental services more than either farm or nonfarm rural residents (Douglass & Cole, 1979; Newman & Anderson, 1972). The most recent national survey showed that the percentage of the population older than two years of age reporting at least one dental visit in the past year was similar—58% for MSA residents and 54% for non-MSA populations. However, the mean numbers of visits in the past year were 2.2 and 1.7, respectively (Bloom, Gift, & Jack, 1992).

Waldman (1990) reported that a smaller percentage of children living in non-MSAs than their metropolitan counterparts had made a visit to the dentist in the previous year, but that the percentage of non-MSA children reporting a dental visit in the past year increased at a faster rate than for MSA children during the 1960s to 1970s and 1970s to 1980s.

Petersen and Pedersen (1984) found that Danish adults who lived in rural areas during childhood and as teens were less likely to demand dental care than their counterparts who had grown up in more urban areas. Similar results were found among Manitoba children, where a significantly higher proportion of urban children had seen a dentist within the previous 12 months (Cageorge, Ryding, & Leake, 1980). In addition, the rural children were less likely to report the reason for seeking dental care to be a "checkup," had a higher prevalence of moderate gingivitis, were more likely to have caries, needed more restorations, and had five times the need for extractions.

As just noted, differences in access to dental care can result in differences in dental service rates. For example, Bader, Scurria, and Shugars (1994) found that, in North Carolina, dentists in the smallest cities reported differences in prosthetic care that reflected more frequent loss of teeth and less frequent replacement of missing teeth. These findings suggest that differences in access may contribute to substantially different oral health outcomes among patients receiving treatment related to tooth loss.

A number of special needs populations face particular problems in accessing oral health services. These include the elderly, homeless persons, migrant and seasonal workers, disabled populations, persons with HIV, veterans, incarcerated individuals, and very young children. As some of these groups are not generally included in national surveys, the magnitude of their oral health needs and the numbers affected have not been ascertained.

Barriers to Access

Availability of Providers

Among the reasons why poor and rural residents receive less dental care than others is the number of dentists in the community. Higher-income areas have two-thirds more dentists per capita than low-income areas. The supply of dentists per capita actually decreased in low- and medium-income areas during the 1980s, while it increased in high-income areas (Center for Health Economics Research, 1993). A recent California study found a clear geographic maldistribution of dentists in the state: 22% of the state's medically underserved areas, containing almost 10% of it's population, had a possible problem with access to dental health services (Mertz, Grumbach, MacIntosh, & Coffman, 2000). The study also found that communities with a shortage of dental professionals tend to have a higher percentage of minority and/or low-income persons.

Rural Residence

Rural residents face a number of barriers to receiving all types of health services. Rates of health insurance in rural areas are lower, reflecting in part the fact that poverty is higher in rural areas than in urban areas, so that rural residents are less able to afford insurance coverage (Chollett, 1987). Rural residents are also more likely to be employed in agriculture and in small businesses, neither of which offer private insurance (medical or dental) as extensively as more urbanized industries. Medicaid coverage tends to be less extensive in rural areas due to variations in coverage between states and the exclusion of coverage for two-parent families in most states (Rowland & Lyons, 1989). Rural areas also have fewer preventive and health-promotion programs than urban areas (Bushy, 1990; Weinert & Long, 1990). A family's not owning a car and not having a telephone—more common in some rural areas—have been found to be detrimental to a young child's dental health status (Thomas & Startup, 1992). Oral conditions were worse among nursing home residents in moderate-size and rural communities in Washington (Kiyak, Grayston, & Crinean, 1993).

In nonmetropolitan counties, the ratio of both physicians and dentists to population decreases with declines in population size, even after controlling for population density and income (Taylor, Puskin, Cooley, & Braden, 1993). Urban residents are more likely to have dental examinations than rural residents, and 11% of rural residents have never visited a dentist (Office of Technology Assessment, 1990). A higher percentage of children residing in nonmetropolitan areas than metropolitan areas are unable to obtain needed dental care (Waldman, 1998).

Among the rural elderly, those with no insurance are less likely to visit the dentist during the year. Visits to the dentist are typically discretionary and the effect of income is expected to be the most pronounced for visits to the dentist, since insurance coverage for such services is typically limited and Medicare does not pay for routine dental services (Kassab, Luloff, Kelsey, & Smith, 1996).

Regular Source of Care

Having a gap in health insurance coverage affects access to medical care in two ways: first, it requires families already having financial difficulties to pay out-of-pocket for service, and second, it makes maintaining a continuous relationship with a primary care physician much more difficult (Berman, 1995). As fewer children have dental insurance than have medical insurance and as dental care is considered a more discretionary service than medical care, it stands to reason that the factors limiting the regular use of medical care will also limit the regular use of dental care. Among children, the extent to which the last dental visit was for a checkup or for preventive care is clearly income-related. Among children from lower-income families without health insurance, approximately 35% reported that their previous dental visit was preventive, whereas this figure was over 60% among those from the higher-income category (Call, 1989).

Having a regular source of care has been found to increase dramatically the likelihood that Medicaid children will use dental services. Those children with a usual source of care were at least 15 times more likely to have had a dental visit in the past 12 months than those without a usual source of care (Venezie, Garvan, Mitchell, Yin, & Conti, 1997). There is also evidence that children are more likely to use dental services if their parents also do, with one study reporting that children whose parents both saw a dentist in the past year were 13 times more likely to see a dentist themselves than children whose parents did not both see a dentist in the past year (Bonito & Gooch, 1992).

Health Insurance

Persons without *health* insurance are not only less likely to receive the health coverage af-

forded by typical health insurance plans but also less likely to get needed *dental* care. Children with no health insurance are three times as likely as privately insured children to be unable to get dental care when they need it (Simpson, Bloom, Cohen, & Parsons, 1997). Working-age adults are four times as likely as their privately insured counterparts to be unable to get dental care when they need it (Bloom, Simpson, Cohen, & Parsons, 1997). And older adults with no health insurance are twice as likely as privately insured older adults to be unable to get dental care when they need it (Cohen, Bloom, Simpson, & Parsons, 1997).

When children from poor families, minority children, and uninsured children were compared with a reference group of children from nonpoor, white, insured families, a higher proportion of children in every group was found to be unable to get needed dental care than was the case for any of the other health care services. In particular, uninsured children were more than twice as likely as children from poor families, more than three times as likely as children from minority families, and almost four times as likely as children from nonpoor, white, insured families to have reported they were unable to get needed dental care. Although poverty and minority status posed significant barriers to gaining access to primary care, the most important barrier in this study was lack of insurance coverage (Newacheck, Stoddard, Hughes, & Pearl, 1997). A California study of rural Hispanic children also found that lack of health insurance was the strongest predictor of not having a dental visit in the past year (Smith, Kreutzer, Goldman, Casey-Paal, & Kizer, 1996).

Dental Insurance

Private dental insurance has been a factor of increasing significance in the use of dental services since the 1970s. By 1989, the most recent year for which a representative national sample is available, 95 million Americans, or about 38% of the total United States population at that time, had private dental insurance (Bloom *et al.*, 1993). Today, dental benefits are the third most common employer-provided health benefit (National Association of Dental Plans, 1997), and in 1995 about 147 million Americans, or 55%

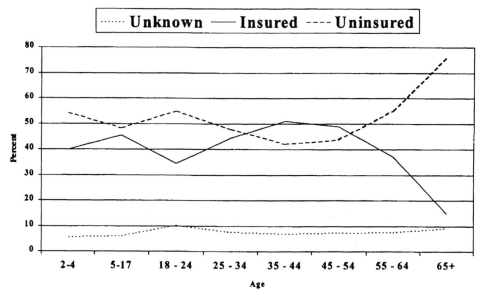

FIGURE 4. Percentage distribution of persons ages two and older by private dental insurance status, United States, 1989. From Bloom et al., 1993.

of the total United States population, had private dental insurance (National Association of Dental Plans, 1999).

People between the ages of 35 and 54 were the most likely group to have dental insurance; males were more likely than females (41.4% and 39.6%, respectively) to have coverage, especially those 45 years of age and older (Figure 4). A larger proportion of White persons than Black persons had coverage, and non-Hispanics were more likely to be covered than Hispanics (Bloom *et al.*, 1992).

Persons with private dental insurance are significantly more likely to have had a recent dental visit, as well as a higher number of dental visits per person per year, than are those without such coverage. These differences existed in most age, sex, and racial groups; however, there were still disparities between those with and without private dental insurance by age, sex, and race. Among children, those with dental insurance had more visits per child, a greater proportion with one or more dental visits, and a greater percentage with three or more visits (Waldman, 1994). More than half of MSA residents had private dental insurance coverage in 1989 compared with 39% for non-MSA residents (Bloom *et al.*, 1992).

The disparities in number of visits between

insured and uninsured persons suggest that the uninsured are not only less likely to have seen a dentist recently but also less likely to be using preventive dental services, less likely to and have all their dental needs addressed, and more likely to make episodic use of the dental care delivery system. For example, in one study of children newly enrolled in a health insurance program, the proportion of children who visited a dentist in the past year increased by nearly 25% (Keane, Lave, Ricci, & LaVallee, 1999). This study also found that financing of health coverage is not enough in itself to assure adequate health care, and that reduced access to care results in decreased opportunities for early intervention.

Medicaid Coverage

By all reasonable measures, Medicaid has failed to live up to its potential and mandate to make dental services available to the poor. In a nation that spends approximately 5% of personal health care expenditures on dental services, less than 1% of Medicaid expenditures go toward this purpose, although the Medicaid population is clearly one with greater dental needs than the general population (Isman & Isman, 1997). It is estimated that less than one-half of 1% of Medicaid expenditures are for children's dental services, the target of Medicaid's Early and Periodic Screening, Diagnosis, and Treatment (EPSDT) program, which is considerably less than Medicaid spending for laundry services in nursing homes (Edelstein, 1997). Fewer than one in five Medicaid children receive any preventive dental services each year (United States Department of Health and Human Services, 1996). Because Medicaid dental services for adults are optional, many states provide coverage only for emergency dental treatment.

Although in theory dental managed care would appear to offer some potential for increasing access to dental care under Medicaid, there is little evidence to support that perspective and some evidence to support the opposite: that utilization of dental services, including preventive services, is lower under dental managed care programs than under fee-for-service arrangements (Isman, 1996).

Financing of Oral Health Services

Unlike most other health services, the vast majority—96%—of oral health services are paid for privately. Table 2 illustrates the major differences between funding for physicians' and dental services (Health Care Financing Administration, 1999). Out-of-pocket expenditures represent almost half (47%) of all oral health expenditures, compared with only 16% of all expenditures for physicians' services. Also, public funding sources account for a far higher percentage of expenditures for physicians' services

than of dental services. In particular, Medicare paid for only 3% of all publicly funded dental expenditures but for two-thirds of all publicly funded physicians' services expenditures.

Dental Managed Care

Enrollment in commercial dental managed care (DMC) plans more than tripled between 1990 and 1997, reaching an estimated 56.3 million persons by the end of 1997 (National Association of Dental Plans, 1999). DMC enrollment is growing faster than medical managed care and is paralleling the growth of medical managed care several years ago. Between 1990 and 1995, medical managed care enrollment increased by 54%, while DMC enrollment increased by 164%. In 1995, 10 states represented three-fourths of the total market for dental HMO enrollment. California, with 6.4 million persons enrolled, outpaced the next four highest states combined.

Growth in the DMC industry is being driven by the cost of care. A survey by a large health benefits consulting firm late in 1995 found that more than half the companies that offered only fee-for-service dental benefits to their employees at the time planned either to switch to DMC or to offer it as an option by the end of 1997 (National Association of Dental Plans, 1997).

The extent to which DMC has affected the availability or delivery of dental services in rural areas is unknown, but it is probably very little. In 1995, less than 8% of the rural population in eight states was enrolled in a commer-

TABLE 2. Percentage of Public and Private Expenditures for Physicians' and Dental Services, 1997

Source of Funding	Dental Services	Physicians' Services
All Sources	100.0	100.0
Private Funds	95.5	67.8
Consumer Payments	95.0	65.8
Out-of-pocket payments	47.1	15.7
Private health insurance	47.9	50.2
Public funds	4.5	32.2
Federal funds	2.6	26.8
Medicare	0.2	21.3
Medicaid	2.2	4.3
State and local funds	1.9	5.4

Note: From *National Health Expenditures by Type of Service and Source of Funds*, by Health Care Financing Administration, 1999.

cial HMO, compared with 26% of the urban population in the same states (Fasciano, Felt-Lisk, Ricketts, & Popkin, 1999), although increasing numbers of urban-based HMOs have expanded their service areas into surrounding rural counties. A recent study of the feasibility of a statewide rural HMO in California, which has one of the highest penetration levels of managed care among all states, found that the prospects for such an HMO were not encouraging—the break-even point would not be reached in five years and the HMO would continue to lose money beyond that time (State of California, Rural Health Policy Council, 1999). On the other hand, in California, the new state children's health insurance program has contracts with four dental managed care firms and has attempted to increase access to dental services in rural areas by providing grants to community clinics to expand their operations and reimbursing dentists in rural networks for their usual and customary fees.

Historically, the limited presence of HMOs in rural areas has been attributed to several factors, including smaller populations, the relatively low number of large employers in many rural areas, resistance of some rural physicians to participation in HMOs, lack of available capital for HMO development, and low Medicare and Medicaid payment rates (Casey, 1999; Voelker, 1998). With the exception of the Medicare rates—which for the most part are not applicable to dentistry because of Medicare's lack of dental benefits—all of these factors are equally applicable to dental managed care in rural settings.

Another reason cited for the slow evolution of managed care in rural areas is risk; that is, how to determine the risk of a small population, and in turn, how to determine rates (Voelker, 1998). This is less of an issue for dental services because dental managed care is more related to prepayment than determining risk of catastrophic events.

Although little is known about the prospects of either commercial or Medicaid dental managed care in rural communities, a number of factors suggest that dentists may be in a better position of being able to resist managed care, especially in rural areas, than their medical counterparts. These include a diminishing supply of dental personnel (Brown & Lazar, 1999b), a minority of Americans with dental insurance, an overall increasing demand for dental services (Brown & Lazar, 1999a), and an aging rural population that generally has a lower demand for dental services. A summary of the experiences of five university-based rural managed care initiatives found that communities in which a majority of physicians are in solo practice seem to have the most difficulty taking the developmental steps toward managed care (Hartley, Jackson, Mueller, Nichols, & Williams, 1999). As a higher percentage of dentists than physicians are in solo practice, this finding does not appear to augur well for rural dental managed care.

Other fundamental differences between medical managed care and dental managed care include dentists' concentration as generalists rather than specialists, their location and business structure in independent offices, their lack of dependency on hospitals and expensive medical technology, their direct dealings with patients with respect to the financing of care, and the nature of their services (Edelstein, 1997).

Prevention of Oral Disease

Caries Prevention

Perhaps the greatest irony surrounding the extensive oral health problems and lack of access to dental care faced by so many Americans is that they are so easily and inexpensively preventable. For no aspect of health care is the old adage "an ounce of prevention is worth a pound of cure" so true as it is for oral health services. In fact, a benefit-cost ratio of 16:1 is exceeded fivefold by one community-based preventive oral health service—community water fluoridation. The Centers for Disease Control and Prevention has estimated that each $1 expenditure for water fluoridation could result in a savings of $80 in dental treatment costs (Centers for Disease Control and Prevention, 1992).

Measures for preventing oral disease are usually characterized as either *community-based*, *self-applied*, or *operator-applied* measures. Community-based measures are those that affect an entire community (e.g., water fluoridation) or groups of individuals (e.g., school-based dental sealant programs); self-applied measures are those performed by an individual (e.g., toothbrushing at home); and operator-applied measures are those performed by a health care provider for an individual (e.g., application of dental sealants in a dental office).

For caries prevention, the quintessential community-based preventive measure is community water fluoridation. Fluoridation has been repeatedly documented to be the most cost-effective preventive measure available for caries. A review of studies on the effectiveness of water fluoridation conducted in the United States during 1979 to 1989 found a range of caries reduction of 8% to 37% among adolescents (mean: 26.5%) and a reduction of enamel caries in adults of 20% to 40% (Newbrun, 1989).

Other effective community-based caries preventive measures include school water fluoridation, school daily fluoride supplement programs (e.g., fluoride tablets), school fluoride mouthrinse programs, and school sealant programs. In addition, fluoride varnish (a sticky solution of fluoride applied to the teeth two to three times a year) is beginning to be more widely used among preschool-age children in community settings, including rural areas served by the Indian Health Service. It should be noted that, with the exception of community water fluoridation, all of these measures are targeted at schoolchildren, for the obvious reason that they represent a "captive audience"—that is, an easy-to-reach population.

Special mention should be made about dental sealant programs. Dental sealants are plastic coatings applied to the chewing surfaces of teeth; they have been shown to be remarkably effective in preventing decay on those tooth surfaces that are benefitted the least by fluorides. The combined and appropriate use of sealants and fluoride has been said to present the prospect of virtually eliminating caries altogether (Burt & Eklund, 1992). In the United States, the application of sealants must be performed by a dentist, dental hygienist, or dental assistant, depending on the provisions of individual state dental practice acts. In recent years, school-based dental sealant programs have come to be the caries preventive measure of choice for children in many communities. Many states now

conduct school sealant programs, and guides to the operation of such programs have been issued by the National Institute of Dental and Craniofacial Research as well as by several state health departments.

The effectiveness of school sealant programs has been reported in the range of 51% to 67%, and the cost per student was estimated in 1989 at $13.07 to $28.37, depending on whether a dentist or dental auxiliary placed the sealant, whether they were paid or volunteers, and the type of equipment used (Burt, 1989). Recent unpublished data from the Ohio Department of Health (M. Siegal, personal communication, December 13, 1999) demonstrate the potential of school-based sealant programs to reach underserved populations. Based on dental screenings of 21,000 children in every Ohio county, low-income children in schools with a sealant program were three times as likely to have received sealants as children in schools without a sealant program. Further, almost three-quarters of the 8-year-olds attending schools that offered a sealant program, and who had received sealants, got them at school.

Prevention of Periodontal Disease

Unfortunately, there is currently no effective public health measure for periodontal disease prevention comparable to community caries prevention measures such as water fluoridation. Periodontal disease is caused by the bacterial colonization of dental plaque, a soft concentrated mass containing a large variety of bacteria that can begin to form on a tooth surface within two hours after it is cleaned. For many years, the regular and consistent mechanical removal of plaque through toothbrushing and the use of dental floss has been the basis for preventing periodontal disease. Plaque can also be controlled with the use of antimicrobial products such as chlorhexidine, dispensed as rinses, sprays, and gels (Mandel, 1994). These approaches depend heavily on individual motivation for success, and for this reason are unlikely ever to be completely effective in preventing periodontal disease in a population (Burt & Eklund, 1992).

At one time, school-based plaque control programs (e.g., "brush-ins") were very popular.

Some of these programs demonstrated that regular thorough plaque removal, *under supervision*, could reduce gingivitis (Suomi, Peterson, Matthews, Voglesong, & Lyman, 1980). However, other studies have found that much of the gain achieved in reducing gingivitis over a school year disappears or is reduced when plaque removal is no longer supervised (Suomi *et al.*, 1980). Also, there is no evidence that mechanical plaque removal without the use of a fluoride-containing toothpaste results in caries reduction.

Prevention of Oral Cancer

The primary risk factors for oral cancers in the United States are use of tobacco and alcohol products, and, for lip cancers, unprotected exposure to the sun. Studies have shown that when smoking is discontinued, the risk for oral cancer, adjusted for drinking, decreases over time to levels similar to those of people who have never smoked (Pendrys, 1998). This suggests that many cases of oral cancer are preventable. However, the science of prevention has far to go before oral cancer can be completely prevented. For the moment, early detection and treatment is the goal, but many cancers are not detected until later stages of development, when treatment is likely to be more invasive and disfiguring.

Despite available knowledge about risk factors for and signs and symptoms of oral cancer, most of the public knows very little about the prevention of oral cancer (Horowitz, Goodman, Yellowitz, & Nourjah, 1996; Horowitz, 1995). In addition, only 14% of United States adults report they have ever had an oral cancer examination (Horowitz & Nourjah, 1996), and dentists and physicians often are not very knowledgeable about oral cancer (Yellowitz & Goodman, 1995). All of these factors make it imperative to implement comprehensive educational interventions, directed at health care providers and the public, about reducing risk factors and promoting early detection (Yellowitz, Goodman, Horowitz, & al-Tannir, 1995).

Prevention of Unintentional Oral-facial Injuries

No single mechanism or program has been proposed to prevent all the different types of unintentional oral-facial injuries. Although no national data for the various causes of oral-facial injuries exist, sports appear to account for a significant proportion (Allukian & Horowitz, 1998). The highest number of unintentional injuries from product-associated sports treated in emergency departments in 1995 were from basketball, followed by bicycles, football, baseball, soccer, and softball (National Injury Information Clearinghouse, 1995).

Protective headgear and mouth guards have been shown to prevent unintentional injuries in sports. For example, the use of face guards and mouth protectors has led to a dramatic reduction in oral-facial injuries in football since 1962 (Allukian & Horowitz, 1998). Although more children are injured in sports outside of school (60%) than in school, and more injuries occur during practice (60%) than in games (National Safe Kids Campaign, 1996; Soporowski, Tesini, & Weiss, 1994), protective equipment is used much less often outside of school and in practice. Regulations, requirements, and guidelines for the use of effective protection in sports should include the mouth. Referees, coaches, parents, school officials, the dental profession, athletic organizations, and local and state health departments should all play a role in protecting the health and safety of children and athletes (Allukian & Horowitz, 1998).

Oral Health Care Workforce and Delivery System Issues

Unlike most health services, most dental services continue to be provided in private practice, with sole proprietorship the norm (O'Neil & Pew Health Professions Commission, 1998). Estimates of the number of dentists in active practice in the United States range from about 138,000 to 141,000, and the ratio of dentists to population increased from 46/100,000 in 1976 to 55/100,000 in 1991, and then dropped to 52/100,000 in 1997 (Brown & Lazar, 1999b). This number is expected to continue to drop due to enrollment and retirement trends in the next 10 years. In fact, dentistry is unique in being the only health care profession that is expected to experience an actual decline in the ratio of professionals to population during the next two decades (Pew Health Professions Commission, 1995). On the other hand, the number of dental specialists, who made up 19% of all dentists in 1997 (Brown & Lazar, 1999b), is projected to increase to 25% by the year 2010 (Institute of Medicine, 1995). The proportion of women in the dental workforce was at almost 13% in 1997 (Brown & Lazar, 1999b) and rising. Minorities account for approximately 10% of the dental workforce. Between 1995 and 1997, the number of non-Hispanic black dentists decreased 8.1% and the number of non-Hispanic American Indian, Eskimo, and Aleutian dentists decreased 1.9%, while the number of Hispanic dentists increased 10.6% and the number of non-Hispanic Asian and Pacific Islander dentists increased 14.6% (Brown & Lazar, 1999b).

Programs to Expand the Dental Workforce

One method used to address barriers to access to health care, whether in isolated rural areas or inner-city neighborhoods, has been to designate such areas as underserved and then target the placement of health care providers in those areas. Two main systems are used to identify such locations: one designates health professional shortage areas (HPSAs), the other medically underserved areas (MUAs). More than half of all United States counties are designated as HPSAs or MUAs, and over another fourth have HPSAs or MUAs somewhere within their borders. In 1995, a federal study concluded that these systems do not effectively identify areas with primary care shortages or help target federal resources to benefit those who are underserved, and there is little assurance that federal funds are used where they are most needed (United States General Accounting Office, 1995a).

The federal government's main program for placing health care providers (including dental care providers) in locations with identified shortages of health professionals is the National Health Service Corps (NHSC). However, the NHSC was found not to distribute provider resources as effectively as it could to alleviate health care needs in the greatest number of eligible shortage areas (United States General Accounting Office, 1995b, 1997).

Federal review of rural health clinics—another program aimed at alleviating access problems—found that the availability of care did not change appreciably for at least 90% of Medicare and Medicaid beneficiaries using the clinics, the federal subsidies had not been used to expand access to underserved portions of the populations, and the clinics did not need the federal subsidies to remain financially viable (United States General Accounting Office, 1997).

Despite these criticisms, community and migrant health centers remain an important entry point for providing medical and dental care to underserved and vulnerable populations (Davis, Collins, & Hall, 1999). Unfortunately, only about 60% of these centers provide dental services (J. Anderson, personal communication, August 22, 1997).

A considerable amount of research and experience shows that employing expanded-function dental auxiliaries to provide some services that state legislation currently restricts to dentists is one way in which the efficiency of the nation's dental care delivery system could be increased, and that needed services could be provided to more people at lower cost (United States General Accounting Office, 1980; Liang & Ogur, 1987). Nevertheless, most states continue to have laws precluding dentists from employing such persons for this purpose. Even the federal government has not established an overall policy requiring or promoting the use of such auxiliaries in federally supported dental care delivery programs.

How the supply of health care providers affects access to health care is a matter of some debate. The traditional approach to workforce planning has been to define the supply requirements based on an assessment of "demand" or "need" for services. However, none of the models developed has been particularly accurate or useful for predicting the supply, demand, or need for dental workers (Crall, 1998). Further, little research has taken the next step—measuring how differing levels of supply actually affect the outcomes of care. This leaves unanswered such questions as these: What ratio of general dentists and dental specialists to population is optimal? What effect does a higher supply of dentists have on the oral health status of a population? Is access to care better in areas with higher proportions of dentists? Does the presence of public and nonprofit community clinics in an area correlate with improved access to care and health outcomes (Isman & Isman, 1997)?

There is some evidence that race and ethnicity are important in explaining differences in physician supply and health outcomes between areas. Grumbach, Seifer, Vranizan, Keane, Osmond, Soffel, Huang, & Bindman (1995) found that people living in low-income, nonminority areas of urban California had more physicians practicing in their neighborhood than people living in higher-income areas with high proportions of African American or Hispanic residents. They concluded that poverty and race, often associated with a lack of health insurance, appear to be much more significant factors influencing access to care and preventable hospitalizations within a community. Therefore, policies aimed at improving access may need to focus particular attention on barriers related to health insurance status, the direct effects of poverty, the ways in which race and ethnicity are associated with disadvantaged health status, and the specific process of care, in addition to considering measures focused on the supply of health care providers in the community.

School-Based Health Centers

Another method that has been proposed to help increase access to dental care, at least for school-age children, is through dental care programs in school-based or school-linked health centers (SBHCs/SLHCs). "School-based" indicates that the services are actually provided in a school facility, whereas "school-linked" refers to services that are linked to schools but provided in off-site facilities—for example, community clinics. SBHCs/SLHCs improve children's access to health care by removing financial and other barriers in the existing health care delivery system. These centers, which take advantage of the fact that children in school settings represent a "captive audience," are a unique delivery system option that gives children, especially those who are poor or uninsured, easy access to services. Providing services in such settings is a particularly effective way to reach adolescents and also yields benefits for younger children.

A study of how SBHCs expand access to health care found that some SBHCs offer or arrange for students to receive dental care. It also implied that, since 50% of children ages 5 to 17 do not have private dental insurance, and for those with insurance, copayments and deductibles may be as high as 50% of the cost of services, SBHCs represent a way of increasing access to dental care for children who lack health insurance and whose parents have difficulty paying for needed health services (United States General Accounting Office, 1994).

Although SBHCs could do much to improve children's access to health care, and to dental care specifically, they cannot provide all needed services to all children. They are not always open during the summer or other times when school is not in session. Relatively few offer dental services. For example, of 41 SLHCs studied in 1995, only 3 offered dental services, and of 144 SBHCs studied in 1994, 11.8% offered dental services (Isman & Isman, 1997). The comprehensiveness of referral networks varies. And SBHCs generally do not serve children who are not in school, such as those younger than age five or adolescents who have dropped out of school. Sometimes, too, students may not be aware of the services offered by their school health centers, or there may be organizational aspects of the center that limit optimal utilization.

SBHCs and SLHCs linked to rural clinics may be a particularly effective mechanism for reaching many rural children with dental services. One recent study noted that SBHCs are increasingly found outside of urban areas, with 26% now in rural areas (Lear, Eichner, & Koppelman, 1999). Other studies have shown that SBHCs increase the likelihood of children receiving an annual dental examination and that persons who reported the SBHC as their most-used health service were significantly more satisfied with their service than those who mostly used community clinics (Kaplan, Brindis, Phibbs, Melinkovich, Naylor, & Ahlstrand, 1999).

Mobile and Portable Dental Care Delivery Systems

Although the vast majority of dental care is provided in private dental offices, mobile and portable dental equipment is increasingly being used to serve individuals and communities that lack access to dental offices either because of geography or a physical condition that limits mobility. The use of mobile clinics as an alternative mode of delivery of dental services dates back as far as 1924 (Murphy, 1996). Mobile dental facilities include both self-propelled vehicles and trailers that must be towed from location to location. Portable dental equipment refers to equipment that is usually lightweight and can be easily transported from site to site in an automobile or small van, and then set up onsite. For example, the Missouri Elks Association operates a program that uses three self-propelled mobile dental units to serve developmentally disabled persons in rural communities (Dane, 1990); a rural hospital has used a trailer dental facility for more than 20 years to bring dental services to children from economically distressed families in rural New York State (Valla & Westcott, 1996); senior dental hygiene students in a dental public health course use portable dental equipment taken to a county health clinic to provide dental disease prevention programs in rural Appalachia (Burger, Boehm, & Sellaro, 1997); and in what is perhaps one of the most novel mobile dentistry applications, dental services have been provided to preschoolers and schoolchildren in remote regions of northern Ontario using dental clinics constructed in two Pullman railway cars ("Railway Dental Car Services," 1969). Probably the most widespread use of portable dental equipment today is in the school-based dental sealant programs that exist in many communities; portable equipment is also used widely to provide care to people in nursing homes and to homebound individuals.

Oral Health System Solutions for Rural Communities

Because the population characteristics and resources of every community are unique, solutions to their rural oral health problems will also be unique. Many of the problems faced by rural communities are also faced by larger communities, so the recommendations that follow should not be considered unique to rural settings.

An Ounce of Prevention

Prevention, especially community-based prevention programs, remains the cornerstone of any effort to make dental care available to more people. Increasing the availability of preventive services will allow more efficient use of the dental workforce and ultimately free more resources to provide more extensive dental care for more people.

The combined use of fluorides and sealants is currently the best means of controlling caries at the community level and has been likened in effectiveness to the ability of childhood immunizations to prevent vaccine-preventable diseases. Without a concerted effort to redirect public monies into fluoridation to serve the entire community and sealant programs to serve underserved children, there will be little progress in fluoridating more communities and sealants will likely remain a privilege of the "haves" in American society. Rural communities present a somewhat greater challenge to fluoridate than urban ones because in many cases the water supplies come from individual wells, which collectively may be more expensive to fluoridate than a surface water system serving an entire community. Nevertheless, many rural and urban communities fluoridate the water from individual wells.

Because the caries process can begin at a very early age, its prevention must likewise begin early—even before the first tooth erupts in children identified as high risk. Unfortunately, there are still few dentists—both general dentists and pediatric dentists—who are willing to see children this early. Further, few health professionals have been trained to provide appropriate preventive services to young children and counseling of parents at and prior to a child's first dental visit. Some ways of addressing this issue include: (1) increase training of primary care providers to provide exams, preventive care, and parental counseling/anticipatory guidance for young children; (2) provide reimbursement for preventive dental counseling and exams for young children; (3) provide on-site day care for families during their appointments, and incorporate a health education–wellness focus into the day care activities; (4) involve parents and members of underserved groups in planning programs for their care; (5) incorporate more preventive dental services into medical HMOs; 6) develop certification programs for dental professionals who wish to improve their skills in working with young children, individuals with chronic medical problems, or other types of special needs; and (7) teach child care providers to assess oral health needs and arrange for palliative care for oral symptoms.

School-Based Dental Services

Although relatively few SBHCs currently offer dental services, the overall number of SBHCs has increased substantially in recent years, and there is no reason that dentistry should be excluded from the services offered by these centers. The availability of such centers with dental components would offer tremendous potential for improving children's access to dental care, especially preventive services. In fact, the vast majority of existing community-based sealant programs are located in schools.

Community, Rural, Migrant, and Native American Health Centers and Other Federal Programs

While only 60% of community, rural, and migrant health centers provided dental services in 1996, they served more than 1 million people. In addition, in 1996, approximately 1.4 million American Indians and Alaska Natives living on or near reservations received clinical dental services at over 430 locations from programs operated by the Indian Health Service (IHS) (F. Martin, personal communication, June 6, 1997). These facilities represent an established and successful model for serving hard-to-reach populations that often will not seek care from private dental providers in a community, even if they are available. In some rural counties in California, clinics have quadrupled Medicaid dental utilization rates. At the same time, federal programs aimed at increasing access to care must improve their focus on access, including

developing better ways of measuring need and evaluating the success of individual programs in meeting this need.

Integration of Oral Health with Primary Care

Serious consideration must be given to better integrating oral health with primary care. The lack of such integration has given us a health care system that routinely excludes the mouth in discussions of so-called comprehensive health care but would never consider excluding other body parts from coverage. Until policymakers recognize the mouth as part of the body, dentistry seems destined to play a minimal role during negotiation of health benefits.

Medicaid And Health Insurance Reform Efforts

Medicaid dental performance falls far short of its promise. By law and regulation, Medicaid entitles one-quarter of all American children to comprehensive dental care, but by administration and implementation it substantially fails these children. If the nation is going to continue to rely on the Medicaid program to serve the poorest Americans, some major reforming of that program will be necessary if services are to be provided through the existing workforce. Some potentially positive changes—such as allowing states to determine eligibility only once a year—have recently been enacted. Other changes that would help increase access include incentives for states to provide dental exams at an earlier age, financial incentives for providing preventive services, adequate reimbursement levels, and broader coverage for adults than many states currently allow. Some evidence already exists that changes such as these can increase access to dental services for Medicaid-enrolled children, such as Washington's Access to Baby and Child Dentistry (ABCD) program (Milgrom, Hujoel, Grembowski, & Ward, 1997).

Workforce Issues

Many ways of addressing dental workforce issues need to be examined. In particular, attention needs to be directed at the already small yet decreasing number of practitioners willing and able to see young children. There appears to be a growing consensus that the way to do this is not by training more pediatric dentists but by training more general dentists in how to care for young children, and by making more efficient use of auxiliary personnel. To the extent that the provisions of state dental practice acts represent barriers to access, restrictions that limit who can provide services must be reexamined. There is ample evidence that expanded-function dental auxiliaries could increase the efficiency of the dental workforce and assure the provision of needed services to more people at lower cost. In addition, the role of nontraditional providers needs further exploration.

Strengthening the Infrastructure

Substantially more oral health–related assessment, policy development, and assurance activities occur in states with full-time dental directors, and such leadership has been identified as essential to ensure that individuals at greatest risk for oral diseases are effectively targeted for preventive intervention. Consequently, all public and private dental organizations should be encouraged to develop, update, and strengthen current policy that advocates for dental public health programs and representation within state and local health departments. This is especially true in predominantly rural states, because resources to address the oral health needs of rural populations are usually even more scarce in those states. Many states now have rural health offices and some are beginning to address oral health issues, but there needs to be better integration between state oral health and rural health activities.

There is also a diminished oral health presence (and rural health presence) in many federal agencies. There needs to be a dental presence within federal government agencies by securing dental leadership involvement on advisory groups, task forces, committees, and panels addressing issues of relevance to oral health. And as is the case with states, there needs to be better coordination between federal oral health and rural health activities.

Need for Multiple Partners

The continuing inability of large segments of our population to realize adequate access to dental services remains a large and complex problem. Some barriers to the utilization of dental services will require long-term social, political, and economic changes. Other barriers are likely only to be adequately addressed through collaborative efforts of the public and private sectors. These might include, for example: (1) forming a national working group on access that includes nondental business, labor, advocacy, and other groups interested in access to oral health; (2) promoting public and private forums to foster collaboration on access issues of mutual interest; (3) assuring a dental presence on state and local advisory groups, rural health task forces, committees, and panels addressing issues of relevance to oral health; and (4) expanding and enhancing support for dental student loan repayment programs for practice in underserved areas and development of new approaches for increasing the number of dental professionals working in underserved areas.

Several states have developed rural dental programs—in particular, placements of dental personnel—through their area health education centers (AHECs). For example, in a collaboration of federal, state, and Cherokee tribal governments, for the past 14 years senior dental students from the University of North Carolina fill and extract teeth, perform routine checkups, and manage dental emergencies for children with advanced tooth decay, allowing more time for public health dentists to staff a remote satellite clinic (North Carolina Area Health Education Centers Program, 1999).

In summary, residents of rural America are faced with a "double jeopardy" situation. First, the oral health needs of rural residents exceed those of their urban counterparts, and second, resources to address those needs are usually fewer. These conditions are not unique to oral health but prevail for virtually all health needs among rural populations. Exacerbating these oral health needs, however, is the undervaluing of oral health by other health care professionals, policymakers, and often the public. Together, these represent formidable obstacles to improving the oral health of rural residents.

At the same time, there are encouraging signs of improvements. The oral health status of all Americans, including rural residents, is continuing to improve. There is growing attention to rural health on the part of federal and state health agencies, including some focus on oral health issues. There is evidence that some mentorship and rural placement programs offered in dental schools are having their intended effect of increasing the size of the rural dental workforce. New technology is bringing improved methods of oral disease prevention. School-based health centers are reaching more rural residents, and more are incorporating a dental component. Plans are under way to increase the dental workforce available through the National Health Service Corps.

Improving oral health for rural residents is largely a matter of improving access. Such improvements will require policies that are based on scientific evidence, reflect differential risk, cast access to dental care as a community health problem rather than a dental problem, recognize access at least in part as behaviorally determined, require that programs to improve access be community-based with performance measured at the community level, and address the need for properly trained personnel, including not only traditional dental providers but also nondental personnel who can help assure access and address prevention and behavioral issues affecting access before dental professional help is sought.

These kinds of policy changes require, more than anything else, political will. Without political will there is unlikely to be an allocation of resources. We do not as a nation lack the knowledge and resources we need to improve the availability of oral health services to rural populations. Once we have garnered the political will to do so, we can look forward to the gradual disappearance of the inequities in oral health between urban and rural Americans.

References

Allukian, M., Jr., & Horowitz, A. M. (1998). Effective community prevention programs for oral diseases. In G. M. Gluck & W. M. Morganstein (Eds.), *Jong's community dental health* (4th ed.). St. Louis: Mosby.

American Cancer Society. (1999). Cancer statistics: Oral cavity and pharynx/uterine cervix. (December 17, 1999); http://www.cancer.org/statistics/cff99/selectedcancers.html#oral/; http://www.cancer.org/statistics/cff99/selectedcancers.html#cervix.

American Society of Plastic Surgeons. (1997). Cleft lip and palate surgery (December 17, 1999); http://www.plasticsurgery.org/profinfo/pospap/cle.htm.

Bader, J. D., Scurria, M. S., & Shugars, D. A. (1994). Urban/rural differences in prosthetic dental service rates. *Journal of Rural Health, 10*, 26–30.

Berman, S. (1995). Uninsured children. An unintended consequence of health care system reform efforts. *Journal of the American Medical Association, 274*, 1472–1473.

Bhat, M, & Li, S. H. (1990). Consumer product-related tooth injuries treated in hospital emergency rooms: United States, 1979–87. *Community Dentistry and Oral Epidemiology, 18*, 133–138.

Bloom, B., Gift, H. C., & Jack, S. S. (1992). Dental services and oral health: United States, 1989. *Vital and health statistics, Series 10(183)*. National Center for Health Statistics.

Bloom, B., Simpson, G., Cohen, R. A., & Parsons, P. E. (1997). Access to health care. Part 2: Working-age adults. *Vital and Health Statistics, Series 10(197)*. National Center for Health Statistics.

Bonito, A. J., & Gooch, R. (1992). *Modeling the oral health needs of 12- to 13-year-olds in the Baltimore MSA: Results from one ICS-II study site*. Paper presented at the American Public Health Association Annual Meeting, Washington, DC, November.

Brown, L. J., & Lazar, V. (1999a). Dental care utilization: how saturated is the patient market? *Journal of the American Dental Association, 130*, 573–580.

Brown, L. J., & Lazar, V. (1999b). Trends in the dental health work force. *Journal of the American Dental Association, 130*, 1743–1749.

Brown, L. J., Brunelle, J. A., & Kingman, A. (1996). Periodontal status in the United States, 1988-91: Prevalence, extent, and demographic variation. *Journal of Dental Research, 75 (special issue)*, 672–683.

Burger, A. D., Boehm, J. M., & Sellaro, C. L. (1997). Dental disease preventive programs in a rural Appalachian population. *Journal of Dental Hygiene, 71*, 117–122.

Burt, B. (1989). Proceedings of the workshop: Cost-effectiveness of caries prevention in dental public health. *Journal of Public Health Dentistry, 49 (special issue)*, 279–289.

Burt, B. A., & Eklund, S. A. (1992). *Dentistry, dental practice, and the community* (4th ed.). Philadelphia: W.B. Saunders.

Bushy, A. (1990). Rural United States women: Traditions and transitions affecting health care. *Health Care for Women International, 11*, 503–513.

Cageorge, S. M., Ryding, W. H., & Leake, J. L. (1980). Dental health status survey of Manitoba children. *Journal of the Canadian Dental Association, 2*, 108–116.

Call, R. L. (1989). Effects of poverty on children's dental health. *Pediatrician, 16*, 200–206.

Caplan, D. J., & Weintraub, J. A. (1993). The oral health burden in the United States: A summary of recent epidemiological studies. *Journal of Dental Education, 57*, 853–862.

Casey, M. M. (1999). Rural managed care. In T. C. Ricketts (Ed.), *Rural health in the United States*. New York: Oxford University Press.

Center for Health Economics Research. (1993). *Access to health care: Key indicators for policy*. Princeton, NJ: Robert Wood Johnson Foundation.

Centers for Disease Control and Prevention. (1992). Public health focus: fluoridation of community water systems. *Morbidity & Mortality Weekly Report, 41*, 372–375, 381.

Centers for Disease Control and Prevention. (1993). Cigarette smoking—attributable mortality and years of potential life lost—United States, 1990. *Morbidity & Mortality Weekly Report, 42*, 645–649.

Chollett, D. (1987). *Uninsured in the United States: The nonelderly population without health insurance*. Washington, DC: Employee Benefit Research Institute.

Cohen, R. A., Bloom, B., Simpson, G., & Parsons, P. E. (1997). Access to health care. Part 3: Older adults. *Vital Health Statistics, 10(198)*. National Center for Health Statistics.

Crall, J. (1998). The dental workforce. In G. M. Gluck & W. M. Morganstein (Eds.), *Jong's community dental health* (4th ed.). St. Louis: Mosby.

Dane, J. N. (1990). The Missouri Elks mobile dental program—dental care for developmentally disabled persons. *Journal of Public Health Dentistry, 50*, 42–47.

Davis, K., Collins, K. S., & Hall, A. (1999). *Community health centers in a changing United States health care system* (policy brief). New York: Commonwealth Fund.

Douglass, C. W., & Cole, K. O. (1979). Utilization of dental services in the United States. *Journal of Dental Education, 43*, 223–238.

Edelstein, B. L. (1997). *Public financing of dental coverage for children: Medicaid, Medicaid managed care, and state programs. A briefing paper prepared for the Reforming States Group*. San Francisco: Reforming States Group.

Edelstein, B. L. (1998). *Fact sheet on children's dental care in CHIP*. Washington, DC: Children's Dental Health Project.

Fasciano, N. J., Felt-Lisk, S., Ricketts, T. C., & Popkin, B. (1999). Preparing rural communities for managed care: Lessons learned. *Journal of Rural Health, 15*, 78–86.

Gift, H. C. (1995). *Dental utilization in the context of dental insurance on other socioeconomic factors, United States, 1988–1991*. Paper presented at a symposium of the 24th annual meeting of the American Association of Dental Research.

Grau, A. J., Buggle, F., Ziegler, C., Schwarz, W., Meuser, J., Tasman, A.-J., Bühler, A., Benesch, C., Becher, H., & Hacke, W. (1997). Association between acute cerebrovascular ishemia and chronic and recurrent infection. *Stroke, 28*, 1724–1729.

Grossi, S. G., & Genco, R. J. (1998). Periodontal disease and diabetes mellitus: A two-way relationship. *Annals of Periodontology, 3*, 51–61.

Grumbach, K., Seifer, S., Vranizan, K. Keane, D., Osmond, D., Soffel, D., Huang, K., & Bindman, A. B. (1995). *Primary care resources and preventable hospitalizations in California*. Berkeley: California Policy Seminar.

Hartley, D., Jackson, J., Mueller, K. J., Nichols, A., & Williams, V. (1999). AHCPR-funded rural managed care centers: Report from the field. *Journal of Rural Health, 15*, 87–93.

Health Care Financing Administration. (1999). *National health expenditures by type of service and source of funds: Calendar years 1960–97*. Baltimore, MD (July 27, 1999); http://www.hcfa.gov/stats/nhe-oact/nhe.htm.

Horowitz, A. M. (1995). The public's oral health: The gaps between what we know and what we practice. *Advances in Dental Research, 9*, 91–95.

Horowitz, A. M., & Nourjah, P. A. (1996). Patterns of screening for oral cancers among United States adults. *Journal of Public Health Dentistry, 56*, 333–335.

Horowitz, A. M., Goodman, H. S., Yellowitz, J. A., & Nourjah, P. A. (1996). The need for health promotion in oral cancer prevention and early detection. *Journal of Public Health Dentistry, 56*, 319–330.

Institute of Medicine (1993). *Access to health care in America*. Washington, DC: National Academy Press.

Institute of Medicine. (1995). *Dental education at the crossroads: Challenges and change*. Washington, DC: National Academy Press.

Isman, R. (1993). *The definition of primary oral health care, how it is part of primary health care, and how it can be integrated into primary health care delivery*. Unpublished paper prepared for the United States Health Resources Services & Services Administration, Bureau of Health Professions, Rockville, MD.

Isman, R. (1996, November 21). *A comparison of Medicaid dental services provided under fee-for-service and dental managed care arrangements*. Paper presented at the 124th annual meeting of the American Public Health Association, New York.

Isman, R., & Isman, B. (1997). *Access to oral health*

services in the United States: 1997 and beyond. Chicago: Oral Health America.

Kaplan, D. W., Brindis, C. D., Phibbs, S. L., Melinkovich, P., Naylor, K., & Ahlstrand, K. (1999). A comparison study of an elementary school-based health center. *Archives of Pediatric and Adolescent Medicine, 153,* 235–243.

Kassab, C., Luloff, A. E., Kelsey, T. W., & Smith, S. M. (1996). The influence of insurance status and income on health care use among the nonmetropolitan elderly. *Journal of Rural Health, 12,* 89–99.

Kaste, L. M., Selwitz, R. H., Oldakowski, R. J., Brunelle, J. A., Winn, D. M., & Brown, J. (1996a). Coronal caries in the primary and permanent dentition of children and adolescents 1–17 years of age: United States, 1988–1991. *Journal of Dental Research, 75 (special issue),* 631–641.

Kaste, L. M., Gift, H. C., Bhat, M., & Swango, P. A. (1996b). Prevalence of incisor trauma in persons 6 to 50 years of age: United States, 1988–1991. *Journal of Dental Research, 75 (special issue),* 696–705.

Keane, C. R., Lave, J. R., Ricci, E. M., & LaVallee, C. P. (1999). The impact of a children's health insurance program by age. *Pediatrics, 104,* 1051–1058.

Kiyak, H. A., Grayston, M. N., & Crinean, C. L. (1993). Oral health problems and needs of nursing home residents. *Community Dentistry & Oral Epidemiology, 21,* 49–52.

Lave, J. R., Keane, C. R., Lin, C. J., Ricci, E. M., Amersbach, G., & LaVallee, C. P. (1998a). The impact of lack of health insurance on children. *Journal of the American Medical Association, 279,* 1820–1825.

Lave, J. R., Keane, C. R., Lin, C. J., Ricci, E. M., Amersbach, G., & LaVallee, C. P. (1998b). The impact of lack of health insurance on children. *Journal of Health & Social Policy, 102,* 57–73.

Lear, J. G., Eichner, N., & Koppelman, J. (1999). The growth of school-based health centers and the role of state policies. *Archives of Pediatric and Adolescent Medicine, 153,* 1177–1180.

Liang, J. N., & Ogur, J. D. (1987). *Restrictions on dental auxiliaries: An economic policy analysis.* Washington, DC: Federal Trade Commission.

Mandel, I. D. (1994). Antimicrobial mouthrinses: Overview and update. *Journal of the American Dental Association, 125,* 2S–10S.

Marcus, S. E., Drury, T. E., Brown, L. J., & Zion, G. R. (1996). Tooth retention and tooth loss in the permanent dentition of adults: United States, 1988–1991. *Journal of Dental Research, 75 (special issue),* 684–695.

Mertz, E., Grumbach, K, MacIntosh, L., & Coffman, J. (2000). *Geographic distribution of dentists in California. Dental shortage areas, 1998.* San Francisco: Center for California Health Workforce Studies, Center for the Health Professions, University of California.

Milgrom, P., Hujoel, P., Grembowski, D., & Ward, J. M. (1997). Making Medicaid child dental services work: a partnership in Washington State. *Journal of the American Dental Association, 128,* 1440–1466.

Murphy, J. E., Jr. (1996). *Mobile dentistry.* Tulsa: PennWell Books.

National Association of Dental Plans. (1997). *Dental marketplace facts.* (July 6, 1997); h t t p : / / www.nadp.org/mktfact.html.

National Association of Dental Plans. (1999). *The dental benefits industry at a glance.* Press release (April 16, 1999); http://www.nadp.org/NEWS/ FrontPageNews/ Dental_April1699.htm.

National Cancer Institute. (1999). *SEER Cancer statistics review, 1973–1996.* Bethesda, MD: United States Department of Health and Human Services, Public Health Service, National Institutes of Health, Cancer Statistics Branch.

National Center for Health Statistics. (1999). *Initiatives and other activities: Healthy people 2000.* Hyattsville, MD (December 17, 1999); http:// www.cdc.gov/nchs/about/otheract/hp2000/ oralhealth/disparitycharts.ppt.

National Injury Information Clearinghouse. (1995). *Estimates for sports injuries.* Washington, DC: United States Consumer Product Safety Commission.

National Institute of Dental Research. (1987). *Oral health of United States adults: The national survey of oral health in United States employed adults and seniors: 1985–1986.* (NIH pub. no. 87-2868). Bethesda, MD: United States Department of Health and Human Services.

National Safe Kids Campaign. (1996). *Sports injury fact sheet.* Washington, DC: National Safe Kids Campaign.

Newacheck, P., Stoddard, J. J., Hughes, D. C., & Pearl, M. (1997). Children's access to health care: the role of social and economic factors. In R. E. K. Stein (Ed.), *Health care for Children: What's right, what's wrong, what's next.* New York: United Hospital Fund of New York.

Newbrun, E. (1989). Effectiveness of water fluoridation. *Journal of Public Health Dentistry, 49,* 279–289.

Newman, J. F., & Anderson, O. W. (1972). *Patterns of dental service utilization in the United States: A nationwide social survey.* Chicago: University of Chicago Press.

North Carolina Area Health Education Centers Program. (1999). *AHEC and rural North Carolina. Dental rotation in Cherokee;* http://www.med.unc.edu/ ahec/ruraldentist.htm

Offenbacher, S., Katz, V., Fertik, G., Collins, J., Boyd, D., Maynor, G., McKaig, R., & Beck, J. (1996). Periodontal infection as a possible risk factor for preterm low birth weight. *Journal of Periodontology, 67,* 1103–1113.

Office of Technology Assessment. (1990). *Health care in rural America.* (Publication no. OTA-H-34).

Washington, DC: United States Government Printing Office.

O'Neil, E. H., & Pew Health Professions Commission. (1998). *Recreating health professional practice for a new century. The fourth report of the Pew Health Professions Commission.* San Francisco: Pew Health Professions Commission.

Pendrys, D. G. (1998). The epidemiology of oral diseases. In G. M. Gluck & W. M. Morganstein (Eds.), *Jong's community dental health* (4th ed.). St. Louis: Mosby.

Petersen, P. E., & Pedersen, K. M. (1984). Socioeconomic demand model for dental visits. *Community Dentistry & Oral Epidemiology, 12,* 361–365.

Pew Health Professions Commission. (1995). *Critical challenges: Revitalizing the health professions for the twenty-first century. The third report of the Pew Health Professions Commission.* San Francisco: Pew Health Professions Commission.

Public Health Service, Bureau of Health Professions. (1991). *Health status of minorities and low-income groups* (3rd ed.). Washington, DC: United States Department of Health and Human Services.

Railway dental car services provided to Northland. (1969). *Journal of the Ontario Dental Association, 46,* 169.

Ries, L. A. G., Miller, B. A., Hankey, B. F., Kasary, C. L., Harras, A., & Edwards, B. K. (Eds.). (1994). *SEER cancer statistics review, 1973–1991: Tables and graphs.* Bethesda, MD: National Cancer Institute.

Rowland, D., & Lyons, B. (1989). Triple jeopardy: Rural, poor, and uninsured. *Health Services Research, 23,* 975–1004.

Scannapieco, F. A., Papandonatos, G. D., & Dunford, R. G. (1998). Associations between oral conditions and respiratory disease in a national sample survey population. *Annals of Periodontology, 3,* 251–256.

Selwitz, R. H., Winn, D. M., Kingman, A., & Zion, G. R. (1996). The prevalence of dental sealants in the United States population: Findings from NHANES III, 1988–91. *Journal of Dental Research, 75 (Special Issue),* 652–660.

Silverman, S., Jr. (1990). *Oral cancer.* Atlanta: American Cancer Society.

Simpson, G., Bloom, B., Cohen, R. A., & Parsons, P. E. (1997). Access to health care. Part 1: Children. *Vital Health Statistics, 10(196).* National Center for Health Statistics.

Smith, M. W., Kreutzer, R. A., Goldman, L., Casey-Paal, A., & Kizer, K. W. (1996). How economic demand influences access to medical care for rural Hispanic children. *Medical Care, 11,* 1135–1148.

Soporowski, N. J., Tesini, D. A., & Weiss, A. I. (1994). Survey of oralfacial sports-related injuries. *Journal of the Massachusetts Dental Society, 43,* 16–20.

State of California, Rural Health Policy Council. (1999). Notes from the Rural Health Policy Council public

meeting, October 1999. *Rural Health Newscast, 3,* 2.

Suomi, J. D., Peterson, J. K., Matthews, B. L., Voglesong, R. H., & Lyman, B. A. (1980). Effects of supervised daily dental plaque removal by children after 3 years. *Community Dentistry and Oral Epidemiology, 8,* 171–176.

Taylor, P., Puskin, D., Cooley, S. G., & Braden, J. (1993). Access. In J. F. Van Nostrand (Ed.), *Common beliefs about the rural elderly: What do national data tell us?* (DHHS publication [no. 93-1412]. Hyattsville, MD: National Center for Health Statistics.

Thomas, J. F. G., & Startup, R. (1992). Some social correlates with the dental health of young children. *Community Dental Health, 9,* 11–17.

University of Medicine and Dentistry of New Jersey. (1996). (December 17, 1999); http://www4.umdnj.edu/~plsurweb/rcpp/introduction.html.

U.S. Department of Health and Human Services. (1996). *Children's dental services under Medicaid: Access and utilization.* (OEI-09-93-00240). San Francisco: U.S. Department of Health and Human Services, Office of Inspector General.

U.S. General Accounting Office. (1980). *Increased use of expanded function dental auxiliaries would benefit consumers, dentists, and taxpayers.* (Publication No. HRD-80-51.) Washington, DC: U.S. General Accounting Office.

U.S. General Accounting Office. (1994). *Health professions education: Role of Title VII/VIII programs in improving access to care is unclear.* (Publication no. GAO/HEHS-94-164). Washington, DC: U.S. Government Printing Office.

U.S. General Accounting Office. (1995a). *Health care shortage areas: Designations not a useful tool for directing resources to the underserved.* (Publication no. GAO/HEHS-95-200). Washington, DC: U.S. Government Printing Office.

U.S. General Accounting Office. (1995b). *Health care: School-based health centers can expand access for children.* (Publication no. GAO/HEHS-95-35). Washington, DC: U.S. Government Printing Office.

U.S. General Accounting Office. (1997). *Health care access: Opportunities to target programs and improve accountability.* (Publication No. GAO/HEHS-97-204). Washington, DC: U.S. Government Printing Office.

Valla, M. E., & Westcott, R. C. (1996). Mobile dental unit brings services to the young and needy. *New York State Dental Journal, 62,* 32–35.

Venezie, R. D., Garvan, C. W., Mitchell, G. S., Yin, M., & Conti, A. J. (1997). *Accessibility and barriers to dental care in the Florida Medicaid program: A report to the Agency for Health Care Administration.* Gainesville: University of Florida, College of Dentistry.

Voelker, R. (1998). Does managed care fit for rural

America? *Advances* (Issue 4). Princeton, NJ: Robert Wood Johnson Foundation.

Vokes, E. E., Weichselbaum, R. R., Lippman, S. M., Hong, W. K. (1993). Head and neck cancer. *New England Journal of Medicine, 328*, 184–194.

Waldman, H. B. (1990). Confirming the continuing potential for pediatric dental services in nonurban areas. *Journal of Dentistry for Children, 57*, 421–423.

Waldman, H. B. (1994b). Pediatric dentistry and national health insurance: A more than favorable opportunity. *Journal of Dentistry for Children, 61*, 361–364.

Waldman, H. B. (1998). More children are unable to get dental care than any other single health service. *Journal of Dentistry for Children, 65*, 204–208.

Weinert, C., & Long, K. (1990). Rural families and health care: Refining the knowledge base. In D. Unger & M. Sussman (Eds.), *Families in community settings. Interdisciplinary perspectives.* Binghamton, NY: Hawthorne.

Winn, D. M., Brunelle, J. A., Selwitz, R. H., Kaste, L. M., Oldakowski, R. J., Kingman, A., & Brown, L. J. (1996). Coronal and root caries in the dentition of adults in the United States, 1988-1991. *Journal of Dental Research, 75 (special issue)*, 642–651.

Yellowitz, J. A., & Goodman, H. S. (1995). Physicians' and dentists' oral cancer knowledge, opinions and practice. *Journal of the American Dental Association, 126*, 53–60.

Yellowitz, J. A., Goodman, H. S., Horowitz, A. M., & al-Tannir, M. A. (1995). Assessment of alcohol and tobacco use in dental schools' health history forms. *Journal of Dental Education, 59*, 1091–1096.

14

Rural Mental Health Services

BRUCE LUBOTSKY LEVIN AND ARDIS HANSON

Health and mental health care in America have come under increasing scrutiny during the last half of the 20th century from a vast array of stakeholders, including consumers, providers, employers, community leaders, policymakers, administrators, educators, as well as lawmakers at the state and federal levels of government. Proposals for national and state health care reform have been prompted, in part, by the need to control the rising costs of health care and to address the obstacles and inequities in accessing health and mental health services. Although the United States Congress did not pass major comprehensive health care reform legislation in the 1990s, significant health care initiatives (particularly in association with entitlement programs) have been proposed and implemented by various individual states.

Historically, individuals who live in rural and frontier areas in America have significant health care needs but experience numerous obstacles in obtaining these services, including lack of accessible services (i.e., social isolation, significant geographical distances, inhospitable climates), a general scarcity of resources and the absence of a human services infrastructure, severe shortages of service providers, the absence of service specialization (availability of ser-

vices), the inappropriate organization of services based upon urban (metropolitan) delivery system models, and inefficient communication (including diversity of languages and subcultures) to disseminate information and coordinate care (Beeson, Britain, Howell, Kirwan, & Sawyer, 1998; Mutel & Donham, 1983; Office of Technology Assessment, 1995; Wagenfeld, Murray, Mohatt, & DeBruyn, 1994; also see Chapters 1 and 4 in this volume).

These rural health care delivery barriers become even more complex with the provision of rural (and particularly frontier) mental health services because mental health service delivery has historically faced problems of stigma (among health providers, consumers, and employers), poor integration with general (or somatic) health services, unique language and cultural challenges to treatment, and substantial reliance on public sector funding (Beeson et al., 1998; Blank, Fox, Hargrove, & Turner, 1995; "Rural Mental Health," 1998; Sawyer & Beeson, 1998; Wagenfeld et al., 1994).

This chapter presents an overview of the major challenges in the provision of rural mental health services in the United States. It also identifies the most important issues facing rural mental health services delivery in the foreseeable future.

It should be noted that this chapter only highlights critical issues in mental health services in rural and frontier areas. For more in-depth information on the major facets of mental health services delivery, see Levin & Petrila (1996) as well as *Mental Health: A Report of the Surgeon General* (U.S. Department of Health and Hu-

BRUCE LUBOTSKY LEVIN • Louis de la Parte Florida Mental Health Institute, College of Public Health, University of South Florida, Tampa, Florida 33612-3807. ARDIS HANSON • Louis de la Parte Florida Mental Health Institute Library, University of South Florida, Tampa, Florida 33612-3807.

Handbook of Rural Health, edited by Loue and Quill. Kluwer Academic/Plenum Publishers, New York, 2001.

man Services, 1999). For important discussions of mental health services delivery in rural and frontier areas, readers should examine Beeson *et al.* (1998), Flax, Wagenfeld, Ivens, and Weiss (1979), and Wagenfeld *et al.* (1994). In addition, individuals interested in accessing papers, publications, and resources on rural mental health services delivery via the Internet should see the Frontier Mental Health Services Resource Network (http://www.du.edu/frontier-mh/), the National Association for Rural Mental Health (http://www.narmh/), and the National Rural Health Association (http://www.nrharural.org/).

Public Mental Health

As we enter the 21st century, mental disorders remain a significant public health problem. According to a recently published report from the U.S. Surgeon General (U.S. Department of Health and Human Services, 1999), mental disorders account for 4 of the 10 leading causes of disability for individuals who are five years and older, with depression the leading cause of disability and suicide one of the leading preventable causes of death in the America. Mental disorders are also significant contributors to the burden of disease, ranking second (to cardiovascular illnesses) in disease burden in the United States.

Approximately one in five Americans has a mental disorder during any given year, with anxiety disorders (e.g., phobias, panic disorder, and posttraumatic stress disorder, among others) found to be the most prevalent mental disorders in adults (see Table 1).

Approximately one in five children and adolescents (ages 9 to 17) has a diagnosable mental disorder during any given year, with 11% of children experiencing significant functional impairment and 5% of children experiencing extreme functional impairment. In addition, at any one time, between 10% and 15% of children and adolescents have symptoms of depression.

Depression is very prevalent among older Americans, affecting 8% to 20% of older adults in the community and affecting approximately one-third of older adults who utilize primary

TABLE 1. Estimate of 1-Year Prevalence Rates Based on the Epidemiologic Catchment Area Study and the National Co-Morbidity Study, Ages 18–54

	ECA Prevalence (Percent)	NCS Prevalence (Percent)
Anxiety disorders[a]	13.1	18.7
Mood disorders[b]	7.1	11.1
All disorders	19.5	23.4

[a]Simple phobia, social phobia, agoraphobia, panic disorder, generalized anxiety disorder, obsessive compulsive disorder, and posttraumatic stress disorder (PTSD).
[b]Unipolar, bipolar I, bipolar II, dysthymia, schizophrenia, nonaffective psychosis, somatization, severe cognitive impairment, antisocial personality disorder (ASP), and anorexia.
Note: From *Mental Health: A Report of the Surgeon General* (Table 2.6), U.S. Department of Health and Human Services, 1999.

health care settings. Depression in older adults often leads to impairments in physical, social, and mental functioning.

Meanwhile, mental health services delivery in America have evolved into a complex array of uncoordinated and fragmented services, programs, and delivery systems, often creating obstacles to accessing these services. The rather large gap between epidemiologic estimates of mental disorders and the actual number of individuals receiving care over the course of a lifetime strongly suggests that many Americans have attempted to cope with their mental health problems either without help and without entering the formal mental health care delivery sector or have received assistance through other health or social service systems, including (primary) health care, welfare, correctional, or long-term care delivery systems (Blanch & Levin, 1998).

In addition, the historical reliance on the public sector for long-term care and on the private sector for acute care has contributed to limited continuity of mental health care (Elpers & Levin, 1996). Although state and federal governments historically funded public mental health care, the financing systems for these services have become considerably more complicated, with a multitude of public and private payors as well as numerous public and private providers of mental health care (Frank & McGuire, 1996). In 1996, total direct costs for mental disorders reached $69 billion, representing in excess of 7% of total health care spending in America. These costs have been conservative, since of the 20% of Americans who have a diagnosable mental disorder, only about 15% have used mental health services during any given year.

Another critical issue in the decision-making process for seeking mental health treatment has been confidentiality of consumer information records. This issue is very important in today's managed behavioral health care marketplace and with recent advancements in information technology. Furthermore, confidentiality of mental health conditions in consumer information databases continues to be of high concern to providers, insurers, and consumers of mental health services because of the considerable and persistent societal stigma associated with use of these services.

Consumer and family movements have played increasingly important roles in the planning, delivery, and evaluation of mental health services as well as in the protection of individual rights of mental health consumers. Consumer organizations have established self-help groups, individualizing services to meet consumer needs, established offices of consumer affairs in state hospitals and state mental health offices, and assisted mental health consumers as employees in mental health and other human service agencies.

The family advocacy movement has been responsible for the inclusion of family participation in service system decision making for children with mental disorders. The family advocacy movement has been represented by three major organizations: the National Alliance for the Mentally Ill, the National Mental Health Association, and the Federation of Families for Children's Mental Health.

Rural Mental Health Services Delivery

Historically, both health and mental health services have been largely concentrated in large urban areas of America. Therefore, it is not surprising that basic organizational models for health and mental health services delivery have been based on urban at-risk populations. In addition, professional and graduate education and training programs for health and mental health practitioners have evolved at universities and hospitals located in major metropolitan locations, with few graduate training programs established with concentrations in rural mental health. Furthermore, similar to the larger field of public health, rural mental health does not have a certification or other credentialing program. Thus far, opportunities for continuing professional development and continuing education in rural mental health have been difficult at best (Sawyer & Beeson, 1998). Nevertheless, recent developments in telemental health technology have begun to address this situation (see the discussion later in this chapter on telemental health communication technologies).

Although urban areas are home to approximately three-quarters of the United States population, rural and frontier areas make up nearly 90% of the actual land mass, with a population base in excess of 62 million people (Sawyer & Beeson, 1998). Furthermore, 15 states in the United States have 50% or more of their population living in rural or frontier areas (Shelton & Frank, 1995). However, social, political, cultural, and economic changes during the last quarter of a century have contributed to significant variability and heterogeneity in rural environments throughout the United States (Ortega, Johnson, Beeson, & Craft, 1994). Thus, every rural community is unique, with its own at-risk populations as well as its underlying economic, political, cultural, and social structures, collectively contributing to diverse patterns of health and mental health problems. Population characteristics and the economic base in rural areas of the Southwest may differ significantly from population characteristics in rural areas of Appalachia, northern New England, the South, the Great Plains, or the frontier West. Moreover, no single organizational model of rural health and mental health services could be expected to serve all rural and frontier areas in the United States. In fact, Sawyer & Beeson (1998) have maintained that there has been more diversity in health and mental health services delivery within rural areas of the United States than between urban and rural areas.

Collectively, rural populations in America

have unique characteristics that affect issues of accessibility and availability of health and mental health services (Office of Technology Assessment, 1990). For example, residents of rural America are more likely to be poorer, older, disabled, less educated, uninsured, and employed by smaller businesses than individuals living in urban areas. Fewer health and mental health practitioners have established practices in rural areas. Thus, few health and mental health services have been available for individuals who have the greatest need.

Hospitals in rural areas tend to be smaller and serve a higher proportion of uninsured or publicly insured individuals than do urban hospitals. Individuals living in rural America have been less likely to have health insurance than were urban residents. In addition, rural populations have historically experienced increased rates of alcohol abuse, child and spousal abuse, and depression. More basic problems, such as insufficient transportation, electricity, water, and communication systems, have only complicated the process of providing and using rural health and mental health services (Beeson *et al.*, 1998; Wagenfeld *et al.*, 1994). Given the higher unemployment, uninsured or underinsured status, and lower income rural populations, rural areas often have a disproportionate number of people dependent on Medicare and Medicaid programs that, in turn, frequently offer unequal coverage for mental health services compared to somatic health services (Office of Technology Assessment, 1990).

Many of the basic service delivery issues and challenges in the organization and delivery of rural mental health services have not been addressed by policymakers and legislators. There has been conflicting evidence about whether there is increased risk for mental disorders for individuals living in urban versus rural America (Sawyer & Beeson, 1998). The following section will briefly present survey findings on the prevalence of mental disorders in rural areas of the United States.

Epidemiology

An estimated 15 million residents of rural areas suffer from one or more behavioral health problems. Symptoms related to anxiety disorders, trauma, cognitive disorders, developmental disorders, and psychotic disorders have been as common among rural residents as among urban residents (Wagenfeld *et al.*, 1994). Furthermore, suicide rates in rural areas have surpassed urban suicide rates. Rural residents who are female, poor, elderly, or belong to a racial or ethnic minority, or who are unemployed, have an increased likelihood of experiencing a mental health problem (Shelton, Merwin, & Fox, 1995).

The stress of ranching and farming has been a major problem in some rural areas of America. The threat of losing the family land, and home, experiencing severe weather problems, and the constant preoccupation with uncertain crop production creates major stressors for many ranch and farm families. Accidents, equipment problems, social isolation, and irregular cash flow can also produce unhealthy emotional reactions, often in association with behavioral or somatic disorders (Ide, Carson, & Araquistain, 1997).

One of the basic problems facing the rural mental health services research field is the estimation of the prevalence of mental disorders in individuals who live in rural and frontier areas as well as subsequent rural versus urban prevalence comparisons. The lack of definitive conclusions and study findings have been attributed, in part, to a variability in definitions (of both rural-urban areas and of mental disorders), sampling design (including potential differences in the age, ethnicity, and racial characteristics of the population), measurement (e.g., treated prevalence versus true prevalence), source of data, and type of instrument utilized in rural mental health studies (Holzer & Ciarlo, 1999; Wagenfeld *et al.*, 1994; Flax *et al.*, 1979).

National studies such as the Epidemiologic Catchment Area Study (Robins & Regier, 1991) found nearly identical one-year prevalence rates for mental disorders in rural and urban areas. In addition, results of the National Comorbidity Study (Kessler, McGonagle, Zhao, Nelson, Hughs, Eshleman, Wittchen, & Kendler, 1994) revealed the prevalence of a diagnosable mental disorder was only about 1% higher (not statistically significant) for individuals living in major metropolitan areas versus nonmetropolitan areas, although the prevalence rates did vary by specific mental disorder. While Ciarlo

& Tweed (1992) found lower prevalence rates of mental disorders in frontier areas than in urban areas, they also found that more densely populated rural areas had similar prevalence rates for mental disorders as selected metropolitan areas. Thus, the definition of what constitutes rural or urban areas has been critical in comparative rates of the prevalence of mental disorders in those residents.

In addition, little is known about the prevalence of comorbid disorders in rural areas. Nationally, people with either a mental health or substance use disorder were more likely to have a co-occurring disorder than the general population (Regier, Farmer, Rae, Locke, Keith, Judd, L. L., & Goodwin, 1990). Therefore, future research in rural mental health services needs to examine the prevalence of co-occurring disorders in individuals treated for substance abuse who have a history of mental disorders as well as individuals treated for somatic disorders who also have a co-occurring mental disorder or addiction.

Services Delivery

The availability of mental health services and service providers, the accessibility of services, the acceptability of these services to rural residents, and the utilization and costs of specialty services have been critical factors in rural mental health services delivery (Shelton et al., 1995).

Availability

Services. It is not surprising that the overall availability and volume of mental health services, programs, and providers increases with the population density of a community or area. Accordingly, the average number of mental health facilities in the most densely populated urban counties of the United States was over 50 times the average number of mental health facilities in the least urbanized counties. Furthermore, in recent years, there has been a gradual increase in the availability of specialty mental health services in metropolitan areas, but a more modest increase in nonmetropolitan areas of the United States. For example, in 1983, approximately 89% of U.S. metropolitan counties (250,000 or more people) had inpatient mental health services. By 1990, this percentage increased to 100. Meanwhile, in 1983, less than 1% of nonmetropolitan counties (populations under 2,500) had inpatient mental health services, increasing to just 1% in 1990 (Goldsmith, Wagenfeld, Manderscheid, & Stiles, 1997). Most rural residents continue to receive inpatient mental health treatment outside of their communities (Wagenfeld et al., 1994).

Thus, the growth of mental health services in rural areas remains limited. Rural America has suffered from continual shortages of available mental health and supportive services. For example, in 1990, while 96% of metropolitan counties in the United States had any mental health services, only 79.5% of nonmetropolitan counties had any mental health services (Goldsmith et al., 1997).

Providers. The availability of specialty mental health services has been partially dependent on the existence and availability of professionally trained mental health providers. Over 60% of rural areas in the United States have been designated as federal mental health professional shortage areas (Office of Technology Assessment, 1990). Furthermore, 55% of the 3,075 rural counties in the United States do not have practicing mental health professionals, including psychiatrists, social workers, and psychologists (National Advisory Committee on Rural Health, 1993). Unfortunately, the sparseness of rural populations as well as geography limit both the number of mental health providers and the diversity of mental health specialists in rural areas. In turn, these shortages in mental health providers and services significantly affect the organization and delivery of rural mental health services.

Holzer, Goldsmith, & Ciarlo (1998) examined the availability of mental health providers in frontier and isolated rural areas through existing national databases. As expected, frontier counties (with less than 7 persons per square mile) had 1.3 psychiatrists per 100,000 population compared with more densely populated counties (over 100 persons per square mile) with 10.5 psychiatrists per 100,000 population.

Because physicians often provide mental health care in the absence of mental health specialty providers, data were examined for all physicians engaged in active patient care. Isolated frontier counties (less than 2 persons per square mile) averaged 31 physicians per 100,000 population, while frontier counties averaged 59 physicians per 100,000 people. The most densely populated counties averaged 180 physicians per 100,000 population.

The number of psychologists with at least a master's degree who worked in health-related settings also increased with population density. Isolated frontier counties had 13 psychologists per 100,000 population, frontier counties had 18 psychologists per 100,000 population, and the most densely populated counties had 29 psychologists per 100,000 population.

For social workers with at least a master's degree who worked in health-related settings, it was interesting to note that isolated frontier counties had nearly 13 social workers per 100,000 population, while frontier counties had only 9 social workers per 100,000 population. The highest-density counties had nearly 24 social workers per 100,000 population. This may or may not be attributed to the variability in the organizational structure and role of county human services and educational settings (social service agencies and schools) where social workers have been traditionally employed.

Hendryx, Borders, & Johnson (1995) found that there was considerable variation in the distribution of mental health providers throughout the state of Iowa. They found that 40% of rural areas had no mental health professionals. They also found that the average rate of urban mental health providers (i.e., psychiatrists, psychologist, social workers, and other counselors) was 75 per 100,000 people, while the average rate of rural mental health providers was 19.4 per 100,000 people. In addition, Hendryx et al. (1995) found that hospitalization rates for individuals with mental disorders were positively related to the physician supply but unrelated to the supply of other mental health professionals.

There have been continuing efforts to recruit, staff, and retain rural mental health professionals from the field of social work, psychology, psychiatry, and psychiatric nursing, but efforts to meet the special needs of these professionals have been isolated and have occurred in relatively few geographic areas in rural and frontier areas of the United States (Wagenfeld et al., 1994).

Recommendations. The Ad Hoc Rural Mental Health Provider Work Group (Pion, Keller, & McCombs, 1997) has outlined a number of major recommendations to enhance the supply and effectiveness of rural mental health professionals:

1. Developing didactic and experiential training for mental health graduate students targeted at competencies needed to practice in rural mental health settings;
2. Encouring graduate training programs in the mental health disciplines to recruit individuals who demonstrate a commitment to practice in rural settings after graduation
3. Increasing interdisciplinary training and service delivery opportunities to enhance the supply and effectiveness of rural mental health providers and improve consumer access to rural mental health providers through increased interdisciplinary practica, internships, and residency placements and through the incorporation of behavioral health services into area health education centers
4. Providing federal and state funds for the training of rural mental health professionals
5. Enhancing the integration of mental health consumers and survivors into rural mental health services delivery
6. Encouraging mental health agencies, funders, and providers to respect and include natural helpers and traditional healers found in rural cultures in order to maximize all available resources in rural communities

New educational initiatives in the general rural health field have slowly begun to surface, although they do not include rural mental health educational initiatives. For example, the first graduate School of Rural Public Health was recently established in the United States at Texas A&M University. In addition, several departmental and program training and research efforts in higher education have surfaced focusing on rural and community health issues.

Provider Challenges

Mental health professionals face a number of challenges, ethical dilemmas, and potential opportunities in the delivery of mental health services in rural communities (Bushy, 1997). Certainly, a rural environment has many lifestyle advantages, including a lower cost of living, outdoor recreational opportunities, less commuting traffic, and perhaps more professional visibility in the community.

However, one of the major challenges for rural mental health professionals is often professional isolation or the lack of peer support from other mental health colleagues. Some people might view it as "living in isolation," while other professionals might view it as an opportunity for "personal solitude." This isolation may also mean a lack of access to continuing education as well as the potential to lose specialty skills because of functioning as a mental health generalist. However, with increasing technological opportunities to participate in continuing education through distance learning initiatives, this may no longer be a critical problem.

Certainly, confidentiality has always been an important ethical issue in behavioral health services. In rural communities, it is often difficult to separate one's professional from one's personal interactions with consumers. This situation of overlapping relationships may place rural mental health professionals in an uncomfortable ethical dilemma, since approximately one-half of ethical complaints about mental health professionals have been related to overlapping relationships. Simon & Williams (1999) have suggested a number of basic treatment boundary guidelines for rural mental health professionals, which include the maintenance of neutrality with the consumer, the minimization of physical contact, and the provision of a professional rural mental health treatment setting.

Accessibility

Accessibility to services refers to whether a rural resident has access to mental health services as well as the ability to purchase needed services (Bushy, 1997). Access to rural behavioral health services (including alcohol, drug abuse, and mental health services) has been problematic for a number of reasons, including geographic challenges, lack of transportation, poor communication equipment, shortage of providers for mental health outreach services, inclement weather, discriminatory reimbursement policies, and inadequate coverage of mental health services under federal and state entitlement programs.

Since approximately 40% of behavioral health professionals are based in rural hospitals (compared to 18% of mental health professionals working in hospitals throughout the United States), the availability of mental health services has been dependent, in part, on the fiscal stability of the rural hospital (Bushy, 1997) as well as the ability to staff mental health units in rural hospitals.

It is not uncommon for individuals living in rural areas in some states (including Arizona, Nebraska, New Mexico, and Wyoming) to travel hundreds of miles to seek inpatient mental health care because of stigma associated with seeking care in their own rural communities or the absence of emergency and 24-hour mental health services in their communities. Although 37% of metropolitan hospitals in the United States offered emergency mental health services, only 19% of nonmetropolitan hospitals in the United States offered emergency mental health services (National Rural Health Association, 1999).

Rural residents often have been unable to advocate on their own behalf (for needed mental health services). Rural mental health providers and agencies, often overextended with large client caseloads, generally do not have the time or expertise to seek additional or supplemental public or private grant support for mental health programs.

In addition, third-party payers have placed restrictions on both the delivery and reimbursement of mental health services (Pion et al., 1997). For rural mental health settings, this has primarily affected Medicare and Medicaid entitlement programs. Although licensed mental health practitioners from various disciplines may be reimbursed for mental health services, physicians continue to have supervisory and medication authority, legal responsibility, and accountability for mental health treatment, despite the severe shortage of physicians trained and/or interested in mental health treatment in rural areas. Furthermore, the particular mental health providers who are "approved" to deliver mental health services vary in terms of the health and mental health service settings, states, and funding sources (Pion *et al.*, 1997). This has been particularly important with the introduction of managed care strategies and developing provider networks in selected rural areas in America.

Recommendations. The Ad Hoc Rural Mental Health Provider Work Group (Pion *et al.*, 1997) has made two further suggestions regarding rural mental health professionals:

1. Training programs and credentialing organizations should identify and remove practice barriers to delivery of rural mental health services.
2. Statutory and regulatory mechanisms should allow rural mental health providers to deliver and receive reimbursement for a more comprehensive range of services.

Acceptability

Acceptability refers to the provision of mental health services in a way that is compatible with the values of the at-risk populations (Bushy, 1997). Rural values, attitudes, and traditions may limit the utilization of mental health services. Given the racial, ethnic, and cultural diversity of rural populations, acceptability of behavioral health services may be difficult to achieve for a number of reasons, including established self-care practices and specific mental health etiologic beliefs, the lack of knowledge about mental health services, gatekeeping, and treatment for these services, and the location of mental health treatment settings.

Acceptability of rural mental health services may also be influenced by the urban education and training orientation of mental health providers (Bushy, 1997). This also can affect issues of trust while the mental health provider–consumer relationship is being established. This relationship directly affects the success of rural mental health outreach and aftercare programs. If the rural mental health outreach providers are

viewed as community outsiders, then the helping relationship will not be established. Thus, careful recruiting and retaining of mental health professionals for work in rural areas is critical.

Community acceptability is also critical to the survival and effectiveness of rural mental health programs (Bushy, 1997). To help ensure that a program is acceptable by a population at-risk for mental disorders, a community needs assessment should be conducted prior to the planning and implementation of a new rural mental health program. Thorough understanding of the cultural data is critical so that the rural mental health services will be made available in a manner consistent with the at-risk populations. Mental health providers should consider a number of factors in a rural mental health needs assessment initiative, including population density, travel time and work-related issues, customs, values, and traditions related to mental health services, and patterns of natural events. Thus, mental health programs will not thrive unless personal, work, cultural, and environmental factors are taken into consideration.

Mohatt (1997b) has suggested that the shortage of rural mental health professionals, the limited availability of mental health services, and the relative dependence on government entitlement programs for the financing of rural mental health services have contributed to several problems among rural communities. These problems include lack of needed services; lack of timely services, potentially increasing the cost, duration, and level of mental health care; and treatment provision in service settings far from the home community.

Health/Mental Health Integration

While rural and frontier areas in the United States face similar obstacles in the delivery of mental health services (including availability, accessibility, service utilization and costs, and provider issues), the organizational models of mental health services delivery are heterogeneous. For example, while some states and communities (e.g., Idaho, North Dakota, Texas) organize mental health services together with substance abuse services in a single agency, other states (e.g., Nevada) have separate agencies for mental health and substance abuse services. In addition, selected states (e.g., Idaho and Montana) house mental health and substance abuse services in an umbrella human services agency (Wagenfeld, 1998a).

Nevertheless, the scarcity of rural mental health services and providers together with continual changes in the organization, financing, and delivery of health and mental health services (through provider networks and managed care) have renewed interest in and provided strong incentives for linking or integrating behavioral health services and primary health care (Mechanic, 1994; Sorensen, 1999). Sorensen (1999) has detailed several models of integration of rural primary and mental health care, including linking of primary and mental health care providers through an integrated provider team and establishing collaborations and partnerships between mental health services and other human services organizations through colocations, site visits, shared facilities, and joint staff activities.

One additional benefit of integrating mental health services with primary health care has been referred to as the medical cost offset effect (Mumford, Schlesinger, Glass, Patrick, & Cuerdon, 1998), or the decrease in medical care utilization and costs after the introduction of an integrated mental health component within a comprehensive health care program (e.g., a health maintenance organization).

Another compelling reason to promote services integration involves the entry point where individuals with mental disorders present themselves. Studies have shown that most Americans seek treatment for mental disorders in primary health care settings (Regier, Goldberg, & Taube, 1979). However, there are problems associated with this gatekeeper approach to mental health care, such as the questionable knowledge base, training, interest, and proficiency of primary care physicians in the diagnosis, assessment, and treatment of individuals with mental disorders. For example, Schulberg (1991) reported that 80% of mental health diagnoses went undetected by primary care providers.

Recommendations. The Ad Hoc Rural Mental Health Provider Work Group (Pion et al., 1997) recommended four strategies for the full integration of behavioral health services:

1. Requiring federally funded rural health programs, as part of their mission, to include behavioral health services
2. Providing incentives to existing rural health networks to incorporate behavioral health services
3. Targeting mental health needs with other high priority needs in rural health demonstration awards
4. Promoting collaboration between primary care and mental health providers to meet the comprehensive health needs of rural residents

Key Issues in the 21st Century

Beeson et al. (1998) suggested that managed care and information technology offer the greatest challenges to as well as potentially the most significant impact on rural mental health services. Change in both managed health care and information technology has been swift and relentless. The remaining sections of this chapter will examine how these two factors are affecting health, mental health, and rural mental health services delivery.

Managed Care

The concept of managing health and mental health care has its historical roots in early 20th-century prepaid group practice plans (Levin, 1992). These organizations, in combination with various health care review, financing, and service coordination organizations, evolved into a variety of alternative health care financing and delivery systems most commonly known as health maintenance organizations (HMOs) and subsequent organizational hybrids (including independent practice associations and preferred provider organizations).

A report from the Office of Technology Assessment (1995) discussed several reasons for the underrepresentation of HMOs in rural areas: (1) scarcity of rural health providers; (2) relative value rural health providers place on autonomy; (3) sparsely populated service areas that are less profitable; and (4) fewer employer-based groups for HMOs to enroll than in urban areas.

Today, managed care has become the most dominant form of health and mental health coverage for individuals with private insurance. This continued growth of managed care "has [increasingly] blurred the distinction between organizations bearing financial risk for health care (insurers), organizations managing care (health maintenance and utilization management organizations), and organizations making clinical treatment decisions (provider groups or individual clinicians)" (Sturm, 1999, p. 362).

Nevertheless, the aggressive and rapid growth of managed care in America has raised concerns that reduction in health and mental health care costs may have resulted in cost shifting to public programs or consumers themselves. In addition, Beeson (1994) has raised a number of concerns about the potential impact of managed care on rural mental health services, including avoidance and neglect of rural populations in general and of individuals with serious mental disorders and comorbidity; a more limited access to mental health care; and the decreased influence of local communities, consumers, and family members in the care of rural residents with mental disorders.

Meanwhile, during the last 15 years, an increasing number of employers and government programs have "carved out" or separated mental health service benefits from general health care benefits through contractual arrangements with specialized vendors that may assume some level of financial risk. These specialized organizations have subsequently emerged under the rubric of "managed behavioral health care organizations" (MBHOs). MBHOs have attempted to reduce the costs of mental health care through the utilization of mental health practitioners at discounted fees, reduction in the length of mental health treatment, decreased use of hospital treatment, and increased use of ambulatory mental health care treatment. Studies have reported significant declines in the costs of mental health care under these MBHOs (Cuffel, Goldman, & Schlensinger, 1999; Goldman, McCulloch, & Sturm, 1998; Grazier, Eselius, Hu, Shore, & G'Sell, 1999; Ma & McGuire, 1998).

At the same time, states have increasingly turned to MBHOs to enroll Medicare and Medicaid populations, with nearly all states having implemented managed behavioral health programs. In recent years, public sector enrollment in managed care plans has dramatically increased, accounting for approximately 13% of the 38 million Medicare beneficiaries and approximately 54% of the 31 million Medicaid beneficiaries (for more information, see http://www.hcfa.gov/medicare/mgdcar.htm).

The complexity of the contractual arrangements between state and local governments and MBHOs has varied considerably (Findlay, 1999). Some states contract directly with MBHOs or subcontract with HMOs, paying a capitated fee to provide mental health services, with the MBHO or HMO assuming the risk. However, other states prefer to retain full risk and contract with MBHOs (or subcontract with HMOs or other managed care plans) to manage mental health or behavioral health benefits. Other MBHOs have been contracted only to conduct utilization review and case management services. However, in some cases, the creation of complex authorization procedures (such as pretreatment assessment, supervision of care, and other reviews) pose serious access questions for rural residents seeking mental health services, particularly if the consumer must obtain a mental health referral from a primary care physician. Furthermore, given the serious shortage of rural health and mental health providers, authorization procedures can create obstacles for rural residents accessing mental health services.

Nevertheless, Mohatt (1997) has suggested that telemental health technology (see the next section of this chapter) may help with preauthorization and assessment procedures as well as with using midlevel health and mental health practitioners. Telecommunications may be a first step to address some of the geographic, personnel, and communication problems.

Recommendations

An issue paper on mental health in rural America by the National Rural Health Association (1999) has suggested that the Medicaid agencies in states that contract with MBHOs should mandate their managed care vendors to monitor the impact of the contractual arrangements on service delivery effectiveness for rural residents under mental health care (i.e., address quality of care issues through accountability measures).

While the integration of managed behavioral health care in rural and frontier areas may create significant challenges, it appears to be inevitable in the current managed health care environment in America. Mohatt (1997b) has proposed five strategies for the delivery of rural mental health services through MBHOs:

1. Developing rural mental health provider networks proactively
2. Developing horizontally integrated rural mental health networks to achieve economies of scale, eliminate administrative and services delivery overlap, and increase efficiency of scarce resources
3. Forming integrative networks of health and mental health providers to provide a better continuum of care
4. Encouraging a public health approach to mental health care through mental health consultations in primary care settings
5. Utilizing telemental health technology to address rural service delivery challenges

Telecommunications

Telemental health services (LaMendola, 1997) and *behavioral telehealth* (Nickleson, 1998) refer to the use of telecommunications technology to overcome geographic limitations in the provision of specialty mental health information and services. These services have included (but are not limited to) prevention, diagnosis, consultation, outreach, case management, education and educational opportunities, treatment, and data management.

Infrastructure Issues

For over 30 years, mental health professionals have been investigating the use of advanced telecommunications and information technologies to improve mental health care. In January 1965 the first "production" in a telepsychiatry program was begun—a microwave-mediated link between Omaha and Norfolk State Mental Hospital, 112 miles away (Wheeler & Allen, 1998). For many rural areas, radio and telephone technologies have remained a critical component in the development of crisis care and community mental health programs. Unfortunately, some rural and frontier areas still have relatively low telephone penetration. In fact, a number of rural and frontier areas do not have any 911 service that relies on digital switches, which are essential for advanced telecommunication services (LaMendola, 1997). With the expansion of communication satellites in the late 1970s, interest in applying new technologies to health and mental health care increased dramatically, particularly with the transition from analog to digital transmission and rapid computer hardware and software development (Parker, 1978). The availability of T-1 and the integrated services digital network (ISDN) fiber optic telephone lines provided the core infrastructure for the Internet.

However, one of telemental health's most significant barriers has continued to be overwhelming costs. In most rural and frontier regions of the United States, telecommunication costs have been far greater than in urban areas. Higher bandwidths, such as ISDN, frame relay, and T-1 (not to mention tremendous geographic challenges) have been so expensive in rural regions that the utilization of these technological advancements is prohibited. As a result, the utilization of telemedicine technology by rural and frontier mental health care providers has been limited. Thus, the rural mental health field is at a distinct disadvantage in 21st-century America.

The Western Governors Association's *Telemedicine Action Report* (1995) recommended that states factor emerging health care applications, such as telemedicine, into state telecommunications and information technology planning and procurement. Their 1998 report concluded that most states have not yet integrated telemedicine applications into the statewide telecommunications network planning process. Alaska is one of the few states that formally looked at telemedicine as part of the entire telecommunications infrastructure (Alaska Telehealth Advisory Committee, 1999). Even fewer states have taken steps to integrate public and private telecommunications networks for the purpose of providing health or mental health services and education. In fact, Texas law prohibits private entities from using the statewide-consolidated telecommunications network (Western Governors Association, 1998).

The *Report on U.S. Telemedicine Activity* (Association of Telemedicine Providers, 1999) indicated that although telemedicine has continued to grow, that does not mean that all consumers or programs have benefited equally. Activity varied greatly by program, state, clinical specialty, and population served. More recently, telemedicine systems have been employed extensively for uses other than health and mental health services delivery. Educational use of systems has been extensive, particularly in the areas of continuing education for mental health providers, psychiatric grand rounds, and supervision and teaching applications. Specialty mental health consultation delivered to rural hospitals has made up only a small fraction of the services. The Joint Working Group on Telemedicine (1997) listed 28 projects that provided mental health services, of which 6 were located in states with significant frontier populations: Alaska, Colorado, Kansas, Montana, Nebraska, and South Dakota (Joint Working Group on Telemedicine, 1997). The Abt study (Hassol, Carol, Gaumer, Puskin, Mintzer, & Grigsby, 1997) found 38 nonfederal rural hospitals and other providers actively using telepsychiatry.

Although interactive video has remained the most common means of delivering mental health care from remote locations, newer technologies are also being used, including a combination of audiographic, store-and-forward, and telemetry technologies.

The Telecommunications Act of 1996 dramatically altered communication rates and services potentially available to telemedicine providers. The federal government has provided $400 million to health providers, libraries, and schools in rural areas to offset telephone line charges incurred in connecting to the Internet via the Universal Service Fund.

Funding and Supporting the Infrastructure

Historically, federal and state budgets appropriated funding for health and mental health programs. How the funds were awarded, the high cost of administering the funds, and the ability to actually meet rural health and mental health needs have been major areas of concern

for rural providers. Usually, health and mental health programs have originated with specific unmet needs in urban areas. Criteria for funds often have been based on criteria relevant to urban areas. Allocation of these funds to rural areas may not cover the administrative requirements of the grant. Categorical funding streams require separate contracts, line item budgets, staffing, statistical reports, financial accounting and reporting, program review, auditing, and an appeals process.

A continuing issue in the use of telecommunications technology is the ongoing expense of time and money for staff training. Training of those who will be using telemental health software and hardware should be incorporated into the payment structure so that it will not be viewed as a "one-time" expense as the infrastructure changes over time. In addition, long-term or start-up monies are necessary for financial or technical support in the development of provider networks integrating mental health delivery systems in rural areas.

Legal and Ethical Issues in Telemental Health

There are additional issues in the provision of telemental health services. First, the technology itself may be unfamiliar to the mental health provider. Accurate transmission, encryption, and reception of data are critical for treatment decisions. With the transmission of data, confidentiality and privacy of client information have also become critical concerns. Electronic storage of client information requires more sophisticated software and hardware solutions (Laske, 1994).

Although state law traditionally protects and holds confidential a patient's medical records, the federal government has also begun to focus on this issue, since current business practices often require the transfer of electronic medical records across state lines. A patient may reside in a state other than where the insurance carrier is located or tests may be analyzed in a state other than where the patient met with his or her primary care physician. Because different states have different laws and different levels of protection for this information, it has been difficult to effectively enforce these laws when information was transferred or used out of state (Gobis, 1997).

On the federal level, Congress passed legislation to move toward the protection of individually identifiable health information—the Health Insurance Portability and Accountability Act of 1996. As part of the act, the Department of Health and Human Services recommended that federal law preempt states only when state law would be less protective than the federal law. The confidentiality protections provided would be cumulative, and the federal law would merely provide a minimum level of protection.

On a state level, California's Telemedicine Development Act of 1996 addresses confidentiality in two ways. First, it provides that state law protects a patient's medical information record transmitted electronically similar to all other medical records. Health and mental health care providers then have certain legal obligations on use, disclosure, confidentiality, retention, maintenance, and access to patient information. Second, the patient must be informed of his or her rights regarding confidential information and the existing legal protections, and verbal and written consent must be obtained from the patient prior to the use of telemedicine. Arizona and Texas have also enacted laws requiring confidentiality of all patient medical records generated through telemedicine and have guaranteed patient access to their medical records resulting from such care.

Liability, Licensing, and Accreditation

Liability, licensing, and accreditation are also issues as consultations now cross state and even international borders (Magenau, 1997). Since the mission of state agencies that regulate professional licensing and practice is to protect the health and safety of their citizens, they have a direct interest in interstate telehealth licensure. From the agency's perspective, this has been most effectively accomplished by requiring a full license for interstate telemedicine practice. A professional could be held to the same standard of care and legal responsibility in every state in which he or she practices telemedicine. Costs for licenses in each state in which a professional could conceivably consult would be prohibitive.

State professional health and mental health associations also have a significant interest in interstate telehealth licensure. In-state health and mental health professionals could lose a significant patient population if barriers to interstate telemedicine licensure were reduced. Therefore, in-state health and mental health professional associations would support full licensure requirements for out-of-state health and mental health practitioners.

Telecommunication carriers and hardware and software vendors may also need to be licensed (Laske, 1997). In the final report of the Alaska Telehealth Advisory Committee (1999), providers were likened to ambulance services whose staff must have specific expertise and credentials and whose equipment must comply with specific regulations, among other elements of service.

There has been a proliferation of state laws and regulations addressing telemedicine licensure for health and mental health professionals. These laws vary widely in their range of options (Schanz, 1998). However, most states have dealt with telemedicine licensure through regulations, not legislation. Between 1994 and 1997, Kansas, California, Hawaii, Nebraska, Nevada, South Dakota, Texas, Utah, and Wyoming all modified existing regulations.

The Association of Telemedicine Service Providers (ATSP) and the Federation of State Boards of Medical Licensure developed model legislation in 1996. The ATSP compact focused on reducing the barriers to practicing interstate telemedicine by utilizing a limited license, mutual recognition model. The federation's model proposed a limited licensing mechanism, only permitting telemedical consultations in remote states. However, with the passage of SB 600 in Oregon (Regulation of Medicine, Podiatry, and Acupuncture, 1999), these earlier models could be superseded. Although SB 600 is focused on out-of-state physicians working with Oregon patients, it also could be considered a possible model for other licensed professions.

Other ethical issues were raised in a white paper issued by the Physicians Insurers Association of America (1998). These ethical issues included the use of e-mail to transmit patient data, "duty of care" and defining the "standard of care," accountability if liability arises from a telehealth consultation, jurisdictional differences in liability cases and how they relate to licensure, inclusion of hardware and software vendors and telecommunications carriers in liability cases, and informed consent (if a state deems telehealth consultations as "experimental" in nature).

Recommendations

The Ad Hoc Rural Mental Health Provider Work Group (Pion *et al.*, 1997) has recommended that creative applications of telecommunications should be utilized to reduce barriers to accessing rural mental health services. Furthermore, they recommended sound evaluations of the effectiveness of the information technology strategies.

Conclusions

The California Rural Health Policy Council (1998) has defined the ideal rural health care delivery system of the future to include the following:

1. fully integrated locally defined health and prevention related services;
2. maintaining broad community involvement, collaboration, and acceptance; and
3. using effective strategic local planning that focuses on measurable outcomes that seek continuous improvement to the overall health status of the entire community (p. 25).

The elements noted only reinforce what mental health providers, consumers, advocates, and researchers have known for some time: although health care in the United States is generally viewed by most in society as a right (of citizenship), behavioral health care is not a part of that right (Shelton, 1995).

The tremendous changes in health and mental health care will continue in the foreseeable future. While challenges remain in addressing severe shortages in rural mental health providers as well as in building successful models of rural managed mental health services delivery, Sawyer & Beeson (1998) have called for a strategic focus on five key elements in rural mental health services delivery:

1. Consumer and family involvement in program, policy, and clinical decision making
2. Clinical, service provision, cultural, and management competence (or rural practice expertise) of rural mental health providers
3. Ability of rural mental health providers to practice within a managed behavioral health care environment
4. Sharing of knowledge and expertise of rural mental health providers with others (i.e., knowledge transfer)
5. Developing collaborative relationships of provider networks, connecting rural mental health consumers and family members with (individual and agency) providers, and developing partnerships between consumers

Through public and private services delivery partnerships, coalitions of consumers and providers, integration of health and mental health providers and services, telecommunication technologies, and targeted as well as experiential education and training programs for practitioners, rural and frontier communities have the potential of building stronger, more vital mental health services.

References

Alaska Telehealth Advisory Committee. (1999). *Final Report*; http://www.hss.state.ak.us/atac/ATAC%20Final%20Report%206-99.pdf.

Association of Telemedicine Providers. (1999). *1999 Report on U.S. Telemedicine Activity*. Portland, OR: Author.

Beeson, P. G. (1994). *Rural mental health in an era of reform*. St. Cloud, MN: National Association for Rural Mental Health and the Center for Mental Health Services.

Beeson, P. G., Britain, C., Howell, M. L., Kirwan, D., & Sawyer, A. D. (1998). Rural mental health at the millennium. In R. W. Manderscheid & M. J. Henderson (Eds.), *Mental health, United States, 1998* (pp. 82–97). (DHHS publication No. [SMA] 99-3285). Washington, DC: Center for Mental Health Services.

Blanch, A., & Levin, B. L. (1998). Organization and services delivery. In B. L. Levin, A. K. Blanch, & A. Jennings (Eds.), *Women's mental health services: A public health perspective* (pp. 5–18). Thousand Oaks, CA: Sage Publications.

Blank, M. B., Fox, J. C., Hargrove, D. S., & Turner, J. T. (1995). Critical issues in reforming rural mental health service delivery. *Community Mental Health Journal, 31*, 511–524.

Bushy, A. (1997). *Mental health and substance abuse: Challenges in providing services to rural clients.* (DHHS publication no. [SMA] 97-3134). Rockville, MD: Center for Substance Abuse Treatment.

California Rural Health Policy Council (1998). *1998 Report on collaboration and innovation in rural health: Part II.* Sacramento: California Rural Health Policy Council.

California Telemedicine Act. (1996). Cal. S.B. 1665 § 2290.5.

Ciarlo, J. A., & Tweed, D. L. (1992). Exploring rural Colorado's need for mental health Services: Some preliminary findings. *Outlook, 2*(3), 29–31.

Cuffel, B. J., Goldman, W., & Schlesinger, H. (1999). Does managing behavioral health care services increase the cost of providing medical care? *Journal of Behavioral Health Services & Research, 26*(4), 372–380.

Elpers, J. R., & Levin, B. L. (1996). Mental health services: Epidemiology, prevention, and service delivery systems. In B. L. Levin & J. Petrila (Eds.), *Mental health services: A public health perspective* (pp. 5–22). New York: Oxford University Press.

Findlay, S. (1999). Managed behavioral health care in 1999: An industry at a crossroads. *Health Affairs, 18*(5), 116–124.

Flax, J. W., Wagenfeld, M. O., Ivens, R. E., & Weiss, R. J. (1979). *Mental health and rural America: An overview and annotated bibliography.* (DHEW publication no. [ADM] 78-753). Rockville, MD: Alcohol, Drug Abuse, and Mental Health Administration.

Frank, R. G., & McGuire, T. G. (1996). Introduction to the economics of mental health payment systems. In B. L. Levin & J. Petrila (Eds.), *Mental health services: A public health perspective* (pp. 23–37). New York: Oxford University Press.

Gobis, L. (1997). An overview of state laws and approaches to minimize licensure barriers. *Telemedicine Today, 5*(6), 14–5,18.

Goldman, W., McCulloch, J. & Sturm, R. (1998). Costs and use of mental health services before and after managed care. *Health Affairs, 17*(2), 40–52.

Goldsmith, H. F., Wagenfeld, M. O., Manderscheid, R. W., & Stiles, D. (1997). Specialty mental health services in metropolitan and nonmetropolitan areas, 1983 and 1990. *Administration and Policy in Mental Health, 24*(6), 475–488.

Grazier, K. L., Eselius, L. L., Hu, T-w, Shore, K. K., & G'Sell, W. A. (1999). Effects of a mental health carve-out on use, costs, and payers: A four-year study. *Journal of Behavioral Health Service & Research, 26*(4), 381–389.

Hassol, A., Carol, I., Gaumer, G., Puskin, D., Mintzer, C., & Grigsby, J. (1997). Rural applications of telemedicine. *Telemedicine Journal, 3*(3), 215–225.

Health Insurance Portability and Accountability Act of 1996, 42 USC, Section 201 (1996).

Hendryx, M. S., Borders, T., & Johnson, T. (1995). The distribution of mental health providers in a rural state. *Administration and Policy in Mental Health, 23*(2), 153–155.

Holzer, C. E. III, & Ciarlo, J. A. (1999). *Mental health service utilization in rural and non-rural areas* (Letter to the field no. 20). Denver: Frontier Mental Health Services Resource Network.

Holzer, C. E. III, Goldsmith, H. F., & Ciarlo, J. A. (1998). *The availability of health and mental health providers by population density* (Letter to the field no. 11). Denver: Frontier Mental Health Services Resource Network.

Ide, B. A., Carson, D., & Araquistain, M. (1997). Development of a farm/ranch stress scale. *Journal of Rural Community Psychology, EI*(1), 1–16.

Joint Working Group on Telemedicine. (1997). Development of a farm/ranch stress scale. *Journal of Rural Community Psychology, EI*(1), 1–16.

Kessler, R. C., McGonagle, K. A., Zhao, S. Nelson, C. B., Hughs, M., Eshleman, S., Wittchen, H. U., & Kendler, K. S. (1994). Lifetime and 12-month prevalence of DSM-III-R psychiatric disorders in the United States. *Archives of General Psychiatry, 51*(1), 8–19.

LaMendola, W. F. (1997). Telemental health services in U.S. frontier areas (Letter to the field no. 3). Denver: Frontier Mental Health Services Resource Network.

Laske, C. (1994). Legal aspects of digital image management and communication. *Medical Informatics, 19*(2), 189–196.

Laske, C. (1997). Health care telematics: Who is liable? *Computer Methods and Programs in Biomedicine, 54*(1–2), 1–6.

Levin, B. L. (1992). Managed mental health care: A national perspective. In R. W. Manderscheid & M. A. Sonnenschein (Eds.), *Mental health, United States, 1992* (pp. 208–216). (DHHS publication no. [SMA] 92-1942), Rockville, MD: Substance Abuse and Mental Health Services Administration.

Levin, B. L., & Petrila, J. (Eds.) (1996). *Mental health services: A public health perspective.* New York: Oxford University Press.

Ma, C. A., & McGuire, T. G. (1998). Costs and incentives in a behavioral health carve-out. *Health Affairs, 17*(2), 53–69.

Magenau, J. L. (1997). Digital diagnosis: Liability concerns and state licensing issues are inhibiting the progress of telemedicine. *Communications and the Law, 19*(4), 25–43.

Mechanic, D. (1994). Integrating mental health into a general health care system. *Hospital & Community Psychiatry, 45*, 893–897.

Mohatt, D. F. (1997a). Access to mental health services

in frontier America (Letter to the field no. 4). Denver: Frontier Mental Health Services Resource Network.

Mohatt, D. (1997b). Rural issues in public sector managed behavioral healthcare. In K. Minkoff & D. Pollack (Eds.), *Managed mental health care in the public sector: A survival manual* (pp. 119–126.). New York: Harwood Academic Publishers.

Mutel, C. F., & Donham, K. J. (1983). *Medical practice in rural communities.* New York: Springer-Verlag.

Mumford, E., Schlesinger, H. J., Glass, G. V., Patrick, C., & Cuerdon, T. (1998). A new look at evidence about reduced cost of medical utilization following mental health treatment. *Journal of Psychotherapy, Practice, & Research,* 7(1), 68–86.

National Advisory Committee on Rural Health. (1993). *Sixth annual report on rural health.* Rockville, MD: U.S. Department of Health and Human Services.

National Rural Health Association. (1999). Mental Health in Rural America. (Issue paper no. 14). Kansas City, MO: National Rural Health Association.

Nickleson, D. W. (1998). Telehealth and the evolving health care system: Strategic opportunities for professional psychology. *Professional Psychology: Research and Practice,* 29(6), 527–535.

Office of Technology Assessment (1990). *Health care in rural America.* Washington, DC: Congress of the United States.

Office of Technology Assessment (1995). *Impact of health reform on rural areas: Lessons from the states.* Washington, DC: Congress of the United States.

Ortega, S. T., Johnson, D. R., Beeson, P. G., & Craft, B. (1994). The farm crisis and mental health: A longitudinal study of the 1980s. *Rural Sociology,* 59, 598–619.

Parker, E. B. (1978). Telecommunication policy and information services. *Bulletin of the American Society for Information Science,* 4(6), 16.

Physicians Insurers Association of America. (1998). *Telemedicine: A medical liability white paper.* Rockville, MD: Author.

Pion, G. M., Keller, P., & McCombs, H. (1997). *Mental health providers in rural and isolated areas.* Rockville, MD: Center for Mental Health Services.

Regier, D. A., Goldberg, I. D., & Taube, C. A. (1979). The de facto U.S. mental health services system. *Archives of General Psychiatry,* 35, 685–693.

Regier, D. A., Farmer, M. E., Rae, D. S., Locke, B. Z., Keith, S. J., Judd, L. L., & Goodwin, F. K. (1990). Comorbidity of mental disorders with alcohol and other drug abuse: Results from the Epidemiologic Catchment Area (ECA) Study. *Journal of the American Medical Association,* 264(19), 2511–2518.

Regulation of Medicine, Podiatry, and Acupuncture. Ore. Stat. § 677. 137–141 (1999).

Robins, L. N., & Regier, D. A. (Eds.) (1991). *Psychiatric disorders in America.* New York: Free Press.

Rural mental health: Familiar problems in a changing world. (1998). *Rural Health News, 4,* 3.

Sawyer, D., & Beeson, P. G. (1998). Rural mental health: Vision 2000 and beyond. National Association for Rural Mental Health; http://www.narmh.org/annfutur.htm.

Schanz, S. J. (1998). State legislatures still debating telemedicine issues. *Telemedicine Today,* 6(5), 17.

Schulberg, H. (1991). Mental disorders in the primary care setting: Research priorities for the 1990s. *General Hospital Psychiatry,* 13(3), 156–164.

Shelton, D. A., & Frank, R. (1995). Rural mental health coverage under health care reform. *Community Mental Health Journal,* 31, 539–552.

Shelton, D. A., Merwin, E., & Fox, J. (1995). Implications of health care reform for rural mental health services. *Administration and Policy in Mental Health,* 23, 59–69.

Simon, R. I., & Williams, I. C. (1999). Maintaining treatment boundaries in small communities and rural areas. *Psychiatric Services,* 50(11), 1440–1446.

Sorensen, J. E. (1999). *Effective management strategies for frontier mental health* organizations (Letter to the field no. 14). Denver: Frontier Mental Health Services Resource Network.

Sturm, R. (1999). Tracking changes in behavioral health services: How have carve-outs changed care? *Journal of Behavioral Health Services & Research,* 26(4), 360–371.

Telecommunications Act of 1996, 47 U.S.C. (1996).

United States Department of Health and Human Services. (1999). *Mental health: A report of the Surgeon General.* Rockville, MD: Substance Abuse and Mental Health Services Administration, National Institute of Mental Health.

Wagenfeld, M. O. (1998a). *Delivering mental health services to the seriously mentally ill in frontier areas: Evidence from five states* (Letter to the field no. 7). Denver: Frontier Mental Health Services Resource Network.

Wagenfeld, M. O., Murray, J. D., Mohatt, D. F., & DeBruyn, J. C. (1994). *Mental health and rural America: 1980–1993: An overview and annotated bibliography.* (NIH publication no. 94-3500), Washington, DC: Office of Rural Health Policy.

Western Governors Association. (1995). *Telemedicine action report* (September 29, 1999); http://www.westgov.org/wga/publicat/actrept.htm.

Western Governors Association (1998). *Health-care on-ramps: A Road Map to Western states' information highways* (September 29, 1999); http://www.westgov.org/wga/publicat/roadrpt.htm.

Wheeler, T., & Allen, A. (1998). Current telepsychiatry activity in the U.S., Australia, Canada, and Norway. *Telemedicine Today Magazine* 6(2), 34–37.

15

Substance Use

L. A. REBHUN AND HELENA HANSEN

Two conflicting stereotypes shape images of drug use in the rural United States. On the one hand, a nostalgic view of rural areas as pastoral landscapes, distant from the modern problems of big cities, shapes the notion that drug use, like other modern urban ills, must be far from agrarian scenes. On the other hand, the stereotype of the Appalachian or Ozark hillbilly with his single-shot rifle and illegal still continues to influence contemporary views of rural alcohol consumption. In truth, rural areas today are neither pastoral havens nor peopled by moonshine-swillling hillbillies. They vary from the isolated arctic villages of northern Alaska to the migrant worker camps of the U.S.–Mexican border, and they include people of every ethnicity, nationality, and level of education. Some rural areas of the United States are major drug-producing areas, especially in the case of marijuana, and others, like the U.S.–Mexico border area, are major corridors for the international drug trade. Rural locales are hardly isolated from urban influences today, and drug problems pervade contemporary agrarian locations, often exacerbated by local conditions. Because rural residents constitute an estimated 20% to 25% (Logan, Schenck, Leukefeld, Meyers, & Allen, 1999; McCoy, Metsch, McCoy, & Weatherby, 1999) of the nation's population and about one

third of its impoverished citizens, they are an important population to study.

Geographical mapping of health problems has been a crucial approach in epidemiology since cholera was traced to the Broad Street pump in London more than a century ago. However, in the case of substance use, researchers are only beginning to use geographic approaches, and most studies have been in urban areas. Those studies that do contrast rural and urban areas in the United States frequently take the form of national or regional surveys, leaving the details of local conditions unexamined. The relative impact of rurality *per se* and of other possible factors in substance use epidemiology remain only lightly studied (Forsyth & Barnard, 1999). Definitions of terms such as "substance use" and even "rural" or "urban" are not standardized in the literature.

Although most people contrast rural and urban as separate concepts, the delineation of one from the other is not simple. Not all nonmetropolitan areas are rural, and community sizes in rural areas vary widely. Many rural areas display internal heterogeneity (Logan *et al.*, 1999). Many researchers use a continuum model, factoring in such characteristics as population density, distance from metropolitan areas, and percentage of population involved in agricultural production (Conger, 1997). The characteristics that define rurality also independently influence substance use and treatment. For example, isolation from metropolitan areas complicates both diagnosis and treatment. Rand Conger (1997) identifies a number of aspects of small community size that affect substance

L. A. REBHUN • Department of Anthropology, Yale University, New Haven, Connecticut 06520-8277. **HELENA HANSEN** • School of Medicine, Yale University, New Haven, Connecticut 06510.

Handbook of Rural Health, edited by Loue and Quill. Kluwer Academic/Plenum Publishers, New York, 2001.

use, including local cultures and traditions, local economies, and the characteristic social structures and styles of interpersonal interactions native to small communities. In some areas, local cultures protect against substance use through often religiously based codes of morality; in other areas, a defiant individualism may encourage illegal behaviors, including the use of illegal drugs (Conger, 1997). Given that the highest mortality and morbidity involved in alcohol use comes from accidents, especially motor vehicle accidents, the long distances between rural households and communities and rural isolation from emergency treatment can also affect the impact of substance use and alcohol abuse on public health.

Finally, a review of the literature that contrasts rural substance use with urban substance use is limited by methodological deficiencies and incompatibilities between data collected in the two contexts. For example, Caetano (1992) points out that the available national substance use data sets tend to oversample urban areas, and tend to sample households, thereby excluding groups such as migrant farmworkers who live in barracks-style housing on a seasonal basis. One must acknowledge these limitations in any use of the literature on rural substance use.

Substance Use

The Diagnostic and Statistical Manual IV (DSM-IV) of the American Psychiatric Association, used to standardize clinical diagnoses, defines substance abuse as "a maladaptive pattern of substance use leading to clinically significant impairment or distress . . . occurring over a 12-month period," and provides a specific list of indicators of impaired social and occupational functioning that constitute "clinically significant impairment," such as failure to fulfill major role obligations, use of substances in situations that are physically hazardous, and recurrent use despite substance-related legal or social problems (American Psychiatric Association, 1994).

This definition provides a standard method for identifying substance use as a clinical problem in individuals and for documenting rates of severe substance use in epidemiological stud-

ies. Alternatively, epidemiological studies use measures of the frequency and quantity of substance use in populations. For individuals, substance use can contribute to heart, liver, kidney, and lung disease and exacerbate any preexisting chronic physical or psychological conditions, as well as make it hard to sustain personal relationships, obtain education, or gain and keep employment. Inebriation interferes with treatment for psychiatric conditions and contributes to accidents as well as to the likelihood of contracting sexually transmitted diseases. Chronic and serious substance use, therefore, has negative consequences for biological health as well as psychological well-being and social success in individuals.

From a public health perspective, however, the DSM-IV list of indicators captures only a small percentage of those for whom substance use poses a danger to health. For instance, in the United States, an estimated 50% of all auto deaths and homicides are alcohol-related (Tomb, 1995), yet most alcohol-related auto accidents occur among moderate drinkers who do not meet the DSM-IV criteria for substance use. Considering the degree to which residents of rural areas rely on automobiles for transportation, the significance of subclinical, or moderate substance use, is clear.

Yet another definition of substance abuse emerges if we consider the differences between illegal, scheduled substances, such as opiates, cocaine, and marijuana, and legal yet highly regulated alcoholic beverages and tobacco cigarettes. From a legal perspective, any use or possession of illegal substances without a permit constitutes abuse. Alcohol and tobacco use, on the other hand, is socially and legally acceptable in some contexts and not in others, and is legally permitted for people over the age of 21, but not for minors. In the case of alcohol, a graded system of regulation based on location (bars versus public parks), age (over or under 21 years), and concurrent activity (eating versus driving) reveals the contextual nature of the legal definition of abuse and its underlying social definition.

Widespread substance use is made possible by an international system of production and distribution. For example, most illegal substances used in the United States, such as opiates and cocaine, are produced in Latin America and enter the United States through border regions such as along the border with Mexico. Exceptions to this include established regions of marijuana production in California and emerging regions of marijuana production in Kentucky and Tennessee. Marijuana is a significant cash crop in the California agricultural economy, and evolving regions of production in the southern United States are those that experienced declines in traditional mining industries for which marijuana production is an alternative. Substance distribution offers economic opportunity in situations of widespread economic dislocation. In examining substance use in rural areas—many of which are experiencing a decline in traditional agricultural production—one must therefore consider it an economically generated problem as well (Clayton, 1995).

In this review we define substance use broadly, as a problem with clinical, public health, legal, and economic dimensions. When literature bearing on all of these dimensions is considered, unique patterns of substance use in rural areas emerge along the lines of rates of diagnosis, rates and modes of treatment, ethnic and class issues, and patterns of drug production and distribution.

Rural versus Urban Substance Use Patterns

Until the mid-20th century, most commentators saw substance use as an urban problem, associated especially with the young, ethnic minorities, and other "sinister" groups. However, historians have found evidence of substance use problems in rural areas since the United States was a British colony. Alcohol was a widespread problem on the Western frontier, associated with much of the violence there, and opium use in the Shenandoah Valley was reported in *The New York Times* as early as 1877, described as one of the reactions of planter-class men to impoverishment as a result of the abolition of slavery following the Civil War. In addition, women in both rural and urban areas used patent medicines that often contained both opium and alcohol (Morgan, 1981).

However, until the mid to late 1970s, study and treatment of drug and alcohol problems were largely confined to urban areas. For example, an NIMH sponsored study in rural Kentucky published in 1969 insisted that alcohol and drug addiction was an urban problem, and that in the rural area it was largely confined to towns and small cities rather than farms (O'Donnell, 1969). But in the 1970s increased awareness of substance use problems in rural areas led to greater scientific and medical attention. In 1975, the National Institute on Drug Abuse sponsored a survey of eight largely rural states that showed both widespread substance use problems and significant difficulties in the provision of medical services in rural areas (Brown, Voskuhl, & Lehman, 1977). Aspects of rural substance use have been of interest to researchers ever since.

A variety of studies in the 1970s, 1980s, and 1990s found differences between patterns of drug use in rural and urban areas. These differences relate to specific features of rural life, including lower population density (Leukefeld, Godlaski, Hays, & Clark 1999), lack of access to health care services and medical insurance (Fitchen, 1991; Logan *et al.*, 1999; Robertson & Donnermeyer, 1997), rural poverty (Beltrame, 1978; Robertson & Donnermayer, 1997), a "frontier" mentality that rejects legal regulation (Clayton, 1995), the existence of culturally specific social structures that influence substance use such as dense and multiply connected social networks (Conger, 1997; Edwards, 1997), the frequency of moving residentially, especially where unemployment is high (Robertson & Donnermeyer, 1997), greater religiosity and social conservatism combined with tolerance for certain kinds of personal eccentricity in rural areas (Beltrame, 1978), distrust of newcomers, including health professionals, and of new ideas (Beltrame, 1978), and a cultural value placed on self-reliance in rural areas, which can interfere with help seeking (Beltrame, 1978; Leukefeld, Clayton, & Myers, 1992; Keller & Murray, 1982).

Another school of thought describes a "rural ghetto" (Davidson, 1990) with substance use problems similar to those in the inner city, and prompted by similar social problems. W. P. O'Hare and B. Curry-White (1992) have shown a similarity between impoverished inner-city and rural areas. They identify four characteristics of the "underclass:" (1) members do not have high school diplomas, (2) majority are supported by public assistance, (3) women tend to be unwed mothers, and (4) men tend to be chronically un- and under-employed. Their research showed 3.4% of inner-city residents displaying these characteristics and 2.4% of rural residents, in contrast to only 1.1% of noninnercity urban residents (cited in Conger, 1997).

Both rural and urban people living in such an underclass are at higher risk than the general population for involvement in substance production, distribution, and use. Illegal substance production and sale often constitutes an underground economy that helps to support those shut out of the legal economy by their lack of education and employment experience. Problematic substance use is positively correlated with emotional problems such as depression, which can result from the many life problems faced by those marginalized and impoverished within the stereotypically prosperous United States economy (Conger, 1997). Members of this underclass are harder to reach through traditional survey research methods, and they also are less likely than the general population to enter drug and alcohol treatment programs voluntarily, which may lead to their undercounting in surveys of substance use.

In general, researchers have found that most substance use problems have a lower incidence in rural areas and that rural residents are more likely than urban residents to report personal and social disapproval of smoking, drinking, and illicit drug use (Logan et al., 1999). However, rates of problematic drug and alcohol use are rising faster in rural than urban areas, as are rates of sexually transmitted diseases (STDs), which may be correlated with certain kinds of drug use, especially crack cocaine (Forney, Inciardi, & Lockwood, 1992).

Alcohol Use

Existing studies of alcohol use have documented some differences between rural and urban populations. A recent comparison of drinking rates among urban and rural residents of six southern states found that rural residents were slightly less likely than urban residents to screen positive for alcohol problems (8.0% versus 8.7%) and that rural residents were much more likely to abstain from alcohol use than urban residents (61.3 versus 49.0%), with women reporting much higher rates of abstinence and fewer maximum drinks when they did drink. No differences in drinking rates were found between white and nonwhite study participants (Booth, Ross, & Rost, 1999).

Adults over the age of 21 in the United States can legally consume alcohol. It is illegal for minors to purchase, possess, or consume it. The legal drinking age has changed over the course of U.S. history, but in the so-called New Temperance period of the 1990s, a national standard was encouraged by the federal government, which also encouraged state compliance through differential access to federal funding. Alcohol use in adolescence is a risk factor for problem drinking in adulthood as well as for illegal drug addiction.

In general, substance users tend to progress from legal to nonlegal and from less powerful to more powerful drugs over their life cycle. For example, a study comparing urban and rural drug-using women in Florida and Georgia found a typical progression from alcohol and tobacco use to marijuana use in adolescence, followed by experimentation with inhalants, hallucinogens, heroin, and so on, and then a progression from powder cocaine to crack (Forney et al., 1992). Minors' use of substances that are legal for adults and the use of marijuana have been identified as risk factors for use of stronger mind-altering substances among those addicted to heroin, cocaine, and so on, although it remains unclear how many people use alcohol, tobacco, and marijuana in adolescence but never pass through the "gateway" to hard drug addiction. Brown et al. (1977) suggest an interesting variation on the gateway hypothesis, positing that community awareness of and willingness to act on drug problems may pass through a trajectory from less to more serious drugs. Communities may be more willing to admit alcohol use problems, and then marijuana use problems, before they are willing to deal with heroin, cocaine, or other hard drug problems. In this sense, recognition of marijuana as a significant problem in the community may be a gateway that must be passed before a community can rally to combat problems with use of other drugs in their area. In rural areas, this lack of recognition of illicit drug use may be even more prevalent, given the image of illicit drug use as an urban problem.

Tobacco Use

The literature on tobacco use is relatively separate from that on alcohol and other drug use. Tobacco does not induce as marked an altered state of consciousness as these other drugs and is therefore not involved in either accident rates or the kinds of social and interpersonal problems caused by mind-altering drug use, but it does have significant negative health consequences for smokers, chewers, and snuffers, including higher rates of lung and cardiovascular disease, and of certain types of cancers, especially lung and maxilofacial cancers. From a public health standpoint, secondhand smoke can cause health problems in those exposed to it. Like alcohol, tobacco is legal for use among persons over the age of either 18 or 21, depending on the state, but it is illegal to sell it to minors and illegal for minors to possess or use it.

Until the invention of a cigarette-rolling machine in 1884 and safety matches in 1889, pipe and cigar smoking and the use of chewing tobacco and snuff were the prevalent forms of tobacco use in the United States. But in the 20th century, the cigarette has ruled (Burns, Lee, Shen, Gilpin, Tolley, Vaughn, & Shanks, 1997). Between 1900 and 1952, chewing tobacco dropped from the product of choice of 52% of tobacco users to 6%. However, in 1991 it had risen to 9% of all tobacco used in the United States, often used in combination with cigarettes (Lewis, Harrell, Deng, & Bradley, 1999).

That tobacco smoking is bad for health has been known since James I of England held a public debate on tobacco in 1605, displaying the blackened lungs of deceased smokers (Jarvik, Cullen, Gritz, Vogt, & West, 1977). In the 20th century, medical science has demonstrated the many malign effects of tobacco on health, especially its connection to lung cancer.

Rates of lung cancer, low at the beginning of the century, have risen in tandem with the popularity of cigarette smoking, and remain highest in those populations most likely to smoke cigarettes. For instance, lung cancer rates among women rose in the 30 years after cigarette advertising began targeting women. Today the highest rates of smoking are among African American males, and since the 1960s rates of lung cancer among African American males has exceeded those among European American males (Burns et al., 1997), although there is some evidence that rates of smoking among African American males are going down (Bachman, Wallace, O'Malley, Johnston, Kurth, & Neighbors, 1991). Many consider smoking to be the major cause of premature death in the nation. Because almost all smokers began smoking before the age of 21, smoking among adolescents and minors is of great concern to those who wish to prevent initiation of smoking. Indeed, some have called smoking-related health problems a "pediatric epidemic" (Sarvela, Cronk, & Isberner, 1997).

Sarvela et al. (1997), in an examination of data from the annual Monitoring the Future project, which surveyed 16,000 high school seniors, found that the highest self-reported smoking rates were among rural European American males and the lowest among urban African American males. Rural males of any ethnicity were more likely to smoke than urban males.

Horn, Dino, and Momani (1999), reporting that predominantly rural West Virginia has the highest national rates of both current and frequent youth smoking, examine the influence of psychosocial stress on male and female adolescent smoking. Surveying 542 fifth- through ninth-graders in West Virginia, they found that although most students did not report smoking, prevalence of ever smoking increased with age, and rates were similar for both males and females. The most significant predictor for smoking was suicidal ideation, especially for girls. The authors call for more extensive and detailed studies to examine the relationship between strong negative feelings and smoking among rural adolescents.

As stated earlier, smokeless tobacco use has risen in popularity in the 1990s, partly in response to the incorrect belief that its use is less unhealthy than smoking. The sharpest rise has been among adolescents, especially females, with a slightly higher prevalence among African American than European American young women, although more males than females use the product. There are some indications that, like smoking, smokeless tobacco use is correlated with depression, suicidal ideation, and low self-esteem in adolescents. High school athletes are significantly more likely to use smokeless tobacco than cigarettes (Lewis *et al.*, 1999).

In a study in rural North Carolina, Lewis *et al.* (1999) found that smokeless tobacco use was also correlated with higher socioeconomic status in European American males, who were twice as likely to use the product than lower-income adolescents, and among females with low self-esteem. They also found a strong correlation between experimental use of smokeless tobacco and having at least one parent who is a current or former smoker. They suggest that prevention programs emphasize the connection between smokeless tobacco use and serious diseases like maxilofacial cancer, and target adolescents at particular risk.

Use of Illegal Drugs

A variety of studies find conflicting evidence on patterns of illegal drug use in rural areas. While some posit that rural drug use patterns change under influence from urban areas (Bowker, 1976), others believe that rural areas have distinctive usage patterns. However, it is hard to draw conclusions from the current literature because findings vary so widely. It does seem clear, however, that while alcohol use has been a problem for a very long time, the use of illegal drugs is newer, although problems with both alcohol and drug use are growing in rural areas (Beltrame, 1978).

For example, evidence on marijuana use varies from studies that show similar rural and urban drug use patterns, to studies that show a greater incidence of marijuana use in rural areas and of opiates in urban areas (Leukefeld *et al.*, 1999), to ones that show greater marijuana use in urban than in rural areas (Heligman, 1973; Tolone & Dermott, 1975). Belyea and Zingraff (1985) point out that since most research on marijuana use is conducted on urban populations, information on rural use is limited, although a general trend toward increase in rural marijuana use throughout the 1970s can be discerned. One possible reason for the conflicting information may be a finding from a national

survey that rural marijuana use increased 40% between 1972 and 1979, whereas it increased by only 15% in urban areas, although the percentage of all rural people surveyed who had lifetime experience with marijuana was 23% as compared to 33% in urban areas. This suggests that rural marijuana use rates, historically lower than urban ones, were rising faster in the 1980s (Social Research Group of George Washington University, cited in Belyea and Zingraff, 1985).

Much of the literature on substance use relies on surveys of students, which do not tell much about possible substance use in older populations. Also, rural studies tend to survey secondary school students whereas urban-based studies tend to focus on college students, because of the greater likelihood of colleges being located in urban areas. It remains unclear what effect on the data this age difference in survey populations has (Belyea & Zingraff, 1985).

Cronk and Sarvela (1977), examining data from the Monitoring the Future project from 1976 through 1992, found that rural students had slightly higher use rates for alcohol and tobacco during the period examined but had lower use rates for illicit substances. In particular, binge drinking rates for both males and females were higher in rural areas. A higher percentage of rural smokers used a pack a day or more. In the case of marijuana and cocaine, although prevalence of use was lower in rural than urban areas throughout the study period, the gap was much smaller in the 1990s than it had been in the 1970s. The authors suggest that substance availability has increased in rural areas, while prevention efforts have been less effective, and that whatever social factors may have protected rural youth from substance use declined from 1976 to 1992.

Brown *et al.* reported in 1977 that patients in rural drug treatment programs were more likely to have used marijuana, sedatives, and amphetamines, whereas urban patients reported problems with opiates such as heroin, although they were unsure whether that was because fewer rural people were using heroin, or because heroin users from both rural and urban areas were entering urban treatment programs. Studies of heroin as well as of cocaine, and especially the less expensive but more powerful crack or rock form of cocaine, have largely focused on inner city areas.

Illegal Drugs and AIDS

When AIDS was first recognized as a disease in the early 1980s, researchers associated it mainly with urban areas in the United States, especially New York and San Francisco. However, in the late 1980s and the 1990s, increasing concern has focused on AIDS rates in rural areas, which seem to be increasing. Unlike the typical profile of young men who have sex with men stereotypically (and increasingly inaccurately) associated with the urban AIDS patient, rural patients are likely to be female and heterosexual and either to have contracted the disease in the rural area in which they reside or to have contracted it elsewhere and then returned home to a rural area upon diagnosis (McCoy *et al.*, 1999).

Sexually transmitted diseases such as AIDS are associated with substance use in two ways: it can be transmitted through contaminated needles used for injecting drugs such as heroin, and it can be transmitted during sexual activities associated with the use of some substances. A steep rise in rates of STDs, including AIDS, in rural areas since the 1980s has led researchers to believe that crack use rates may also be going up, since female users so frequently trade sex for drugs. The rise in STD rates has been alarming. For example, studies in Georgia report that syphilis cases in southeast Georgia rose 800% between 1986 and 1989, as compared to 68% nationally, with the greatest prevalence among African American women. New AIDS cases rose from 510 in 1987 to 1,223 in 1990 (Forney *et al.*, 1992).

Forney *et al.* (1992), in a comparison of rural and urban women in Florida and Georgia, found that crack usage was similar among the compared populations; however, the urban Florida women began using marijuana at a younger age and the rural Georgia women who used "speedball" (a mixture of cocaine and heroin) began at a younger age than did speedball using women in Miami. The authors note that their findings on patterns of crack usage, of trading sex for crack, and of infection with HIV were strikingly similar for regions as diverse as rural Georgia and urban Florida. They argue that patterns of crack usage, including bartering sex for crack, are not dependent on rural or urban locale but rather reflect something about the culture of crack usage itself.

McCoy *et al.* (1999) found that rural Belle Glade, Florida, had the highest cumulative per capita rate of AIDS in the continental United States. The researchers found that migrant workers in their study area (including also Immokalee, in southern Florida, and Miami County) had sex partners from 26 U.S. states and 13 Latin American and Caribbean countries (Weatherby, McCoy, Forney, Bletzer, Inciardi, McBride, McCoy, Akin, Mainster, Polowski, & Petska, 1995), suggesting a great possibility for widespread transmission of HIV. They also found that correlates of HIV serostatus differed between rural and urban study participants. In more urban Miami, HIV seropositivity was significantly correlated with being between 25 and 44 years of age, not having completed high school, unemployment, previous drug user treatment, especially for injection drug or speedball usage, African American or Hispanic ethnicity, exchange of sex for drugs, and a history of treatment for other sexually transmitted diseases. In more rural Belle Glade, the variables most correlated with HIV seropositivity were being female and having used alcohol in the last 30 days, whereas in very rural unincorporated Immokalee, HIV positive subjects were female, African American, had not completed high school, and had used crack cocaine during the previous 30 days. Women were 3.38 times more likely than men to be seropositive for HIV, and alcohol-using women were 6.2% more likely than nonalcohol-using women to be seropositive. In general, subjects in Miami were more likely to be HIV positive than those in Belle Glade, and those in Belle Glade more than those in Immokalee (McCoy *et al.*, 1999).

These findings suggest that HIV, while more prevalent in more urban areas, is growing in rural areas. The significant number of HIV-positive people who are infected in urban areas but migrate back to rural hometowns in search of social support, a healthier lifestyle, and work or educational opportunities may be contributing to this growth (Cohn, Klein, Mohr, van der Horst, & Weber, 1994). Overall, the growth in rural HIV infection rates is particularly prevalent among rural women. McCoy *et al.* (1999) posit that while in Miami the high rates of HIV seropositivity (81.8 per 100,000) can be attributed to the popularity of injection drug use in that community, in rural Florida HIV initially introduced by injection drug-using migrants is currently being spread rapidly through heterosexual activity. The authors theorize that among the reasons for high rates of HIV seropositivity among women is the prevalence of the practice of trading sexual favors for drugs among female crack users. These findings have serious implications for HIV prevention strategies, most of which are targeted at young men who have sex with men and/or women, and suggest that condom distribution and needle exchange programs will not be sufficient to slow down the rapid transmission of HIV in the rural United States.

Substance Production and Transportation

Production of Alcohol and Tobacco

In 1792, President George Washington sent General "Light Horse Harry" Lee to put down the Whiskey Rebellion, in which whiskey producers in rural Pennsylvania, Kentucky, Virigina, and Tennessee had refused to pay excise taxes to the newly formed U.S. federal government on their alcohol production, and tarred and feathered revenue officials in the bargain (Glaser, 1976; Klein, 1976). Since that time, both state and federal governments have imposed taxes on alcohol products in the United States, and rural people in some areas have continued to try to produce and distribute alcohol without telling local revenue service officials. Such "moonshine" production has historically been strong in Appalachia, constituting areas of Virginia, West Virginia, Tennessee, and especially Kentucky (Ayers, 1984; Logan *et al.*, 1999), historically both impoverished and culturally distinct from the surrounding region. Research by Logan *et al.* (1999) showed that 21% of rural Kentucky residents surveyed believed that bootlegging of alcohol had increased in their communities. Lower population density

within the rural counties was correlated with higher rates of reporting moonshining activity, suggesting that illegal distilling of alcohol is a continuing as well as an historical problem in small rural communities.

A number of legal breweries and distilleries also operate in rural areas. No strong relationship has been found between legal alcohol production and usage rates in the local area: Jack Daniels, for example, distills its whiskey in a "dry" county where alcohol is not sold for consumption. And national surveys have found "dry" counties to have the lowest alcohol consumption rates (Room, 1971).

Kentucky is the world's largest producer of burley tobacco, and its economy is largely dependent on that production (Clayton, 1995; Logan *et al.,* 1999). Kentucky residents also report the highest tobacco use rate of any state at 40% (Farabee & Leukefeld, 1999). Economic dependence on the tobacco industry may make some smokers less receptive to an antitobacco public health message. Similarly, Farabee and Leukefeld (1999) suggest that Kentucky's longstanding history with marijuana production (see below) may lead to local ambivalence about the acceptability of marijuana use and consequently about the use of other drugs.

Production of Illegal Substances

The most commonly produced illegal substance in the United States is marijuana, produced from the *cannabis sativa, cannabis indica,* or hemp plants. Hemp has been cultivated in what is now the United States as a source of fiber since the earliest European settlement, as well as for medicinal use, especially as a sedative and appetite stimulant (Clayton, 1995). Today, the cultivation of these plants is illegal, and most growers are trying to produce marijuana for use as an intoxicant. In 1979, the Drug Enforcement Administration established a special Domestic Cannabis Eradication/Suppression Program. At first concentrating on major production areas in California and Hawaii, today, this program targets growers all over the United States. Most marijuana is grown in rural areas, but in response to federal suppression efforts many growers have turned to a variety of indoor growing techniques in urban areas as well (Clayton, 1995).

Although throughout the 1970s and 1980s the major marijuana producers were clustered in California and Hawaii, increasingly rural Appalachia, and especially Kentucky, has been the site of major marijuana production (Clayton, 1995; Leukefeld *et al.,* 1999; Logan *et al.,* 1999). Correspondingly, the literature on illegal marijuana production has focused on Appalachia as an emerging region of production. The decline of the coal mining industry has encouraged newly unemployed miners to seek alternate sources of employment, scarce in the depressed economy of the former coal states. Leukefeld *et al.* (1999) call marijuana a "major cash crop" in contemporary Appalachia. Marijuana production, estimated based on units of marijuana destroyed by federal officials, is highest in Appalachian Kentucky, also where poverty rates are highest in the region. Here, marijuana provides an economic opportunity not available in the legitimate economy, in the same way that urban cocaine sales provide economic opportunity in the inner city for those otherwise shut out of the mainstream economy.

Richard Clayton points out that economic necessity is not the only motivation for marijuana cultivation. Growing marijuana illegally has historically been attractive for people who prefer illegal to legal activities, and for those attracted by its high profit ratios. Historically, tiny communities in Appalachia, built in small "hollows" in the mountains or in mining camps, have lived in proud isolation from mainstream society (Beltrame, 1978). The economic decline of Appalachia has not created the marijuana industry, it has merely added a third group to the ranks of growers: those with economic necessity, because of chronic un- and underemployment. Clayton (1995) estimates that this group is the largest of the three, based on arrest records (although arrest rates may be biased in favor of those with the fewest resources).

The relationship between production and consumption of marijuana is unclear, although Logan *et al.* (1999) found that 53% of their rural Kentucky residents reported that marijuana was the easiest drug to obtain in their communities, suggesting that local production may increase local availability. Increased marijuana production in Appalachia has other effects on public health. On the one hand, in some counties it has very much improved the economic situation, benefiting not only growers but also local merchants. On the other hand, the need of growers to keep both thieves and potential government informers off their illegal plots increases the already high rates of interpersonal violence in the area (Clayton, 1995).

Specific Populations

In addition to variation in size and local cultures among rural communities, the same ethnic, class, religious, and regional issues that obtain in urban areas affect rates and styles of substance use in rural areas. Research has also noted often marked differences in substance use between men and women, between older and younger people, and among members of different occupational groups.

Ethnic and Regional Issues

Several studies have shown that patterns of alcohol use and details of inebriate behavior are cultural phenomena, which vary with social group (MacAndrew & Edgerton, 1969; Spradley, 1970). Researchers have found distinctive patterns of substance use in a variety of ethnic groups as well as for specific regions of the United States. For example, the Appalachian and Ozark area has been characterized by small populations living in isolated hollows, the making of "moonshine" alcohol, and recently, the growing of marijuana. The U.S. Southeast in general has higher populations of conservative Protestants, whose faith forbids the use of intoxicants, than other areas of the country. In California, Texas, and other areas of the U.S. Southwest, migrant farm labor and the presence of large numbers of Latinos, both immigrant and native-born, shape patterns of substance use. Many Native American reservations, with their often severe alcohol problems, exist in the U.S. West and in Alaska. All of these regional and ethnic differences contribute to the patterns researchers have found as they map substance use.

African Americans, Latinos, and European Americans

Numerous researchers have identified specific substance use patterns in particular ethnic populations. For example, Jews have been found to have different drinking patterns than Protestants (Flasher & Maisto, 1984), and such ethnic groups as Italian Americans (Blane, 1977; Lolli, Serianni, Golder, & Luzzatto-Fegiz, 1958), African Americans (Herd, 1985, 1991), Latinos (Gordon, 1985; Gilbert, 1985; Caetano 1991), and Asian Americans (Kitano, Hatanaka, Yeung, & Sue, 1985; Sue, Kitano, Hatanaka, & Yeung, 1985) all display culturally specific drinking and drug use patterns. Some researchers have looked at regional patterns in substance use and at differences in substance use, especially alcohol use, among practitioners of differing occupations (Mandell, Eaton, Anthony, & Garrison, 1992; Parker & Hartford, 1992).

Although stereotypes of substance use suggest that ethnic minorities have more prevalent and problematic usage patterns than the European American majority in the United States, research has not supported this image. For example, Robertson and Donnermayer (1997) discovered two significant factors that predicted the prevalence of drug-related mental health problems in the rural populations they studied: ease of access to cocaine and residence in an ethnically heterogeneous community. They suggest that living in a relatively culturally homogeneous community protects against substance use and mental health problems.

Another study, this one of drug use patterns among adolescents in rural Mississippi, found that African American male and female adolescents were significantly less likely to smoke tobacco, drink alcohol, get drunk, and use marijuana than European American male and female adolescents, with the difference more pronounced for females than males. Differences in usage rates of amphetamines and sedatives were not statistically significant (Allen & Page, 1994).

These findings are not unusual, although as the authors point out, African Americans make up a large percentage of those in drug treatment programs, under law enforcement custody for drug offenses, or admitted to hospitals with alcohol- and drug-related problems, despite constituting only about 12% of the national population. While some of the differences in research findings may reflect patterns of difference in how willing respondents of different ethnicities are to answer survey questions honestly, many researchers believe the findings reflect genuine phenomena rather than simply report bias.

It appears, then, that though overall prevalence of substance use may be similar among ethnic groups, the patterns and consequences of substance use vary along ethnic lines. The literature on African American and Latino substance use, though largely focused on urban populations, bears out this general point. For instance, in his review, Kane (1981) notes that African Americans who drink tend to drink more heavily and to experience more alcohol-related health problems and social consequences than their white counterparts. Similarly, Latino men who drink tend to drink larger quantities in one sitting. Kane refers to sociological and cultural explanations for these patterns (see also MacAndrew & Edgerton, 1969, and Spradley, 1970). Among African Americans, he notes the historical encouragement of extremes of consumption by white society, through cycles of prohibition and alcohol promotion. He points to the current high density of liquor stores and bars in minority neighborhoods, and to the function of taverns as African American social institutions. Among Latinos, he refers to a culture of "machismo," which idealizes a high tolerance for alcohol, and to the psychological effects of extreme economic deprivation among impoverished Latino subgroups such as Puerto Ricans (Kane, 1981).

Possible reasons for the differences need further research. In particular, a finding that alcohol, tobacco, and illicit drug use among African American adults surpasses that among European American adults, while adolescent use is lower (Bachman et al., 1991) needs further research and explication. The suggested possible influence of membership in conservative Protestant churches as an ameliorating factor in African American substance use (Watts & Wright, 1986–87) also needs further investigation.

Robertson and Donnermayer (1997), examining data from the national Household Survey on Drug Abuse, found that non-Hispanic blacks were less likely to report mental health problems related to substance use than either whites or nonblack Hispanics, that people in relatively ethnically homogeneous neighborhoods report fewer mental health and substance-use problems, and that minority members living in areas with low minority populations are more likely to report such problems than those living in areas with a greater minority–majority balance of ethnicity. This suggests that being a member of an ethnic minority is in itself a risk factor for mental health and substance-use problems, where a small minority population lives among a much larger majority. Their data also suggest, but do not prove statistically, that people living in rural areas were both more likely to be non-Hispanic whites and less likely to report mental health and substance-abuse problems than people living in more urban areas. They found that people working in blue-collar job categories were more likely to report substance use–related mental health problems than either white-collar workers or unemployed people. They suggest that a "complex hierarchy of personal and community-level factors define risk of self-reported problems" (p. 479) but state that much more research needs to be done to tease out the various factors in this hierarchy.

Migrant Farmworkers

Migrant farmworkers, many of whom are undocumented immigrants from Mexico or other Central American and Caribbean countries, and most of whom have ancestral ties to these countries, represent a large population about whom substance use data is scarce. Current U.S. Department of Labor statistics estimate the number of migrant farmworkers in the United States at 2.2 million (Inciardi, Surratt, Colon, Chitwood, & Rivers, 1999). Caetano (1992), in a review of existing literature and databases examining alcohol and substance abuse among migrant farmworkers, points out that the majority of such workers are young males with low educational attainment. Alcohol abuse is high at 22% to 24% among males and 7% to 11% among females, with the highest rates among 18-to-39 year old high school

dropouts who are first-generation Mexican Americans or born in Mexico. Alcohol use is highest in the Eastern migration corridor, where farmworkers are more likely to be single men living in barracks-style housing. Illegal drug use is also comparatively high among migrant farmworkers; cross-sectional surveys have shown that 3% of Latino farmworkers currently inject drugs as opposed to 1.6% of all Latinos who report any drug injection in their lifetimes (Caetano, 1992). In a recent study of drug use among migrants along the Eastern corridor, almost all had a history of marijuana use, greater than 50% had tried crack cocaine, 9.9% had a history of injection drug use, and 40% had traded sex for money or drugs in the past (Inciardi et al., 1999). A study of migrant workers in Florida found that crack cocaine use among men and women was positively related to involvement in crime and commercial sex work (Weatherby, McCoy, Metsch, Bletzer, Mckoy, & de la Rosa, 1999).

In the United States, the highest prevalence of drug use is among Latinos of Mexican or Puerto Rican descent who speak English as their primary language. Estimates of the prevalence of drug use among rural Latinos is difficult to make from national databases, however, because most of their sampling occurs in urban areas and migrants living in camps may be excluded in surveys of households (Caetano, 1992).

Native Americans

A large body of literature exists on substance abuse among Native Americans in particular because of the severity of the problem on reservations and because reservations are legally separate entities from the United States. Substance use, especially alcohol abuse, is a major problem on most Native American reservations (Heath, 1985; Kunitz & Levy, 1994; Leland, 1976; Lurie 1979; Stillner, Kraus, Leukefeld, & Hardenbergh, 1999; Weibel-Orlando, Long, & Weisner, 1982; Whittaker, 1982). On some reservations, the majority of morbidity and mortality is alcohol- and drug-related. For example, one study of an Ojibwa community in Canada found that only about one-quarter of all deaths were from causes other than alcohol-related violence, suicide, or accidents (Shkilnyk, 1985); however, the type and severity of substance use problems vary widely among different tribes as well as within specific tribes (May, 1982; Stubben, 1997; Topper, 1985).

Studies among Alaska Natives have found high incidences of problem drinking, with the alcohol-related death rate at 33.7 per 100,000 (the U.S. general alcohol-related death rate is 14 per 100,000), and many Alaska Natives have been found to begin drinking heavily as young as age 10—despite the legally dry status of many Alaska Native areas and the difficulty of bringing alcohol illegally into the remote tundra (Stillner et al., 1999). Rates of marijuana and injection drug use are high among Alaskan Native people. In response, an Alaska state-wide native sobriety movement has become very active in the area, and many native people surveyed express strong concern over substance use problems in their communities (Stillner et al., 1999).

Some studies have found that marijuana and inhalant use has gone up, especially among young native people, while rates of alcohol abuse have held steady. Cocaine, crack, and LSD use are also problems among Native American youth, possibly related to the casino trade on reservations (Stubben, 1997). Rates of both marijuana and inhalants have been found higher among Native American youth than among nonnative U.S. youth (Edwards & Edwards, 1989; Stubben, 1997).

Reasons identified for high rates of problematic substance use on reservations include psychological problems deriving from cultural destruction and status as a minority, the stresses of poverty and unemployment, genetic predispositions (Dozier, 1966), a sense of powerlessness due to political domination, and permissive cultural attitudes toward inebriation (Stubben, 1997). Some researchers have also traced the history of alcohol use among Native Americans, pointing to the lack of distilled liquors in the Americas prior to contact and the use of "Indian Whiskey" as a trade good in the colonial U.S. (Parker & Rebhun, 1995). Alcohol, conquest, epidemics, and massacres all descended upon tribes at the same time, and the cultural and personal sequelae remain tied up with substance use to this day.

Gender and Substance Use

Numerous researchers have noted differences between men and women in substance use (Roman, 1988; Wilsnack, Wilsnack, & Klassen, 1984). Gender affects substance use in a variety of ways. Because average body weight and the relationship of lean body mass to body fat vary between the sexes, men and women have different biologically based capacities to tolerate specific quantities of alcohol and other substances. Cultural attitudes toward substance use among men are different from attitudes about substance use among women in most groups that have been studied. In particular, the widespread idea that substance use leads to disinhibition, especially sexual disinhibition, leads to a more negative valuation of women's alcohol and drug use than of men's, on moral grounds (Morgan, 1987). Women are at greater risk of sexual assault when using drugs and alcohol and more likely than men to engage in trade of sex for money or drugs to support substance use habits. Women's generally greater responsibility for children, and positioning as moral arbiter in families, encourages greater disapproval of women's substance use than of men's. In fact, one study of cocaine use among rural women found living with children to be negatively related to crack cocaine use (Weatherby et al., 1999). Substance use by pregnant women can have devastating consequences for their fetuses, leading to miscarriage, neonatal death, and serious birth defects. For all of these reasons, substance use is often considered a more serious problem among women than among men, even where prevalence rates are lower (see specific studies comparing women's with men's substance use rates in the preceding section on rural and urban substance use patterns).

Age and Substance Use

Adolescents have long been a special concern of those who study substance use. Rebelliousness, a tendency toward experimentation, and peer pressure all can encourage adolescents to try illegal substances. Cultural associations of the use of both legal and illegal drugs with adulthood make smoking, drinking, and drug use desirable in the eyes of many adolescents. Adolescents who use both legal and illegal drugs can be more likely to overdose and to cause accidents related to their use than older users because of their inexperience. A general lack of exacerbating health problems also makes it easier for younger people to consume more without feeling sick. And adolescents are engaged in a process of choosing behaviors that will become patterns in later life (Hawkins, Catalano, & Miller, 1992). All of these reasons make their substance use of particular concern to researchers.

National surveys published in 1994 and 1997 found few differences in usage patterns of alcohol and illegal drugs between rural and urban adolescents (Conger, 1997; Cronk & Sarvela, 1997), although Brown *et al.* (1977) found that the client base in rural area substance use treatment programs was significantly younger than that in urban areas, with 62.2% of admissions to rural programs of patients under the age of 21, as opposed to 18.5% of urban patients. From a national sample comparing across generations in rural regions, Room (1971) found younger men and women more likely to drink than their older counterparts. Yet rural adolescent substance use can change in either direction with successive cohorts; Winfree and Griffiths (1984) found in their study of rural 13- and 16-year-olds between 1975 and 1982 that respondents reported significant declines in rates of use and a general trend toward conservatism in attitudes toward drug use within the space of seven years.

Yet another study comparing urban and rural high school students in Ohio showed significantly higher drug use among urban boys and posited that rural boys may experience more surveillance by family members than urban boys as they tend to be employed within their family and encounter a higher number of family members in their daily activities (Falck, Siegal, Wang, & Carlson, 1999). Finally, Roundtree and Clayton (1999) found heterogeneity of drug use rates among rural adolescent populations, which they related to features of the local school environment. It appears, then, that generational variation in rural substance use is multifactorial and not unidirectional.

Religion and Substance Use

Membership and participation in an organized religious group can be a protective factor for substance use. Many Protestant churches prevalent in rural areas of the United States, including Baptists, Evangelicals, and Pentacostals, as well as the Church of Jesus Christ of Latter Day Saints, strongly disapprove of the use of psychoactive substances and generally foster conservative social mores. In an early national sample, Room (1971) found conservative Protestants to be more likely to abstain from alcohol and less likely to drink heavily than other respondents. On a regional level, Room (1971) found that alcohol abstention was most common in rural, southern, and midwestern regions that had prohibition policies and were almost totally composed of conservative Protestants. Because of the strong religiosity of many rural residents, employment of clergy in substance-use treatment programs may increase efficacy (Beltrame, 1978).

Treatment and Prevention Services in Rural Areas

The existing data indicate a severe shortage of substance abuse treatment services in rural areas. Mick, Morlock, Salkever, deLissovoy, Malitz, and Jones (1993) found that less than one in five rural hospitals in a national survey (19%) offered alcohol and chemical abuse services of any kind, despite the fact that rural populations have a similar level of need for such services as urban populations. Those rural hospitals that offered substance abuse treatment tended to serve fewer clients and offer a more limited scope of services performed by a less professionally accredited staff.

Factors associated with the presence of such services in rural hospitals included location in counties that were more densely populated, had a higher per capita income, and had more physicians per 1,000 population. Hospitals that were in New England, Mid-Atlantic, East North Central census divisions, and had a large number of beds as well as psychiatric personnel, were also more likely to offer treatment for substance abuse. Of these associated factors, the authors emphasize the scarcity of psychiatric personnel in rural areas as a major reason for the paucity of substance abuse treatment in rural hospitals (Mick *et al.*, 1993).

In a study comparing rural and urban drug users in Florida, Metsch and McCoy (1999) found that urban users were 2.57 times more likely to have been in treatment than their rural counterparts. Study participants cited the un-availability of treatment slots and their ineligibility for treatment benefits as reasons for not entering treatment. The structural barriers to treatment for rural substance abusers appear to be formidable. The effects of the economic re-structuring of health care services due to the growth of managed care and changes in federal reimbursement policies on substance abuse treatment in rural areas remain to be seen. Mick *et al.* (1993) note that while many rural hospitals are downsizing or changing their service mix as a result of such changes, for the time being this has not translated into a reduction in substance abuse services in rural hospitals. Instead, it has been accompanied by a number of expanded or newly established substance abuse treatment programs in rural hospitals.

However, Rivers, Komoroff, and Kibort (1999) found in a study of treatment services in rural and urban Florida that as they adapt to managed care, service managers report that short-term economic constraints are forcing clients into inappropriate treatment modalities such as less expensive outpatient programs and programs based on a medical rather than social support model. This leads to a higher relapse rate and higher long-term social and economic costs. Service managers report that indigent patients are getting squeezed out of available public programs as managed care clients exhaust their (more limited) private benefits and are transferred to public programs (Rivers *et al.*, 1999).

Treatment services in rural areas are complicated by the long distances patients need to travel, by a possibly greater stigma associated with treatment seeking in small communities, and by a tendency toward both poverty and lack of insurance coverage in rural areas, as well as a shortage of doctors practicing in regions of the country with low population density

(Robertson & Donnermeyer, 1997). An ethic of self-reliance can make residents suspicious of medical personnel; what researchers such as Leukefeld *et al.* (1999) have identified as a "'keepin' to self' attitude" that encourages both illegal behavior and avoidance of medical treatment for such problems as substance use. As Robertson and Donnermeyer (1997) have pointed out, experiencing problems does not necessarily lead to seeking help.

Low population density makes it hard to provide specialized medical care like substance use treatment economically (Human & Wasem, 1991). Doctors unfamiliar with local folklore may misunderstand patients (Conger, 1997). And the combination of unavailability of hospitals and clinics and lack of access to medical insurance makes it difficult for many rural residents to access substance use treatment (Robertson & Donnermeyer, 1997). Robertson and Donnermeyer suggest that research into barriers to treatment utilization might be more useful to more potential patients than more research into patterns of substance use problems in rural areas.

Some researchers call for more research on rural–urban drug use differences, claiming, based on their research, that therapies developed in use with patients from urban areas must be modified to adapt to rural patients. These therapies would take into account both characteristics of the user's life and aspects of the community in which he or she lives (Leukefeld *et al.*, 1999).

Psychiatric diagnoses ranging from depression to psychosis often co-occur with substance use disorders, complicating treatment (Robertson & Donnermeyer, 1997). Beltrame (1978) suggests that cultural differences between medical personnel and local residents may complicate substance abuse treatment. He states that mental health personnel working in rural areas should focus on the specific mental health or substance use problems at hand rather than try to modify clients' social conservatism, religiosity, and tendency toward cultural isolation. Metsch and McCoy (1999) suggest that existing substance treatment in rural areas may be culturally unacceptable to clients due to their fears of lack of privacy, the stigma of their illness, the prominent role of religion and community norms, a rural work ethic that stresses self-reliance and the importance of continuing work, as well as a rural tradition of reliance on extended families and neighbors instead of social service institutions.

Similarly, a number of problems plague substance use prevention programs. Many programs targeting youth take a punitive approach. For example, Horn et al. (1999) report that the West Virginia schools they studied tended to take a "scared straight" approach, directing students caught smoking into substance use education as an alternative to suspension or other punishment. They tended to employ inadequately trained personnel as instructors, and the correlations among depression, suicidal ideation, and smoking they found suggest that punitive approaches directed at adolescents may be counterproductive. Prevention programs that target the stresses underlying adolescent lifestyle choices might be more effective than those focusing on the future health effects of smoking.

The Centers for Disease Control recommends that schools prohibit use of tobacco by faculty, staff, parents, and visitors, as well as by students on school property and during school sponsored events. They recommend early drug prevention education, focused on middle school and junior high. Sarvela et al. (1997) add that such programs should include education targeted specifically at particular genders and ethnic groups, and including local issues rather than attempting a one-size-fits-all approach. Given the disparity of use rates in rural areas outlined above along the lines of socioeconomic status, ethnicity, and gender, these recommendations seem particularly appropriate for rural regions.

Efforts to prevent drug use in ethnic minority rural communities may falter because members of these communities have yet to recognize drug use prevention as a pressing need. Plested, Smitham, Jumper-Thurman, Oetting and Edwards (1999), in their national study of readiness for drug use prevention in rural communities, found that while one-third of primarily nonminority communities had prevention programs in place, only 2% of the Native American and Mexican American communities surveyed had drug use prevention programs of any kind. For some ethnic populations, such as Native Americans, culturally specific treatment and

prevention programs may be needed. Patterns of drinking vary by cultural context, and in many Native American communities abstinence–binge cycles predominate that may not fit DSM IV definitions of alcoholism. Some researchers have found that Alcoholics Anonymous and similar programs do not work well among some Native American groups because of their emphasis on the individual rather than the family, the style of public confessional, and the Protestant religious basis of the twelve-step program. Some native religions involve the use of mind-altering substances, such as peyote, in a religious context, necessitating an approach that separates acceptable ceremonial from problematic secular use (Stubben, 1997).

Stillner et al. (1999) describe difficulties in alcohol abuse prevention in remote Alaska Native villages, where alcohol problems were a major concern. The researchers also found that over 41% of those surveyed used smokeless tobacco (compared to a U.S. norm of 4.4%), that smoked tobacco use was one and a half times the national norm, and that marijuana use was three times more frequent than that found in national surveys. A survey of local school teachers turned up complaints of students as young as third and fourth grade using snuff and cigarettes, and 11- and 12-year-olds coming to school inebriated. Residents also complained of large numbers of children unsupervised in public late at night because their parents were drinking, with high incidence of sexual acting out and physical violence among teenagers. Police complained of drug- and alcohol-related violence, the need to patrol for drunks freezing to death in snowbanks, and the constant battle with bootleggers.

In these villages, formal systems of government, imposed by the state, conflict with local informal patterns of negotiation on political issues among elders of extended families. Because local mayors, city managers, and city council members all had conflicting loyalties to their towns as defined by the state of Alaska and to their families as defined by local tribal customs, because the style of leadership required in a mayor and in a family elder are very different, and because some local politicians were themselves problem drinkers or involved in the bootleg alcohol business, enforcement of village alcohol prohibition was very difficult. Stillner and his colleagues (1999) contrast the situation in one village where local leaders had a history of opposition to bootlegging with that in a neighboring village where locals reported that the bootleggers themselves were in control of the town. The vagaries of local politics in this area were very influential in prevention of alcohol access, availability of treatment for alcohol problems, and community attitudes toward how to deal with alcohol. Stillner and colleagues call for greater attention to how to create programs that target specific problems contributing to substance use in local communities, recognizing the complexity of local conditions, and taking advantage of local people dedicated to helping their communities prevent substance abuse problems.

Direction for Further Research

Clayton's work on marijuana cultivation in Appalachia (1995) suggests that more research is needed on the relationship between poverty and illegal industries like drug production, as well as on the relationships among marijuana production, consumption, and public health problems like accident rates and violence. Edward's (1997) demonstration of the variation in adolescent substance use in three different rural communities and her detailed study of the relationship between the density of adult social relationships and their ability to guide adolescents away from substance use suggest important areas for further research in a greater number of rural communities to identify protective as well as predisposing social factors with regard to substance abuse.

Not enough is known about patterns of alcohol and drug use in ethnically defined communities in the United States. The findings of researchers such as Allen and Page (1994), Bachman et al. (1991), and Watts and Wright (1986–87) among others, suggest that patterns of substance use throughout the life cycle may be different for African Americans than for other U.S. populations, but more research is needed on this intriguing possibility, as well as on the validity of suggested reasons for it, such as the influence of religious group membership.

Although there has been extensive research on alcohol use among Native Americans, more research of a nonbiological nature is needed, especially research on the similarities and differences among various tribes. Not enough is known about patterns of other drug use, nor has the impact of gambling and other vice industries on reservations been studied in any detail (Stubben, 1997). Suggestions that cultural revival programs might ameliorate problem substance use, while intriguing, have yet to be established by careful research. The research of Stillner *et al.* (1999) suggests that substance use prevention programs would also benefit from better understanding of local politics and the varieties of social practice in native communities. Their call for programs tailored to the specificities of local conditions mandates not only generalized research into the problems they denote but also detailed qualitative as well as quantitative studies of individual communities as a precondition for setting up prevention and treatment programs in local areas.

Research in rural Florida by McCoy *et al.* (1999) and Forney *et al.* (1992) suggest that the spread of HIV is a rapidly growing and serious problem and that the demographics of HIV seropositivity are different in rural than in urban areas of the United States. In particular, the epidemic seems to be spreading more rapidly among women than men and to be strongly correlated with the use of crack cocaine. More research is needed to see if this pattern holds for other rural areas of the United States, as well as to design prevention programs targeted to women and drug users.

Despite many studies on substance use in specific ethnic and occupational groups, in different age groups and genders, in particular regions, and among members of certain ethnic groups, not enough is known about how these various factors interact in the substance use behaviors of individuals (Ames & Rebhun, 1996) or how they fit in with rural–urban differences. Belyea and Zingraff (1985) call for more studies that compare similar age, ethnic, and socioeconomic groups in rural and urban areas, instead of the more common simple rural–urban comparison without adjustment for these other variables. They call for more longitudinal studies that can capture the trajectory of drug and alcohol use over the life cycle. The components and structure of Robertson and Donnermeyer's "complex hierarchy" (1997) remain incompletely identified and explicated.

Although poverty has been identified as a factor in patterns of substance use in rural communities, not enough is known about the details of the types, patterns, and effects of poverty, and the relationship between experiencing personal poverty and living in a generally impoverished region. The loss of jobs in the mining industry has been correlated with a rise in marijuana production in Kentucky and other Appalachian states by a number of researchers (Clayton, 1995; Leukefeld *et al.*, 1999) although how that affects marijuana use remains unclear.

Robertson and Donnermeyer (1997) point out that the economic well-being of rural residents has been affected by the farm crisis of the 1980s, as well as by changes in other industries prevalent in rural areas, such as logging and mining, and by the seasonal pattern of labor availability in some rural areas. These not only affect income levels but also affect access to health insurance and therefore to medical care. The loss of industries also affects the tax bases of local communities, leading to problems in funding public health care services and higher rates of hospital and clinic closures as well as lower rates of road building and repair and public funding of transportation services. In the 1990s, federal funding to many rural substance abuse prevention programs was cut by the U.S. Congress (Paz, 1998), exacerbating the crisis of health care for rural substance abusers. This more detailed consideration suggests that the problem of rural isolation from health care is getting worse, not better, and shows the importance of considering the nature and effects of industrial change and economic dislocation in more detail.

Davidson's (1990) concept of a rural underclass and its role in high rates of drug and alcohol use deserves closer consideration. McCoy *et al.'s* (1999) research on HIV seropositivity in rural Florida found high rates among people who fit Davidson's criteria for underclass membership. In particular, the relationship between low rates of high school completion and chronic unemployment, unwed parenthood, and dependence on public assistance remains to be elucidated. More research into educational failure, what causes it, its consequences, and how

to combat it can only help populations largely unreached by secondary public education.

In general, the drug and alcohol research field is dominated by quantitative, survey-based studies. More qualitative research is needed to flesh out the broad outlines provided by regional and national survey research, to help generate explanatory hypotheses for quantitative study, and to provide insights into the experiences of the individuals who form the groups sampled by survey research. A better balance of regional and local, and of quantitative and qualitative, studies in the literature would help in the definition of terms, detection of patterns, and formulation of theories. A greater attention to standardization of terms such as "rural," "urban," "substance abuse," and so on would help to make different studies more easily comparable.

The field of substance use prevention is littered with programs that sound great but do not work as predicted. Not enough is known about the specifics of why people use and what will help them stop. The differences noted in the literature for people living in rural and urban areas, for males and females, and for members of different ethnic, religious, and age groups suggest that much more work needs to be done to discover how to tailor programs to the specific needs of a diverse population. It is probable that substance use rates can be affected by programs not directly targeting them: for example, improvements in economic status, educational attainment, and mental health in general could reduce the numbers of people who decide to use substances or who use them excessively.

The findings of researchers working in rural areas have important implications for all who strive to reduce the considerable personal and public health problems caused by substance use. As Rand Conger points out, "A special quality of rural places is that they provide a research setting in which the multiple facets of social, economic, psychological, historical, and cultural experiences and characteristics can be studied in relatively pure form as they relate to the risk for alcohol, drug, and tobacco abuse" (Conger, 1997, p. 47).

Research on drug and alcohol use patterns in rural communities promises insights into problems and treatments that will benefit the U.S. population at large. The broad outlines of patterns and issues have been identified in the current literature, but the details remain to be filled in.

References

Allen, O., & Page, R. M. (1994). Variance in substance use between rural black and white Mississippi high school students. *Adolescence, 29*(114), 401–405.

American Psychiatric Association. (1994). *Diagnostic and statistical manual of mental disorders* (4th ed., DSM-IV). Washington, DC: American Psychiatric Association.

Ames, G. M., & Rebhun, L. A. (1996). Women, alcohol and work: Interactions of gender, ethnicity and occupational culture. *Social Science and Medicine, 43,* 1649–1663.

Ayers, E. L. (1984). *Vengeance and justice: Crime and punishment in the 19th century American South.* New York: Oxford University Press.

Bachman, J. G., Wallace, J. M., O'Malley, P. M., Johnston, L. D., Kurth, C. L., & Neighbors, H. W. (1991). Racial/ethnic differences in smoking, drinking, and illicit drug use among American high school seniors, 1976–1989. *American Journal of Public Health, 81,* 372–277.

Beltrame, T. F. (1978). Meeting the special needs of Appalachian alcoholics. *Hospital and Community Psychiatry, 29,* 792–793.

Belyea, M. J., & Zinngraff, M. T. (1985). Monitoring rural-urban drug trends: An analysis of drug arrest statistics, 1976–1980. *The International Journal of the Addictions, 20,* 369–380.

Blane, H. T. (1977). Acculturation and drinking in an Italian-American community. *Journal of Studies on Alcohol, 3,* 1324–1346.

Booth, B. M., Ross, R. L., & Rost, K. (1999): Rural and urban problem drinkers in six southern states. *Substance Use & Misuse, 34,* 471–493.

Bowker, L. H. (1976). The incidence of drug use and associated factors in two small towns: A community survey. *Bulletin on Narcotics, 28,* 17–25.

Brown, B. S., Voskuhl, T. C., & Lehman, P. (1977). Comparison of drug abuse clients in urban and rural settings. *American Journal of Drug and Alcohol Abuse, 4,* 445–454.

Burns, D. M., Lee, L., Shen, L. Z., Gilpin, E., Tolley, H. D., Vaughn, J., & Shanks, T. (1997). Cigarette smoking behavior in the United States. In L. Garfinkel (Ed.), *Changes in cigarette-related disease risks and their implication for prevention and control.* (NIH monograph no. 8, publication no. 97-4213). Washington, DC: National Institutes of Health, National Cancer Institute.

Caetano, R. (1991). Findings from the 1984 national survey of alcohol use among U.S. Hispanics. In W. Clark & M. Hilton (Eds.), *Alcohol in America* (pp. 293–307). Albany: State University of New York Press.

Caetano, R. (1992). *Epidemiology feasibility study: Alcohol and drug abuse among migrant farmworkers in California.* Unpublished manuscript, Alcohol Research Group, Berkeley, CA.

Clayton, R. R. (1995). *Marijuana in the "Third World:" Appalachia, U.S.A.* Boulder, CO: Lynne Rienner Publishers.

Cohn, S. E., Klein, J. D., Mohr, J. E., van der Horst, C. M., & Weber, D. J. (1994). The geography of AIDS: Patterns of urban and rural migration. *Southern Medical Journal, 87,* 599–606.

Conger, R. D. (1997). The special nature of rural America. In E. B. Robertson, Z. Sloboda, G. M. Boyd, L. Beatty, & N. J. Kozel (Eds.), *Rural substance abuse: State of knowledge and issues* (NIDA research monograph 168; pp. 37–52). Washington DC: U.S. Department of Health and Human Services.

Cronk, C. E., & Sarvela, P. D. (1997). Alcohol, tobacco, and other drug use among rural/small town and urban youth: A secondary analysis of the monitoring the future data set. *American Journal of Public Health, 87,* 760–765.

Davidson, O. G. (1990). *Broken heartland: The rise of America's rural ghetto.* New York: Free Press.

Dozier, E. F. (1966). Problem drinking among American Indians: The role of sociocultural deprivation. *Quarterly Journal of Studies of Alcohol, 27,* 72–87.

Edwards, R. W. (1997). Drug and alcohol use among youth in rural communities. In E. B. Robertson, Z. Sloboda, G. M. Boyd, L. Beatty, & N. J. Kozel, (Eds.), *Rural substance abuse: State of knowledge and issues* (NIDA research monograph 168; pp. 53–79). Washington DC: U.S. Department of Health and Human Services.

Edwards, D. E., & Edwards, M. E. (1989). Alcoholism prevention/treatment and Native American youth: A community approach. In D. J. Pittman & C. R. Snyders (Eds.), *Alcohol problems of minority youth in America.* Lewiston, NY: Edwin Mellon Press.

Falck, R. S., Siegal, H. A., Wang, J., and Carlson, R. G. (1999). Differences in drug use among rural and suburban high school students in Ohio. *Substance Use and Misuse, 34,* 567–577.

Farabee, D., & Leukefeld, C. G. (1999). Opportunities for AIDS prevention in a rural state in criminal justice and drug treatment settings. *Substance Use and Misuse, 34,* 617–631.

Fitchen, J. (1991) *Endangered spaces, enduring places: Change, identity, and survival in rural America.* Boulder, CO: Westview Press.

Flasher, L. V., & Maisto, S. A. (1984). A review of theory and research on drinking problems among Jews. *Journal of Nervous and Mental Diseases, 172,* 596–603.

Forney, M. A., Inciardi, J. A., & Lockwood, M. A.

(1992). Exchanging sex for crack-cocaine: A comparison of women from rural and urban communities. *Journal of Community Health, 17,* 73–85

Forsyth, A. J. M., & Barnard, M. (1999). Contrasting levels of adolescent drug use between adjacent urban and rural communities in Scotland. *Addiction, 94,* 1707–1718.

Gilbert, M. J. (1985). Mexican-Americans in California: intracultural variation in attitudes and behavior related to alcohol. In L. A. Bennett & G. M. Ames (Eds.), *The American experience with alcohol* (pp. 255–278). New York: Plenum.

Glaser, F. B. (1976) Alcoholism in Pennsylvania—A bicentennial perspective. *Pennsylvania Medicine, 123,* 12–16.

Gordon, A. J. (1985). Alcohol and Hispanics in the Northeast: A study of cultural variability and adaptation of alcohol use. In L. A. Bennett & G. M. Ames (Eds.), *The American experience with alcohol* (pp. 297–314). New York: Plenum.

Hawkins, J. D., Catalano, R. F., & Miller, J. Y. (1992). Risk and protective factors for alcohol and other drug problems in adolescence and early adulthood: Implications for substance abuse prevention. *Psychological Bulletin, 112,* 64–105.

Heath, D. B. (1985). American Indians and alcohol: epidemiological and sociocultural relevance. *Alcohol use among U.S. ethnic minorities.* (HHS research monograph no. 18). Rockville, MD: Health and Human Services.

Heligman, A. C. (1973). A survey of drug use in a rural Minnesota senior high school. *Drug Forum, 2,* 173–177.

Herd, D. (1985). Ambiguity in black drinking norms: an ethnohistorical interpretation. In L. A. Bennett& G. M. Ames (Eds.), *The American experience with alcohol* (pp. 149–170). New York: Plenum.

Herd, D. (1991). Drinking patterns in the black population. In W. Clark & M. Hilton (Eds.), *Alcohol in America* (pp. 308–328). Albany: State University of New York Press.

Horn, K., Dino, G., & Momani, A. (1999). Smoking and stress among rural adolescents: The gender factor. *American Journal of Health Studies, 14*(4), 183–193.

Human, J., & Wasem, C. (1991). Rural mental health in America. *American Psychologist, 46*(3), 232–239.

Inciardi, J. A., Surratt, H. L., Colon, H. M., Chitwood, D. D., & Rivers, J. E. (1999). Drug use and HIV risks among migrant workers on the DelMarVa Peninsula. *Substance Use and Misuse, 34,* 653–666.

Jarvik, M. E., Cullen, J. W., Gritz, E. R., Vogt, T. M., & West, L. J. (1977). *Research on Smoking Behavior.* (NIDA monograph 17). Washington DC: Department of Health, Education, and Welfare, Public Health Service, Alcohol, Drug Abuse and Mental Health Administration, National Institute on Drug Abuse.

Kane, G. P. (1981). *Inner city Alcoholism: An ecological analysis and cross-cultural study.* New York: Human Services Press.

Keller, P. A., & Murray, J. D. (1982). Rural mental health: An overview of the issues. In P. A. Keller & J. D. Murray (Eds.), *Handbook of rural community mental health* (pp. 3–19). New York: Human Sciences Press.

Kitano, H. L., Hatanaka, H., Yeung, W. T., & Sue, S. (1985). Japanese-American drinking patterns. In L. A. Bennett & G. M. Ames (Eds.), *The American experience with alcohol* (pp. 335–358). New York: Plenum.

Klein, R. M. (1976). A nation of moonshiners. *Natural History, 85,* 23–31.

Kunitz, S. J., & Levy, J. E. (1994). *Drinking careers: A twenty-five year study of three Navajo populations.* New Haven, CT: Yale University Press.

Leland, J. (1976). *Firewater myths: North American Indian drinking and alcohol addiction.* New Brunswick, NJ: Rutgers Center for Alcohol Studies.

Leukefeld, C. G., Clayton, R. R., & Myers, J. A. (1992). Rural drug and alcohol treatment. *Drugs and Society, 7,* 95–116.

Leukefeld, C. G., Godlaski, T. M., Hays, L. R., & Clark, J. (1999). Developing a rural therapy with big city approaches. *Substance Use and Misuse, 34,* 747–762.

Lewis, P. C., Harrell, J. S., Deng, S., & Bradley, C. (1999). Smokeless tobacco use in adolescents: The Cardiovascular Health in Children (CHIC II) Study. *Journal of School Health, 69,* 320–326.

Logan, T. K., Schenck, J. E., Leukefeld, C. G., Meyers, J., & Allen, S. (1999). Rural attitudes, opinions, and drug use. *Substance Use and Misuse, 34,* 545–565.

Lolli, G., Serianni, E., Golder, G., & Luzzatto-Fegiz, P. (1958). *Alcohol in Italian culture: Food and wine in relation to sobriety among Italians and Italian-Americans.* Glencoe, IL: Free Press.

Lurie, N. O. (1979). The world's oldest ongoing protest demonstration: North American Indian drinking patterns. In M. Marshall (Ed.), *Beliefs, behaviors, and alcoholic beverages* (pp. 127–145). Ann Arbor, MI: University of Michigan Press.

MacAndrew, C., & Edgerton, R. (1969). *Drunken comportment: A social explanation.* Chicago: Aldine.

Mandell, W., Eaton, W. W., Anthony, J. C., & Garrison, R. (1992). Alcoholism and occupations: A review and analysis of 104 occupations. *Alcoholism: Clinical and Experimental Research, 16*(4), 734–746.

May, P. A. (1982) Substance abuse and American Indians: Prevalence and susceptibility. *International Journal of the Addictions, 17,* 1185–1209.

McCoy, C. B., Metsch, L. R., McCoy, H. V., & Weatherby, N. L. (1999). HIV seroprevalence across the rural/urban continuum. *Substance Use and Misuse, 34,* 495–615.

Metsch, L. R., & McCoy, C. B. (1999). Drug treatment

experiences: rural and urban comparisons. *Substance Use & Misuse, 34,* 763–784.

Mick, S. S., Morlock, L. L., Salkever, D., deLissovoy, G., Malitz, F., & Jones, A. S. (1993, July). Rural hospital-based alcohol and chemical abuse services: Availability and adoption, 1983–1988. *Journal of Studies in Alcohol,* pp. 488–501.

Morgan, H. W. (1981). *Drugs in America: A social history, 1800–1980.* Syracuse, NY: Syracuse University Press.

Morgan, P. (1987). Women and alcohol: the disinhibition rhetoric in an analysis of domination. *Journal of Psychoactive Drugs, 19,* 129–133.

O'Donnell, J. A. (1969). *Narcotics addicts in Kentucky.* Chevy Chase, MD: Department of Health, Education, and Welfare, Public Health Service, Health Services and Mental Health Administration, National Institute of Mental Health.

O'Hare, W. P., & Curry-White, B. (1992). *The rural underclass: Examination of multiple-problem populations in urban and rural settings.* Louisville, KY: Population Reference Bureau, University of Louisville.

Parker, D. A., & Harford, T. C. (1992). The epidemiology of alcohol consumption and dependence across occupations in the United States. *Alcohol Health Research World, 16,* 97–106.

Paz, J. (1998). The drug-free workplace in rural Arizona. *Alcoholism Treatment Quarterly, 16,* 133–145.

Plested, B., Smitham, D. M., Jumper-Thurman, P., Oetting, E. R., & Edwards, R. W. (1999): Readiness for drug use prevention in rural minority communities. *Substance Use & Misuse, 34,* 521–544.

Rivers, J. E., Komaroff, E., & Kibort, A. C. (1999). Access to health and human services for drug users: An urban/rural community systems perspective. *Substance Use & Misuse, 34,* 707–725.

Robertson, E. B., & Donnermeyer, J. F. (1997). Illegal drug use among rural adults: Mental health consequences and treatment utilization. *American Journal of Drug and Alcohol Abuse, 23,* 467–484.

Roman, P. (1988). *Women and alcohol use: A review of the research literature.* Rockville, MD: U.S. Department of Health and Human Services.

Room, R. (1971). Drinking in the rural south: some comparisons in a national sample. In J. A. Ewing & B. A. Rouse (Eds.), *Law and drinking behavior* (pp. 79–105). Chapel Hill, NC: Center for Alcohol Studies.

Roundtree, P. W., & Clayton, R. R. (1999). A contextual model of adolescent alcohol use across the rural-urban continuum. *Substance Use and Misuse, 34,* 495–519.

Sarvela, P. D., Cronk, C. E., & Isberner, F. R. (1997). A secondary analysis of smoking among rural and urban youth using the MTF data set. *Journal of Public Health, 67,* 372–377.

Spradley, J. P. (1970). *You owe yourself a drunk: An ethnography of urban nomads.* Boston: Little, Brown.

Stillner, V., Kraus, R. F., Leukefeld, C. G., & Hardenbergh, D. (1999). Drug use in very rural Alaskan villages. *Substance Use and Misuse, 34,* 579–593.

Stubben, J. (1997). Culturally competent substance abuse prevention research among rural Native American communities. In E. B. Robertson, Z. Sloboda, G. M. Boyd, L. Beatty, & N. J. Kozel, (Eds.), *Rural substance abuse: State of knowledge and issues* (NIDA research monograph no. 168; pp. 459–483). Washington DC: U.S. Department of Health and Human Services.

Sue, S., Kitano, H. L., Hatanaka, H., & Yeung, W. T. (1985). Alcohol consumption among Chinese in the United States. In L. A. Bennett & G. M. Ames G. M. (Eds.), *The American experience with alcohol* (pp. 359–374). New York: Plenum.

Tolone, W. J., & Dermott, D. (1975). Some correlates of drug use among high school youth in a midwestern rural community. *International Journal of the Addictions, 10,* 761–777.

Tomb, D. (1995). *Psychiatry.* (House Officer Series). Baltimore: Williams and Wilkins Publishers.

Topper, M. D. (1985) Navajo 'alcoholism': Drinking, alcohol abuse, and treatment in a changing cultural environment. In L. A. Bennett & G. M. Ames (Eds.), *The American experience with alcohol* (pp. 227–254). New York: Plenum.

Watts, T. D., & Wright, R. (1986–87). Prevention of alcohol abuse among black Americans. *Alcohol Health and Research World, 2,* 40–41.

Weatherby, N. L., McCoy, H. V., Forney, M .A., Bletzer, K., Inciardi, J. A., McBride, D. C., McCoy, C. B., Akin, R., Mainster, B., Polowski, J., & Petska, M. (1995). Sexual activity and HIV among drug users: Migrant workers and their sexual partners in southern Florida. *Florida Journal of Public Health, 7,* 22–26.

Weatherby, N. L., McCoy, H. V., Metsch, L. R., Bletzer, K. V., McCoy, C. B., & de la Rosa, M. R. (1999). Crack cocaine use in rural migrant populations: Living arrangements and social support. *Substance Use & Misuse, 34,* 685–706.

Weibel-Orlando, J. C., Long, J., & Weisner, T. S. (1982). *A comparison of urban and rural Indian drinking patterns in California.* Los Angeles: UCLA Neuropsychiatric Institute, Alcohol Research Center.

Whittaker, J. O. (1982). Alcohol and the Standing Rock Sioux Tribe: A twenty-year follow-up study. *Journal of Studies on Alcohol, 4,* 191–200.

Wilsnack, R .W., Wilsnack, S. C., & Klassen, A. D. (1984). Women's drinking and drinking problems: Patterns from a 1981 national survey. *American Journal of Public Health, 74,* 1231–1238.

16

No Safe Place to Hide

Rural Family Violence

SUSAN MURTY

People in the United States who choose to live in urban or suburban environments retain nostalgic and rosy views of rural life. They imagine small towns and rural areas as places where neighbors are friendly and helpful, where families are close and caring, and where children can grow up without witnessing violence. Unfortunately, although rural communities have many postive characteristics, they are not immune to the types of violence that threaten the peace of urban and suburban communities. In particular, family violence is a serious problem in rural areas just as it is in urban areas. This chapter examines the problems of spouse abuse, child abuse, and elder abuse in rural areas, and the rural services available for families who are affected by these types of violence. The emphasis of the chapter is on spouse abuse and violence against women, but the occurrence of the other forms of family violence is discussed as they relate to the overall theme of family violence.

Public awareness of family violence has been hampered by the confusion about the meaning of the terms abuse and neglect (Harbison & Morrow, 1998). Elders and children are considered vulnerable because they may not be able

to provide for their own needs. Therefore, reported cases of child and elder neglect are investigated and reported along with cases of physical abuse. In the case of elder abuse, the situation is even more confused because elders who do not care for themselves are identified as cases of "self-neglect" even when the neglect may be due to isolation and lack of community resources (Wiehe, 1998). In this chapter the term *abuse* will be used to refer specifically to physical abuse. The topic of neglect, although important, is not addressed in this chapter on family violence.

Public Awareness of Family Violence

Child Abuse

Child abuse was the first of the forms of family violence to receive public recognition. The battered child syndrome was identified by Kempe, Silverman, Steele, Droegemueller, and Silver (1962). The number of cases reported and substantiated has risen dramatically in the decades since that time. The increase may be due to increased public awareness among professionals and the general public and more consistent data collection at the state level (Wiehe, 1998). Research based on reported and confirmed child abuse suffers from many methodological problems because it does not allow for comparisons with a population that is not re-

SUSAN MURTY • School of Social Work, University of Iowa, Iowa City, Iowa 52242.

Handbook of Rural Health, edited by Loue and Quill. Kluwer Academic/Plenum Publishers, New York, 2001.

ported or investigated for child abuse. Many episodes of child abuse are never reported and the incidence of child abuse cannot be determined based on public records. Straus and Gelles (1990a) estimate that there are between 3.4 and 16 times more physically abused children in the United States than suggested by the rate based on Child Protective Service records.

In order to overcome these methodological problems, a random sample from the population must be surveyed. The National Family Violence Resurvey carried out by Straus and Gelles in 1985 was based on a national probability sample of 4,032 households. Respondents from these households were interviewed by telephone. Straus and Gelles make clear the importance of the problem of child abuse with their findings that 10.7% of the parents interviewed reported using severe violence against their children aged 3 to 17 in the previous year (Straus & Gelles, 1990b).

A widespread system of services has developed to respond to the problem of child abuse. In 1970 Parents Anonymous was established. The Child Welfare League of America and the American Association for Protecting Children, the children's division of the American Humane Society, have been active in treatment and prevention efforts. In 1974, federal legislation was passed that required states to enact child abuse and neglect laws and to establish procedures for reporting and investigating child abuse if they wished to receive federal funds to address the problem of child maltreatment. The National Center on Child Abuse and Neglect and the National Clearinghouse on Child Abuse and Neglect Information were also established by this legislation (Wiehe, 1998). Legislation passed in 1980 established a national program of family based social services to strengthen families and reduce the need for foster placement and adoption in cases of child abuse and neglect. Public child protective services are responsible for child abuse and neglect investigations and services in all states in the nation.

Spouse Abuse

The problem of battered women and spouse abuse was recognized more slowly. Battered women's shelters were established in England and the United States in the early 1970s (Wiehe, 1998; Schechter, 1982). As awareness grew in the 1980s, many states began to enact mandatory arrest laws in cases of spouse abuse, indicating that they considered it a crime, not a private matter. Nevertheless, arrests in incidents investigated by the police are still rare (Kantor & Straus, 1990). Estimates of the annual incidence of serious violence in adult intimate relationships by Straus and Gelles's National Family Violence Resurvey based on reports of respondents to that random survey vary from 3.0% to 4.8%. Based on couples as the unit of analysis, the estimates are that serious violence occurs in 6% of couples each year (Straus, Gelles, & Steinmetz, 1980; Straus & Gelles, 1990b; Straus & Smith, 1990b).

In the 1990s, interest at the national level became focused on the issue of spouse abuse (Klein, Campbell, Soler, & Ghez, 1997; Crowell & Burgess, 1996; Wilt & Olson, 1996). In 1992, national resource centers on domestic violence were opened with federal support. In 1994, Congress passed the Violence Against Women Act (VAWA), which provided support for services and criminal justice interventions on behalf of women who have been battered as well as for women who have been raped. In 1995, the Centers for Disease Control and Prevention (CDC) began to focus attention on domestic violence as a public health problem and to fund research investigating incidence, prevention, and treatment (Schechter, 1996).

The response to domestic violence has continued to focus on women as victims of violence. More than 1 million women seek medical assistance each year for injuries sustained at the hands of an intimate partner (Centers for Disease Control, 1990) and cost projections for health care alone are about $44 million per year (McLeer & Anwar, 1989). A recent national survey reported that 22% of women reported being physically assaulted by an intimate partner in their lifetime and that 1.3% of women reported being physically assaulted by an intimate partner in the last 12 months (Tjaden & Thoennes, 1998). These rates are significantly higher for women than for men, and the injury rates for women are much higher. Researchers agree that all figures are underestimates (Gelles & Straus, 1988).

Elder Abuse

The problem of elder abuse was the last to gain recognition. An amendment to the Older Americans Act in 1987 mandated states to formulate protocols for receiving and investigating elder abuse reports and to develop educational programs and outreach programs in order to identify cases. Congress appropriated $3 million for these activities in 1990. In 1992, another amendment to the Older Americans Act created Title IV, an elder rights title that includes directives for legal assistance, the long-term care ombudsman, and elder abuse prevention services. The Administration on Aging (AoA), through Title IV of the Older Americans Act, provides funding for research and project evaluation (Quinn & Tomita, 1997). Adult protective service divisions are now located in public social service agencies throughout the country. National advocacy groups have also championed the cause of elder abuse prevention. The Older Women's League (OWL), the National Organization of Women (NOW), and the American Association of Retired Persons (AARP) have been instrumental in lobbying for elder abuse prevention and awareness programs (Wiehe, 1998).

According to Wiehe (1998), in 1996 the number of reported cases of domestic elder abuse in the United States was 293,000. Of these reported cases, neglect was the most prevalent type of abuse reported (55%). Physical abuse made up 15% of these reported cases and sexual abuse .3%. However, as in the case of the other forms of family violence, the reported cases do not provide data on the problem as a whole. Even though there has been an increase in the rate of elder abuse reporting, according to Hudson (1997) only one of every eight cases of elder abuse is reported to authorities.

Tatara (1990) states that the true prevalence or incidence of elder abuse is not known. Pillemer and Finkelhor (1988) report results of a random survey of 2,020 community-dwelling elders ages 65 or older in the metropolitan area of Boston. Two percent reported experiencing physical abuse. Sixty percent of the perpetrators were spouses, and the remainder were children, grandchildren, siblings, and boarders. In a report prepared for the Administration on Aging (AoA) and the Department of Health and Human Services, estimates of the prevalence of elder abuse in the United States range between 1% and 10% of the elder population (Tatara, 1990). Variations in the definition of elder abuse and the methodology used may account for this variability.

The National Center on Elder Abuse reported that in 1996, 66% of elder abuse victims were women (Tatara & Kuzmeskus, 1997). This is partly due to the fact that women live longer than men. There are other factors involved, however. Women tend to have fewer assets in old age than men, and from a feminist perspective, power and control over women by men may contribute to the victimization of women (Wiehe, 1998).

Relationships Between Types of Family Violence

Research has shown that spouse abuse, child abuse, and elder abuse are associated in several ways. There is evidence that some elder abuse is a continuation of spouse abuse that has been occuring for many years (Van Hightower & Gorton, 1998; Cupitt, 1997; Brandl & Raymond, 1997). The negative impact of domestic violence on children has been established.

In the 1970s research began on the effects of violence on child witnesses (Copping, 1996). It has been estimated that between 3 million and 10 million children in the United States witness violence between the adults in their homes (Edelson, 1999; McNeal & Amato, 1998; Peled, 1998; Silvern & Kaersvang, 1989; Stephens, 1999). Copping (1996) reports that children were present as observers in 68% of 2,910 cases in which charges were filed for domestic assault against wives. These children are caught in an environment that is detrimental to their physical and emotional well-being (Erikson & Henderson, 1992).

Children who witness domestic violence experience a wide range of symptoms and are at increased risk for physical and psychological health problems (Cummings, Pepler, & Moore, 1999). External behavior problems such as aggression and antisocial behavior, hyperactivity, delinquency, and defiance may result, as well as internalized behaviors such as fear and depression, withdrawal, anxiety, and somatic disturbances (Stephens, 1999; Edelson, 1999). There is evidence that girls who witness abuse are more likely to have internalizing symptoms such as depression and somatic complaints, whereas boys are more prone to externalizing behaviors, such as aggression and hostility (Coppling, 1996; Edelson, 1999; Jouriles & Norwood, 1995). Among children exposed to domestic violence, difficulties in school and low self-esteem also develop at a higher rate than for children from nonviolent homes (Graham-Bermann, 1996). Symptoms of posttraumatic stress may also result (Graham-Bermann & Levendosky, 1998; Kilpatrick & Williams, 1998). Children who have witnessed domestic violence have a greater acceptance of violence as a coping mechansm in dealing with interpersonal conflict (Eriksen & Henderson, 1992; Hedeen, 1997).

There is an increased risk of child abuse by adult partners who are violent toward each other (Moffitt & Caspi, 1998; Straus & Smith, 1990b). Children are often the victims of abuse themselves when their mother is assaulted. Children may be used as a hostage during the conflict, or as a physical weapon against the mother; they may be forced to participate in the abuse (Edelson, 1999). Copping (1996) reports that in a longitudinal study of 75 children in five women's shelters, almost two-thirds of the children were also direct victims of abuse. Peled (1997) estimates that between 28% and 70% of children of battered women have been physically or sexually abused.

There is considerable evidence to support the hypothesis of the intergenerational transmission of violence. A large proportion of abusive husbands and abused wives experienced violence in their families of origin (McNeal & Amato, 1998; Ericksen & Henderson, 1992; Hedeen, 1997; Egeland, 1993; Straus & Smith, 1990a). Children from violent families are more likely to grow up to engage in violent marital or cohabiting relationships. Therefore, spouse abuse is important not only for the adults involved but also for its consequences for the children in the family and for the transmission of a culture of violence.

Rural Family Violence

Although research on various forms of family violence has increased dramatically in recent years, very little of it has focused on family violence in rural communities. Few studies have compared prevalence of domestic violence in urban and rural areas. The recent National Violence Against Women Survey did not compare the reports of rural and urban women, for example (Tjaden & Thoennes, 1998). Research generally focuses on the more densely settled areas of the United States, even though approximately one-quarter of the population—those living in nonmetropolitan areas—can be considered to be rural. Most of the surveys on family violence have been based on representative population samples that include small numbers of respondents who live in rural areas. In addition, the difficulties associated with different ways of measuring rurality have made research on the topic challenging. A considerable amount of further research on the various types of rural family violence remains to be carried out.

Prevalence of Rural Child Abuse

Very little research has compared urban and rural child abuse, although by the 1980s child abuse was recognized as a serious problem in rural areas (McKenzie, 1989; Andrews & Linden, 1985; Northwest Indian Child Welfare Institute, 1984; Frederick, 1982; Leistyna, 1980; Sefcik & Ormsby, 1980). Child sexual abuse was also identified as an important concern in rural areas (Hagen & McKinley, 1992; Ray & Murty, 1990; Kleven, 1988; Halseth & Hein, 1982). The National Family Violence Resurvey described earlier gathered some data on rural child abuse from a population-based random sample (Straus & Smith, 1990b). A three-category measure of urbanization was used. Households were categorized by the population size of their residence: 1 = cities with population of 100,000 or more; 2 = cities with population between 2,500 and 100,000; 3 = rural communities with population under 2,500. Although the rate of child abuse was higher in the most rural areas, the rate was also associated with demographic variables such as race and family income. On the average, income rates are lower in rural areas, for example. There was no statistically significant difference in child abuse rates among the different categories from urban to rural when all the other significant variables were held constant. These findings suggest that child abuse should be considered as serious a problem in rural communities as in urban areas.

Prevalence of Rural Spouse Abuse

A similar situation exists with rural spouse abuse. Data from a variety of different researchers provide evidence that spouse abuse is a serious problem in rural areas (Derk & Reese,1998; Websdale, 1998; Van Hightower & Gorton, 1998; Websdale & Johnson, 1997; Johnson, & Elliott, 1997; Bachman & Saltzman, 1995; Monsey, Owen, Zierman, Lambert, & Hyman, 1995; McGuire, Rice, & Tabor, 1994; Gagne, 1992; Peterson & Olday, 1992; Rural Justice Center, 1991; Rural Task Force of the National Coalition Against Domestic Violence, 1991; Bogal-Allbritten & Daughaday, 1990; Andrews, 1987). However, few research studies have compared rural spouse abuse rates with urban rates. The validity of data based on police reports is subject to question. Only a small proportion of violent incidents between husbands and wives or intimate partners is reported to the police (Kantor & Straus, 1990). As in the case of child abuse, only random samples from the population offer data that are free from some of these methodological problems. In addition to data on child abuse, the 1975 National Family Violence Survey and the 1985 National Family Violence Resurvey gathered data on violence between spouses and intimate partners. The findings of these surveys and other research suggest that there is a statistically significantly higher rate of spouse abuse in urban households and lower rates in rural areas (Straus & Smith, 1990b; Byrne, 1979; Murty, Zwerling, Stromquist, Merchant, & Burmeister, 1999a). Other surveys based on random samples, however, have found no difference between husband-to-wife violence in metropolitan and nonmetropolitan areas (Rodgers, 1994; Buehler, Dixon, & Toomey, 1998).

Although some rural areas in the United States have low proportions of ethnic minority groups, there are significant rural populations of color. There is evidence that spouse abuse is

an important problem in these populations. For example, there are battered rural Latina women (Florida Coalition Against Domestic Violence, 1999; Van Hightower & Gorton, 1998), African American women (Florida Coalition Against Domestic Violence, 1999), and Native American women (Florida Coalition Against Domestic Violence, 1999; Wolk, 1982). Rural migrant labor and immigrant communities are at risk (Florida Coalition Against Domestic Violence, 1999).

Prevalence of Rural Elder Abuse

As in the case of the other types of family violence, there is very little literature specifically on elder abuse in rural populations. The 1990 United States Census showed that 32.7% of older Americans live in rural communities (Griffin, 1994). In a 1988 study carried out by the National Aging Resource Center on Elder Abuse (NARCEA), elder abuse in rural states was reported as lower, at 2.60 reports per 1,000 elders compared to urban states, which reported 3.77 reports per 1,000 elders (Tatara, 1990). The difference in reported cases may be due to geographic isolation and lack of services. In a study of elder abuse in Australia, Cupitt (1997), found the type and prevalence of elder abuse in rural areas and metropolitan areas to be very similar. In a study that looked at the factors affecting the rate of elder abuse reporting to a state protective services program in Massachusetts, Wolf and Donglin (1999) found that the incidence of elder abuse was no different in rural and urban areas.

Summary

The findings on rural family violence indicate that further research is needed. Nevertheless, research carried out so far confirms that family violence is a serious problem in rural areas as well as in urban areas. The illusion of a peaceful rural family life has been shattered by evidence of rural family violence.

Recent Research on Rural Spouse Abuse

Previous research on rural family violence has suffered from inadequate measurement of rurality. Several studies compare metropolitan to nonmetropolitan counties (Buehler *et al.*, 1994). The comparison of rates from metropolitan areas to nonmetropolitan areas is misleading since there are rural areas within metropolitan counties and there are relatively urban areas within nonmetropolitan counties. The three-point scale used in the 1985 National Family Violence Resurvey offers a slightly more specified method of comparing residence from urban to rural; however, the intermediate point on the scale covers a vast range, from places with as few as 2,500 people to places with a population up to 100,000. The most rural category used in this survey does not distinguish places with low populations that are close to and far from metropolitan areas. More refined measurement of degree on the urban-to-rural continuum is essential for increasing our understanding of rural family violence.

Because further research on rural family violence was needed, the author carried out a statewide survey of women in Iowa on domestic violence that was funded by the Iowa Social Science Institute. A telephone survey of women in Iowa used a stratified random sample to ensure an equal number of women from four strata from rural to urban. The sampling strategy was based on the ordinal system of 10 categories developed by the United States Economic Research Service to differentiate counties on the urban-to-rural continuum (Butler & Beale, 1994). These codes are commonly referred to as the "Beale Codes." Counties are categorized by the aggregate size of their urban population and also by adjacency to a standard metropolitan statistical area. The counties designated as most urban are in metropolitan areas as identified by the Census Bureau. The counties designated as most rural have no town with a population as great as 2,500 people and also are not located adjacent to a metropolitan area. (For technical details, see Butler & Beale, 1994.) Based on these codes, four complete lists of the counties of Iowa were developed. The first list was made up of the metropolitan counties (Beale Codes 0-2), the second of counties intermediate on the rural-to-urban continuum (Beale Codes 3-6), the third of counties that are moderately rural (Beale Codes 7-8); and the fourth of the most extremely rural counties (Beale

Code 9). Ten counties were randomly selected from each of these lists, for a total of 40 counties. Since there are only 10 metropolitan counties in Iowa, all were selected.

Telephone numbers were randomly selected using computer-assisted telephone interviewing technology until approximately 30 interviews were completed from each county. Respondents were women 18 years or older who were married, had been married, or were currently living with or had lived with a man as an intimate partner. There were approximately 300 interviews completed with women from each of the four strata on the urban-to-rural continuum for a grand total of 1,238 respondents. (For more detailed information on the study, see Murty, Whitten, Zwerling, & Burmeister, 1999b.)

In addition to using the county-level codes to measure the urban-to-rural continuum, respondents were asked to provide their zip code to allow more precise classification of residence on the rural-to-urban continuum. An alternative analysis used the population density of the zip code area as a measure of rurality at a subcounty level.

The Conflict Tactics Scale was used to measure physical abuse reported as inflicted by the women's intimate partner. As recommended by Straus (1979, 1990), the five most severe items on the scale were used to measure severe physical abuse: kicking, biting, hitting with a fist or with an object, beating up, and either threatening to use or actually using a knife or gun. The percentage of women who reported any severe abuse in the last 12 months on the CTS was 2.9%. For lifetime experience of severe wife abuse, it was 13.5%. There were no statistically significant differences among the counties categorized as more or less rural for abuse reported in the last 12 months or for abuse ever experienced with the current partner or a previous partner. The results were similar when the population density of zip code area was used as the measure of rurality. The results concerning domestic violence across the urban-to-rural continuum were sustained in the multivariable environment. There were no statistically significant differences in reported abuse across the urban-to-rural continuum when controlling for the effects of the demographic variables.

Women who were divorced, separated, or

never married were much more likely to report experiencing abuse than women who were married or widowed. These findings confirm results of previous research (Stets & Straus, 1990). No associations with age, income, or education were found in the multivariable analyses.

Overall, the findings indicate that the prevalence of domestic violence reported by women does not differ significantly between rural and urban areas. These findings confirm some previous research (Buehler et al., 1998; Rodgers, 1994) and do not confirm previous studies (Straus & Smith, 1990b; Byrne, 1979) that reported lower rates of domestic violence in rural areas.

An additional interesting finding of this study of women in Iowa had to do with help-seeking behavior. All the women were asked whom they would turn to for help if they were abused by their husband or partner. Multiple-choice responses were provided, including informal community sources of help such as family, neighbors, and friends and formal service providers such as doctors, hospitals, law enforcement, lawyers, social workers, and battered women's programs. The only statistically significant difference across the urban-to-rural continuum was on seeking help from clergy. The women from urban environments were less likely to seek help from clergy than women in the more rural areas. This finding has implications for the delivery of prevention and intervention services, which will be discussed later in the chapter.

The Experience of Family Violence in the Rural Environment

Since there is already considerable evidence to suggest that family violence is a serious problem in rural areas just as it is in urban areas, it is important to determine whether the experience of victims of family violence is different in rural and urban areas.

The literature on rural spouse abuse makes clear that there are unique characteristics of the rural environment that affect the response to victims of abuse. This literature includes a range of different kinds of reports, varying from anecdotal reports and small-scale qualitative interviews to more comprehensive surveys of particular rural communities and states. It seems reasonable to assume that these factors affect the response to child and elder abuse in similar ways. Because of the sparse population, there are barriers that prevent victims of abuse from seeking and obtaining help. There is striking consistency in the reported findings concerning the barriers that rural victims experience.

Geographical Isolation

Many residents of rural areas are geographically isolated (Fishwick, 1998; Websdale, 1998; Rubinstein, 1996; Edelson & Frank, 1991; Rural Task Force of the National Coalition Against Domestic Violence, 1991; Rural Justice Center, 1991). Some live many miles from main roads; dirt roads may be impassable due to floods, mud, and snow. Lack of means of transportation adds to the problem. Many women, especially older women, do not have a driver's license; frequently, victims of abuse do not have access to a vehicle and are dependent on the abuser for transportation. There is often no public transportation of any kind; if there is any, it is accessible only far from the isolated rural home. Many rural households still do not have telephone service, and even when they do, communicating by phone usually involves expensive long-distance toll charges. In addition, the abuser may restrict access to the telephone or cut off telephone lines. Especially for elderly victims and women with children, escape from an abusive relationship may be almost impossible. Neighbors may be five or more miles away and they may not be supportive; if the closest neighbors are relatives of the abuser, they may be unwilling to help. Even if a victim of abuse can reach the nearest small town or village, limited resources, judgmental attitudes, and lack of anonymity create additional barriers.

Lack of Anonymity

An important aspect of communities with small populations is that the residents tend to be acquainted with each other in multiple ways and have very little privacy from each other. Although this is a positive aspect of rural communities in some ways, the lack of anonymity can be a barrier to women who seek escape from abuse (Fishwick, 1998; Websdale, 1998; Rubinstein, 1996; Edelson & Frank, 1991; Rural Task Force of the National Coalition Against Domestic Violence, 1991). Rural women are hesitant to seek help because of the reactions of relatives and neighbors. Even going to the emergency room at the hospital, for example, will result in staff finding out about the abuse, and some of these people may be acquaintances, friends, neighbors, relatives of the abuser, or members of community organizations of which the abuser is a member. Frequently when battered women seek help, people who know the abuser do not believe them, because they believe the abuser would not be capable of committing violent acts. Often the abused woman is blamed for raising suspicions about the abuser.

Rural Attitudes

Traditional attitudes are still more common in rural areas. Domestic violence is often considered a private matter; interference by outsiders would seem inappropriate (Fishwick, 1998; Websdale, 1998; Rodriguez, 1998; Rural Justice Center, 1991; Rural Task Force of the National Coalition Against Domestic Violence, 1991). Women are still expected to submit to their husbands and physical abuse is commonly considered necessary for discipline of children and even for women. Rural communities engage in active denial of the abuse that occurs in families (Ray & Murty, 1990; Halseth & Hein, 1982).

Members of rural communities are expected to avoid conflict and to keep family problems private. Attitudes of rugged individualism are common, and rural residents are often hesitant to ask for help or admit that they have problems. The church is very important to many rural women, but they often feel that they cannot discuss abuse in church or with the clergy. Outsiders to a rural community are treated with suspicion and it is considered inappropriate to go to formal service providers for assistance (Rubinstein, 1996).

Inadequate Response from Law Enforcement

The literature on rural spouse abuse is consistent in identifying poor law enforcement response as a serious problem in rural areas (Rubinstein, 1996; Bell, 1989). Websdale (1998) carried out an excellent ethnographic study of battered women in rural Kentucky. This study makes clear that in spite of mandatory arrest laws, rural police and the local criminal justice system frequently fail to intervene to protect battered women. Because of geographical isolation and inadequate staffing of rural law enforcement, especially sheriff's departments, there may be long delays before the arrival of law officers. Attitudes of law enforcement personnel make them ineffective at confronting violence against women. Women are often hesitant to call the police because they know that the officers are friends of the abuser. The "old boys network" operates to pressure officers who are relatives and acquaintances of abusers not to take the violence seriously and to avoid arresting the perpetrator. In some cases, the complicity of law enforcement officers in illegal activities makes it difficult for them to enforce the law against abusers.

Poverty

Poverty frequently limits the options for victims of family violence (Rubinstein, 1996; Rural Justice Center, 1991). On the average, rural households have lower incomes than those in urban areas; many rural households live at or below the poverty level, even when both parents work (Garrett & Lennox, 1992; Bedics, 1987). Many rural communities are suffering from the recurring rural and farm crises that have affected many small towns and have caused many local businesses to close or move away (Jacobsen & Albertson, 1987). Unemployment and seasonal employment are common, and the jobs that are available are often low-paying jobs (Bedics, 1987). Employment opportunities are especially bleak for women in rural areas (Martinez-Brawley & Durbin, 1987). Poverty is also a serious problem for many of the elderly in rural areas (Coward, 1987). It is difficult to escape from pockets of poverty located in rural areas (Fitchen, 1987). Because seeking help often involves expenses for transportation and long-distance phone calls, poverty can exacerbate barriers in rural areas.

The Rural Service Delivery System

In addition to the barriers listed above, victims of abuse in rural areas are less likely to be able to obtain the services they need. All types of social and health services are sparse in rural areas. Victims of family violence are frequently unable to obtain services they need (Rubinstein, 1996; Rural Justice Center, 1991). Many of the kinds of services that are taken for granted in urban areas are not available or are available only on limited schedules or after long delays. Domestic violence services and shelters may be among these services, but frequently a whole range of other services is also inaccessible such as child care, legal aid, affordable housing, and job training. Even essential services such as health care services are often inadequate. Many rural counties do not have a hospital, some have no doctor, and rural medical clinics may be open only a few days a week. For many medical services, rural residents are expected to travel long distances to service providers in population centers. Applying for public assistance, for Medicaid, and for food stamps usually requires traveling to the office in the county seat and even there the applicant may be placed on a waiting list. Under the new laws for welfare reform, requirements for welfare recipients to find employment are being enforced more strictly, even though employment opportunities in rural communities are rare, public transportation is absent, and child care is often unavailable.

Recent Survey of Domestic Violence Service Providers

Although the previous literature on rural domestic violence identified barriers and gaps in service delivery, it was based on a variety of anecdotal reports, small-scale qualitative studies, and surveys of women and service providers in limited areas. In order to provide more comprehensive data concerning rural domestic violence, a national survey was conducted by the author and Susan Schechter, funded by the Administration for Children and Families, Department of Health and Human Services (Murty & Schechter, 1999). The findings confirm the previous reports of barriers experienced by battered women and gaps in the services for victims of rural family violence.

Four methods were used to gather data. We began by surveying the directors of the state domestic violence coalitions using a mailed questionnaire to collect information describing the types of services available in rural areas, the barriers to service delivery, and rural innovative responses to domestic violence.

We next obtained more detailed county-level data from state agencies and domestic violence coalitions in six case study states: Alabama, Iowa, Nevada, New Mexico, Tennessee, and Wisconsin. These were selected to represent states with rural populations in different regions of the United States and to include states with rural populations of African Americans, Latinos, and Native Americans. Before making the final selection of states, we contacted the state domestic violence coalition to determine that staff there would be willing and able to help us obtain local and statewide data. For each of the case study states, we attempted to obtain data on the location of domestic violence services, the number of victims seeking help from each county, the number of protection orders filed and granted in each county, and the number of incidents and arrests reported by law enforcement.

In order to get more in-depth information at the local level, we also carried out a telephone survey of local domestic violence programs serving a sample of 60 rural counties, 10 from each of the six case study states. We asked the informants from these local programs to give us information about specific barriers to service delivery in these counties and about relationships with other organizations and community resources in the county.

Finally, we located some of the most innovative rural service delivery and community coordination projects in different regions of the country. Several of these programs have successfully involved rural women of color. Using telephone interviews and obtaining written reports and descriptions, we gathered detailed information from nine of these innovative programs (Correia, 1999). Some of these are described in the following section on innovative rural programs.

The findings of this multiple-level survey

confirm previous research that a wide range of barriers prevents rural battered women from obtaining help when they need it. A basic infrastructure of services is missing in many rural communities. Basic needs of battered women are not met in areas such as employment, housing, transportation, and child care. Without public transportation, telephone service, and access to child care and medical services, for example, it is difficult for women in crisis to take the first steps toward obtaining help for themselves and their children. Lack of privacy and confidentiality create acute dilemmas for battered women seeking services in rural communities. Insufficient and inaccessible domestic violence services also limit the options open to rural battered women. Lack of community awareness and an inadequate response from law enforcement, courts, and health and social service providers further discourage battered women from seeking help.

The findings of the survey also support the previous research with convincing evidence that domestic violence services are less accessible to battered women in rural areas. In spite of the efforts of the state domestic violence coalitions and local programs, many isolated rural counties have no local services. Respondents at the local programs that we interviewed reported that they are interested in providing more comprehensive services to the rural counties that we selected. Lack of funds and staff limit what they can do, and without additional resources they do not feel that they can improve services to the outlying parts of their service areas.

Seventy-eight percent of the rural counties in our telephone survey had no local domestic violence program located within their borders. Many rural counties receive services only infrequently from another county. The extremely rural counties have no safe refuge for battered women. In the western regions of the nation, the service areas of domestic violence programs are thousands of square miles in size, making access to services even more difficult. Many of the services that urban battered women turn to are not available to rural women unless they can travel long distances to a metropolitan or urban area. Women in the rural counties we studied must drive average distances between 30 and 98 miles one way to reach a battered women's shelter. Counties in the West cover such immense geographic areas that even programs located within the county may be many hours' drive away.

In addition, few of the rural counties studied have a batterers' intervention program located within the county. Because batterers' intervention programs are frequently inaccessible, it is difficult for rural communities to hold perpetrators accountable and put a stop to the abuse.

The survey made clear that there are special needs among various underserved populations. Forty-one of the 45 states reported rural lesbian and bisexual women in their states, indicating that the needs of these rural women must be addressed as well. Respondents commented that the issues are different for this group. They mentioned that homophobia, fear of being forced to come out ("outing"), and the problem of everyone knowing everyone are common barriers for this rural population. For lesbians, additional problems are that the programs focus on men as batterers, that female abusers may also have access to shelters, and that laws on domestic violence don't always recognize same-sex abuse.

The situation of women of color and other underserved groups is also difficult. The respondents reported that women of color and other underserved groups are found in most of the rural regions of the United States. Thirty-seven of the states reported having Latina women in the rural areas of their states, 35 reported rural African American women, and 34 reported rural Native American women. Thirty (67%) of the states reported Native American reservations, villages, or tribal communities within their borders. The number of native groups reported varied from 1 for Alabama to 107 for Alaska.

Thirty-five of the states reported that they have rural women who are migrant farmworkers and that they have undocumented rural women (illegal immigrants) who are especially isolated. These findings are important since access to services and legal remedies are limited for these women due to their transient living arrangements, their legal status, and the cultural and language barriers they encounter. Immigration issues and fear of deportation make it difficult for these battered women to seek help. Many barriers prevent them from obtaining the services they need. Few rural areas have domestic violence services that are culturally appropriate to reach African American women, Latinas, Native American women, and other groups of underserved women such as farmworkers and recent immigrants.

Innovative Rural Programs

A report on the innovative rural programs identified in the national survey (Murty & Schechter, 1999) describes nine innovative programs (Correia, 1999). Each of these programs has developed strategies designed to meet the needs of particular rural communities. Each of them uses a community-based approach that involves community organization and local coordination of services along with planning processes that include local women who have experienced abuse. Seven of these programs are listed below. For more information on each of these programs, see Correia (1999).

- Stop Abusive Family Environments, Inc. (SAFE), West Virginia, provides housing and economic opportunities for rural battered women.
- The Massachusetts Rural Domestic Violence and Child Victimization Project serves a rural area of Massachusetts that was selected because it had a very high rate of restraining orders issued per capita. It provides services to children who have witnessed family violence and it provides community training to improve collaboration among organizations serving families experiencing violence.
- Seeley-Swan Talk Education and Prevention (SSTEP) serves a small-town and very rural portion of a county in Montana. It provides education to clergy, schools, and the community at large. It also trains local advocates and has established a crisis help line.
- Family Crisis Center, Kotzebue, Alaska, and Cangleska, Inc., Pine Ridge Reservation, South Dakota, provide services that are designed to serve Native American women and families. Both draw on uniquely Native American cultural traditions in their programs.

- Lideres Campesinas, a grassroots program of farmworker women, serves 12 communities in California. The organization addresses domestic violence and sexual assault, pesticides and field sanitation, HIV/AIDS, and economic development. In addition to a small paid staff, the program uses many volunteer *lideres* (leaders) from the local communities served.

Community education and prevention services are a high priority for rural communities. Excellent model community education programs have been developed in Florida and West Virginia that can be adapted for use in other rural areas (Florida Coalition Against Domestic Violence, 1999; National Resource Center on Domestic Violence, 1999).

There are other examples of model programs designed for rural communities. A study of 31 programs serving rural areas in Minnesota was carried out by Edelson and Frank (1991). These small-scale low-budget programs have been resourceful in providing services. They have relied on effective use of informal networks and coalitions with other agencies in their community, including leaders on Indian reservations in their areas. Personal contacts with key people were essential in building these relationships.

The Canadian Farm Women's Network (Fletcher, Lumm, & Reith, 1996) is another interesting rural program that helps rural communities develop local strategies to prevent domestic violence. The national advocacy group promotes information-sharing and education. It developed a video called "Fear on the Farm," which is used to educate rural and farm communities about domestic violence. It also distributes community kits that are used to help communities develop local action groups and plans to address the problem of spouse abuse.

Recommendations

Because of their low population density and inadequate funding, rural communities may find that the methods used to deliver family violence services in urban areas may not be the best strategies for them. Perhaps it is not realistic and cost-effective to attempt to establish an autonomous program and a shelter in every sparsely populated rural county. In addition, some people believe that shelters for battered women are not well-suited to rural communities because confidentiality is so difficult to maintain. Alternative approaches may be more promising for delivering services in rural areas. Safe homes, motel and hotel emergency housing, outreach programs, satellite offices, local community advocates, local rural community task forces, and partnerships with local rural service providers are all examples of approaches to family violence services that are being used in rural areas and should be evaluated for their effectiveness.

Innovative programs have been identified that have been successful at serving rural communities. These programs can provide models and stimulate other rural communities to develop their own programs. They should draw on the unique strengths of rural communities and use informal support networks and also service providers who are available locally. Especially important in rural areas are rural congregations and clergy, as was suggested by the survey of women in Iowa (Murty et al., 1999b). Local community education and training on domestic violence would help to ensure that victims of violence will be responded to appropriately. Local service providers could also include visiting and public health nurses, staff of rural health clinics and hospitals, family support workers, and county extension workers. Collaboration with other agencies is essential (Pryke & Thomas, 1998). It should include law enforcement agencies and public child protective service agencies. Greater collaboration with child protective services has been recommended recently, even though in the past the battered women's movement has limited communication with these agencies because of a justifiable concern about blaming battered women for the abuse of their children. If domestic violence and child protective service programs can build effective partnerships that are respectful of their respective missions, they can work together to protect both abused women and abused children (Peled, 1997; Schechter, 1996, 1995, 1994). Together they can develop long-term solutions to the problems of family violence. This approach may be especially important in rural areas where programs and services and trained staff are limited, making collaboration essential.

Rural women are likely to stay or return to abusing partners because of traditional attitudes, the lack of viable alternatives, and ties to the local community. Recently a controversial approach to working with abused women has been proposed focused on empowering women to make their own choices. The approach is critical of programs that assume that the only solution is for battered women to leave the abusive situation (Peled, Eisikouits, Enash, & Winstock, 2000); see also related proposals in Hadley, Short, Lezin, and Zook (1995) and Wolk (1982). This approach may be one that should be evaluated in rural areas, because it is respectful of abused women if they decide to stay and try to change their situation from within the family. This approach may be especially important to encourage rural women to take the time they need to make their decision and to develop trust with service providers.

Ensuring the safety of rural women and their children in potentially violent households may require a willingness to consider innovative approaches rather than assuming that refuge in a women's shelter is necessarily the best step for every woman. Safety planning can be adapted to the kinds of conditions in which many rural women live (Florida Coalition Against Domestic Violence, 1999). Rubinstein (1996) reports on some types of help that rural battered women themselves suggested. These include local volunteers going door to door, working with churches to fill unmet family needs, especially needs for food, and providing child care and transportation. Support groups should be available locally but should not be identified with domestic violence services. Instead they should offer information on women's health and parenting. A van to take women to support groups would be very helpful. Rubinstein (1996) describes a program in upstate New York that used a staff member, a van, and a CB radio. The staff person went to rural women who requested assistance and tried to provide what they needed.

Further research is needed to document the prevalence of rural family violence and to gather information about the specific difficulties encountered by abused children, intimate partners, and elders. We need to gather information directly from those who experience family violence about the context in which they live and the factors that affect their lives. Data must also be gathered from service providers, advocates, law enforcement, and community leaders in particular rural areas. Private and public funders should support in-depth qualitative studies in a sample of rural counties from different regions of the United States. Open-ended interviews should include members of populations of color and other underserved groups. The respondents should be encouraged to communicate their stories in their own voices, using their words.

In order to serve rural battered women of color and the perpetrators of violence from these populations, domestic violence services should be funded that draw on the strengths and traditions of ethnic minority communities. Such programs are most likely to be *culturally competent* if they include members of these communities in planning and providing services. In rural areas, these groups include Latino, African American, Native American, immigrant, refugee, and migrant labor families.

The large number of states with native populations shows that culturally relevant services for Native American women should be a high priority throughout the United States. There is a severe shortage of programs, shelters, and outreach services for native battered women on reservations, in tribal villages, and native settlements. Additional services and improved communication between native groups and state and local domestic violence coalitions should improve the situation of Native American battered women in rural areas.

Larger amounts of demonstration funding for the targeted development of rural service models must be made available by federal and state governmental agencies and private funders. An important start has been made with the Rural Domestic Violence and Child Abuse Enforcement Grants funded under the Violence Against Women Act. Funds should be targeted to develop and implement creative models for rural service delivery that make services more available in rural areas. These model programs must target services for victims, perpetrators, and children in a variety of rural environments, including extremely isolated rural areas. Funding should be made available to allow family vio-

lence programs to collaborate with service providers and community leaders in the small towns throughout their service areas and work to overcome the many barriers that rural battered women face. Public education and training programs are especially important to improve the awareness and response in rural communities.

New technology offers some exciting new approaches for rural communities. Rural women can be encouraged to develop the skills they need to contact other rural women by means of the Internet to share experiences and resources (Kelly & Lauderdale, 1996). Service providers can also benefit from these new methods to overcome the isolation of rural communities. The new technology can be especially important for isolated rural women; distance education using Internet and other advanced technologies is now making educational opportunities available to rural areas (Morris, 1996). In order to take advantage of these new opportunities, private and public funding must be used to make computers accessible to residents of rural communities, or they will be left behind in the technological revolution.

Conclusion

Child abuse, spouse abuse, and elder abuse all occur in rural areas. Rural communities must intervene to prevent family violence and to provide assistance to family members who have experienced abuse. They will be more successful if they develop their own programs and strategies to meet their needs rather than attempt to imitate programs designed for urban environments. Because they have fewer resources and formal service providers and need to cover large sparsely settled areas, rural family violence programs must be resourceful. Because the infrastructure of basic services is inadequate in many rural areas, programs will need to provide a wide range of services to families experiencing abuse. Collaboration with local leaders and community organizations appears to be effective in addressing family violence in rural communities. Innovative rural programs have been developed and can serve as models to be adapted for use in any particular rural community. Although the challenge is great, there are many promising ways in which rural communities can respond to children, women, and elders who have been abused and collaborate to create communities where family violence is no longer tolerated.

References

Andrews, J. (1987). A support group for rural women survivors of domestic violence. *Human Services in the Rural Environment, 11*(2), 39–42.

Andrews, D., & Linden, R. R. (1985). The role of volunteers in preventing rural child abuse. In W. H. Whitaker (Ed.), *Social work in rural areas: A celebration of rural people, place, and struggle* (pp. 149–162). Orono: University of Maine, Department of Sociology and Social Work.

Bachman, R., & Saltzman, L. (1995). *Violence against women: Estimates from the redesigned survey.* Washington, DC: Bureau of Justice Statistics.

Bedics, B. (1987). The history and context of rural poverty. *Human Services in the Rural Environment, 10*(4)/*11*(1), 12–14.

Bell, D. J. (1989). Family violence in small cities: An exploratory study. *Police Studies, 12*(1), 25–31.

Bogal-Allbriten, R., & Daughaday, L. R. (1990). Spouse abuse program services: A rural-urban comparison. *Human Services in the Rural Environment, 14*(2), 6–10.

Brandl, B., & Raymond, J. (1997). Unrecognized elder abuse victims: Older abused women. *Journal of Case Management, 6*(2), 62–68.

Buehler, B., Dixon, B., & Toomey, K. (1998). Lifetime and annual incidence of intimate partner violence and resulting injuries—Georgia, 1995. *Morbidity and Mortality Weekly Report, 47*(40), 849–853.

Butler, M. A., & Beale, C. L. (1994). *Rural-urban continuum codes for metro and nonmetro counties, 1993.* Washington, DC: U.S. Dept. of Agriculture, Economic Research Service.

Byrne, J. K. (1979). *Social integration, conflict, and violence in rural and urban families.* Unpublished master's thesis, Wilmington College, Wilmington, OH.

Centers for Disease Control. (1990). *Healthy people 2000: National health promotion and disease prevention objectives.* Washington, DC: U.S. Public Health Service, National Institutes of Health.

Copping, V. A. (1996). Beyond over-and-under-control: Behavioral observations of shelter children. *Journal of Family Violence, 11*(1), 41–57.

Correia, C. (1999). *Innovative rural responses to domestic violence: A description of nine programs.* Iowa City: University of Iowa, School of Social Work.

Coward, R. T. (1987). Poverty and aging in rural America. *Human Services in the Rural Environment, 10*(4)/*11*(1), 41–47.

Crowell, N. A., & Burgess, A. W. (Eds.) (1996). *Understanding violence against women.* (Panel on Research on Violence Against Women, Committee on Law and Justice, Commission on Behavioral and Social Sciences and Education, and the National Research Council). Washington, DC: National Academy Press.

Cummings, J. G., Pepler, D. J., & Moore, T. E. (1999). Behavior problems in children exposed to wife abuse: Gender differences. *Journal of Family Violence, 14*(2), 133–156.

Cupitt, M. (1997). Identifying and addressing the issues of elder abuse: A rural perspective. *Journal of Elder Abuse and Neglect, 8*(4), 21–30.

Derk, S., & Reese, D. (1998). Rural health-care providers' attitudes, practice, and training experience regarding intimate partner violence—West Virginia, March 1997. *MMWR, 47*(32), 670–673.

Edelson, J. L. (1999). Children's witnessing of adult domestic violence. *Journal of Interpersonal Violence, 14*(8), 839–870.

Edelson, J. L., & Frank, M. D. (1991). Rural interventions in woman battering: One state's strategies. *Families in Society, 72*(9), 543–551.

Egeland, B. (1993). A history of abuse is a major risk factor for abusing in the next generation. In R. J. Gelles & D. R. Loseke (Eds.), *Current controversies on family violence* (pp. 197–208). Newbury Park, CA: Sage.

Erikson, J. R., & Henderson, A. D. (1992). Witnessing family violence: The children's experience. *Journal of Advanced Nursing, 17,* 1200–1209.

Fishwick, N. (1998). Issues in providing care for rural battered women. In J. C. Campbell (Ed.), *Survivors of abuse: Health care for battered women and their children* (pp. 280–290) Thousand Oaks, CA: Sage.

Fitchen, J. M. (1987). When communities collapse: Implications for rural America. *Human Services in the Rural Environment, 10*(4)/*11*(1), 48–57.

Fletcher, S., Lunn, D., & Reith, L. (1996). Fear on the farm: Rural women take action against domestic violence. *Women and Environments, 38,* 27–29.

Florida Coalition Against Domestic Violence. (1999). *Domestic violence in rural America: A resource guide for service providers.* Tallahassee: Author.

Frederick, C. J. (1982). Violent behavior in rural areas. In P. A. Keller & J. D. Murray (Eds.), *Handbook of rural community mental health* (pp. 74–84). New York: Human Sciences Press.

Gagne, P. L. (1992). Appalachian women: Violence and social control. *Journal of Contemporary Ethnography, 20*(4), 387–415.

Garrett, P., & Lennox, N. (1992). *Rural families and children in poverty.* Chapel Hill, NC: Frank Porter Graham Child Development Center, University of North Carolina.

Gelles, R. J., & Straus, M. A. (1988). *Intimate violence.* New York: Simon & Schuster.

Graham-Bermann, S. A. (1996). Family worries: Assessment of interpersonal anxiety in children from violent and nonviolent families. *Journal of Clinical Child Psychology, 25*(3), 280–287.

Graham-Bermann, S. A., & Levendosky, A. A. (1998). Traumatic stress symptoms in children of battered women. *Journal of Interpersonal Violence, 13*(1), 111–128.

Griffin, L. (1994). Elder maltreatment among rural African-Americans. *Journal of Elder Abuse and Neglect, 6*(1), 1–27.

Hadley, S., Short, L. M., Lezin, N., & Zook, E. (1995). WomanKind: An innovative model of health care response to domestic abuse. *Women's Health Issues, 5*(4), 189–198.

Hagen, B. H., & McKinley, K. (1992). Using family crisis groups to treat rural child sexual abuse. *Human Services in the Rural Environment, 16*(1), 15–19.

Halseth, J. H., & Hein, N. J. B. (1982). Group work with teenage victims of incest. In G. M. Jacobsen (Ed.), *Nourishing people and communities through the lean years: Selected papers of the Seventh National Institute on Social Work in Rural Areas* (pp. 91–97). Iowa City: University of Iowa Printing Services.

Harbison, J., & Morrow, M. (1998). Re-examining the social construction of 'elder abuse and neglect': A Canadian perspective. *Ageing and Society, 18*, 691–711.

Hedeen, F. (1997). The legacy of domestic violence: Effects on the children. *Women & Therapy, 20*(2), 111–118.

Hudson, M. (1997). Elder mistreatment: Its relevance to older women. *JAMWA, 52*(3), 142–147.

Jacobsen, G. M., & Albertson, B. S. (1987). Social and economic change in rural Iowa: The development of rural ghettos. *Human Services in the Rural Environment, 10*(4)/*11*(1), 58–65.

Johnson, M., & Elliott, B. A. (1997). Domestic violence among family practice patients in midsized and rural communities. *Journal of Family Practice, 44*, 391–400.

Jouriles, E. N., & Norwood, W. D. (1995). Physical aggression toward boys and girls in families characterized by the battering of women. *Journal of Family Psychology, 9*(1), 69–78.

Kantor, G. K., & Straus, M. A. (1990) Response of victims and the police to assaults on wives. In M. A. Straus & R. J. Gelles (Eds.), *Physical violence in American families: Risk factors and adaptations to violence in 8145 families* (pp. 473–487). New Brunswick, NJ: Transaction Books.

Kelly, M. J., & Lauderdale, M. L. (1996). The Internet: Opportunities for rural outreach, exchange and resource development. *Human Services in the Rural Environment, 19*(4), 4–9.

Kempe, C. H., Silverman, F. N., Steele, B. B., Droegemueller, N., & Silver, H. K. (1962). The battered-child syndrome. *Journal of the American Medical Association, 181*, 17–24.

Kilpatrick, K. L., & Williams, L. M. (1998). Potential mediators of post-traumatic stress disorder in child witnesses to domestic violence. *Child Abuse & Neglect, 22*(4), 319–330.

Klein, E., Campbell, J., Soler, E., & Ghez, M. (1997). *Ending domestic violence: Changing public perceptions/ Halting the epidemic.* Thousand Oaks, CA: Sage.

Kleven, S. (1988). Southwestern Alaska Council for prevention of child sexual abuse. *Human Services in the Rural Environment, 12*(1), 32.

Leistyna, J. A. (1980). Advocacy for the abused rural child. In H. W. Johnson (Ed.), *Rural human services: A book of readings* (pp. 92–96). Itasca, IL: Peacock.

Martinez-Brawley, E., & Durbin, N. (1987). Women in the rural occupational structure: The poverty connection. *Human Services in the Rural Environment, 10*(4)/*11*(1), 29–39.

McGuire, L., Rice, K., & Tabor, M. (1994). *Final report of the Supreme Court Task Force on Courts' and Communities' Response to Domestic Abuse.* Des Moines: Supreme Court of Iowa.

McKenzie, B. (1989). Child welfare: New models of service delivery in Canada's Native communities. *Human Services in the Rural Environment, 12*(3), 6–11.

McLeer, S. V., & Anwar, R. (1989). A study of battered women presenting in an emergency department. *AJPH, 79*, 65–66.

McNeal, C. & Amato, P. R. (1998). Parent's marital violence: Long-term consequences for children. *Journal of Family Issues, 19*(2), 123–139.

Moffit, T. E., & Caspi, A. (1998). Annotation: Implications of violence between intimate partners for child psychologists and psychiatrists. *Journal of Child Psychology and Psychiatry, 39*(2), 137–144.

Monsey, B., Owen, G., Zierman, C., Lambert, L., & Hyman, V. (1995). *What works in preventing rural violence: Strategies, risk factors, and assessment tools.* St. Paul, MN: Amherst H. Wilder Foundation.

Morris, L. C. (1996). Facilitating participation of rural women in distance education through use of gender-friendly interactive technologies. *Human Services in the Rural Environment, 19*(4), 23–27.

Murty, S., & Schechter, S. (1999). *Reaching rural communities: A national assessment of rural domestic violence service needs.* (Administration for Children and Families, Department of Health and Human Services, grant no. 90EVO152/01). Iowa City: University of Iowa, School of Social Work.

Murty, S., Zwerling, C., Stromquist, A., Merchant, J., & Burmeister, L. (1999a). *Spouse Abuse in a Rural County* (unpublished manuscript). Iowa City: University of Iowa, Injury Prevention Research Center and School of Social Work.

Murty, S., Whitten, P., Zwerling, C., & Burmeister, L. (1999b). *Intimate partner violence against women in Iowa in rural and urban communities* (unpublished manuscript). Iowa City: University of Iowa, School of Social Work.

National Resource Center on Domestic Violence. (1999). *Getting the word out: Domestic violence awareness in rural communities.* Harrisburg, PA: Author.

Northwest Indian Child Welfare Institute. (1984). *Heritage and helping: A model curriculum for Indian child welfare practice.* Portland, OR: Parry Center for Children.

Peled, E. (1997). The battered women's movement response to children of battered women. *Violence Against Women, 3*(4), 424–466.

Peled, E. (1998). The experience of living with violence for preadolescent children of battered women. *Youth & Society, 29*(4), 395–430.

Peled, E., Eisikovits, Z. Enosh,G., & Winstok, Z. (2000). Choice and empowerment for battered women who stay: Toward a constructivist model. *Social Work, 45*(1), 9–25.

Peterson, S., & Olday, D. E. (1992). "How was your date last night?" Intimate relationship violence among high school students. *Human Services in the Rural Environment, 16*(2), 24–30.

Pillemer, K., & Finkelhor, D. (1988). The prevalence of elder abuse: A random sample survey. *The Gerontologist, 28,* 51–57.

Pryke, J., & Thomas, M. (1998). *Domestic violence and social work.* Aldershot, England: Ashgate.

Quinn, M., & Tomita, S. (1997). *Elder abuse and neglect: Causes, diagnosis, and intervention strategies.* New York: Springer.

Ray, J., & Murty, S. A. (1990). Rural child sexual abuse prevention and treatment. *Human Services in the Rural Environment, 13*(4), 24-29.

Rodgers, K. (1994). Wife assault: The findings of a national survey. *Statistics Canada Catalogue 85-002 Service Bulletin, 14*(9), 1–22.

Rodriguez, R. (1998). Clinical interventions with battered migrant farm worker women. In J. C. Campbell (Ed.), *Survivors of abuse: Health care for battered women and their children* (pp. 271–279). Thousand Oaks, CA: Sage.

Rubinstein, P. G. (1996). The development of battered women's services in rural areas. *Human Services in the Rural Environment, 19*(2/3), 29–33.

Rural Justice Center. (1991). *Not in my county: Rural courts and victims of domestic violence.* Montpelier, VT: Author.

Rural Task Force of the National Coalition Against Domestic Violence. (Eds.). (1991). *Rural resource packet.* Washington, DC: National Coalition Against Domestic Violence.

Schechter, S. (1982) *Women and male violence: The visions and the struggles of the battered women's movement.* Boston: South End Press.

Schechter, S. (1994, June). *Model initiatives linking domestic violence and child welfare.* Briefing paper presented at the conference on Domestic Violence and Child Welfare: Integrating Policy and Practice for Families. Racine, WI.

Schechter, S. (1995, March). *The battered women's movement in the United States: New directions for institutional reform.* Paper presented at the International Study Group on the Future of Intervention with Battered Women and Their Families. Haifa, Israel.

Schechter, S. (1996). *Improving the response to domestic violence: Recommendations to federal agencies.* (Grant #R13 CCR 711883-01, National Center for Injury Prevention and Control, Centers for Disease Control and Prevention). Iowa City: University of Iowa, School of Social Work and Injury Prevention and Research Center.

Sefcik, T. R., & Ormsby, N. J. (1980). Establishing a rural child abuse/neglect treatment program. In H. W. Johnson (Ed.), *Rural human services: A book of readings* (pp. 97–104). Itasca, IL: Peacock.

Silvern, L., & Kaersvang, L. (1989). The traumatized children of violent marriages. *Child Welfare, 4,* 421–436.

Stephens, D. L. (1999). Battered women's view of their children. *Journal of Interpersonal Violence, 14,* 731–746.

Stets, J. E., & Straus, M. A. (1990). The marriage license as a hitting license: A comparison of assaults in dating, cohabiting, and married couples. In M. A. Straus & R. J. Gelles (Eds.), *Physical violence in American families: Risk factors and adaptations to violence in 8145 families* (pp. 227–244). New Brunswick, NJ: Transaction Books.

Straus, M. A. (1979). Measuring intrafamily conflict and violence: The Conflict Tactics (CT) Scale. *Journal of Marriage and Family, 41,* 74–85.

Straus, M. A. (1990). Measuring intrafamily conflict and violence: The Conflict Tactics (CT) Scales. In M. A. Straus & R. J. Gelles (Eds.), *Physical violence in American families: Risk factors and adaptations to violence in 8145 families* (pp. 29–47). New Brunswick, NJ: Transaction Books.

Straus, M. A., & Gelles, R. J. (1990a). How violent are American families? Estimates from the National Family Violence Resurvey and other studies. In M. A. Straus & R. J. Gelles (Eds.), *Physical violence in American families: Risk factors and adaptations to violence in 8145 families* (pp. 95–112). New Brunswick, NJ: Transaction Books.

Straus, M. A., & Gelles, R. J. (1990b). Societal change and change in family violence from 1975 to 1985 as revealed by two national surveys. In M. A. Straus & R. J. Gelles (Eds.), *Physical violence in American families: Risk factors and adaptations to violence in 8145 families* (pp. 113–131). New Brunswick, NJ: Transaction Books.

Straus, M. A., & Smith, C. (1990a). Family patterns and child abuse. In M. A. Straus & R. J. Gelles (Eds.), *Physical violence in American families: Risk factors and adaptations to violence in 8145 families* (pp. 245–261). New Brunswick, NJ: Transaction Books.

Straus, M. A., & Smith, C. (1990b). Violence in Hispanic families in the United States: Incidence rates and structural interpretations. In M. A. Straus & R. J. Gelles (Eds.), *Physical violence in American families: Risk factors and adaptations to violence in 8145 families* (pp. 341–367). New Brunswick, NJ: Transaction Books.

Straus, M. A., Gelles, R. J., & Steinmetz, S. K. (1980). *Behind closed doors: Violence in the American family.* New York: Doubleday/Anchor.

Tatara, T. (1990). *Elder abuse in the United States: An issue paper.* (Prepared for the Administration on Aging and the Department of Health and Human Services). Washington, DC: National Aging Resource Center on Elder Abuse.

Tatara, T., & Kuzmeskus, L. (1997). *Summaries of the statistical data on elder abuse in domestic settings for FY 95 and FY 96.* Washington, DC: National Center on Elder Abuse.

Tjaden, P., & Thoennes, N. (1998). Prevalence, incidence, and consequences of violence against women: Findings from the National Violence Against Women Survey. *Research in Brief.* Washington, DC: National Institute of Justice, Centers for Disease Control and Prevention.

Van Hightower, N. R., & Gorton, J. (1998). Domestic violence among patients at two rural health care clinics: Prevalence and social correlates. *Public Health Nursing, 15*(5), 355–362.

Websdale, N. (1998). *Rural woman battering and the justice system: An ethnography.* Thousand Oaks, CA: Sage.

Websdale, N., & Johnson, B. (1997). The policing of domestic violence in rural and urban areas: The voices of battered women in Kentucky. *Policing and Society, 6,* 297–317.

Wiehe, V. (1998). *Understanding family violence: Treating and preventing partner, child, sibling, and elder abuse.* Thousand Oaks, CA: Sage.

Wilt, S., & Olson, S. (1996). Prevalence of domestic violence in the United States. *Journal of the American Women's Medical Association, 51*(3), 77–82.

Wolf, R., & Donglin, L. (1999). Factors affecting the rate of elder abuse reporting to a state protective services program. *The Gerontologist, 39*(2), 222–228.

Wolk, L. E. (1982). *Minnesota's American Indian battered women: The cycle of oppression: A cultural awareness training manual for non-Indian professionals.* St. Paul, MN: St. Paul American Indian Center.

17

Theories, Models, and Methods of Health Promotion in Rural Settings

JOHN P. ELDER, GUADALUPE X. AYALA,

MARION F. ZABINSKI, JUDITH J. PROCHASKA,

AND CHRISTINE A. GEHRMAN

"We steered by the stars not the light of each passing ship." General Omar Bradley

Introduction

Health promotion interventions are evaluated on both the amount of individual behavior change achieved and the extent to which broader generalizations can be made to other behavior change efforts. This is largely a function of whether the interventions and evaluation methods employed are theory-driven (Elder, Geller, Hovell, & Mayer, 1994). Yet many theories and models current in the field have limited applicability to rural populations since the underlying theories are generally predicated on more urban notions of individual autonomy and purpose, with potentially less relevance for populations in smaller and more traditional communities. In addition, many theories imply detailed, thorough individual measurement, making them

less practical for people not accustomed to such instrumentation or with limited literacy, or for programs with no resources for such measurement. Despite these limitations, individually oriented theories form the basis of health behavior programs and their evaluation. They provide the departure point for the conceptualization of broader psychosocial, social network, and community change theories and models. This chapter presents a few prominent theories current in the field, from the individual to the community level. The suitability or adaptability of these theories and models in rural settings is also discussed.

Definitions and Populations

In 1990, the rural[1] American population numbered 61,656,386 (U.S. Census Bureau, 1990), constituting 24.8% of the total population, living on 97% of the nation's land (Luloff &

JOHN P. ELDER, GUADALUPE X. AYALA, MARION F. ZABINSKI, JUDITH J. PROCHASKA, AND CHRISTINE A. GEHRMAN • San Diego State University, Graduate School of Public Health and SDSU–UCSD Joint Doctoral Program in Clinical Psychology, San Diego, California 92123.

Handbook of Rural Health, edited by Loue and Quill. Kluwer Academic/Plenum Publishers, New York, 2001.

*There is some confusion about the use of an urban–rural distinction versus a metropolitan–nonmetropolitan distinction (Clarke & Miller, 1990; Fuguitt, 1995). These terms, however, are not interchangeable. According to the U.S. Census Bureau (1990), the definition of a metropolitan area is based on the county. Counties or groups of counties that include large cities and their suburbs are considered metropolitan; all others are con-

Swanson, 1990; Ricketts, Johnson-Webb, & Randolph, 1999). These numbers are based on criteria established by the U.S. Census Bureau, which uses one of the following to define a rural[2] setting: a territory outside an urban area, any incorporated area located outside an urban area having fewer than 2,500 residents, or any place outside an incorporated area (U.S. Census Bureau, 1990). Rural places are further subdivided into rural farms and rural nonfarms, with rural farms consisting of places from which $1,000 or more of agricultural products were sold in 1989. Hart (1995) argues, however, that the use of a cutoff of 2,500 residents to classify an area as rural fails to consider numerous factors that distinguish rural places from urban places and types of rural environments from each other. Galston & Baehler (1995) contrast the "dairy farms of New England and the humid poverty of the Delta; the midwestern farming communities and the forbidding semi-aridity of the mining Southwest; the moist timber-dependent Northwest and the ranching of the West" (p. 3). They suggest that rural places differ widely as a function of their geography, climate, history, and the manner in which people make a living. According to Clarke & Miller (1990), the U.S. Department of Agriculture provides further specificity to the definition of rural by considering the economic dependencies of the area. The seven classes of nonmetropolitan counties based on the dependencies are these: (1) farming-dependent; (2) manufacturing-dependent; (3) mining-dependent; (4) spe-

cialized government; (5) persistent poverty; (6) federal land; and (7) retirement. These distinctions, as well as the fact that mass media, transportation, and technological advances are modernizing rural communities, suggest that merely classifying a particular region as rural informs us little about the types of health promotion approaches that may be effective in these communities.

Additional characteristics that are important to consider when selecting health behavior change strategies to implement in rural settings include sociodemographic variables such as age, education, and ethnicity. Rural areas tend to have a higher proportion of people who are younger than 15 and older than 64 (Fuguitt, 1995). Researchers have documented an outmigration of younger, more-educated adults to urban areas in pursuit of higher-paid employment (Clarke & Miller, 1990). Considering ethnic distributions, with the exception of American Indians (50% living on or near reservations), rural areas are less ethnically diverse than urban areas (Fuguitt, 1995). Pockets of large ethnic populations, however, do exist in certain rural places. For example, the cotton, peanut, and tobacco-growing areas of the South have a large population of African Americans, and the southwestern states include a large concentration of Hispanics.

Galston & Baehler (1995) argue that there are three fundamental dimensions of rural places, which suggest a multilevel approach to health promotion and health behavior change. These dimensions concern the individual's relationship to nature, community members, and family and community history. Individuals living in rural areas often have a more intimate relationship with nature and a greater appreciation for its valuable resources. Individuals living in rural places generally get to know one another more intimately and support each other during times of need. There is a connection with a larger community to which one both gives to and receives from for sustenance and quality of life. Social networks with community members foster a "high density of acquaintanceship" that provides support and functions to regulate the individual's behavior (Salamon, 1995, p. 353). With the exception of migrant communities, rural places are often more stable, or less transient, than urban

---

sidered nonmetropolitan. Using this definition, nearly half of the rural population is metropolitan and 11% of the urban population is nonmetropolitan (Fuguitt, 1995). The authors of this chapter chose to use the rural–urban distinction consistent with the title of this handbook.

†According to Clarke and Miller (1990), the National Rural Health Association further divided the rural-urban distinction into four categories: (1) adjacent rural areas—counties next to or within metropolitan areas; (2) urbanized rural areas—counties with populations of greater than or equal to 25,000 but not attached to a metropolitan area; (3) frontier areas—counties with a population density of less than or equal to 6 persons per square mile; and (4) countryside rural areas—remaining rural areas not covered by the three preceding definitions.

environments. Individuals are not only linked to one another in the present, through reciprocity and mutual dependence, but also linked to their community because of their personal and family history. Rural people are more likely to live and die where they were born. According to Galston & Baehler (1995), there is a shared memory between individuals of different generations. These three characteristics, typical of most rural places, suggest that any approach to health care and health education for people living in rural areas must consider aspects within the individual, within the family, and within the community.

Health Issues of Rural Populations

Health issues specially identified with rural populations tend to be associated with occupational risks and by-products of the local economy. For example, coal miners are at greater risk of developing lung cancer and black lung disease (Galston & Baehler, 1995). Farming-dependent communities are at increased risk of having a contaminated water supply as a result of the pesticides and toxic chemicals used in farming (Rochín & Marroquin, 1997). The farmers' dilemma often is whether to use pesticides in the face of increased health and safety risks. Other occupational risks include farming machinery accidents, mining accidents, and manufacturing accidents (Clarke & Miller, 1990). There is evidence to suggest that although farmers believe farm accidents to be dangerous, they don't believe they are vulnerable to such accidents (Witte, Peterson, Vallabhan, & Stephenson, 1993). Teens working on farms report common injuries such as insect stings, cuts, burns, and falls (Schulman, Evensen, Runyan, Cohen, & Dunn, 1997). Galston & Baehler (1995) noted that many of the industries involving natural resources (e.g., farming, food manufacturing, and forestry) are considered some of the most dangerous jobs in this country, having the second highest rate of occupational injuries and illnesses (Galston & Baehler, 1995). Notwithstanding the depiction of rural employment consisting primarily of farming, mining, forestry, and manufacturing jobs, there are still others who argue that rural environments are in a state of transition. According to Hart (1995, p. 63):

> The traditional concept of rural Americans conjoined people and place, and was based on the fact that people in certain occupations (e.g., farming, forestry, and mining) lived in the sparsely populated open countryside, because their livelihood required relatively extensive areas of land. The association between occupation and the open countryside is no longer as compelling as it once was, however, for increasing numbers of people with other occupations have been moving to sparsely populated places, and one can no longer assume that people who live in the open countryside have traditional rural occupations.

This suggests that researchers should look beyond the health risk factors traditionally observed in rural communities and examine other occupational and environmental factors that place the individual at greater risk for injury, illness, and death. Theories of behavioral and community change are key elements of that examination.

Health Behavior Change Theories

A review of the major health behavior change theories is presented here to familiarize the reader with the theoretical constructs and their operationalizations. As noted in the introduction, the health promotion field is dominated by theories that assume individual autonomy and purpose. This review includes theories with an individual focus as well as theories with a family and community focus. Suitability and applicability of these theories will be discussed in subsequent sections of this chapter. In addition, Table 1 provides a summary of the major theories, their underlying assumptions, the focus of health behavior interventions, and the types of interventions emphasized by each theoretical orientation.

The Theory of Reasoned Action and the Theory of Planned Behavior

The theory of reasoned action (TRA) and theory of planned behavior (TPB) were developed by researchers in the fields of personality and social psychology, and focus on motivational factors within the individual as determi-

Table 1. Theories of Health Behavior Change

Health Behavior Theory	Underlying Assumptions	Focus of Health Behavior Interventions	Types of Interventions Emphasized
Theory of reasoned action /Theory of planned behavior	Attitude and subjective norms influence intentions, which influences behavior. TPB also accounts for perceived behavioral control as a determinant of intention.	Motivational factors within an individual.	For behaviors that are of voluntary control.
Transtheoretical model	Individuals proceed through cognitive–behavioral stages of change, from precontemplation to maintenance.	Individual.	Increase "pros" of making a change and decrease "cons"; tailor the intervention to the specific stage in which the person starts.
Communication–persuasion model	Individuals proceed through stages based on type of communication to which they are exposed.	Individual–communication interactions.	Design communication that will increase exposure, attention, acceptance, or behavior change, depending on what stage audience is in.
Applied behavioral analysis	Behavior is a product of its physical and social consequences. The relationship between the environment and behavior is known as "contingencies of reinforcement."	Person–behavior–environment interactions.	Increase positive reinforcement for and reduce barriers to engaging in healthy behaviors; if needed, reduce reinforcement for and increase barriers to engaging in unhealthy behaviors.
Social learning/ Cognitive theory	Behavior interacts with "person" (e.g., attitudes and knowledge) and environment in a process called *reciprocal determinism*.	Person, environment, and behavior.	Increase self-efficacy and outcome expectations related to the desired behavior change; allow opportunities for vicarious learning.
Problem behavior theory	Accounts for personality, environment, and behavior in determining proneness, or risk, that a problem behavior will occur.	Adolescent problem behavior and unconventionality.	Emphasizes the need to work with the individual as well as the family structure.
Family systems theory	Agencies and individuals influence the choices available to the individual (e.g., family, church, health departments, media, policymakers).	Individual within family system.	Useful in therapeutic setting as approach emphasizes situational and interpersonal factors.
Social ecology model	Individual behavior is a function of the larger social context.	Individual and community.	Combines individual change with modification of physical and social environments.
Media advocacy	Health communication efforts need to be less narrow and focus on broader societal topics, such as illness industries.	Perpetrators of problems, policymakers.	Publicity used both as carrots and sticks.
Community self-control	Communities proceed through a process of self-directed change, much in the same way as do individuals.	Small, self-identified communities.	Early adopters work with change agent to select targets, set goals, decide on interventions, monitor progress, and reinforce success.

nants of behavior. TRA was first introduced in 1967 and was designed to predict behaviors over which people have a high degree of volitional control (Fishbein, 1967). The theory of planned behavior evolved from the TRA to take into account barriers and constraints to performing a behavior (Ajzen, 1985).

The TRA is made up of the following constructs: intention to perform the behavior, attitude toward the behavior, and subjective norm (Fishbein & Ajzen, 1975). *Intention* to perform a behavior is the construct theorized to be most closely and directly related to the corresponding behavior. *Attitude* toward the behavior, the degree to which the behavior is favorably or unfavorably evaluated by the individual, and *subjective norm*, the perceived social pressure to perform or not perform the behavior, act indirectly through intention to predict the occurrence or nonoccurrence of a behavior. According to the TRA, any variable other than attitude and subjective norm can affect intention and behavior only indirectly, by influencing one of these two predictors (Ajzen, 1987). Attitude is determined by beliefs about attributes of performing the behavior and evaluations of those behavioral outcomes. The TRA distinguishes itself from previous models, which demonstrated low correspondence between attitudes and behaviors. In the TRA, attitude toward the specific behavior is measured rather than attitude toward an object or outcome. For example, attitude toward cigarette smoking is measured, rather than attitude toward lung cancer. Subjective norm is determined by normative beliefs and motivation to comply with those referents.

The theory of planned behavior is an extension of the theory of reasoned action (Ajzen, 1985; Ajzen & Madden, 1986). TPB maintains the original constructs of TRA but adds a third direct antecedent of intention, *perceived behavioral control*. This factor refers to the perceived ease or difficulty of performing the behavior and is related to past experience as well as anticipated barriers. Determinants of perceived behavioral control are control beliefs and perceived power. When there is agreement between perceived and actual behavioral control, perceived behavioral control is believed to have a direct influence on behavior (Ajzen, 1987). The addition of perceived behavioral control as a

direct determinant of intention, independent of attitudes and subjective norms, was found to improve prediction of the model (Ajzen & Madden, 1986). TPB includes the motivational factors of TRA but also takes into account constraints to performing a behavior. This contrast between motivational factors and perceived control is quite similar to Bandura's (1977b) distinction between outcome beliefs and self-efficacy beliefs in social learning theory.

The predictive value of the TRA has been evaluated in experimental and naturalistic settings to help understand health behaviors and to develop interventions. Generally, the TRA has demonstrated applicability as long as the behavior under study is clearly of voluntary control (Ajzen, 1987). The TRA has been successfully applied in studies of smoking, drinking, contraceptive use, testicular and breast self-exam, mammography screening, flu vaccine use, exercising, seat belt use, and safety helmet use behaviors (Fishbein, 1993; Moore, Barling, & Hood, 1998). These studies have generally demonstrated that, as hypothesized, attitudes and subjective norms predict intentions to perform a behavior, and intentions in turn predict the actual behavior.

Godin and Kok (1996) reviewed all studies published since 1985 that applied the theory of planned behavior to understand health-related behaviors. Their conclusion was that the theory performs very well for the explanation of intention, with attitude toward the action and perceived behavioral control being the strongest predictors. Prediction of behavior was lower, but still significant. Intention was the most important predictor of behavior, with perceived behavioral control significantly adding to the prediction in half of the studies reviewed. The authors noted that predictive power of the theory, however, varied among health-related behavior categories. Blue (1995) examined the predictive capacity of the TRA and the TPB specifically in exercise research. As compared to the TRA, the TPB was suggested as a more promising framework for the study of exercise because it includes assessment of perceived behavioral control over factors that may facilitate or hinder the performance of exercise.

The theories of reasoned action and planned behavior provide theoretical frameworks to conceptualize, measure, and identify factors that determine behavior. The TRA focuses on cognitive factors (beliefs and values) that determine motivation (intention). With the addition of perceived behavioral control, the TPB extends the TRA to address constraints to performing a behavior. Of note, these theories were developed to explain behavior, not to predict behavior change.

Transtheoretical Model

The transtheoretical model (TTM) has proven useful for characterizing the process of behavior change and for guiding intervention design and evaluation (Prochaska, Redding, Harlow, Rossi, & Velicer, 1994). Developed in the area of smoking cessation, it has also been shown to be relevant to alcohol and drug dependence, exercise adoption, diet and weight control, sun exposure behaviors, diabetes self-management, HIV risk behaviors, partner violence, and cancer screening practices (Prochaska et al., 1994).

The TTM was originally developed through observations of how people quit smoking on their own. It was observed that smokers move through a series of stages of change in their efforts to quit (DiClemente & Prochaska, 1982; Prochaska & DiClemente, 1983). "Stage" is the temporal dimension that represents when particular changes occur (Prochaska, 1992). Stages also represent a continuum of motivational readiness to take and sustain action (see Prochaska & DiClemente, 1998, for more information on stages). In this model, individuals move sequentially through the following stages: precontemplation, not intending to change; contemplation, intending to change within six months; preparation, actively planning change within the next 30 days; action, overtly making changes; and maintenance, taking steps to sustain change and resist temptation to relapse (Prochaska et al., 1994). The TTM conceptualizes change as a dynamic, nonlinear process, with the majority of people relapsing and returning to earlier stages of change before successfully reaching maintenance (Prochaska & DiClemente, 1998).

Stage of change is one component within the larger framework of the TTM, which also includes the processes of change, self-efficacy,

and decisional balance. Processes of change are covert and overt experiences that mediate the transition through the stages of change (Prochaska & DiClemente, 1983). Numerous studies have shown that successful self-changers employ a common set of processes traditionally associated with such theoretically diverse psychological models as social learning theory, psychodynamic theory, and behavior modification (Prochaska, 1979). The 10 processes of change are consciousness raising, counterconditioning, dramatic relief, environmental reevaluation, helping relationships, reinforcement management, self-liberation, self-reevaluation, social liberation, and stimulus control. Multiple techniques, methods, and interventions can be used to promote the different processes. For example, the process of consciousness raising—increasing one's level of awareness of the target problem—can be achieved through reading articles, searching the Web, or speaking with a physician, therapist or loved one. Research has supported the hypothesized relationships between the stages and the processes of change, with individuals in the later stages of change making greater use of the more experiential processes (e.g., helping relationships, stimulus control; DiClemente, Prochaska, Fairhurst, Velicer, Velasquez, & Rossi, 1991; Gottlieb, Galavotti, McCuan, & McAlister, 1990; Prochaska & DiClemente, 1983). Successful progression through the stages of change has been associated with use of specific processes at the appropriate stages. For example, consciousness raising is viewed as critical for moving an individual from precontemplation to contemplation, but engaging in consciousness raising during preparation can delay steps toward action.

Adapted from work by Janis & Mann (1968, 1977), decisional balance refers to the relative weight given to the pros and cons of changing behavior. Velicer, DiClemente, Prochaska, and Brandenburg (1985) allied the decisional balance construct with the stages-of-change model in studying the pattern of cognitive and motivational shifts in the change process. Studies across different problem behaviors have suggested that the positive aspects (pros) of changing a problem behavior begin to outweigh the negative aspects (cons) of change early in the contemplation stage (Prochaska *et al.*, 1994). In the TTM, self-efficacy has been operationalized in two ways: situational confidence in changing behavior and situational temptations to engage in problem behavior (DiClemente *et al.*, 1991; Velicer, DiClemente, Rossi, & Prochaska, 1990). The amount of confidence one has in making a behavior change has been shown to be directly correlated with stage (Prochaska, Velicer, Guadagnoli, Rossi, & DiClemente, 1991).

Some researchers (e.g., Herzog, Abrams, Emmons, Linnan, & Shaddel, 1999) have questioned whether processes of change and the decisional balance actually predict progressive movement toward behavior change in longitudinal designs in contrast to demonstrating associations in cross-sectional studies. Relationships among the model's constructs, however, have been supported in prospective, retrospective, cross-sectional, and longitudinal studies (Prochaska *et al.*, 1994). Stage-based interventions have also demonstrated effectiveness in promoting behavior change for smoking cessation (Dijkstra, De Vries, Roijackers, & van Breukelen, 1998; Prochaska, DiClemente, Velicer, & Rossi, 1993), mammography screening (Rakowski *et al.*, 1998), exercise (Marcus, Bock, Pinto, Forsyth, Roberts, & Traficante, 1998), and diet (Greene & Rossi, 1998).

Communication–Persuasion Model

Parallel to the TTM is another stage-based system, McGuire's communication–persuasion model (McGuire, 1989). McGuire considers how communication can effect change in individual attitudes and behaviors. The communication–persuasion model can be conceptualized in terms of an input–output matrix to describe stages (outputs) leading to behavior change, and how progress through these stages is aided by communication in its various forms (inputs).

The inputs represent qualities of the communicated message that can be manipulated and controlled by campaign designers, whereas outputs represent the information-processing steps that must be stimulated in those receiving the message. Specifically, the inputs address "who says what, via what medium, to whom, directed at what kind of target" (McGuire, 1989, p. 45).

This translates into information regarding the "source," the "message," the "channel," the "receiver," and the "destination." Source characteristics refer to the communicator of the message. Persuasive impact may be influenced by such factors as age, gender, ethnicity, credibility, and socioeconomic status. Message refers to the information that is communicated, and important factors include delivery style, content organization, length, and repetition. Channel is the mode of communication, including face-to-face, print (e.g., newspaper, brochures), broadcast, and electronic media (e.g., computer, Internet). Receiver characteristics include such variables as age, education, intelligence, and demographic variables considered when creating a public health campaign. Finally, the destination describes the targeted behaviors and issues to be considered, including long-term versus short-term change and specific versus general behaviors.

Outputs reflect the temporal process and stages of change, from initial exposure to communication to long-term maintenance of change within the intended receiver. The 12 output steps progress as follows: exposure, attention, liking, comprehension, skill acquisition, attitude change, memory storage, information search and retrieval from memory, decision based on retrieval, behaving in accordance with decision, reinforcement, and consolidation. All are necessary for a given communication to be effective, and the theory assumes that these output processing steps are contingent on each other and, therefore, must occur in the specified sequence.

A strength of McGuire's theory is that it lends itself both to program design and to evaluating specific changes related to a communication effort. More than any other theory, McGuire's conceptualization has guided the field of public health communication, which uses a variety of techniques but specifically emphasizes a few practical and simple messages through as many "channels" as possible. The success of a communication program is determined by a variety of factors including: (1) how much access the target audience has to the information (e.g., does a large percentage of the target audience own television sets and telephones?); (2) whether people were actually exposed to the media advertisement (e.g., did a poster in a clinic stay up long enough for people to see it?); (3) whether the target audience acquired sufficient knowledge and skills to perform the target behavior (e.g., is the amount of exposure to the campaign sufficient to result in behavior change?); (4) whether the target audience actually has the opportunity to perform the behavior (e.g, new physical activity skills should be taught with reference to the appropriate season); and (5) whether this trial and short-term adoption can be reinforced naturally through subsequent communication approaches.

More than any other health promotion techniques, communication is the process of sharing information between two or more persons via mass media, face-to-face exchanges, or other channels using words, pictures, music, and other audiovisual or symbolic approaches. A related applied field, social marketing, is defined as the application of communication and marketing concepts to the design, implementation, and management of social change programs, such as health and safety promotion. Social marketing can serve a variety of purposes. Applied specifically to health promotion, it has been used to: (a) create awareness of a health issue, problem, or solution; (b) create demand for health services or support for individual or community action (see the following section "Media Advocacy"); (c) teach skills; and (d) prompt and reinforce the maintenance and generalization of beneficial behavior change (U.S. Department of Health and Human Services, 1989). Social marketing can be used to target any of McGuire's output variables, especially the initial stages of getting people's attention and improving knowledge about a health issue.

Applied Behavior Analysis

Staged-based health communication and social marketing techniques are held to be valuable and effective procedures for altering protective or risk-related behavior. Indeed, marketing strategies may be very useful in prompting an initial behavior change. However, marketing should not be expected to sustain behavior change except where the new behavior is reinforced by consequences intrinsic to the task or available in the environmental set-

ting. Most health communication campaigns attempt to change the consumer's attention, attitude, knowledge, or beliefs. The theoretical assumption underlying these campaigns is that new cognitive processes will lead to "informed" decisions to change behavior since they have changed their beliefs with respect to the behavior. From a behavior modification or operant psychology perspective, the tactics used to change knowledge, attitudes, and beliefs are largely antecedent-oriented educational procedures. In other words, they represent stimuli that set the stage for the occurrence of the behavior through forging antecedent-behavior or A-B links. Procedures derived from applied behavior analysis (Miller, 1980; Skinner, 1953), in contrast, emphasize behavior-consequence ("B-C") associations or "contingencies."

Contingency management has been defined as "the systematic application of principles derived from learning theory to altering environment–behavior relationships in order to strengthen adaptive and weaken maladaptive behaviors" (Elder et al., 1994; p. 128). Consequences can be applied, removed, or discontinued, resulting in a strengthening or weakening of a behavior. Applying a pleasant consequence or removing or discontinuing unpleasant ones will strengthen behaviors through the processes of positive reinforcement, negative reinforcement, or response facilitation, respectively. Removing a pleasant consequence, applying an aversive consequence, or discontinuing a pleasant consequence will weaken behaviors. The first two of these latter contingencies are forms of "punishment", whereas the latter is referred to as "extinction" (Elder et al., 1994; pp. 129–131). Although not all six of these contingencies are tools of public health promotion, understanding the processes of how behaviors are formed or eliminated is critical to developing campaigns, policies, and other behavior change interventions.

The HealthCom Project (Academy for Educational Development, 1995) identified six different criteria for selecting target behaviors: the health impact of the behavior, its perceptible positive reinforcers, any punishers or barriers to its performance, whether the behavior is compatible with and similar to existing practices, and the ease or complexity of engaging in the behavior in general and specifically at the rate and duration required to alleviate a health problem. Program planners can weight these criteria differentially to design campaigns, environmental interventions, or policies that promote adaptive or weaken unhealthy behavioral alternatives. At times health behavior change efforts need to go beyond the establishment of appropriate contingencies to strengthen healthy behaviors or at times weaken unhealthy ones. Less-than-optimal levels of behavior may result from either a "performance" or "skill" deficit. In the former case, contingency management procedures are in order, whereas when skill deficits are present, additional training with appropriate supervision would be indicated (Graeff, Elder & Booth, 1993).

Applied behavior analysis has broad general applicability to public health promotion. Generally, it can be used to understand why healthy behaviors do or do not exist, and to develop environments and policies that promote health and in some cases reduce unhealthy behaviors and their causes. ABA, however, is not widely accepted among more cognitively oriented behavioral scientists because it places less emphasis on the link between cognitions and behaviors and more emphasis on environmental influences of behavior.

Social Learning Theory and Social Cognitive Theory

With his book *Behavior Modification*, Albert Bandura (1969) initially estalished himself as a social psychologist in the applied behavior analysis mode. Less than a decade later, however, he drifted to a more cognitive orientation within learning theory. His development of social learning theory (SLT; 1977) emphasized the interaction of internal and external factors in human behavior. SLT stems partially from B. F. Skinner's experimental analysis of behavior, suggesting that behavior was explained largely in terms of its consequences. Bandura blended Skinner's ideas with his own, emphasizing that both consequences of an action and one's perceptions of the consequences determine one's ultimate behavior.

In his theory, Bandura posited that personal (cognitive and physiological) and environmental (social and physical) factors do not function as independent determinants but rather determine each other. He states that "people are not simply reactors to external influences; they select, organize, and transform the stimuli that impinge upon them" (Bandura, 1977, p. 9). As such, SLT goes beyond individually oriented models of human behavior to consider both the social and physical environment, and the person's active role in them. It is largely through their own actions that people produce the environmental conditions that affect their behavior in a reciprocal fashion (Bandura, 1977). This conception portrays people neither as powerless objects controlled by environmental forces nor as entirely free agents who can become whatever they choose. Both people and their environments are reciprocal determinants of each other. The relative influences exerted by these interdependent factors differ in various settings and for different behaviors. There are times when environmental factors exercise powerful constraints on behavior and other times when personal factors modify the course of environmental events. According to Bandura, a theory that denies that cognitions can regulate actions does not lend itself readily to the explanation of complex human behavior.

Three key components of SLT include observational learning, outcome expectancies or consequences, and self-efficacy. Vicarious or observational learning refers to learning through observing the topography of a response and the consequences others (role models) experience as a result of the behavior. The more complex the behavior, the more times one must observe it being executed and practice what has been observed. One forms a conception of how new behavior patterns are performed by observing others, and then these modeled images serve as guides for action on later occasions (Bandura, 1977). Much of human behavior is acquired through modeling.

Outcome expectancies refer to the perceived consequences of a given behavior. The individual's belief that a specific response will follow a specific action is a salient determinant of behavior. In this way, the expected outcome or consequence serves as a reinforcer for subsequently engaging in the desired behavior. Consequences serve as a way of informing performers what they must do to gain beneficial outcomes and to avoid punishing ones. Responses to new behavior patterns serve an informative function: people notice the effects of their actions, and the acquired information serves as a guide for future action. Because learning by response consequences is largely a cognitive process, consequences generally produce little change in complex behavior when there is no awareness of what is being reinforced. Even if certain responses have been positively reinforced, they will not increase if individuals believe from other information that the same action will not be rewarded on future occasions. By observing the differential effects of their own actions, individuals discern which responses are appropriate in which settings and behave accordingly (Dulany, 1968). Thus, according to Bandura, the reinforcing effects of an expected outcome serves principally as an informative and motivational operation rather than as a mechanical response strengthener, as proposed in behavior analysis.

Self-efficacy, or one's confidence for success in a given situation, is an important determinant of whether one will attempt to initiate or maintain a behavior or make changes in one's environment (Bandura, 1986). Actions are based not only on expectancies of reinforcement but also on self-evaluation of competency. Moreover, self-efficacy determines not only whether we will engage in a particular behavior but also the extent to which we will maintain the behavior in the face of adversity. Low self-efficacy can hamper both the frequency and quality of behavior–environment interactions, and high self-efficacy can facilitate both.

In 1986, Bandura further distanced himself from learning theory by recasting his research as social cognitve theory (SCT). According to SCT, it is necessary to remove not only real but perceived barriers, as well as to heighten awareness of environmental cues to promote the desired behavior (Dishman, 1991). People can benefit from self-directed behavior change when they understand how personal habits contribute to their well-being, are taught how to modify them, and have the confidence in their capabilities to perform the desired behaviors (Bandura, 1986). Individuals need to be provided not only with reasons to change but also with the means

to do it. Effective self-regulation of behavior requires certain skills. People have to learn how to monitor the behavior they seek to change, how to set proximal goals to motivate and guide their efforts, and how to arrange incentives for themselves to put forth the necessary effort.

The strength of SLT/SCT stems from the reciprocal determinism that allows for mutual influences between environment and behavior while accounting for an individual's cognitions and thoughts. The interactive structure makes no suggestion about the relative strength or dominant direction of influence since it will vary for each individual (Bandura, 1986). In addition, SCT allows for temporal ambiguity among factors by recognizing that influences and effects may not happen simultaneously. It may take time for a causal factor to have an effect within an individual. From the health behavior perspective, SCT implies that one can change behavior through personal influences (such as outcome expectancy and self-efficacy) or environmental influences. SCT promotes specificity of interventions by assessing important personal determinants of behavior and mediators of change for each individual and has been successful in multiple health domains.

Problem Behavior Theory

Sharing many elements in common with social learning theory is problem behavior theory. Problem behavior theory was developed in order to predict and explain adolescent problem behaviors, such as alcohol and drug abuse, in a psychosocial context (Jessor, Donovan, & Costa, 1991). In general, a problem behavior is defined as one that departs from social and legal norms of society, potentially resulting in negative reactions and attempts at social control from authority institutions. Although there are subgroups and communities with social norms that are at odds with society at large and potentially detrimental to health behaviors (e.g., Ku Klux Klan), this theory is based on an underlying assumption that the given society is "healthy" and, therefore, problems can be operationally defined as above.

To explain adolescent behavior, the psychosocial perspective extends beyond medical or genetic rationales and considers the psychological aspects of the individual, the influences of the environment, and the situational attributes in which the behavior takes place (Donovan, Jessor, & Costa, 1991). Within each of these three systems (personality, environmental, behavioral), influences can have different effects. While some variables may make a problem behavior more likely, others may reduce its occurrence. Taken together, these concepts define the *proneness* of an individual to a behavior, or the risk that a problem behavior will occur. Proneness can be determined by many variables within the personality, environmental, and behavioral systems. Some variables are more proximal and exert more influence over behaviors, whereas other variables are more distal and their connection with a given behavior is less obvious. Personality factors are sociocognitive and reflect social values, attitudes, expectations, and beliefs. For example, personality proneness to problem behavior for adolescents might include lower academic achievement, lower expectations of attaining goals, lower value on achievement, and higher independence (Donovan *et al.*, 1991). Environmental characteristics refer to expectations of others and systems of support, influence, and control. Therefore, environmental proneness may result from lower parental support, lower parental control, and higher friend influence. Finally, the behavior system can be divided into problem (or unconventional) behaviors and conventional behaviors based on the adolescent's conceptualization. For example, problem behaviors may include drinking, cigarette smoking, and sexual activity, whereas conventional behaviors may refer to church attendance and academic performance (Jessor, 1987, 1991). The psychosocial perspective looks at the interaction of these variables in order to predict particular actions. Problem behaviors have diverse meanings for different adolescents as they perform different functions. For some, these behaviors may provide an outlet for expressing opposition to socially accepted norms. Problem behaviors may also serve as a coping mechanism for dealing with strong emotions such as anxiety or frustration. A common and important function of many problem behaviors rests on the goal of independence in the transition to adulthood. Therefore, it is important to consider the sub-jective experience of adolescents when interpreting their behavior and to be aware that many of the problem behaviors are connected to the fulfillment of important developmental goals.

Problem behavior theory has been applied to a wide variety of adolescent behaviors, including drug use, sexual intercourse, alcohol abuse, and general delinquency (Bingham & Crockett, 1996; Jessor, 1987; Jessor & Jessor, 1973). In addition to being applied to unconventional behavior, this theory has been successfully applied to other behavioral domains including physical and mental health and health-compromising behaviors such as sedentary activity, overeating, dental hygiene, and sleep patterns (Donovan *et al.*, 1991). In general, this theory has been useful in explaining unconventional or problem behaviors as it has been shown to account for between a third and a half of the variance in studies assessing relevant psychosocial variables.

Family Systems Theory

The family has long been considered an important context in which human behavior develops. As such, it forms the basis of a theoretical orientation that focuses on the influential effects of the interrelatedness of family member behavior. As early as the 1920s, family systems theorists viewed the family as having both protective and maladaptive influences on individual behavior as a result of our mutual involvement with others. Although family systems theory (FST) originally began with a psychodynamic focus and considered only the maladaptive effects of this interrelatedness, it has since followed a very divergent path (Guerin & Chabot, 1997).

Numerous researchers have contributed to the development of the FST. In the early 1950s, Dr. Sullivan (1953) recognized that people were the product of their relatively enduring patterns of recurrent interpersonal situations. Gregory Bateson and his colleagues investigated the context and communication patterns of families with a schizophrenic family member (Bateson, Jackson, Haley, & Weakland, 1956). The concept of a "double-bind communication" that followed from this line of research sparked investigations focusing on role relationships and communication, and the eventual development of maladaptive behaviors. Haley (1987), among others in the "strategic movement," emphasized the importance of defining "rules" within the family that determine the roles and behaviors of each of the members. Bowen´s family systems model was a clinically-derived theoretical model that evolved directly from psychoanalytic principles and practice, which included such ideas as differentiation of self, triangles, family projection process, emotional cutoff, and sibling position (Bowen, 1966). Salvador Minuchin formed his model based on the family as a relationship system and emphasized roles, rules, and boundaries (Minuchin, 1974; Minuchin, Lee, & Simon, 1996). Although these viewpoints appear considerably varied, common ideas are shared between the various contributors to the family systems framework. Most theorists agree that the family is a system and has properties that are characteristic of systems in general. Systems are generally described in the following ways: (1) consisting of interrelated components; (2) dynamic and constantly changing; (3) functioning in a nonlinear, cyclic manner; and (4) having a whole that is different from the sum of its parts. Its behavior can only be understood by the interrelatedness of its parts. In this sense, the family system is viewed as an organized and durable living system, consisting of a network of related parts that together constitute an entity larger than the simple sum of its individual members. Attempting to explain the interactional nature of the family system and individual behavior, Ackerman (1984) asserted that a change in behavior in any one entity is a function of the sum of the behaviors of the other entities. Thus, a change in behavior in any one family member is a function of the behavior of all other family members. The behavior of individuals "within the family is related to and dependent upon the behavior of all others" (Denton, 1990, p. 115). Conversely, change in the family system can affect change on any one individual member of the family.

Family systems theory appears reasonable as a conceptual framework for understanding individual behavior within a family context. This perspective has led to several different therapeutic approaches to treat individuals with emotional and behavioral problems within the family. The family therapy movement was fueled by a shift away from an emphasis on individual therapy and intrapsychic processes to more situational and interpersonal factors. Family systems therapy, and especially behavioral family systems therapy, has shown promise in treating alcoholism (Bessey & Borduin, 1986; Bowen, 1991; Joanning, Quinn, Thomas & Mullen, 1992; Rohrbaugh, Shoham, Spungen, & Steinglass, 1995; Shoham, Rohrbaugh, Stickle, & Jacob, 1998) and other addictions (Walitzer, 1999), anorexia nervosa (Robin, Bedway, Siegel, & Gilroy, 1996), chronic pain (Roy, 1986), domestic violence (Combrinck-Graham, 1990), coping with unplanned pregnancy (Barnett & Balak, 1986), and juvenile diabetes (Wysocki, Harris, Greco, Harvey, McDonell, Caroline, Bubb, & White, 1997). A related construct, social support, has received far more empirical support in the health behavior change arena. For example, social support showed a strong relationship to exercise habits in a study by Sallis, Hovell, Hofstetter, and Barrington (1992). In this study, more people met the American College of Sports Medicine guidelines for recommended amounts of exercise if they had more social support, fewer perceived barriers, and greater self-efficacy. Thus, tied to a focus on families is the broader issue of sources and types of social support and their effects on health behavior change. During the 1970s, the War on Poverty resulted in large-scale interventions that included preschool programs for children at risk, an emphasis on maternal health, and a proliferation of support groups. This broader approach considered individual behavior within multiple contexts, including the family.

FST aims to intervene on a broader level by examining individuals within a larger context, the family. Taking into account the effects of one individual on another within the system has made it useful in the therapeutic setting as well. Practically speaking, it is reasonable to assume that an individual is highly affected by the surrounding environment and other people in it. The importance of defining roles and appropriate behaviors is crucial for developing communication skills and support for behavior change, specifically within the health domain.

Social Ecology Model

In addition to the theoretical orientations to modifying an individual's behavior that reflect varying degrees of cognitive, affective, behavioral, and familial processes, ecological and community approaches are receiving more attention in the field of health behavior change (Stokols, 1996). Given the communal nature of rural settings, community and ecological models may be of special relevance to rural populations.

Social ecology recognizes that individual behavior is often a function of the larger social context of the individual's life (Breslow, 1996). A person's desire to modify his or her own behavior may be impeded by economic, social, and cultural constraints (Stokols, 1996). Control over one's health can be exercised "individually or collectively, the former for one's own self and the latter for the community" (Breslow, 1996; p. 253). Thus, in order to engage in health promotion, the social ecological approach suggests combining individually focused efforts at change with modifications of the physical and social surroundings. Early social ecological researchers delineated the various levels of the environment that interact with individual factors that ultimately affect health behavior. These levels of stratification were developed primarily because the size and complexity of the system as a whole appeared too daunting to approach scientifically (Richard, Potvin, Kishchuk, Prlic, & Green, 1996). Bronfenbrenner (1979), identified the following three levels: (1) microsystem—interpersonal relationships in various settings such as the home, school, and work; (2) mesosystem—interactions between these various settings; and (3) exosystem—large social systems including the impact of economic and political forces. Moos (1979), outlined four sets of environmental factors that apply to health promotion: (1) physical settings—features of the natural environment; (2) organizational—size and function of the organization; (3) human aggregate—sociodemographic or sociocultural characteristics of the population in a given region; and (4) social climate—aspects of the environment that provide an indication of the amount of social support in the environment.

As outlined in the previous sections, most health promotion theories currently employed by researchers and practitioners address the interactional nature of the individual in his or her environments. The social ecology approach takes it one step further by arguing that any effort at health promotion must target behavior change at multiple levels and create a health-promoting climate in the social environment in which people make health-related decisions. Breslow (1996) asserts that efforts should be directed at "breaking into these microsocial [e.g., peer groups, family] and macrosocial [e.g., public health departments, churches] environments . . . and creating a milieu in which people readily can, and often do, adopt behaviors that are favorable to health" (p. 256). He noted two classic examples of environmental deficiencies—fluoridating the water and adding potassium iodide to salt—to illustrate the importance of social ecology in improving the quality of the individual's health. However, he also illustrated that health-compromising behaviors such as tobacco consumption and obesity are also affected by the social milieu. Using a social ecological approach, efforts to eradicate cigarette use would target the individual's behavior (in the form of smoking cessation programs), the community (removing cigarette machines), and the government (laws against smoking in restaurants).

Despite the development of models promoting multilevel change, there is evidence to suggest that most health promotion efforts continue to focus only on the intrapersonal level. Richard and colleagues (Richard et al., 1996) evaluated the extent to which the ecological approach was integrated into 44 different health promotion programs. They specifically examined whether change was targeted at the individual, interpersonal, organizational, political, or community level. Their results suggest that despite evidence to the contrary, health promotion practitioners and researchers continue to target intrapersonal determinants of health rather than unhealthy aspects of the environment (Richard et al., 1996). Most researchers acknowledge the difficulty of testing hypotheses, focusing interventions, and measuring change due to intervention using a social ecological approach (Green, Richard, & Potvin, 1996). Notwithstanding these limitations, sustained health behavior change is unlikely to occur in an environment that does not promote and reinforce such behavior.

Media Advocacy

Although not developed as a theory or model *per se*, media advocacy bridges the gap between health communication and applied behavior analysis theories and models of community change. Wallack (1990) asserts that the media usually represents health as an individual responsibility rather than the product of societal forces. Media role models and advertising add to the promotion of instant gratification and the minimization of risks associated with this gratification. Wallack states that since "mass media generally serve to reinforce existing arrangements and not stimulate social change, this perspective on health promotion represents a challenge to public health professionals and the mass media to rethink basic assumptions" (p. 148). Decrying the power of tobacco, alcohol, and other forces of illness in our society, he calls for more creative and aggressive approaches in health promotion's use of the media.

Wallack and Dorfman (1996) suggest a reorientation away from traditional antecedent-oriented health communication approaches toward a methodology that promotes public agenda setting away from individual and toward societal responsibility for health. Media advocacy maintains a "behavior change" focus— only in this case, the behavior of policymakers rather than individual citizens. Members of the legislative and executive branches of government at all levels are responsible for structuring environments that reinforce healthy behaviors and make unhealthy ones less appealing. Policymakers are unlikely to fund universal child health care, raise taxes on tobacco and alcohol, pass clean indoor air acts, control gun sales, or promote conservation without pressure from the public to do so.

Describing social marketing and other efforts to change individual behaviors as too narrow, Wallack notes that appeals to change health behavior in exchange for a reinforcer that is delayed until the distant future will have little success in maintaining that behavior change. Media advocacy thus integrates the antecedent-oriented techniques of social marketing and health communication with policy changes and other methods that make up contingency management. Media advocacy implies the use of both positive and negative reinforcement as an integral part of health communication efforts. These efforts often emphasize confronting "illness industries": manufacturers of tobacco, alcohol, weapons, and other products that contribute to the population's morbidity and mortality.

Community Self-Control

Social ecological approaches to understanding behavior imply broad-based behavior change efforts sufficient to realize a public health impact. Yet maintenance of such change may still require intensive efforts on a community-by-community basis. Complementing social ecology are *locality development* (Rothman, 1968) and community self-control models that parallel individual models of behavior change. Anticipating many of the key elements of social learning theory, Frederick Kanfer (1975) suggested that for individual behavior change to be effective, self-control must be achieved through mechanisms of monitoring self, setting achievable goals, experimenting with the behavior change, evaluating self, and reinforcing self. Roland Bunch (1982), a specialist in agricultural extension, outlined a community organization approach to achieving effective and responsible change in rural communities that incorporates Kanfer's individual self-control processes as well as key elements of applied behavior analysis, social learning theory, and the transtheoretical model.

Bunch's approach, scaled to small groups or small communities of farmers, serves as a model not only for agricultural settings but for health and other sectors as well. For example, Bunch asserts that sustained efforts for community improvement will only occur if there are recognizable successes. Therefore, initial targets must be achievable and accomplished with technology that is affordable and available. The amount of participation in a community program will depend on the enthusiasm that is created through setting appropriate, achievable goals, as well as other factors: starting a program at a small and simple level involving only individuals in the action stage who are initially enthusiastic about it; initially conducting small-scale trials rather than trying to conquer an entire community or region at once; and constantly monitoring the participation in the program by the entire community.

Community Self-Control Processes

Once an area is selected for the program, the planning process begins, with community participation as part and parcel of this process. The planning process, according to Bunch, consists of five basic stages: (1) gathering information; (2) establishing goals and objectives; (3) developing a work plan; (4) preparing the budget; and (5) monitoring. Information gathering will occur with respect to many of the same factors discussed above. In this case, however, the local residents themselves should be doing the information gathering. The data gathered during this phase will then inform the goals and objectives that are established. Goals should be established in a consensus fashion, much in the same way that individual efforts of behavior change negotiate a contingency contract with a professional. Once specific objectives are decided on, constant monitoring of a program's activities is essential to maintain a continuing flow of feedback for purposes of self-correction or reinforcement.

Selecting Early Adopters and Target Behaviors

Once goals and objectives are established, the intervention procedure may begin. For example, participants may choose protection from pesticides as a priority. The health planner would work with them to identify the most appropriate technology for accomplishing this. Once this technology is identified, however, the program should be launched with only a small number of individuals already in the action stage. Once success is achieved with this smaller group, expansion to the larger community will prove much easier.

Behavioral Trials and Vicarious Learning

Before the developer promotes widespread adoption of a new behavior, participants should be encouraged to engage in small-scale, time-limited experimentation with it. They then can experience for themselves how much effort is required as well as what costs are incurred and what benefits are produced. Perceived health improvement will serve as a feedback mechanism for adjusting the participant's behavior or for reinforcing it and promoting the vicarious learning to others. Written behavioral contracts developed with the early adopters may increase their commitment to staying with the new technologies, and should it be successful, teaching them to many of their neighbors. Mass media can be used to back up the face-to-face communication messages as well.

Although many theories focus on the individual as the unit of change, interventions aimed at affecting a larger group or community are crucial for broad-scale intervention and health enhancement. By incorporating many of the tenets of individually based theories (e.g., goal setting, evaluation, reinforcement, monitoring), community-based programs hold much promise. In addition to a solid theoretical framework, it is necessary to focus attention on the process of implementation. Following Bunch's (1982) approach of starting small and gradually expanding to a community wide effort will also increase chances of successful health promotion.

Suitability for and Adaptability of Theories, Models, and Methods to Rural Settings

The preceding presentation of 10 health promotion theories is clearly not an exhaustive list of theories available for intervention development and analysis. Space considerations required us to select specific theories with some demonstrated utility in the field of health promotion and with potential suitability for rural settings. In addition, much more information is available on each of the theories presented in this chapter than space would permit. (Readers should consult the appropriate references for more information.)

Several of the theories identified have been employed in rural settings, or at minimum suggest some degree of suitability. Application of the TRA in rural settings is limited. Martin and

Newman (1990) applied the TRA to understand seat belt safety with a sample of urban and rural women. Differences were found in attitudes and subjective norms between intenders and nonintenders to use seat belts. DeBarr, Ritzel, Wright, & Kittleson (1998) measured constructs in the TRA to identify the single best predictor of adolescents' behavioral intention regarding safe farm tractor operation. Subjects were 215 Future Farmers of America students (15 to 18 years old) from 10 schools in Illinois. The single strongest predictor of adolescents' behavioral intention was the TRA construct subjective norm. More recent studies have used the TPB to understand rural health behavior. Lee, Jenkins, & Westaby (1997) used the TPB to identify factors that influence parents' decisions to expose children to major hazards on family farms. The study was conducted in Wisconsin with 1,255 dairy farm fathers. Attitudes, subjective norms, and perceived control were found to account for 75% of the variance in fathers' behavioral intentions. Behavioral beliefs were stronger predictors of behavioral intentions than subjective norms or perceived control.

Findings from a number of studies support the applicability of the stages of change model to rural settings: dietary change (Campbell, Symons, Demark-Wahnefield, Polhamus, Bernhardt, McClelland, & Washington, 1998; Kristal, Goldenhar, Muldoon, & Morton, 1997), smoking behavior (Schorling, Roach, Siegel, Baturka, Hunt, Guterbock, & Steward, 1997), mammography (Mah & Bryant, 1997), and exercise (Potvin, Gauvin, & Nguyen, 1997). Most of the applications of the TTM to rural health behaviors have been cross-sectional in design. More studies are needed to evaluate the efficacy of stage-based interventions for promoting rural health. Existing studies suggest the usefulness of evaluating stage progression; movement in intention to change is not tapped by traditional outcome measures, thereby obscuring intervention effects.

Several of the theories are less well developed in the health promotion research, let alone in rural health settings. Nevertheless, the extended kin and close family ties that typically characterize rural families make family systems theory one of several appropriate models to consider when examining health behaviors in rural settings. Roles within the family have the potential to influence health behaviors. Community organizing has the potential to build community-based alternatives to health care that are currently lacking in rural areas (Denham, Quinn, & Gamble, 1998) and to provide the foundation for intercommunity collaborations where resources are limited (Chang-Yit, Lippert, & Thielges, 1992). The social ecology approach suggests targeting the interconnectedness of an individual's existence to his or her environment, thus fitting nicely into a prominent feature of rural settings—man's connection with the land, the family, and the community. More than any other theory, McGuire's communication–persuasion theory has guided the field of public health communication, while media advocacy has served as a vehicle for change. This holds special relevance for health promotion in rural settings, where mass media must be relied on to a greater extent than where populations are concentrated and can be contacted relatively easily. In addition, McGuire's theory is much more relevant for complex and more risky rural behaviors such as the safe operation of farm machinery than for relatively simple ones such as bringing a child in for immunizations.

An intriguing new model has been suggested and evaluated in rural communities that builds on an individually focused model (i.e., transtheoretical model) and a community-based model. As the name suggests, "community readiness" refers to the extent to which a community is ready to address a particular concern (Plested, Smitham, Jumper-Thurman, Oetting, & Edwards, 1999). Nine stages of community readiness have been examined in the context of drug use prevention: no awareness, denial, vague awareness, preplanning, preparation, initiation, stabilization, confirmation-expansion, and professionalism. Similar to the transtheoretical model, rural settings at different levels of readiness require different types of interventions. For example, those in the earlier stages require more information about how the behavior fits into the existing social milieu. If, as many of the theories suggest, individual behavior change cannot be maintained without some type of environmental, familial, or other support, then an imperative need is to understand whether the "community" is ready to support those changes.

References

Academy for Educational Development. (1995). *A tool box for building health communication capacity*. Washington DC: Author.

Ackerman, N. J. (1984). *A theory of family systems*. New York: Gardner Press.

Ajzen, I. (1985). From intentions to actions: A theory of planned behavior. In J. Kuhl & J. Beckmann (Eds.), *Action-control: From cognition to behavior* (pp. 11–39). Heidelberg: Springer.

Ajzen, I. (1987). Attitudes, traits, and actions: Dispositional prediction of behavior in personality and social psychology. In L. Berkowitz (Ed.), *Advances in experimental social psychology* (Vol. 20; pp. 1–63). San Diego: Academic Press.

Ajzen, I., & Madden, T. (1986). Prediction of goal-directed behavior: Attitudes, intentions, and perceived behavioral control. *Journal of Experimental Social Psychology, 22*, 453–474.

Bandura, A. (1969). *Principles of behavioral modification*. New York: Holt, Rinehart & Wintston.

Bandura, A. (1974). Behavior theory and the models of man. *American Psychologist, 29*, 859–869.

Bandura, A. (1977). *Social learning theory*. Englewood Cliffs, NJ: Prentice-Hall.

Bandura, A. (1986). *Social foundations of thought and action. A social cognitive theory*. Englewood Cliffs, NJ: Prentice-Hall.

Barnett, P., & Balak, D. W. (1986). Unplanned pregnancy in young women: Managing treatment. *Social Casework, 67*(8), 484–489.

Bateson, G., Jackson, D., Haley, J., & Weakland, J. (1956). Toward a theory of schizophrenia. *Behavioral Science, 1*, 251–264.

Bessey, J. L., & Borduin, C. M. (1986). Application of behavioral principles within family systems therapy: A conceptual framework for the treatment of alcoholism. *Deviant Behavior, 7*(4), 357–369.

Bingham, C. R., & Crockett, L. J. (1996). Longitudinal adjustment patterns of boys and girls experiencing early, middle, and late sexual intercourse. *Developmental Psychology, 32*, 647–658.

Blue, C. L. (1995). The predictive capacity of the theory of reasoned action and the theory of planned behavior in exercise research: an integrated literature review. *Research in Nursing and Health, 18*, 105–121.

Bowen, M. (1966). The use of family theory in clinical practice. *Comprehensive Psychiatry, 7*, 345–374.

Bowen, M. (1991). Alcoholism as viewed through family systems. *Family Dynamics of Addiction Quarterly, 1*(1), 94–102.

Breslow, L. (1996). Social ecological strategies for promoting health lifestyles. *American Journal of Health Promotion, 10*(4), 253–257.

Bronfenbrenner, U. (1979). *The ecology of human development: Experiments by nature and design*. Cambridge, MA: Harvard University Press.

Bunch, R. (1982). *Two ears of corn: A guide to people-centered agricultural improvement*. Oklahoma City: World Neighbors.

Campbell, M. K., Symons, M., Demark-Wahnefried, W., Polhamus, B., Bernhardt, J. M., McClelland, J. W., & Washington, C. (1998). Stages of change and psychosocial correlates of fruit and vegetable consumption among rural African-American church members. *American Journal of Health Promotion, 12*, 185–191.

Chang-Yit, L., Lippert, M., & Thielges, I. (1992). Model for rural collaboration for AIDS education: A case study. *Family & Community Health, 15*(3), 62–69

Clarke, L. L., & Miller, M. K. (1990). The character and prospects of rural community health and medical care. In A. E. Luloff & L. E. Swanson (Eds.), *American rural communities* (pp. 74–105). Boulder, CO: Westview Press.

Combrinck-Graham, L. (1990). Developments in family systems theory and research. *Journal of the American Academy of Child & Adolescent Psychiatry, 29*(4), 501–512.

DeBarr, K. A., Ritzel, D. O., Wright, W. R., & Kittleson, M. J. (1998). Friends and family: Implications for youth tractor safety. *Journal of Safety Research, 29*, 87–95.

Denham, A., Quinn, S. C., & Gamble, D. (1998). Community organizing for health promotion in the rural south: An exploration of community competence. *Family & Community Health, 21*(1), 1–21.

Denton, W. (1990). A family systems analysis of DSM-III-R. *Journal of Marital and Family Therapy, 16*(2), 113–125.

DiClemente, C. C., & Prochaska, J. O. (1982). Self-change and therapy change of smoking behavior: A comparison of processes of change in cessation and maintenance. *Addictive Behaviors, 7*, 133–142.

DiClemente, C. C., Prochaska, J. O., Fairhurst, S. K., Velicer, W. F., Velasquez, M. M., & Rossi, J. S. (1991). The process of smoking cessation: An analysis of precontemplation, contemplation, and preparation stages of change. *Journal of Consulting and Clinical Psychology, 59*, 295–304.

Dijkstra, A., De Vries, H., Roijackers, J., & van Breukelen, G. (1998). Tailoring information to enhance quitting in smokers with low motivation to quit: three basic efficacy questions. *Health Psychology, 17*, 513–519.

Dishman, R. K. (1991). Increasing and maintaining exercise and physical activity. *Behavior Therapy, 22*, 345–378.

Donovan, J. E., Jessor, R., & Costa, F. M. (1991). Adolescent health behavior and conventionality-unconventionality: An extension of problem-behavior theory. *Health Psychology, 10*, 52–61.

Dulany, D. E. (1968). Awareness, rules, and propositional control: A confrontation with S-R behavior theory. In T. R. Dixon & D. L. Horton (Eds.), *Verbal behavior and general behavior theory*. Englewood Cliffs, NJ: Prentice-Hall.

Elder, J., Geller, G., Hovell, M., & Mayer, J. (1994). *Motivating health behavior.* New York: Delmar.

Fishbein, M. (1967). *Readings in attitude theory and measurement.* New York: Wiley.

Fishbein, M. (1993). Introduction. In D. J. Terry, C.Gallois, & M. McCamish (Eds.), *The theory of reasoned action: Its application to AIDS preventive behaviour.* Oxford, England: Pergamon Press.

Fishbein, M., & Ajzen, I. (1975). *Belief, attitude, intention and behavior: An introduction to theory and research.* Reading, MA: Addison-Wesley.

Fuguitt, G. V. (1995). Population change in non-metropolitan America. In E. N. Castle (Ed.), *The changing American countryside: Rural people and places* (pp. 77–100). Lawrence: University of Kansas Press.

Galston, W. A., & Baehler, K. J. (1995). *Rural development in the United States: Connecting theory, practice, and possibilities.* Washington, DC: Island Press.

Godin, G., & Kok, G. (1996). The theory of planned behavior: A review of its applications to health-related behaviors. *American Journal of Health Promotion, 11,* 87–98.

Gottlieb, N. H., Galavotti, C., McCuan, R. A., & McAlister, A. L. (1990). Specification of a social-cognitive model predicting smoking cessation in a Mexican-American population: A prospective study. *Cognitive Therapy and Research, 14,* 529–542.

Graeff, J., Elder, J., & Booth, E. (1993). *Communications for health behavior change: A developing country perspective.* San Francisco: Jossey-Bass.

Green, L. W., Richard, L., & Potvin, L. (1996). Ecological foundations of health promotion. *American Journal of Health Promotion, 10*(4), 270–281.

Greene, G. W., & Rossi, S. R. (1998). Stages of change for reducing dietary fat intake over 18 months. *Journal of the American Dietetic Association, 98,* 529–534.

Guerin, P. J., & Chabot, D. R. (1997). Development of family systems theory. In P. L. Wachtel & S. B. Messer (Eds.), *Theories of psychotherapy* (pp. 181–225). Washington, DC: American Psychological Association.

Haley, J. (1976). *Problem-solving therapy.* San Francisco: Jossey-Bass.

Hart, J. F. (1995). "Rural" and "farm" no longer mean the same. In E. N. Castle (Ed.), *The changing American countryside: Rural people and places* (pp. 63–76). Lawrence: University of Kansas Press.

Herzog, T. A., Abrams, D. B., Emmons, K. M., Linnan, L. A., & Shaddel, W. G. (1999). Do processes of change predict smoking stage movements? A prospective analysis of the transtheoretical model. *Health Psychology, 18*(4), 369–375.

Janis, I. L., & Mann, L. (1968). A conflict-theory approach to attitude change and decision making. In A. Greenwald, T. Brook, & T. Ostrom (Eds.), *Psy-chological foundations of attitudes* (pp. 327–360). New York: Academic Press.

Janis, I. L., & Mann, L. (1977). *Decision making: A psychological analysis of conflict, choice, and commitment.* New York: The Free Press.

Jessor, R. (1987). Problem-behavior theory, psychological development, and adolescent problem drinking. *British Journal of Addiction, 82,* 331–342.

Jessor, R. (1991). Risk behavior in adolescence: A psychosocial framework for understanding and action. *Journal of Adolescent Health, 12,* 597–605.

Jessor, R., & Jessor, S. L. (1973). A social psychology of marijuana use: Longitudinal studies of high school and college youth. *Journal of Personality and Social Psychology, 26,* 1–15.

Jessor, R., Donovan, J. E., & Costa, F. M. (1991). *Beyond adolescence.* New York: Cambridge University Press.

Joanning, H., Quinn, W., Thomas, F., & Mullen, R. (1992). Treating adolescent drug abuse: A comparison of family systems therapy, group therapy, and family drug education. *Journal of Marital & Family Therapy, 18*(4), 345–356.

Kanfer, F. H. (1975). Self-management methods. In F. H. Kanfer & A. P. Goldstein (Eds.), *Helping people change* (pp. 309–316). New York: Pergamon.

Kristal, A. R., Goldenhar, L., Muldoon, J., & Morton, R. F. (1997). Evaluation of a supermarket intervention to increase consumption of fruits and vegetables. *American Journal of Health Promotion, 11,* 422–425.

Lee, B. C., Jenkins, L. S., & Westaby, J. D. (1997). Factors influencing exposure of children to major hazards on family farms. *Journal of Rural Health, 13,* 206–215.

Luloff, A. E., & Swanson, L. E. (1990). Introduction. In A. E. Luloff & L. E. Swanson (Eds.), *American rural communities* (pp. 1–18). Boulder, CO: Westview Press.

Mah, Z., & Bryant, H. E. (1997). The role of past mammography and future intentions in screening mammography usage. *Cancer Detection and Prevention, 21,* 213–220.

Marcus, B. H., Bock, B. C., Pinto, B. M., Forsyth, L. H., Roberts, M. B., & Traficante, R. M. (1998). Efficacy of an individualized, motivationally-tailored physical activity intervention. *Annals of Behavioral Medicine, 20,* 174–180.

Martin, G. L., & Newman, I. M. (1990). Women as motivators in the use of safety belts. *Health Values, 14,* 37–47.

McGuire, W. J. (1989). Theoretical foundations of campaigns. In R. E. Rice & C. K. Atkin (Eds.), *Public communication campaigns* (2nd ed.; pp. 43–65). Newbury Park, CA: Sage Publications.

Miller, L. K. (1980). *Principles of everyday behavior analysis.* Monterey, CA: Brooks/Cole.

Minuchin, S. (1974). *Families and family therapy.* Cambridge, MA: Harvard University Press.

Minuchin, S., Lee, W., & Simon, G. M. (1996). *Mastering family therapy: Journeys of growth and transformation*. New York: Wiley.

Moore, S., Barling, N., & Hood, B. (1998). Predicting testicular and breast self-examination behaviour: A test of the theory of reasoned action. *Behaviour Change, 15*, 41–49.

Moos, R. H. (1979). Social ecological perspectives on health. In G. C. Stone, F. Cohen, & N. E. Alder (Eds.), *Health psychology—a handbook: Theories, applications, and challenges of a psychological approach to the health care system* (pp. 523–547). San Francisco: Jossey-Bass.

Plested, B., Smitham, D. M., Jumper-Thurman, P. Oetting, E. R., & Edwards, R. W. (1999). Readiness for drug use prevention in rural minority communities. *Substance Use and Misuse, 34*(4&5), 521–544.

Potvin, L., Gauvin, L., & Nguyen, N. M. (1997). Prevalence of stages of change for physical activity in rural, suburban, and inner-city communities. *Journal of Community Health, 22*, 1–13.

Prochaska, J. O. (1979). *Systems of psychotherapy: A transtheoretical analysis*. Homewood, IL: Dorsey Press.

Prochaska, J. O., & DiClemente, C. C. (1983). Stages and processes of self-change in smoking: Towards an integrative model of change. *Journal of Consulting and Clinical Psychology, 51*, 390–395.

Prochaska, J. O., Velicer, W. F., Guadagnoli, E,, Rossi, J. S., & DiClemente, C. C. (1991). Patterns of change: Dynamic typology applied to smoking cessation. *Multivariate Behavioral Research, 26*, 83–107.

Prochaska, J. O., & DiClemente, C. C. (1998). Towards a comprehensive, transtheoretical model of change: Stages of change and addictive behaviors. In W. R. Miller & N. Heather (Eds.), *Treating addictive behaviors* (2nd ed.; pp. 3–24). New York: Plenum Press.

Prochaska, J. O., DiClemente, C. C., Velicer, W. F., & Rossi, J. S. (1993). Standardized, individualized, interactive and personalized self-help programs for smoking cessation. *Health Psychology, 12*, 399–405.

Prochaska, J. O., Redding, C. A., Harlow, L. L., Rossi, J. S., & Velicer, W. F. (1994). The transtheoretical model of change and HIV prevention: A review. *Health Education Quarterly, 21*, 471–486.

Rakowski, W., Ehrich, B., Goldstein, M. G., Rimer, B. K., Pearlman, D. N., Clark, M. A., Velicer, W. F., & Woolverton, H. III. (1998). Increasing mammography among women aged 40–74 by use of a stage-matched, tailored intervention. *Preventive Medicine, 27*(5, Pt. 1), 748–756.

Richard, L., Potvin, L., Kishchuk, N., Prlic, H., & Green, L. W. (1996). Assessment of the integration of the ecological approach in health promotion programs. *American Journal of Health Promotion, 10*(4), 318–328.

Ricketts, T.C. III, Johnson-Webb, K. D., & Randolph, R. K. (1999). Populations and places in rural America. In T. C. Ricketts (Ed.), *Rural health in the United States* (pp. 7–24). New York: Oxford University Press.

Robin, A. L., Bedway, M., Siegel, P. T., & Gilroy, M. (1996). Therapy for adolescent anorexia nervosa: Addressing cognitions, feelings, and the family's role. In E. D. Hibbs & P. S. Jensen (Eds), *Psychosocial treatments for child and adolescent disorders: Empirically based strategies for clinical practice* (pp. 239–259). Washington, DC: American Psychological Association.

Rochín, R. I., & Marroquin, E. (1997). *Rural Latino resources: A national guide*. East Lansing, MI: Julian Samora Research Institute.

Rohrbaugh, M., Shoham, V., Spungen, C., & Steinglass, P. (1995). Family systems therapy in practice: A systemic couples therapy for problem drinking. In B. M. Bongar, & L. E. Beutler (Eds), *Comprehensive textbook of psychotherapy: Theory and practice* (Vol. 1; pp. 228–253). New York: Oxford University Press.

Rothman, J. (1968). Three models of social work practice. In National Conference on Social Welfare (Ed.), *Social work practice: Proceedings*. New York: Columbia University Press.

Roy, R. (1986). A problem-centered family systems approaching treating chronic pain. In A. D. Holzman & D. C. Turk (Eds.), *Pain management: A handbook of psychological treatment approaches*. Pergamon general psychology series (Vol. 136; pp. 113–130). New York: Pergamon Press.

Salamon, S. (1995). The rural people of the Midwest. In E. N. Castle (Ed.), *The changing American countryside: Rural people and places* (pp. 352–368). Lawrence: University of Kansas Press.

Sallis, J. F., Hovell, M., Hofstetter, C. R., & Barrington, E. (1992). Explanation of vigorous physical activity during two years using social learning variables. *Social Science Medicine, 34*(1), 25–32.

Schorling, J. B., Roach, J., Siegel, M., Baturka, N., Hunt, D. E., Guterbock, T. M., & Stewart, H. L. (1997). A trial of church-based smoking cessation interventions for rural African Americans. *Preventive Medicine, 26*, 92–101.

Schulman, M.D., Evensen, C.T., Runyan, C.W., Cohen, L.R., & Dunn, K.A. (1997). Farm work is dangerous for teens: Agricultural hazards and injuries among North Carolina teens. *The Journal of Rural Health, 13(4)*, 295-305.

Shoham, V., Rohrbaugh, M. J, Stickle, T. R., & Jacob, T. (1998). Demand-withdraw couple interaction moderates retention in cognitive-behavioral versus family-systems treatments for alcoholism. *Journal of Family Psychology, 12*(4), 557–577.

Skinner, B. F. (1953). *Science and human behavior*. New York: Macmillan.

Stokols, D. (1996). Translating social ecological theory into guidelines for community health promotion.

American Journal of Health Promotion, 10(4), 282–298.

Sullivan, H. S. (1953). *Interpersonal theory of psychiatry.* New York: W.W. Norton.

U.S. Census Bureau. (1990). *Statistical abstract of the United States.* Washington, DC: Government Printing Office.

U.S. Department of Health and Human Services. (1989). *Making health communication programs work: A planner's guide.* (NIH publication no. 89-1493). Washington, DC: U.S. Government Printing Office.

Velicer, W. F., DiClemente, C. C., Prochaska, J. O., & Brandenburg, N. (1985). A decisional balance measure for predicting smoking cessation. *Journal of Personality and Social Psychology, 48,* 1279–1289.

Velicer, W. F., DiClementi, C. C., Rossi, J. S., & Prochaska, J. O. (1990). Relapse situations and self-efficacy: An integrative model. *Addictive Behaviors, 15,* 271–283.

Wallack, L., & Dorfman, L. (1996). Media advocacy: A strategy for advancing policy and promoting health. *Health Education Quarterly, 23*(3), 293–317.

Wallack, L. (1990). Two approaches to health promotion in the mass media. *World Health Forum, 11*(2), 143–154.

Witte, K., Peterson, T. R., Vallabhan, S., & Stephenson, M. T. (1993). Preventing tractor-related injuries and deaths in rural populations: Using a persuasive health message framework in formative evaluation research. *International Quarterly of Community Health Education, 13*(3), 219–251.

Wysocki, T., Harris, M. A., Greco, P., Harvey, L. M., McDonell, K. D., Caroline, L. E., Bubb, J., & White, N. H. (1997). Social validity of support group and behavior therapy interventions for families of adolescents with insulin-dependent diabetes mellitus. *Journal of Pediatric Psychology, 22*(5), 635–649.

18

Health Education

Community-Based Models

GAIL E. SOUARE

In 1997, approximately 54 million Americans lived in rural areas (Beale, 1999), and over 22 million rural Americans lived in areas that are designated primary care health professional shortage areas (Health Resources and Services Administration, 1998). In 1996, only 53.7% of residents in rural areas had private health insurance, while 62.5% of urban residents had such coverage (Vistnes & Monheit, 1997). According to the Agency for Health Care Policy and Research, 28% of the adult rural population reported their health status as fair to poor (Health Care Financing Administration, 1995). Chronic conditions were also more prevalent in rural areas, with 46.7% of rural adults reporting a chronic condition compared with 39.2% of the urban population (Braden & Beauregard, 1994). These data underscore the need for community health education programs that can improve awareness, promote changes in health behavior and increase access to rural health care.

The U.S. government defines "rural" as places of 2,500 or more inhabitants outside of urbanized areas or counties outside the boundaries of metropolitan areas that have no cities larger than 50,000 residents (Rickers, Johnson-Web, & Taylor, 1998). There are also a number of counties and areas that are more sparsely populated.

Places with six or fewer persons per square mile are considered frontier counties or communities, and 383 counties, excluding Alaska boroughs, met these criteria in 1995 (Ricketrs *et al.*, 1998). These areas have unique problems in health service delivery and access to health care.

Whites make up almost 83% of the rural population (Beale, 1999), African Americans make up 9%, and Hispanics 5.4% (Rogers, 1999). Median household income is generally lower in rural areas ($18,527) compared with urban areas ($25,944) (Ghelfi, 1999). More than 25% of rural counties had poverty levels of 20% or more in each census from 1960 through 1990 (Beale, 1996). Twenty-four percent of rural children live in poverty (Dagata, 1999). This high incidence reflects inadequate income among African American, Hispanic, and American Indian and Alaska Native residents (Native Americans). Although poverty rates have dropped substantially in counties where most of the poor are African American, much less progress has been made in the Hispanic and Native American areas (Beale, 1996).

The level of black poverty is over 50% in more than 100 rural counties that which are predominantly African American (Beale, 1996). Likewise, there are many persistently poor Hispanic rural areas. Although Hispanics have a relatively high employment rate compared with other rural groups, limited full-time year-round work for men, incomplete high school educa-

GAIL E. SOUARE • Alliance Healthcare Foundation, San Diego, California 92123.

Handbook of Rural Health, edited by Loue and Quill. Kluwer Academic/Plenum Publishers, New York, 2001.

315

tion, and early childbearing are factors that contribute to persistent poverty (Beale, 1996).

Among Native Americans in 35 counties and Alaskan county equivalents, there is high overall poverty stemming from chronically low income levels. Native Americans are the least numerous of the persistent-poverty groups, with a total population of 558,000. The average poverty rate for Native Americans is 51%, and over three-fourths of the poor households are severely impoverished with incomes less than 75% of the official poverty level. In Native American areas, poor children outnumber poor seniors by four to one (Beale, 1996).

Private health insurance coverage is less available through employment in rural areas due to the characteristics of the rural employment market. Farm families are less likely than other working families to work for employers who contribute toward health insurance (Frenzen, 1994).

Elderly people, ages 65 or older, make up 18% of the rural population compared with 15% of the urban population (Rogers, 1999). Thus, Medicare is a significant source for funding rural health care. Medicare beneficiaries are somewhat more likely than the general population to reside in rural areas. According to the Health Care Financing Administration (1995), while approximately 20% of the general population lived in rural areas, over 23% of Medicare beneficiaries resided in rural areas.

Most rural hospitals are small, with fewer than 100 beds (American Hospital Association, 1997) and are heavily dependent on Medicare revenues (Project HOPE, 1998). From 1980 to 1991, a total of 363 rural hospitals closed (American Hospital Association, 1992) followed by another 77 hospitals between 1991 and 1997 (Georgia Department of Health and Human Services, 1998). Although the number of hospitals has declined, the number of rural health centers (RHCs) has increased. RHCs are located in underserved areas and are entitled to Medicare and Medicaid reimbursement at a higher rate than other health care providers. From 1990 to 1997, 2,600 new RHCs were certified (Cheh & Thompson, 1997). In addition, 60% of all federally funded community health centers, which provide primary health care services in medically underserved areas, are located in rural areas (Bureau of Primary Care, Health Resources and Services Administration, 1999).

Challenges to Rural Community-Based Health Education Programs

Factors affecting the development and delivery of rural community-based health education programs are complex. To improve health, individuals must modify preventive health practices and increase their use of health care services. According to Konyha (1975), "modifications will be made only when (a) rural people are aware of the behavioral changes that need to be made, (b) learn how to make these changes, (c) perceive both the economic and social incentives for doing so, (d) and have access to adequate health treatment services and facilities when they are needed" (p. 340).

Effective interventions in rural health care encounter a number of barriers. These include the difficulty of maintaining confidentiality and anonymity in small communities, diverse cultural makeup, numerous languages, and overwhelming distances (Crown, Duncan, Hurrell, Ootoova Trembly, & Yazdanmehr, 1993). In addition, in communities where economic survival is the key priority, some diseases are not given high priority (Hooks, Ugarte, Silsby, Brown, Weinman, Fernandez, Foxwell, Newton, & Connally, 1996).

In many rural communities, language is a great barrier (Hooks et al., 1996). Often, the educator and the client do not speak a common language. This is marked in work with Native American populations. Also, there is an absence of a common language about some diseases, such as HIV/AIDS, in populations where a native language is spoken at home and English is taught in school. This may create a communication barrier between generations (Crown et al., 1993).

Many rural residents are employed in agricultural production. Barriers to providing agricultural health and safety education include the absence of effective regulations; distrust of those investigating an injury or illness; long working hours, often dawn until dusk; and the unpredictability of the agricultural cycle (Randolph & Migliozzi, 1993; Hooks et al., 1996).

Providing health education to seasonal farmworkers faces additional problems. Often it is difficult to identify seasonal farmworkers. The number and size of camps may be overwhelming and difficult to penetrate. Conversations must be conducted in person rather than over the telephone or by mail. Bilingual and bicultural translators are scarce. Support from growers in gaining access to seasonal farmworkers is also a challenge (Hooks *et al.*, 1996).

Cultural backgrounds of Native American populations are not readily apparent to casual observers and it is not easy to describe cultural values (Dignan, Sharp, Blinson, Michielutte, Konan, Bell, & Lane, 1994). Many Native Americans, especially those on reservations, live in a distinct culture. They tend to value the group and extended family over the individual. They are oriented toward the present rather than the future, and they emphasize cooperation and sharing as opposed to competition and individual ownership. Native Americans have a holistic view of health and illness, with health a balance between the mental, spiritual, and physical (Dignan *et al.*, 1994).

Diversity of Rural Populations

Although all persons living in rural areas may face the same barriers to receiving health care, such as distance, a lack of transportation, and isolation, rural communities are not homogeneous. Most documented rural health education programs have targeted ethnic minority groups, such as Native Americans or African Americans, although the majority of the rural population is Caucasian. Although whites may face the same health risks, they too have cultural preferences that are important.

At-risk youth

Much of the literature on health education models targeting rural youth concerns agricultural production and occupational safety. While agricultural safety is important for rural youth, many other issues need to be addressed. Rural youth are often at-risk for many of the same health problems as adolescents in urban areas, such as HIV/AIDS, sexually transmitted diseases (STDs), substance abuse, teen pregnancy, and violence.

Seniors

Seniors living in a rural environment confront a special set of problems. In addition to the health care issues that result from the natural aging process, seniors do not have access to services available to urban dwellers, such as home health care, assisted living facilities, education and support for caregivers, and support for independent living. In addition, senior day care facilities, which offer respite to caregivers of seniors affected by Alzheimer's or dementia, may not be available. Rural seniors may be more vulnerable to substance abuse and problems with prescription medications. And because of their isolation, they may be more vulnerable to financial, physical, and emotional abuse by caregivers and family members.

Immigrant Populations

Immigrants have long been a critical part of agricultural production in rural communities. Many are employed as agricultural workers who migrate from place to place to seek seasonal agricultural employment. These groups are primarily Mexican, Haitian, and Puerto Rican. Factors that affect the health behavior and needs of these immigrants are complex. Barriers to health care include poverty, poor living conditions, educational barriers, limited English language skills, lack of transportation, limited office hours at clinics, and frequent relocation. Immigrants also have different cultural perceptions about health, including how and where to seek health care services and the use of traditional medicine (Candelaria, Campbell, Lyons, Elder, & Villaseñor, 1998).

Developing Rural Health Education Models

Components of Effective Models

To be effective, a good rural health education model must gain buy in and ownership from the community. Rural health education programs should focus on the community rather than the individual workplace (Randolph & Migliozzi, 1993), keeping in mind the social interactions that exist in small communities (Nelson, 1993). In Native American cultures, this might mean presenting to elders and tribal councils for approval. In African American communities, this could mean involving church and community leaders. In rural farming communities, working with established and trusted organizations or community groups, such as the U.S. Cooperative Extension Service agents, agricultural dealers, and rural health care providers, may be necessary. It is important first to conduct a community analysis to determine who are the community leaders that can bring support and lend credibility to a program.

During a community analysis, it is important to engage other resources that have credibility in the community, such as the U.S. Cooperative Extension Service, 4-H groups, women's groups, church groups, and schools. Program implementers should recruit the participation of influential community leaders, such as agricultural nurses, cooperative extension leaders, local health departments, physicians, farming implement dealers, and elected officials as well as interested community members.

Who Is Delivering Health Education?

Rural hospitals have the potential to make significant contributions to the health promotion needs of the community. Some have established primary prevention strategies, thereby lowering community health care costs (Dorresteyn-Stevens, 1993). Other organizations can also participate in community health education activities. Some of these include the U.S. Cooperative Extension Service, schools, and nonprofit organizations, either through direct education or recruiting community members as lay health advisers.

U.S. Cooperative Extension Service

The U.S. Cooperative Extension Service (CES) is a government-supported agency, established in 1914, to take knowledge directly to the people of rural America by providing health education to rural communities (Konyha, 1975).

It maintains a network of agents to serve as educators for rural people in their communities and farms (Chapman, Schuler, Skolaas, & Wilkinson, 1995a). The CES is a unique partnership of federal, state, and county governments. The system has survived and grown because of its objectivity and its ability to adapt short-range priorities to longer-range public needs. Its strength is its ability to use research findings to develop effective rural health care education programs (Konyha, 1975).

CES educational activities are designed to respond to locally identified needs and objectives. The CES is also a neutral agency that can provide a forum on rural health issues. CES educators support health care professionals by providing leadership in several areas of health education: occupational health and safety; nutrition; preventive health; screening for cancer, hypertension and diabetes, drug abuse; STDs; community health services and facilities; and the safer use of pesticides. CES also provides educational activities through 4-H groups, extension homemaker clubs, agricultural producers, special interest groups, forums, and local community decision makers (Konyha, 1975).

Schools

In schools, agricultural education instructors working in general or comprehensive high schools and often collaborating with CES agents teach tractor and machinery safety to farm youth working in production agriculture. Classes emphasize hazard recognition, identification, and prevention. Instructors use both classroom teaching and laboratory-based instruction, conducting on-site visits and hazard inspections, continuing education classes, and safety-related public events. One strength of this approach is that the instructors are well established in the communities and committed to the issues. The classes often involve farmers, farm equipment dealers, agricultural suppliers, and medical personnel in the teaching activities (Chapman, Schuler, Wilkinson, & Skjolaas, 1995b).

Nonprofit Organizations

One nonprofit organization is Farm Safety 4 Kids, whose mission is to prevent farm-related childhood injuries, health risks, and fatalities. According to McNab (1998), farm injuries and accidental deaths of children fall into three categories: (1) accidents involving machinery; (2) accidents involving livestock; and (3) accidents involving recreation and play. The organization provides brochures and videos and offers teaching ideas on farm safety. Some examples of teaching ideas include coordinating a farm safety camp that demonstrates tractor accidents, livestock safety, and farm hazards; hosting a "safety sleuth hazard hunt" on a local farm and demonstrating ways to prevent those hazards; and developing farm safety slogans or stickers (McNab, 1998). Other nonprofit organizations include churches and local chapters of state and national organizations.

Lay Health Advisers

Providing access to health care services for the hard-to-reach rural population is a challenge. Eng, Parker, and Harlan (1997) describe the hard-to-reach population as "people who are hard for health care providers to find, meet, talk with, and consequently, serve" (p. 413). One way to overcome this difficulty is to use lay health advisers (LHAs). Lay health advisers are individuals who are indigenous to their community and who consent to serve as a link between community members and the service delivery system (Service & Salber, 1979). Examples of terms used for LHAs in health promotion and disease prevention programs are community health advisers, community health workers, health aides, natural helpers, navigators, paraprofessionals, peer educators, promoters, and outreach workers (Eng & Young, 1992).

Ideally, LHAs should be recruited from the target population. They should be persons who are well respected by the community and able to reach the target population. If delivered by a community member, the health education messages may be in a more culturally appropriate format. LHAs should be able to communicate with community members in their own language and at their level. During development of educational materials, input from LHAs is important to ensure that the materials are culturally appropriate. Last, because they are members of the community and recognized experts, they

may continue to serve as an important community resource even if the program ends.

The LHA approach is guided by the assumption that behavior is influenced by social norms. LHAs can comfort people who know and trust them, providing a community-based system of care and social support that complements formal systems of care. And given that LHAs share the language, religious beliefs, and other social and ethnic characteristics, they may be more successful in reaching underserved, ethnic minority populations (Eng et al., 1997).

LHA interventions do, however, have some inherent limitations. They do not equally benefit all members of the target community. Persons who are unaccustomed to or fearful of asking for assistance, who are unaware of where to seek help, who value privacy and independence, or who are social isolates have limited opportunities for contact with LHAs. Concern that LHAs may divulge personal information may deter some individuals. In addition, because LHAs are not professionals, some people may not consider their advice to be reliable (Earp, Viadro, Vincus, Altpeter, Flax, Mayne, & Eng, 1997).

Health Behavior Change Models

When developing rural health education programs, it is important to incorporate behavioral health models during both the planning and implementation stages. Six models are commonly used in developing health promotion strategies (Elder, Apodaca, Parra-Medina, & Zuñiga de Nuncio, 1998): the health belief model (Becker, 1974; Janz & Becker, 1984), the PRECEDE model (Green, 1984; Green & Kreuter, 1991), the social cognitive theory (Bandura, 1986, 1989, 1991), the theory of reasoned action (Ajzen & Fishbein, 1980; Fishbein, 1980; Fishbein & Azjen, 1975), behavior analysis (Elder, Geller, Hovell & Mayer, 1994; Skinner, 1953), and the transtheoretical or stages of change model (Prochaska & DiClemente, 1983). For a more detailed overview of these models, see "Strategies for Health Education: Theoretical Models" in the *Handbook of Immigrant Health* by Elder et al. (1998).

Although the six models are different, all have

similarities. They maintain that to effect behavior change, an individual must: (1) have a positive intention or predisposition to change behavior; (2) face a minimum of environmental barriers to the change; (3) possess the necessary skills to make the change; (4) believe the change will have positive outcomes; (5) believe that the change conforms to accepted societal norms; (6) believe that the behavior is consistent with his or her self-image; (7) believe that the behavior change will have a positive effect; and (8) receive appropriate cues or enablers to act on the changes (Elder *et al.*, 1998).

Examples of Innovative Rural Health Programs

The following are some examples of innovative rural health education programs covering a broad spectrum of health issues and incorporating a variety of behavioral change models. The programs, targeting a broad spectrum of populations, incorporate cultural competency as an underlying framework for program design. The examples included in this chapter demonstrate examples of the lay health adviser model, culturally appropriate programs targeting African American and Native American women for breast or cervical cancer screening, programs using the media to reach rural communities, programs for Native Americans that use traditional communication methods, peer educator models, occupational safety programs and a school-based dental health education.

The Save Our Sisters Project

The Save Our Sisters Project (SOS), conducted by the School of Public Health at the University of North Carolina (UNC), was a pilot demonstration project to increase annual mammograms among older African American women. The target population was 2,600 African American women between the ages of 50 and 74 residing in a rural county in North Carolina. SOS recruited and trained 64 African American women who were identified as "natural helpers" to act as lay health advisers (Eng, 1993).

SOS used the PRECEDE model, which focuses on perceived and actual barriers to behavior change as the theoretical basis for the intervention. The barriers identified included costs, physicians not ordering exams, personal fears about mammograms, lack of self-efficacy to ask the physician for a mammogram, and lack of confidence in the accuracy of radiology. The implementation model used was the social change model, which stresses increasing community competence.

First, SOS hired a coordinator. The coordinator was identified in the community as a natural helper and had lived in the county for more than 50 years. She, in turn, formed a community advisory group to identify groups to which the women belonged. Second, the program conducted a communitywide survey, followed by a telephone survey and focus groups to identify perceived needs. Third, they used the focus groups to identify existing resources and assets in the community. Last, the program trained natural helpers after determining that women turned to other women they knew for advice. The trained natural helpers, called community health advisers (CHAs), easily identified by lapel pins, went out into the community to educate other women about breast cancer. They contacted women through personal acquaintances, at church meetings and in the workplace. The most frequently discussed topics were mammograms, how to become a community health worker, cervical cancer, and Pap tests.

One month after graduation, the first group of CHAs met with the project coordinator and UNC staff to develop an annual action plan. They decided to organize five committees to: (1) train more CHAs; (2) obtain financial sponsorship from African American churches to fund one mammogram a month for women who could not afford to pay; (3) promote understanding of the regulations of the health care system and assist women in accessing health care services; (4) offer support groups for African American women with breast cancer; and (5) establish a speakers' bureau. The CHAs also produced a breast cancer screening video for older black women. After four groups had graduated, the training committee concluded that the number of CHAs was adequate and recruiting was discontinued. Evaluation of the program was limited to process evaluation; no outcome evaluation was found in the literature.

The North Carolina Breast Cancer Screening Program

The North Carolina Breast Cancer Screening Program (NC-BCSP) was also developed by the University of North Carolina (UNC) to reach older African American rural women and increase the use of mammography screening. The target population was African American women ages 50 and older in five rural counties in eastern North Carolina (Earp, Altpeter, Mayne, Viadro & O'Malley, 1995).

Like the Save Our Sisters Program, the NC-BCSP used the PRECEDE model to design the intervention but added the social ecological perspective, which recognizes that health-related behaviors have mutually influencing and multiple reinforcing determinants. In this case, the program looked at multiple influences that are barriers to seeking mammograms. These included predisposing factors such as attitudes, knowledge, and beliefs; enabling factors related to the health care system and access to services; and reinforcing factors such as encouragement, support, and social norms of the community.

The health belief and the stages of change models were used to design the intervention. The health belief model focused on susceptibility, severity, perceived barriers, perceived benefits, and cues to action. The stages of change model focused on moving clients through the stages of precontemplation, contemplation, preparation, action, and maintenance.

NC-BCSP formed a collaboration of state and local public health agencies and universities under the direction of a team at the University of North Carolina Lineberger Comprehensive Cancer Center. The team consisted of 40 full- and part-time staff and students from three universities. NC-BCSP followed the Community Health Advocacy Program and Save Our Sisters models to identify and train community members to act as lay health advocates.

The NC-BCSP program had three complementary intervention components: InReach, OutReach, and Access. The first component, InReach, addressed the enabling factors that had been identified. These included the need to re-structure clinic policies and procedures, offer continuing provider education, reorganize inefficient mammography referral patterns, and remove organizational barriers that prevented referrals. Program staff visited local providers and health departments, collected data, gave recommendations, and identified leaders in the medical community.

The second component, OutReach, focused on predisposing and reinforcing factors and addressed attitudes and perceptions about screening and cancer. By using community outreach specialists (lay health advisers), the program attempted to enhance awareness and generate community support for screenings. They conducted focus groups to identify concerns about breast cancer; printed messages tailored to the population, which addressed the different stages women go through when getting mammograms; and formed community advisory groups of influential community members. The program hired and trained three full-time community outreach specialists. These were older women who lived in the counties and shared the same background as the target population. The community outreach specialists were supervised by local health departments and community health centers. In each county, the program established lay health adviser networks, formed local community advisory groups, and developed culturally appropriate stages of change messages.

The third component, Access, concentrated on building the capacity of local agencies. Efforts were aimed at overcoming barriers by providing linkages with local groups to provide transportation, increasing the quality of mammograms, lowering the price of mammograms, and providing low-cost or free screening. They formed connections with state agencies responsible for health among women and minorities. The program established a 25-member advisory committee with representatives from health departments, volunteer breast cancer and health advocacy groups, and professional and government organizations. The advisory committee reviewed program progress, offered advice and recommendations, identified methods of generating resources, and developed strategies for institutionalizing the program.

Results from baseline data collected in 1994 and follow-up interviews in 1996 suggest that the lay health advisers made a difference in breast cancer screening rates. From 1994 to 1996, self-reported mammography use increased 17% in intervention counties compared with 11% in comparison counties. The intervention appeared to have the greatest effect among older African American women with family incomes under $12,000 per year. Older low-income women reported a 22% increase in mammography screenings from 37% in 1994 to 59% in 1996 compared with 11% in comparison counties (Earp, O'Malley, & Rauscher, 1999; "What Difference?" 1999).

The North Carolina Native American Cervical Cancer Prevention Project

The North Carolina Native American Cervical Cancer Prevention Project was a five-year National Cancer Institute–funded public health education program designed to reduce mortality from cervical cancer among Native American women (Dignan *et al.*, 1994). The target population was women, ages 18 and older, from the Cherokee and Lumbee tribes in North Carolina. These are two distinct tribes with no common background. Although the Cherokees are a rural tribe, both geographically and culturally isolated, the Lumbees live in mixed urban and rural areas and are assimilated into the diverse communities.

The goal of the program was to increase screening and follow-up of abnormal Pap smears. To accomplish this, the program developed an individualized health education program guided by the health belief model, social learning theory, self-efficacy theory, and the PRECEDE model.

Following the planning phase, which used the PRECEDE model, the program conducted a community analysis through focus groups and key informant interviews. The focus groups, through which information about the emotional reactions to cervical cancer prevention was collected, had different results in the two populations. The Lumbee focus groups were easier to recruit and their discussions were more open and free-flowing. The program encountered difficulties organizing focus groups among Cherokee women. There was also considerable hesitation in the focus groups, possibly because open

criticism of others is not accepted in the Cherokee culture. However, the results of the focus groups showed that both groups shared values, including family, and believed that good health is important for parenting. Health care providers were considered helpful and professional but ineffective in treating cancer. Early detection of cancer was viewed negatively because of the resulting emotional turmoil. Also, both communities made it clear that telling success stories about women with cancer in the target population would be valuable to the education program.

Key informants, including tribal leaders, business owners, managers, workers, elected officials, teachers, and health care professionals were also interviewed. The findings showed that awareness of cervical cancer was limited, the population was skeptical of the value of treatment, and many were fearful of harm resulting from treatment. The health care providers identified barriers to treatment that included the isolated rural environment and the need to travel out of town to receive specialty care.

Based on the results of the community analysis, the education program was designed to be delivered in a face-to-face format in the participants' homes by local Native American lay health educators. Using local Native American women increased the likelihood of mutual trust between health educator and participants. The lay health educators helped to ensure that Native American cultural values were respected. In addition, using Native American lay health educators allowed the program to integrate subtle communication patterns, which were not apparent to outsiders, into the program. The design allowed the program to be individualized, increased personal interaction, and provided a relaxed atmosphere where women would be more likely to ask questions.

The program delivered the following messages: (1) cervical cancer can be cured; (2) cervical cancer can be detected early with a Pap smear; and (3) the earlier cervical cancer is detected, the easier it is to cure. To ensure cultural appropriateness, tribal officials reviewed and approved all the education materials. One female lay health educator was hired from each target population. Both were given the title "project guides" which conveyed the message that they were there to guide women through the process of learning about cervical cancer and Pap smears and taking action to obtain screenings. The project guides were also required to observe a Pap smear procedure at a local medical center. Following one week of training, each guide was observed in the field to guarantee that the program could be effectively translated to a field setting. The project guides also provided feedback in the development of education materials and presentation.

Each participant received two in-home visits by a project guide. During the first visit, participants completed a health risk appraisal that had been designed by the Centers for Disease Control (CDC) for the Native American population. The guides then asked a series of questions about perceived barriers. They used portable video players to show a video, which was introduced with a story, followed by a discussion. At the end of the visit, the guides provided a personalized folder with printed educational materials and set up a second appointment. On the second visit, the guides reviewed the information presented in the first visit, conducted a process evaluation of printed materials given at the first visit, and asked women about scheduling a Pap smear. If follow-up was needed, the guides contacted the project office and further action was developed. To reinforce the program, guides sent periodic reminders about Pap smears and cards for birthdays and special events.

Conclusions drawn from this program indicate that the cultural backgrounds of Native American populations were not readily apparent to casual observers and it was not easy to describe cultural values. Therefore, it was important to develop a culturally sensitive program using focus groups, key informant interviews, involvement of tribal officials in the review of educational materials, and the participation of resident women in the design and implementation of the intervention. There were marked differences between and within the two target populations. Older women tended to remain passive during the first visit and waited for the second to ask questions, whereas younger women responded during the initial visit.

An evaluation of the Cherokee population program found that the educational program had positive effects on knowledge and the behavior of participants (Dignan, Michielutte, Blinson,

Wells, Case, Sharp, Davis, Konen & McQuellon, 1996). Although there was no difference between the control and intervention groups for intent to get a Pap smear, women who participated in both the pretest survey and intervention were more likely than control subjects to report receiving a Pap smear in the past year (71% versus 65%). Among the women who participated only in the intervention, 76% reported a Pap smear in the past year versus 62.5% of the control group. Therefore, whether they participated in the pretest or not, women participating in the intervention were more likely than the control group to report a Pap smear in the past year.

The Forsyth County Project

The Forsyth County Project was a five-year community-based health educational program on cervical cancer targeting 25,000 African American women, 18 years of age and older, in Forsyth County, North Carolina. The program had two components. The first involved using mass media to increase awareness of cervical cancer as a means to motivate women to seek Pap smears. The second supplemented the media campaign by providing direct education to groups of women about cervical cancer and the importance of prevention and screening (Dignan, Beal, Michielutte, Sharp, Daniels, & Young, 1990).

To develop the direct education component, the program began with an assessment that involved a community analysis, focus groups, a leadership survey of the African American community, and a random digit–dialed telephone survey. The results indicated that women felt fearful and fatalistic about cancer. Little hope was held for those with cancer, and divine intervention was viewed as the most likely cure. The focus groups, which were led by African American female professionals, found that women valued health, especially as it related to their families. Most women knew about the Pap smear but had little knowledge about its role in early detection of cervical cancer. Although they expressed fear and fatalism about cancer, with no difference between types of cancer, the women agreed that early diagnosis and treatment were important. Some of the barriers identified during the community analysis included competing financial obligations and transportation. Women were more likely to make appointments for specific complaints than for preventive screening, disliked the waiting time for non-acute problems, and viewed physicians as bearers of bad news.

The authors (Dignan et al., 1990) developed and pretested the program in urban and small rural communities as well as with a focus group from rural Forsyth County. The pretest revealed that although participants were fearful, apprehensive, and had a fatalistic view of cancer, they wanted to learn more about prevention. There was also significant misinformation about Pap smears and cancer prevention. Following the pretest, the authors found it was necessary to adjust the reading level and refine the printed materials to avoid unfamiliar and difficult technical terms.

The program developed a flip chart and instructional packet, which were used as teaching aids for the educational program. They chose the flip chart format over 35mm slides because it was easily portable and did not require cumbersome technical equipment. The instructional packet included an assortment of pamphlets dealing with reproductive health issues; a booklet explaining Pap smears, cervical cancer diagnosis, and treatment; and a postage-paid card to request additional materials. The educational program included a session on healthy lifestyles; another on the importance of early detection, female reproductive anatomy, key points about cervical cancer and the Pap smear, a description of the Pap smear and pelvic exam, and an explanation of the results; and a third on the barriers to obtaining Pap smears. The presentations were made to civic, social, and church groups across the county.

The program was successful, with the majority of women who participated and who had not had a recent Pap smear reporting they planned to get one. It was also found that women who feared cancer experienced increased anxiety when they attended the program, especially those who had not had a Pap smear for many years. Women who had hysterectomies, postmenopausal women, and those who were no longer sexually active often believed they no longer needed Pap smears and were hesitant to attend workshops, assuming the materials did not pertain to them. To include high-risk women over 50, it was necessary to make greater efforts to reach women in the workplace, retirement centers, and senior citizen groups, as well as the socially isolated.

Health Is a Community Affair Campaign/Door-to-Door Project

The Health Is a Community Affair Campaign, also known as the Door-to-Door Project, is an innovative way to promote HIV/AIDS prevention in the Canadian Northwest Territories (NWT). The NWT face several unique barriers: they cover an area larger than the country of India; most communities are accessible only by air; and the population is culturally diverse, with various Inuit, Dene, Metis, and nonnative groups. One of the major health issues identified in the NWT was sexually transmitted diseases (STDs), especially HIV/AIDS (Crown et al., 1993).

Although the government had a strong HIV/AIDS component in the school curriculum, it was not consistently followed in all schools. In addition, for persons living with AIDS or HIV (PLWAs/HIV), specialized support systems were extremely limited due to immense distances and the sparsely populated areas. Many PLWAs/HIV left the northern territories due to lack of services while some southern PLWA/HIV sought refuge and anonymity in NWT communities.

The campaign involved using community health representatives (CHRs), community committees, and teleconferences to bring HIV/AIDS information to communities across the NWT. The CHRs were specially trained to deliver health information and training programs in three communities. Elsewhere, approximately 65 community members (canvassers) were hired and trained only to deliver health information messages and pamphlets on AIDS and STD prevention.

Health education materials were culturally relevant, written in simple language, and translated into local languages. They included illustrations to deliver the message. In addition to accurate translations, the authors found that using someone from the community who spoke the native language added credibility to the message. In Dene communities, protocol was an important issue; therefore, tribal chiefs and councils were informed about the campaign and their approval was requested. In all communities, canvassers went first to homes of seniors to gain support from the elders before approaching the council.

The program leaders developed five pamphlets in English, French, and four different Inukitut languages. They also produced cassettes with text translated into Dene, a language that is primarily oral. Later, at the request of the communities, cassettes were also produced in Inukitut. Due to time constraints and varying educational levels of the canvassers and the CHRs, the three-day training sessions were tailored to fit their needs more closely. The training covered the history and goals of the campaign, the role of the canvassers and CHRs, the information in the campaign packages, concerns about health issues, and skill development to facilitate delivery of the campaign messages door-to-door. At a time when no one in the NWT disclosed HIV status, a PLWA assisted with the training.

In addition to door-to-door health education, community radio stations informed the public, canvassers and CHRs gave community and school presentations, and posters were displayed. In the northern communities, an Inuit woman living with AIDS spoke to groups and on the radio. Because her storytelling was so powerful, the canvassers documented her presentations in local reports.

Evaluation showed that because the CHRs and canvassers were able to communicate in the local languages and were members of the community, they were crucial to the organization and implementation of the program. For these rural communities, use of the media to reinforce the community presentations was also very important. Showing respect for elders and gaining appropriate support from local councils promoted community ownership and receptivity. Last, by associating a face and a story of a PLWA, the message became more real to the community.

Community Health Promotion Grants Program

In 1990, the Kaiser Family Foundation funded the Community Health Promotion Grants Program (CHPGP), a major initiative to foster community-based health promotion activities (Cheadle, Pearson, Wagner, Psaty, Diehr, & Koepsell, 1995). One of the grantees, an unnamed Native American reservation in one of the plains states, listed alcohol abuse, particularly among youth, as its primary target for intervention. The reservation had a population of 21,900, with 2,200 youth between the ages of 12 and 17. Ninety-one percent of the residents were Native American, the unemployment rate was 70%, and 35% lived below the federal poverty level. The initial impetus for the program was an epidemic of suicides—more than 20 times the national rate in 1985.

The overall goal of the program was to reduce the rate of alcohol and drug use among youth ages 21 and younger. Specific goals were all alcohol- related: (1) to reduce the reported prevalence of binge drinking; (2) to delay the reported onset of first use of alcohol by one year; and (3) to decrease the number of 12th graders who drove a vehicle after drinking. The community formed a coalition that included representatives from the health department, schools, private nonprofessional organizations, and government. Interventions, which targeted youth, parents, and the community as a whole, included classes, skills development programs, alcohol- and drug-free events, and public campaigns.

The components of the program included:

- *Children are People:* educational support groups for children, ages 6 to 12, from alcoholic and drug-dependent families
- *Home Education Parties:* small-group gatherings in individual homes to discuss and learn about healthy life choices
- *Just Say No Club:* a national club for children, ages 7 to 14, who pledge to lead a drug-free life
- *Preparing for the Drug-Free Years:* an education program for parents of children in grades four to seven
- *School-Based Prevention Program:* prevention education and skill-building programs provided by program staff on request from local school districts
- *STEP:* educational programs for parents of children in three age groups: ages five and younger, 6 to 12, and adolescents

- *SMILE:* skill-building activities for junior and senior high school students
- *Summer Youth Employment Program:* a hiring program among students to assist with summer youth activities
- *Super Tots:* healthy living skills for 3- to 4-year-olds through structured play activities
- *Youth Leadership Training:* one-day sessions providing information, education, and training for local students on current issues
- *Proud to be Drug-Free Carnival:* an annual carnival supported by local school districts to raise community awareness about substance-abuse issues
- *Community Fun Days:* fun activities for families implemented by neighborhood committees

A self-administered school survey was used to examine the effectiveness of the program in reducing the rate of substance use, particularly alcohol, by adolescents. The results showed that alcohol, marijuana, and smokeless tobacco use declined substantially among Native Americans living on the reservation. Two of the three substance use measures targeted by the program—binge drinking and driving after drinking—showed an absolute decline nearly twice the overall average. However, the declines for alcohol use were not significantly greater than in the comparison groups. In smokeless tobacco, the decline among participants was both large and statistically significant. However, evaluating the success of the program had some limitations, which included the inability to identify a true control community, small sample sizes, and difficulty assessing behaviors of high school dropouts, typically high substance users.

Pathways

Pathways was a culturally appropriate obesity prevention intervention for third-, fourth-, and fifth-grade Native American schoolchildren and their families, which promoted increased physical activity and healthful eating. The intervention was developed in 1993 through a collaboration of universities and Native American nations, schools, and families. It focused on individual, behavioral, and environmental

factors, combining the social learning theory with Native American customs and practices (Davis *et al.*, 1999).

The program established five principles for developing the components of the intervention. Each component was: (1) culturally acceptable; (2) complementary; (3) successful using strategies identified during the feasibility stage; (4) sustainable; and (5) standardized. The collaborative team also identified seven indigenous learning modes: (1) storytelling; (2) metaphoric; (3) holistic; (4) trial and error; (5) play; (6) cooperation; and (7) reflection. The curriculum was based on the social learning theory model and used seven of the major theoretical concepts: modeling, social support, opportunities, knowledge, self-efficacy, skill building, and reinforcement.

Pathways developed a comprehensive curriculum to meet three goals: develop high levels of activity for all children regardless of skill level, promote aerobic activities and development of skills necessary for sports, and be practical and easy to implement. The program was implemented by developing a classroom curriculum, increasing exercise during physical education classes, educating family members, and providing low-fat food choices through the school food service.

The children were provided with activities and stories that followed the journeys of two fictional Native American children. The children could relate to the fictional characters who served as models for a healthier lifestyle. The curriculum combined cultural stories, indigenous learning modes, hands-on activities, and games. To gain teacher support, Pathways created an instructor's manual designed to coordinate the intervention. The manual contained an outline of the project and a series of detailed lesson plans that complemented core subjects such as social studies and language arts. The lessons were designed to run twice a week for six weeks in both the fall and spring. Pathways staff provided the teachers with training in use of the curriculum.

The program increased the children's activities and energy expenditure by increasing the frequency and quality of physical education and activity breaks, including recess periods. The program also encouranged positive attitudes toward physical activity and developing motor skills through lessons that promoted motor skill development and traditional physical fitness. During a "Personal Best Day," the children tested and monitored their improvement in fitness. With the assistance of the Native American advisory group, Pathways also developed games that were derived from traditional games of each of the participating nations, which were incorporated into the curriculum.

The program leaders also involved families by informing them of the program goals and intervention strategy, and worked with families to reinforce behaviors through school-based events and sadvisory groups.

Last, the program worked with the school nutrition program to lower the amount of fat in the school meals. Pathways staff developed nutrient guidelines that complied with the U.S. Department of Agriculture school meal regulations. They also provided training for school service workers, including skill-building techniques for food service workers in planning, purchasing, preparing, and serving lower-fat meals, and visited the school kitchens to demonstrate how to best implement specific behavioral guidelines.

Evaluation of this program revealed that there were limitations to using a standardized intervention across cultures and a need for flexibility in program implementation in different settings. Although there was an increase in teachers' satisfaction with the lessons, students' enjoyment of the lessons, and attainment of knowledge and skills as the weeks advanced, some teachers neglected to follow the complete lesson plans. They reported that although they enjoyed teaching the curriculum, the lessons were too long and they wanted more flexibility in how to teach the curriculum.

American Indian Women's Talking Circle

The American Indian Women's Talking Circle was a cervical cancer screening and prevention program conducted at eight Native American clinics in California in 1994. California is home to 242,000 Native Americans, the second-largest number residing in any state. The target population was Native American women, 18 years and older. The intervention was conducted at eight sites, four rural and four urban, with 400 women, half of whom served as controls (Hodge, Fredericks, & Rodriguez, 1996).

The goals of this program were to increase cancer prevention knowledge, establish positive attitudes toward screenings, reduce risk factors, increase the proportion of women receiving cervical cancer screening at clinics, increase the percentage of postmenopausal women receiving regular cervical cancer screening, and increase the percentage of Native American women who receive appropriate follow-up services for abnormal Pap examinations.

The program was based on the talking circle format, a method of intragroup communication that is well known in traditional Native American communities. In talking circles, small groups meet periodically to share information, provide support, or solve problems. A facilitator opens the session with a traditional story followed by discussion. An arrow, feather, or talisman is passed around the circle and the person holding it has the floor with no fear of challenge or interruption. The facilitator builds on the use of traditional oral narrative, using stories, legends, or myths. For this intervention, the facilitator began with a traditional story, introduced a health topic, and then opened the floor for discussion.

The program conducted a community analysis by facilitating 10 focus groups, both urban and rural, to determine health beliefs, barriers to screening, experiences with Pap smears, and patterns of patient–physician communication. The findings from the focus groups confirmed less frequent use of cancer prevention measures and cultural barriers. Modesty, taboos, and use of traditional healing practices were important elements in the Native American culture. Witching, evil spirits, and elements beyond an individual's control were believed to be possible causes of cancer. Barriers to follow-up that were identified included beliefs about illness, educational levels, concepts about disease, communication styles, and fear of cancer treatment. Preventive health was found to have a low priority compared with economic needs.

Although multiple tribal affiliations make it difficult to design culture-specific intervention programs, some common traits were identified through the focus groups. These included the importance of family, community, cooperation, and harmony with nature. Native language, native healers, and reliance on traditional ceremonies were considered important in the healing process. Native American women reported they went to traditional healers for "female problems" associated with pregnancy and childbirth.

One barrier identified through the focus groups was that cancer is a relatively new illness in the Native American population and has only recently received recognition as a health problem requiring intervention (American Indian Health Care Association, 1989; Rhoades, Hammond, Welty, Handler, & Amber, 1987). In addition, both race and poverty affect survival rates due to lack of access to adequate care and the lack of culturally appropriate screening and intervention programs (McWhorter, Schatzkin, Horm, & Brown, 1988).

The focus group placed a high value on cultural sensitivity in the patient–provider relationship; however, this was complicated by communication problems and health care system barriers that included lengthy delays between screening and referrals for follow-up. Other issues were staff turnover and long waits for clinic appointments. Cultural differences between the non-Indian providers and Indian patients were also perceived as a barrier. Reportedly, providers either did not understand or ignored the issue of modesty and interpreted the indirect communication style of Native Americans as an unwillingness to participate in their own care. Community members viewed providers as too busy or uncaring to listen to symptoms.

The educational program used the talking circle format, mixed with traditional Native American stories, as a vehicle to provide cancer education and to improve adherence to cancer screening. The results indicated that women who participated in the intervention displayed more consistent and substantial improvement in their levels of knowledge of cervical cancer and cancer in general compared with the control groups. The evaluation also indicated that differences between the intervention and control groups were generally consistent among urban and rural women. Findings showed that women responded favorably to the culturally framed education project. The health-related information was accepted, and the women reported tak-ing action because the information was viewed as meaningful and culturally appropriate (Hodge, Stubbs, & Fredericks, 1999).

Volunteer Peer Counselors to Increase Breast-Feeding Duration Among Rural Low-Income Women

A volunteer peer-counseling program designed to increase the duration of breast-feeding targeted 143 rural low-income pregnant and postpartum women in Iowa who qualified for the Women, Infants, and Children (WIC) program. The intervention was designed to match participants one-on-one with volunteer peer support during pregnancy and postpartum (Schafer, Vogel, Viegas, & Hausafus, 1998).

The volunteers, who received nine hours of training, were recruited from the community. Requirements for the volunteer peer counselors included a successful breast-feeding experience of at least three months, willingness to attend ongoing training, and availability to work with participants in person and by phone. Their training covered general nutrition, advantages of breast-feeding, basic management of breast-feeding, confidentiality and record-keeping skills, home visit skills, listening and communication skills, and goal setting. Educational materials for use with clients included small flip charts on breast-feeding, five nutrition lessons from the state's Expanded Food and Nutrition Education Program, and six extension pamphlets on feeding babies and breast-feeding.

The program was overseen by a state coordinating committee that included the program director, a lactation consultant, two representatives from the state WIC office, nutrition and health specialists, WIC directors, and local project coordinators from each county. Other collaborating members included hospital and clinic-based medical personnel, social service staff, and members of the target communities.

A total of 94 volunteers were trained and worked with clients. Local WIC clinics referred 241 potential participants, of which 143 requested a peer counselor. Eighty-two percent of the intervention group compared with 31% of the control group women initiated breast-feeding. Mean duration of breast-feeding for the intervention group was 5.7 weeks; it was 2.5

weeks for the control group. At four weeks, 56% of intervention and 10% of the control group women were still breast-feeding.

Wisconsin Farmers' Cancer Control Program

The Wisconsin Farmers' Cancer Control Program was a peer-educational program targeting white rural third-graders about the importance of sun protection against skin cancer. Farmers and their families, due to the nature of their occupations, have high exposure to the sun and are therefore at a higher risk of developing skin cancer. By educating third-graders, the program hoped the message would reach the entire family (Reding, Fischer, Gunderson, Lappe, Anderson, & Calvert, 1996).

Through the Future Farmers of America association (FFA), teenagers were trained as peer facilitators to provide sun protection education to third-graders. The FFA is a national association of high school agriculture students who are preparing for careers in agriculture or related fields. The FFA often uses peer education to teach younger children agricultural principles. A one-day peer educator training was given to 217 teen peer educators in 39 FFA chapters throughout Wisconsin. The peer educators learned about the anatomy of skin, skin cancer, the sun, sun damage, and the importance of protecting skin from the sun.

During the months of April and May 1993, the peer educators gave presentations to over 2,000 third-graders using "The Children's Guide to Sun Protection K–3," developed by the American Academy of Dermatology and the American Cancer Society. There was information on the anatomy of skin, skin cancer, and the importance of protecting skin from the sun. Third-graders received two 30- to 40-minute sessions in a one-week period. The students were given sun protection activity sheets that could be taken home along with other materials to share with the family. A survey, which included 20 knowledge-based questions, was given to the children to follow up on the educational sessions.

The survey was administered to 3,142 third-graders and completed by 85% of them. It found no difference between the control and intervention groups on presurvey questions; however, the postintervention surveys found that the latter had an increase in knowledge on 90% of the questions.

The change in behavior and attitude of the peer facilitators was also assessed at the end of the one-day training session and again six months later. It was found that 30% of the peer educators improved their overall scores on the knowledge questions even though the majority of the teens were already familiar with the information. On behavior change questions, there was an increase in the percentage of peer educators who reported they were likely to practice the desired behavior.

A Hearing Conservation Program for Wisconsin Youth Working in Agriculture

The Hearing Conservation Program was a multicomponent educational intervention to increase use of hearing protection devices (HPD) by adolescents. The target population was identified as at risk for hearing loss because adolescents who live and work on farms may be exposed to loud noise from farm equipment and other equipment on a regular basis. The program was conducted at 34 schools in rural Wisconsin with 753 students who were randomly assigned to either the intervention or the control group (Knobloch & Broste, 1998).

The students received an educational intervention that spanned four school years, from 1992 to 1996, including three summers. The design of the educational program was based on the health belief model, especially the "cues to action" necessary to begin a health-related behavior, and on the theory of self-efficacy, which states that one must believe in one's ability to perform a behavior. The cues to action included giving the students hearing protection devices to try out during the first two years as well as yearly hearing tests. Based on the theory of self-efficacy, students were given time to try out and correctly fit the hearing protection devices so they could become proficient at the intended behavior.

In addition to the HPDs and hearing tests, the program offered classroom-style education, including the basics of anatomy and physiology of the ear, taped testimonials from young farmers, and demonstrations of music that was missing certain frequencies. Additional "cues to action" included periodic school visits, direct mailings, and noise-level assessments conducted by the students at their own home.

The results of the evaluation showed that 81% of the intervention students would use HPDs compared with 43% of the control group. Students reported that three factors had the most influence in their decisions to use HPDs: the free HPDs, the yearly exams, and the educational materials mailed to their homes. The final surveys revealed that 87.5% of youth in the intervention used hearing protection devices (HPDs) at least some of the time, compared with 45% of control students.

An Educational Intervention Program for Prevention of Occupational Illness in Agricultural Workers

The Educational Intervention Program for Prevention of Occupational Illness in Agricultural Workers was a five-year program to study the efficacy of education and consultation in reducing the hazards in the swine confinement industry. The confinement system applies the principles of mass production to livestock production. As the swine are confined to a small, enclosed area, the potential for workers' exposure to airborne hazards increases. Exposed workers have a higher prevalence of respiratory syndromes. Participants were 198 Iowa farmers who conducted swine containment operations. The health education program sought to change knowledge, attitudes, and behaviors in the confinement environment and to increase the use of personal protective equipment, such as a dust mask (Ferguson, Gjerde, Mutel, Donham, Hradek, Johansen, & Merchant, 1989).

The theoretical model used to design the intervention was the health belief model. This model suggested "that individuals who believed strongly they could develop respiratory disease to occupational exposure presumably would take measures to protect themselves, while those who believed the risk to be minimal would not" (Ferguson et al., 1989, p. 36). It was anticipated "that swine confinement workers who recognized the short-term and long-term benefits gained from wearing a dust mask would be more

likely to wear an effective dust mask. Conversely, those who perceived barriers associated with dust mask use, such as cost, inconvenience, or discomfort, would be less likely to wear a mask" (Ferguson et al., 1989, p. 37). The health belief model also states knowledge is necessary but not sufficient to change behavior.

The educational component included six written units mailed to participants at two-week intervals. Participants completed a pre- and posttest for each unit. The units covered six topics: (1) confinement dusts and gases; (2) confinement and human health; (3) hog health and confinement; (4) measuring confinement dusts and gases; (5) reducing confinement dusts and gases; and (6) using respirators in confinement.

Besides providing the written materials, the program also held group meetings to facilitate discussion and to demonstrate equipment. Since the farms were scattered over great distances, the meetings were held within 40 miles of each participant's farm. The meetings consisted of a meal and social time, demonstration of testing equipment and respirators, and group problem-solving discussions related to the confinement environment. Participants were given the opportunity to try the equipment themselves. Case studies were used to generate discussion about problems associated with implementing the program's recommendations. These discussions encouraged participants to apply information they had received in the written materials.

Pre- and posttest analysis showed substantial gain in knowledge about the hazards and use of protective equipment. When tested about the recommended levels of various substances, 28% to 55% answered correctly on the pretest compared with 88% to 100% on the posttest. Participants learned that good ventilation would not solve most air-quality problems (28% pretest versus 76% posttest) and that it was wise to wear a respirator when feeding animals (62% pretest versus 100% posttest).

In follow-up among nonresponders, it was reported that the two-week interval between units was too short, despite the effort to plan the mailing to avoid the planting and harvesting seasons. However, participants who completed evaluations felt the written materials were readable and not too technical and that the pacing of the educational components was appropriate. Many reported that they planned to use dust masks more, and some planned to make environmental or housekeeping changes.

The authors concluded that, although farmers are very busy, most had read the written materials and were interested in changing their behaviors because the recommendations were relevant and the economic and health benefits were linked.

The Rural Dental Health Program

The Rural Dental Health Program, initiated in 1975 and completed in 1979, was a joint effort between the rural school district of Juniata County, Pennsylvania, and the University of Pennsylvania School of Dental Medicine (Bentley, Feldman, & Oler, 1989). The program was designed to improve the oral health status of children living in a rural underserved area. It included three components: (1) delivery of professional services; (2) preventive activities in the schools; and (3) evaluation. The effectiveness of dental public health programs is particularly important in rural areas, where access to dental care is often limited. The program identified two basic approaches to improving the oral health status of children living in areas with limited or no dental care services. Children can be treated in school-based dental practices, or communities can implement school-based health education programs that teach proven methods of improving oral health, such as hygiene, dietary management, and appropriate use of professional dental care. The high cost of preventive dentistry delivered in a professional practice environment and the lack of professional care available in many rural areas makes the first option unfeasible. Therefore, it follows that if school-based dental health programs can produce tangible health improvements, they may be particularly useful in rural areas.

Since dental public health programs are designed to prevent disease, an effective dental health program must, over the long run, contain dental disease at a level below what it otherwise would be in a target population. Proponents of school-based dental health instruction expect effective programs to gradually reduce the levels of dental caries over time.

The Rural Dental Health Program was a con-trolled, clinical program to measure the effects of a school-based dental health program on the oral health status and dental health beliefs, attitudes, and practices of rural children. The dental health education component consisted of 83 lesson plans that integrated information and principles of oral health with regular academic subjects. The oral hygiene component provided a place in the classroom for children to keep a toothbrush and floss and encouraged the children to brush daily. Teachers were allowed to implement all or part of the program components on a voluntary basis, and two health educators were available to assist the teachers, if requested.

In 1975, the Rural Dental Health Program enrolled 725 students, from kindergarten through second grade. In 1985, 463 students, 64% of the participants, were examined for dental health status and tested for dental knowledge and current health behaviors. Baseline data collected in 1975 on 262 students who were not examined in 1985 showed that this group averaged roughly the same number of deciduous decayed surfaces as the 463 who were followed-up in 1985. The results from the follow up study showed that after a six-year period, the school-based dental health program had a positive effect on oral health in a population of 15- to 19-year-old high school students' gums and lowered need for orthodontic treatment. The authors concluded that oral hygiene instruction and reinforcement and an increase in the students' ability to understand their treatment needs were key components to this effective school-based dental health education program.

Conclusions and Recommendations

Despite the seemingly large number of agencies providing rural health education, there is a dearth of published information about these programs. Many of the programs cited in this chapter were developed at the University of North Carolina, which has been very active in designing rural health education models.

The types of health issues addressed are also very limited; many published articles focus on breast and cervical cancer education or agricultural safety. Other education programs for health issues that are not adequately documented include alcohol abuse, HIV/AIDS, communicable disease (e.g., tuberculosis, hepatitis), mental health, gay and lesbian health, and nonagricultural unintended injuries. Although over 80% of the rural population is Caucasian, most published articles, with the exception of those on agricultural safety, focus on ethnic minorities. Published articles on providing health education for seasonal migrant farmworkers are virtually nonexistent. And although seniors make up 18% of the population, there are very few published articles on successful health education models for seniors and none addressing programs targeting ethnic minority elders.

Rural populations face the same social health issues as urban areas; however, these issues are exacerbated by distance and isolation. Substance abuse is not exclusive to urban areas; however, little attention has been given to health education about the risks involved with tobacco, alcohol and other drugs. In many rural areas, tobacco is a cash crop that provides income for rural families. There is little in the published literature on education programs about the dangers of alcohol, especially when driving on rural, isolated, and often dangerous roads. Few programs address the development of treatment modalities that overcome the barriers rural residents face when accessing recovery programs. The manufacture, trafficking, and abuse of drugs are increasing exponentially in rural areas; they have become the new markets for hard drugs. Growing competition and effective law enforcement in large cities is forcing drug manufacturers to relocate to remote areas to evade detection and to exploit potential consumers. As a result, methamphetamine and crack cocaine are becoming increasingly popular in rural areas. The majority of methamphetamine labs seized by law enforcement agencies are located in rural areas throughout the country (O'Dea, Murphy, & Balzer, 1997).

To improve the delivery of rural health care services, it is necessary to reduce barriers; however, many of the barriers are complex. Distance, lack of transportation, and language and cultural differences create challenges to health care providers. One way to break down some of these barriers is by providing culturally appropriate health care education to rural residents where they live and socialize.

Many of the programs cited incorporated the lay health adviser model. The use of indigenous health workers contributes to the success of rural health education programs by offering culturally sensitive outreach and support to the community. As members of the target population, LHAs possess the language skills to build trust and to disseminate culturally appropriate health care messages. And by educating community members, the LHA model increases the capacity and exchange of knowledge of community members, increasing the sustainability of programs. Using LHAs in rural health education programs also has the potential to increase outreach efforts while maintaining costs.

One of the shortcomings of the LHA model in rural settings is that much of the literature on the model focuses on ethnic minorities. Because most of the rural population is Caucasian, more research needs to be conducted on the success of this model with that population. Researchers also need to document how the model can be modified to develop health education programs for other groups, such as youth, seniors, and agricultural workers.

Finally, when designing rural health education interventions, programs should include a formative evaluation process, which may include community analysis, focus groups, key informant interviews, and pilot testing of the intervention. This process provides a framework for designing culturally appropriate and acceptable programs in the community. Involvement in the development and subsequent implementation of the program can engender long-term commitment of community members in program activities or services.

Many of the programs cited were of relatively short duration. More research must be dedicated to following longer-term programs and documenting their outcomes. No literature was found that evaluated what happens to a community when a program ends. Although the programs are designed with sustainability as an outcome, the lack of follow-up leaves a gap in their documentation. There may be unexpected long-term challenges and successes to rural health education programs that can only be addressed through surveillance of interventions over time.

References

American Hospital Association. (1992). *Hospital closures 1980 through 1991: A statistical profile*. Chicago: American Hospital Association.

American Hospital Association. (1997). *A profile of nonmetropolitan hospitals, 1991–1995* (Table 1). Chicago: AHA Center for Health Care Leadership, Section for Small or Rural Hospitals.

American Indian Health Care Association. (1989). *Urban Native American women's cancer prevention project*. St. Paul, MN: American Indian Health Care Association.

Azjen, I., & Fishbein, M. (1980). *Understanding attitudes and predicting social behavior*. Englewood Cliffs, NJ: Prentice-Hall.

Bandura, A. (1986). *Social foundations of thought and action: A social cognitive theory*. Englewood Cliffs, NJ: Prentice-Hall.

Bandura, A. (1989). Perceived self-efficacy in the exercise of personal agency. *Psychologist: Bulletin of the British Psychological Society, 10*, 411–424.

Bandura, A. (1991). A social cognitive approach to the exercise of control over AIDS infection. In R. DiClemente (Ed.), *Adolescents and AIDS: A generation in jeopardy* (pp. 1–20). Beverly Hills, CA: Sage.

Beale, C. L. (1996). The ethnic dimension of persistent poverty in rural and small-town areas. In L. L. Swanson (Ed.), *Racial/ethnic minorities in rural areas: Progress and stagnation, 1980–90* (pp. 26–32). (Agricultural economic report No. 731). U.S. Department of Agriculture: Rural Economy Division, Economic Research Service.

Beale, C. (1999). Nonmetro population rebound: Still real but diminishing. *Rural Conditions and Trends, 9*(2), 20–27, 46–51.

Becker, M. (1974). The health belief model and personal health behavior. *Health Education Monographs, 2*, 324–508.

Bentley, J., Feldman, C., & Oler, J. (1989). The rural dental health program: The long-range effect of a school-based enriched dntal health program on children's oral health. *The Journal of Rural Health, 5*(3), 231–245.

Braden, J., & Beauregard, K. (1994). Health status and access to care of rural and urban populations. *National Medical Expenditure Survey Research Findings 18*. (AHCPR pub. no. 94-0031). Rockville, MD: Public Health Service, Agency for Health Care Policy and Research.

Bureau of Primary Health Care, Health Resources and Services Administration. (1999). Community health center program. (September, 1999). [http://www.bphc.hrsa.dhhs.gov/]

Candelaria, J., Campbell, N., Lyons, G., Elder, J. P., & Villaseñor, A. (1998). Strategies for health education: Community-based methods. In S. Loue (Ed.), *Handbook of immigrant health*. New York: Plenum Press.

Chapman, L. J., Schuler, R. T., Skjolaas, C. A., & Wilkinson, T. L. (1995a). Agricultural work safety efforts by Wisconsin Extension agricultural agents. *Journal of Rural Health, 11*(4), 295–304.

Chapman, L. J., Schuler, R. T., Wilkinson, T. L., & Skjolaas, C. A. (1995b). Farm-work hazard prevention efforts by school-based agricultural education instructors. *American Journal of Industrial Medicine, 28*(4), 565–577.

Cheadle, A., Pearson, D., Wagner, E., Psaty, B. M., Diehr, P., & Koepsell, T. (1995). A community-based approach to preventing alcohol use among adolescents on an American Indian reservation. *Public Health Reports, 110*(4), 439–447.

Cheh, V., & Thompson, R. (1997). Rural health clinics: Improved access at a cost. Princeton, NJ: Mathematica Policy Research, November 25.

Crown, M., Duncan, K., Hurrell, M., Ootoova, R., Tremblay, R., & Yazdanmehr, S. (1993). Making HIV prevention work in the North. *Canadian Journal of Public Health, 84*(suppl. 1), S55–S58.

Dagata, E. M. (1999). The socioeconomic well-being of rural children lags that of urban children. *Rural Conditions and Trends, 9*(2), 85–90.

Davis, S. M., Going, S. B., Helitzer, D. L., Teufel, N. I., Snyder, P., Gittelsohn, J., Metcalfe, L., Arviso, V., Evans, M., Smyth, M., Brice, R., & Altaha, J. (1999). Pathways: A culturally appropriate obesity-prevention program for American Indian schoolchildren. *American Journal of Clinical Nutrition, 69*(suppl.), 796S–802S.

Dignan, M. B., Beal, P. E., Michielutte, R., Sharp, P. C., Daniels, L. A., & Young, L. D. (1990). Development of a direct education workshop for cervical cancer prevention in high risk women: The Forsyth County project. *Journal of Cancer Education, 5*(4), 217–223.

Dignan, M., Sharp, P., Blinson, K., Michielutte, R., Konen, J., Bell, R., & Lane, C. (1994). Development of a cervical cancer education program for Native American women in North Carolina. *Journal of Cancer Education, 9*(4), 235–242.

Dignan, M. B., Michielutte, R., Blinson, K., Wells, H. B. Case, L. D., Sharp, P., Davis, S., Konen, J., & McQuellon, R. P. (1996). Effectiveness of health education to increase screening for cervical cancer among eastern-bank Cherokee Indian Women in North Carolina. *Journal of the National Cancer Institute, 88*(22), 1670–1676.

Dorresteyn-Stevens, C. (1993). The rural hospital as a provider of health promotion programs. *The Journal of Rural Health, 9*(1), 63–67.

Earp, J. A., Altpeter, M., Mayne, L., Viadro, C. I., & O'Malley, M. S. (1995). The North Carolina breast cancer screening program: Foundations and design of a model for reaching older, minority, rural women. *Breast Cancer Research and Treatment,* *35,* 7–22.

Earp, J. A., Viadro, C. I., Vincus, A. A., Altpeter, M., Flax, V., Mayne, L., & Eng, E. (1997). Lay health advisors: A strategy for getting the word out about breast cancer. *Health Education & Behavior, 24*(4), 432–451.

Earp, J, O'Malley, M., & Rauscher, G. (1999). *Increasing mammography use among older, rural, African-American women.* Presentation at the American Public Health Association Conference, UNC Lineberger Comprehensive Cancer Center University of North Carolina, Chapel Hill.

Elder, J. P., Geller, E. S., Hovell, M. H., & Mayer, J. A. (1994). *Motivating health behavior.* New York: Delmar.

Elder, J. P., Apodaca, J. X., Parra-Medina, D., & Zuñiga de Nuncio, M. L. (1998). Strategies for health education: Theoretical models. In S. Loue (Ed.), *Handbook of immigrant health* (pp. 567–585). New York: Plenum Press.

Eng, E., & Young, R. (1992). Lay health advisors as community change agents. *Journal of Family and Community Health 15*(1), 4–40.

Eng, E. (1993). The Save Our Sisters Project: A social network strategy for reaching rural black women. *Cancer, 72*(suppl.), 1071–1077.

Eng, E., Parker, E., & Harlan, C. (1997). Lay health advisor intervention strategies: A continuum from natural helping to paraprofessional helping. *Health Education & Behavior, 24*(4), 413–417.

Ferguson, K. J., Gjerde, C. L., Mutel, C., Donham, K. J., Hradek, C., Johansen, K., & Merchant, J. (1989). An educational intervention program for prevention of occupational illness in agricultural workers. *The Journal of Rural Health, 5*(1), 33–47.

Fishbein, M. (1980). A theory of reasoned action: Some applications and implications. In H. Howe & M. Page (Eds.), *Nebraska symposium on motivation, 1979* (pp. 65–116). Lincoln: University of Nebraska Press.

Fishbein, M., & Azjen, I. (1975). *Belief, attitude, intention, and behavior: An introduction to theory and research.* Boston: Addison-Wesley.

Frenzen, P. D. (1994). Health care: Premiums and coverage in rural areas. *Agricultural Outlook AO-209* (pp. 22–25), Washington, DC: U.S. Department of Agriculture, Economic Research Service.

Georgia Department of Health and Human Services. (1998, January). *Hospital closure: 1997.* Atlanta, GA: Office of Inspector General.

Ghelfi, L. M. (1999). Rural per capita income grows slightly faster than urban. *Rural Conditions and Trends, 9*(2), 63–65.

Green, L. W. (1984). Modifying and developing health behaviors. In L. Breslow, J. A. Fielding, & L. B. Lave (Eds.), *Annual review of public health* (Vol. 5; pp. 215–236). Palo Alto, CA: Annual Reviews.

Green, L. W., & Kreuter, M. W. (1991). *Health promotion planning: An educational and environment approach* (2nd ed.). Mountain View, CA: Mayfield.

Health Care Financing Administration. (1995). *HCFA current beneficiary survey, 1995.* [www.hcfa.gov/]

Health Resources and Services Administration. *Selected statistics on health professional shortage areas: As of December 31, 1998.* Washington, DC: Department of Health and Human Services, Division of Shortage Designation, Bureau of Primary Health Care.

Hodge, F. S., Fredericks, L., & Rodriguez, B. (1996). American Indian Women's Talking Circle: A cervical cancer screening and prevention project. *Cancer Supplement, 78*(7) 1592–1597.

Hodge, F. S., Stubbs, H. A., & Fredericks, L. (1999). Talking Circles: Increasing cancer knowledge among American Indian women. *Cancer Research Therapy and Control, 8,* 103–111.

Hooks, C., Ugarte, C., Silsby, J., Brown, R., Weinman, J., Fernandez, G., Foxwell, J., Newton, N., & Connally, L. B. (1996). Obstacles and opportunities in designing cancer control communication research for farmworkers on the Delmarva Peninsula. *The Journal of Rural Health, 12*(4), 332–342.

Knobloch, M. J., & Broste, S. K. (1998). A hearing conservation program for Wisconsin youth working in agriculture. *Journal of School Health, 68*(8), 313–318.

Konyha, M. E. (1975). Cooperative Extension Service's potential to meet the needs in rural health education and in rural institutional development. *Public Health Reports, 90*(4), 340–343.

McNab, W. L. (1998). Incorporating farm safety into the health education curriculum. *Journal of School Health, 68*(5), 213–215.

McWhorter, W. P., Schatzkin, A. G., Horm, J. W., & Brown, C. C. (1988) Contribution of socio-economic status to black/white differences in cancer incidence. *Cancer, 63,* 982–987.

Nelson, D. (1993). AIDS prevention programs in a smaller community. *Canadian Journal of Public Health, 84*(suppl. 1), S39–S41.

O'Dea, P. J., Murphy, B., & Balzer, C. (1997). Traffic and illegal production of drugs in rural America. In E. B. Robertson, Z. Sloboda, G. M. Boyd, L. Beatty, & N. J. Kozel (Eds.), *Rural substance and abuse: State of knowledge and issues* (NIDA Monograph no. 168; pp. 79–89). Arlington, VA: U.S. Department of Health and Human Services.

Prochaska, J., & DiClemente, C. (1983). Stages and processes of self-change in smoking: Toward an integrative model of change. *Journal of Consulting and Clinical Psychology, 51,* 390–395.

Project HOPE. (1998). *Financial dependence of rural hospitals on outpatient revenue.* Bethesda, MD: Project Hope.

Randolph, S. A., & Migliozzi, A. A. (1993). The role of the agricultural health nurse. *American Association of Occupational Health Nurses Journal, 42*(9), 429–433.

Reding, D. J., Fischer, V., Gunderson, P., Lappe, K., Anderson, H., & Calvert, G. (1996). Teens teach skin cancer prevention. *Journal of Rural Health, 12*(4), 265–272.

Rhoades, E. R., Hammond, J., Welty, T. K., Handler, A. O., & Amber, R. W. (1987). The Indian burden of illness and future health interventions. *Public Health Report, 102*(4), 361–368.

Ricketts, T. C., Johnson-Webb, K. D., & Taylor, P. (1998, July 1). *Definitions of rural: A handbook for health policy makers and researchers.* Washington, DC: U.S. Department of Health and Human Services, Federal Office of Rural Health Policy, Health Resources and Services Administration.

Rogers, C. C. (1999). Socioeconomic circumstances of minority elderly differ from those of wWhite elderly. *Rural Conditions and Trends, 9*(2), 35–41.

Schafer, E., Vogel, M. K., Viegas, S., & Hausafus, C. (1998). Volunteer peer counselors increase breastfeeding duration among low-income women. *BIRTH, 25*(2), 101–106.

Service, C., & Salber, E. (Eds.) (1979). *Community health education: The lay health advisor approach.* Durham, NC: Duke University Health Care System.

Skinner, B. F. (1953). *Science and human behavior.* New York: Macmillan.

Vistnes, J. P., & Monheit, A. C. (1997). Health insurance status of the civilian noninstitutionalized population. Medical Expenditure Panel Survey (MEPS) Research Findings, Number 1, Agency for Health Care Policy and Research Pub. No. 97-0030.

What difference do lay health advisors make? Initial results from NC-BCSP's outcome evaluation (1999). *North Carolina Breast Cancer Screening Program, 14,* 4–5.

19

Recruiting, Training, and Retaining Rural Health Professionals

JAMES ROBINSON III AND JEFFREY J. GUIDRY

Introduction

Since the United States was founded, the country's population has shifted from what was once overwhelmingly rural—95% in 1790—to what is now predominantly urban, reported as 75% in 1990. During the 1970s there was a movement toward rural living; it became known as the "rural renaissance." The country witnessed a loss of rural population in the 1980s, but data indicate there may be another turnaround to increased rural population in the years to come (Ricketts, Johnson-Webb, & Randolph, 1999).

Rural areas have numerous characteristics that clearly distinguish them from urban environments. For example, rural communities have less well-developed economies, lower population density, and a higher percentage of elderly people in the population. Health status in rural areas is another circumstance that is somewhat different from health status in urban settings. When controlled for age and gender, the health status (as measured by mortality and severe morbidity) of rural Americans does not differ substantially from urban residents. However, rural individuals often describe their health as poor to fair. It appears this response is due to the level of care they receive and the timeliness with which they receive it (Ricketts et al., 1999).

Some of these conditions have stimulated increased interest in the health of rural populations. Politicians and citizens are aware of the need for quality health services in rural as well as urban environments. Numerous funding sources and agencies have been created by the federal government to address the health needs of rural populations. For example, the Health Resources and Services Administration (HRSA) created the Office of Rural Health Policy in 1987 and the Consolidated Health Centers Program in 1998 with $826 million in funding. Over the years, the number of rural health clinics created by the Rural Health Clinic Program in 1980 has risen from 285 to more than 3,500 clinics since the program went into effect (Ricketts, 1999). Federal funding to improve rural health has increased in the past decade—for example, the Department of Health and Human Services' Rural Health Outreach Grant Program was authorized in 1991 and there was increased funding for Area Health Education Centers ($32 million) in 1998. The U.S. Centers for Disease Control and Prevention currently support public health leadership programs at various state and regional locations nationwide. The public

JAMES ROBINSON III • Department of Social and Behavioral Health, School of Rural Public Health, Texas A&M University System, Health Science Center, College Station, Texas 77843-1266. **JEFFREY J. GUIDRY** • Department of Health and Kinesiology, Texas A&M University, College Station, Texas 77843-4243.

Handbook of Rural Health, edited by Loue and Quill. Kluwer Academic/Plenum Publishers, New York, 2001.

health leadership institutes are designed to improve the knowledge and skills of public health practitioners, who in turn are expected improve public health infrastructures and services nationwide.

Health Care and Rural America

The agencies and organizations that are established to promote and maintain health in rural areas are distinctly different from their counterparts in the cities. The demographic profile of rural America, its health care infrastructure, and its health promotion needs reflect the conditions in rural towns. The most pronounced of them are these:

Population Characteristics

Rural communities are diverse and have widely distributed populations. Elements of diversity include race and ethnicity, gender, age, and socioeconomic status. The population in rural areas is growing more slowly than the population in more urban areas, and compared with urban areas, the population is older, lower in socioeconomic status, and more likely to be below poverty level (Ricketts *et al.*, 1999). As a result, rural populations are not only more vulnerable to various health threats but also have specific access problems. Health care for an aged rural resident, for example, becomes compromised when that person becomes too old to drive, has no access to public transportation, and has relatives living miles away. The barrier of isolation becomes more pronounced the further from town people live; the more isolated they are, the more removed they will be from social support networks that can help with their access needs.

Limited Access to Health Care

Rural communities lack the mechanisms to generate financial resources to fund health promotion and health care programs. Communities are small and tend to lack the population density and commercial enterprises that would generate sufficient tax dollars and private-sector revenues. Moreover, rural residents are more likely to be self-employed or work for small businesses; consequently, employee health benefits are scarcer and less generous than the benefits available in urban settings. Only about 54% of rural residents have insurance coverage through their employer compared with 63% of urban residents, and the rate of uninsured rural residents (20%) is higher than urban residents (16%) (Shur & Franco, 1999). People in rural areas have less income and are less likely to have a third-party payer for their hospital services (Gay, 1990). It is not uncommon for services or programs to be dependent on federal, state, or county support. The dearth of financial support has led to the closing of many rural health care facilities.

There is clear evidence that rural residents face greater hardships when traveling to health facilities due to lack of transportation and distance. Only 12% of communities with fewer than 2,500 residents have public transportation systems (Shur & Franco, 1999).

Scarcity of Qualified Practitioners

The lack of strong economic support creates an environment where health practitioners can ill afford to practice. Trained professionals, given the choice, locate in the more urban environments where they can earn more money. Rural areas are likely to have incomplete health care and public health workforces. For example, Kennedy (1996) reports that of 211 public health service agencies surveyed in Texas, 63% had professional personnel shortages in the areas they serviced. Nurses and physicians were in greatest demand. A national study of physician assistants (Larson, Hart, Goodwin, Geller, & Andrilla, 1999) discovered that PAs who started their careers in rural settings were likely to leave for urban locations within the first five years (41%), and of the PAs who started their careers in rural locales only 59% were still in rural settings at the time of the survey. Larson and colleagues also found that there was higher retention among generalist PAs in rural areas of states that had more favorable PA practice environments—that is legal status, reimbursement, and prescriptive authority.

Provider shortages are currently being addressed by programs such as the National Health

Services Corps, which provide educational loan repayment for health professionals who agree to serve in health professional shortage areas (HPSA) for at least two years (Ricketts, 1999). Funding to the Health Service Corps was reduced dramatically in 1985 but revitalized in 1990. The revitalization contributed to a significant increase in the number of physician assistants and nurse practitioners (Ricketts, 1999). There are also state programs, such as Texas Health Find, that work with rural communities to develop financial packages to recruit health professionals. However, programs such as these tend to be very new and the effects have not yet been well evaluated.

Limited Opportunities for Resource Sharing

Geographical isolation has an important effect on health care delivery. Resource sharing becomes important to rural isolated communities because the equipment, facilities, and consultations are too expensive for each small town to purchase. Yet the distance between communities impedes pooling of resources among providers.

Health delivery organizations in rural areas thus face unique management challenges. Employers are likely to emerge from regional or county public health offices, branches of voluntary health agencies, community health centers, local health clinics, and so on. But the characteristics of rural areas described above require nontraditional ways of developing a qualified and stable health professions workforce. Health care organizations need to look inward to the community for assessments to guide the structure of health services and the personnel who will be charged with delivering health promotion programs and services. Rural areas have complex health care needs that demand complex and creative solutions.

Staffing Challenges in Rural Areas

An administrator in a rural health agency or organization will find recruiting, hiring, and training challenges unlike those experienced by administrators in urban organizations. There is

a defined set of principles in management science regarding best practice procedures for acquiring new personnel. Although some can be applied to rural settings, there will be some need for modification. A number of conditions, characteristic of the rural workforce, will affect recruitment, the hiring process, and retention of personnel.

Shortage of Trained Individuals

The limited resources of rural counties and towns do not enable them to attract the highly trained and qualified practitioners who may be available in and around urban areas. Well-trained individuals, wanting to make the best possible living, tend to seek out opportunities in more urban environments. The health needs of a dense urban population and the financial base to support programs to promote or maintain health result in a financial reward system that makes urban health practice more attractive. In addition to the financial rewards, there exists a larger pool of community resources and professional collaborators. A less qualified practitioner may not be hired in an urban area because of the strong competition from other highly qualified candidates, but the same practitioner may find a position in a rural area because there won't be as much highly qualified competition.

An examination of health professional shortage area (HPSA) designation data reveals that the actual number of full-time equivalent (FTE) shortages appears more numerous among metropolitan designations. The interpretation of this information may be misleading, however. The HPSA shortages are related to the number of practitioners according to the population, and rural area populations are spread out over a large geographical area. The area for one practitioner in a city may be two square miles, whereas in a rural town the catchment area may be 50 square miles (Health Resources Services Administration, 2000). Simply put, low population density and the high cost of services often make rural medical practice economically unfeasible, or at best, difficult (LeBlanc, Simon, & Garard, 1997). Due to the necessity for 24-hour on-call coverage in rural areas, and due to difficulties encountered by internists and pediatricians trying to cover each other's practice, internists and pediatricians are unlikely to practice in areas where they will be the only practicing member of their specialty (Rosenblatt & Hart, 1999). The difficulty in attracting and retaining physicians makes it more likely that rural residents will change providers (Shur & Franco, 1999).

Limited Labor Pool

For every position advertised in a rural community, there will be fewer potential applicants than for a similar position in the city. As already mentioned, there will also be fewer *trained* applicants. These applicants will be spread out over a large geographical area. The number of potential applicants may also be limited because of networks through which recruiting takes place. The professional networks in rural locations are fewer and less dense than in and around urban centers, thus contributing to fewer referrals for certain positions.

Less Competitive Salaries

Salaries in rural areas are less competitive than they are in the cities. The limited financial resources available to rural communities and the lack of highly trained persons create conditions whereby the rural communities can, must, and do advertise positions with a lower salary. However, the job requirements may be less rigorous than for a similar position in the city. For example, a rural area far removed from any urban region that is interested in hiring someone to plan and deliver a health promotion program is likely to hire someone with a bachelor's degree; a similar agency in the city where will have the luxury of seeking and finding someone who is prepared at the master's level.

Health organizations must work together with community members to develop a comprehensive recruitment plan. Rural communities need to go beyond merely putting a job advertisement in the local paper. If health care and prevention services are important to a community, the community members must be active participants in the recruitment process. Many rural communities are now forming recruitment committees to attract health professionals. These committees include chamber of commerce members, clergy, local politicians, residents, and so on, and work

toward "selling" the virtues of the local area. They may even pool resources to develop incentive packages to attract professionals.

Although health professionals will find themselves working in areas where salaries are lower than in urban settings, other incentives can be appealing. Some professionals are attracted to rural settings by virtue of their remote, quiet, and relaxed atmosphere. In many instances the culture of the community itself can be attractive to potential recruits. The culture includes the close-knit nature of the community, heritage, and community ownership of problems and solutions. Some people are attracted to the recreational opportunities that rural areas often have to offer. The astute recruiter will want to capitalize on these nonfinancial rewards when seeking new personnel.

Determining Needs

Organizational growth or long-range planning can lead to the necessity of hiring personnel. New public health initiatives that arise from disease epidemics or emerging health threats may bring financial resources for new programs. The closing of hospitals and health agencies due to lack of funds may also influence personnel needs. In such cases, new staffing patterns will be created. Careful planning and stakeholder involvement are necessary if the organization is to attract and retain health professionals in the area.

Data are needed to construct an accurate assessment of personnel needs. The organization will want to conduct an analysis of the internal environment (mission, organizational culture, policies, procedures, financial resources and personnel, and so on) and the external environment, especially the community health needs, social policies, and culture that may have an effect on the community's health. Data can be collected from reports, from employees, or directly from organizational stakeholders. A stakeholder is any "individual or group with a 'stake' in the organization" (Hernandez, Fottler, & Joiner, 1998, p. 6). There are three types of stakeholders: those who are *external* to the organization (e.g., clients, third-party payers, and patients); *internal* stakeholders (e.g., staff, managers, and maintenance); and *interface* stakeholders. Interface stakeholders are those who may be external to the organization but who work closely with personnel and programs within the organization. Interface stakeholders include board members, equipment vendors, personnel from collaborating agencies, and subcontractors.

External Needs Assessment

In rural areas, communities and organizations must work together to determine the depth and breadth of personnel needs. Data from the local area and surrounding areas can be used to ensure that resources are allocated correctly. If the community or agency is to spend money on new personnel, it should be clear that the money will be used to support a needed position and that the money spent will result in a cost-effective hire for the position. Local needs assessment data can be used along with HPSA data or state health department data to assure that new personnel will best meet the needs of everyone. For example, the community may need an OB-GYN physician but not have the capacity to provide the appropriate resources for such a person. Analysis of data and discussion with local residents and business leaders may reveal that there is OB-GYN support at the next closest community, and so a decision may be made to hire a nurse practitioner or physician assistant instead. The nurse practitioner or the physician assistant then can provide needed services to the local community with input and support from the OB-GYN physician in the nearby community.

A number of information sources can help organizations plan appropriately for increases in personnel. Rural communities do not have their own data management systems. As a result, many states have data systems that are available to support the development of rural health care (Slifkin, 1999). These databases can be used to analyze the unmet needs in local communities and shape recommendations for new personnel, policy development, and mechanisms to assure access to health care. The data can also be helpful in exposing areas that require special attention in the recruitment and retention of practitioners (Slifkin, 1999).

Community members can be valuable resources in the recruitment process. Because they have an ongoing investment in the community, they can help identify key characteristics essential to the position to be advertised. They can help create incentive packages to attract personnel to the community. Community members can serve as members of recruitment committees, and they can be essential links, helping the newly hired professional connect to the community once that individual is hired.

Internal Needs Assessment

A internal needs assessment is the first in a series of steps an organization will undertake to foster effective change (McArdle, 1996). A needs assessment that identifies the knowledge, skills, and experience required for the new position is essential. The needs assessment must also relate to the mission and goals of the organization, and it is the foundation upon which planning decisions are made. Figure 1 illustrates the steps in the human resource planning process.

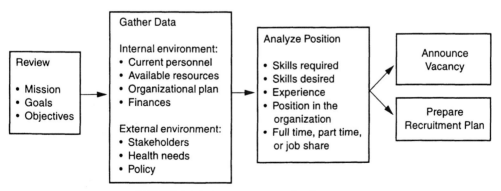

FIGURE 1. The human resources planning process.

Following review of the mission, goals, and objectives, data can be collected from reviews, production outcomes, financial reports, and so on, and organized to help with decision making. The creation of a new position may necessitate a modification of planning objectives. Planning of any kind, whether it is short-term (i.e., for next year), long-term (i.e., for two or more years), or strategic (in response to the competitive environment) must relate back to the mission and goals of the organization (Hernandez, 1998). Conversely, a review of planning objectives may lead to a rethinking and modification of the intended qualifications needed for the position.

In smaller organizations, such as those in rural areas, turnover does not occur with any predictable regularity. When of one employee leaves a small organization it has a much greater effect than when the organization is large. This factor is compounded when the organization is located in a rural community. Organizations are well advised to plan their personnel needs carefully in order to maximize retention.

Technology has a significant on staffing patterns. In today's workplace, technology is indispensible. Organizations try to plan for technological advances and their impact on doing business, but technological advancements are unpredictable. In fact, the more technologically dependent an organization is, the greater the technological effect on planning is likely to be (Rabin, Teasley, Finkle, & Carter, 1985). Technology skills and training needs should be considered when developing staffing needs.

In some cases, focus groups can be conducted to ascertain qualitative opinions during needs assessment (McClelland, 1994). These focus groups can be conducted with both organizational personnel and community members. In the absence of a trained and qualified consultant to conduct focus groups in rural areas, any individual can learn enough about focus group practice to conduct groups on his or her own. Morgan (1997) offers an easy-to-follow primer for conducting focus groups, for example.

After data have been gathered and analyzed in light of the organization's goals and objectives and the community's needs, the data can be used to frame the job analysis. The elements of the job analysis will be used to create the vacancy announcement to advertise the position.

Creative Staffing Options

As discussed previously, a rural area probably will not have a large pool of potential employees. Thus administrators must think creatively about responding to their needs when staffing their organizations and programs. Some possible alternative staffing patterns include:

Job Sharing

Rural organizations tend to be small, so an organization may not be large enough to support a number of full-time staff positions. It may be possible to create two (or three) smaller positions that could be staffed on a part-time basis. Doing this would permit a number of tasks to be completed for the organization using multiple employees who together total one full time equivalent (i.e., 40 hours a week). This would be especially important if the needed tasks were so diverse that one person could not be found to perform all duties.

Outsourcing/Contracting

Not always are the skills of one individual needed for 40 hours a week every week. For example, an organization may need an auditor or a program evaluator, but on an infrequent basis. It will be less expensive to hire someone on contract work to complete those tasks than to invest in an annual salary to have a person on staff full-time. Contract employees offer other advantages. As a rule, they are not eligible for benefits as is the case with full-time employees.

Volunteers

Perhaps some jobs can be covered with volunteer staff. Volunteers can perform many of the tasks that can be performed by regular staff, such as education, clerical functions, fundraising, interactions with clients, and so on (Gamm & Kassab, 1982). This is especially true if the organization is a voluntary health agency such as the American Heart Association or American

Cancer Society. In communities where there are retired professionals, retirees often look for ways to serve their communities and make worthy use of their time. Before using volunteers, however, it is important to check on liability issues.

Interorganizational Hiring

Another way to address personnel shortages in rural areas is for agencies to join together and hire someone to perform the same or similar duties for more than one organization on a part-time basis for each. This approach is especially useful if the organizations deliver similar types of services or products.

Determining Qualifications for the Position

When an organization or community group begins the hiring process, it is an opportunity for it to engage in organizational planning, including a job analysis. Job analysis is the process by which the organizational objectives, needs assessment, and other data are used to clarify the job skills needed for the new position. The skills can be defined by the organization or the organization may use contemporary professional and community standards. A number of methods can be used to conduct a job analysis (Graham & Bennett, 1998), including:

- Direct observation
- Job-holder interview
- Supervisor interview
- Review of work records
- Questionnaires

It is suggested that the organization collect as much data as possible from as many sources as possible to obtain a valid set of findings to finalize the characteristics of the new position. The job analysis will result in a description of the various tasks, duties, and qualifications that would be needed for successful job performance.

Recruitment and Retention

The limited labor pool will be a concern in rural areas, so it is helpful to include anything that might motivate potential candidates to apply for positions in recruitment materials. Consideration of *structural incentives,* such as "a flexible comp time policy," "ongoing training and development programs," "family leave program," "paid vacation time beginning the first year," or *environmental incentives,* such as "a quiet community to raise a family," "one of the best school systems in the county," or "just hours away from the finest recreation facility in the state," can be as attractive as salary to many people. As mentioned previously, many states are now offering loan repayment programs to attract physicians and other professionals to serve in medically underserved areas, and the National Health Service Corps provides loan repayment for physicians, physician assistants, nurse practitioners, dental professionals, and mental health providers if they agree to practice in health professional shortage areas. Other forms of special incentives to attract new personnel can be created by the community search committee. Such incentives could include support for continuing education, travel stipends, shared resources or equipment with local businesses, and professional support networks. One emerging area of professional development that can be explored as a recruitment incentive is distance learning. If a community is able to "teleconnect" with a state agency or institution of higher education to receive continuing education or professional development coursework, it may have an edge on recruiting and retaining new personnel.

The recruitment process begins when the organization undertakes a job analysis as part of an internal needs assessment to determine what type of person is needed for the position. Once the position and the qualities of the candidate are defined and a vacancy announcement is prepared, recruiting can begin. There is a difference between recruiting and advertising when looking for someone to fill the position. Simply sending announcements out through professional networks, journals, or newspapers is a means of *advertising.* When the process involves planning, implementation, and evaluation, the art of *recruiting* begins (Landau & Abelson, 1998).

The recruiting plan in rural health organizations includes the development of an organized strategy that evolves in response to a couple of important questions:

- *From where will the candidates be recruited?* Ideally candidates should emerge from local pools. It may also be possible to take a local person and train him or her in the needed skills. Internal candidates have familiarity with the organization and are likely to perpetuate organizational plans, values, and culture (Landau & Abelson, 1998), but external candidates are likely to bring fresh ideas and perspectives. If the organization is serious about recruiting, it will need to identify places where recruitment can take place.
- *When will the process begin so that the successful candidate is found in a timely fashion?* If the organization knows by when the new position must be filled, a calendar should be developed to help manage the process. A time line should be determined and a date advertised that specifies when applications will be reviewed.

The characteristics of the position and the potential labor pool may determine whether the search for the successful candidate will be conducted locally, regionally, or nationally. The more far-reaching the search, the more expensive it will be, but there is a greater likelihood of a stronger pool of applicants. On the other hand, the more far-reaching the search, the greater the probability that applicants will be dissimilar from the community members and their health beliefs and practices.

Essential to the recruiting process is the vacancy announcement. The formulation of a vacancy announcement engages the organization in the process of clarifying the job analysis and the responsibilities that go along with it. The vacancy announcement is also useful for those individuals who are responsible for identifying the successful candidate. It becomes a template against which the applicants' qualifications can be compared. There is no standard format for writing vacancy announcements. The essential elements of an announcement are shown in Figure 2.

The vacancy announcement can also be used as a guide to performance once the candidate is hired. The vacancy announcement describes the elements of that person's tasks in the organization, so it can become the framework for performance appraisal. For example, if an organization is looking for someone who has the training and experience to plan and evaluate health promotion programs for the work site and it expects that person also to manage budgets, these skills should be specified in the vacancy announcement. Once the person is on the job, he or she must be able to successfully demonstrate these skills. If the employee fails to do so, the vacancy announcement can be used to justify a poor performance review or dismissal or to defend the justification during any subsequent litigation.

Legal Considerations

Any organization that receives funds, directly or indirectly, from a federal source is obligated to hire individuals in a nondiscriminating manner. Federal guidelines require businesses not only to conduct searches for new employees according to specific guidelines, but also make special accommodations for applicants and employees who need them. Two specific laws merit attention:

Affirmative Action/Equal Opportunity

The basic concept of affirmative action stems from the old English legal concept of equity. Affirmative action does not relate to legal rules *per se*; rather it is the simple administration of justice according to what might be fair in a given situation (Skrentny, 1996). The current scope of affirmative action is best understood as an outgrowth of our national effort to remedy the historical subjugation of racial or ethnic minorities and women. Other significant pieces of affirmative action legislation include those on age discrimination, Vietnam-era veterans' protection, treatment of maternity as a disability, and the Americans with Disabilities Act (Higgins, 1991). Although AA/EO is accomplishing what it was intended to, there is evidence that some of the racial and gender stratification of jobs that existed in the 1960s still exists today (Newman, 1997).

Director, Behavioral Health Division

Salary: $43,240-$52,889   Closing Date: February 1, 2000

The ABC County Health Department is seeking a Director for the Behavioral Health Division to join our senior management team. ABC County is located in central Texas. The department is governed by Board of Health and appointed by an elected County Board. The department provides public health services to a diverse population of approximately 70,000 including both urban and rural settings. The department employs a 70 FTE professional and support staff, 8 of whom are in the Behavioral Health Division.

The successful candidate will manage programs with the primary objective of developing and managing numerous health promotion programs to safeguard public health. Duties include planning, developing and administering programs, grants, policies, and goals. The director must contribute pertinent and/or specialized information at internal and external meetings to identify and resolve problems, assess overall community needs, and ensure effectiveness of environmental programs. This position also manages quality control measures for content and delivery of information to community groups, contractors, residents, and business operators. The director performs supervisory responsibilities including program oversight, performance evaluation, training and coaching of a staff 7. The director will also participate in strategic planning and resource acquisition for the division and the department.

Candidates must have a master's degree in public health promotion, health education, or related field and five years of related experience in health promotion or equivalent combination of education and experience. Prior program management experience, including staffing, planning, budgeting, and supervision also required. Certification as a Health Education Specialist is desired.

Entry in the position with a salary range of $43,240-$52,889 is based on experience and qualifications. Excellent benefits.

Interested candidates should submit a cover letter describing interest with an updated resume emphasizing education and work experience.

For further information, contact . . .

An AA/EO Employer

FIGURE 2. Sample vacancy announcement.

Affirmative action policies aside, the actual concern should be the development of a diverse workforce. Ideally, the workforce should reflect the racial composition of the rural community. The reality is, however, this will remain a challenge for rural organizations. Urban areas must follow AA/EO guidelines as well, and the organizations in those areas have more resources to lure minority professionals to their locales. Until such time that rural communities have strong incentive packages or are able to develop "homegrown" talent, true diversity will remain an ideal for them.

Americans with Disabilities Act

The Americans with Disabilities Act (ADA) was enacted in 1990 and took effect July 26, 1992. The ADA regulations apply to all companies with 15 or more employees (U.S. Equal Opportunity Commission, 1997). The act prohibits employers from discriminating against qualified individuals who have disabilities. Furthermore, employers cannot discriminate against any individual who has a relationship with a disabled person. A qualified employee or applicant with a disability is an individual who, with or without reasonable accommodation, can perform the essential functions of the job in question. Reasonable accommodation may include, but is not limited to:

- Making existing facilities used by employees readily accessible to and usable by persons with disabilities
- Restructuring jobs, modifying work schedules, reassigning to a vacant position
- Acquiring or modifying equipment or devices, adjusting or modifying examinations, training materials, or policies, and providing qualified readers or interpreters

Thus, the ADA requires employers to focus on an applicant's ability to perform certain job tasks rather than on the applicant's medical condition.

An employer is required to make an accommodation to the known disability of a qualified applicant or employee if it would not impose an "undue hardship" on the operation of the business. Rural health organizations may have knowledge of the ADA legislation in basic and general terms, but their greatest challenge will be in knowing the specific interpretations and applications of the law. For example, an organization could be unaware that it is not required to make an accommodation for a disability until it is told by the applicant or the employee that an accommodation is needed. The organization may also not know that tax credits and deductions are available to offset the costs of accommodation (U.S. Department of Justice, 1992). Employers who are not sure of the compliance issues in a given circumstance should contact the ADA for clarification. Information can also be obtained from the ADA Web site itself (http://www.usdoj.gov/crt/ada/).

Finding the Successful Candidate

Once applications arrive, the local search committee will conduct a preliminary screening to sort the applicants. All applications should be reviewed for completeness and responsiveness to the vacancy announcement. Applicants who do not meet the required training and skills specified in the announcement should be set aside and not included for further review. Individuals associated with the hiring process will eventually sort the pool and identify the leading candidates. The following guidelines may be helpful after the pool is delimited.

Conducting the Interview

Often the most critical part of the hiring process is the interview, but quite often the interview is the weakest link in the search for the best employee in the applicant pool (Higgins, 1991). The interview for positions in rural areas will be very important, especially if the candidate is not from within the community. There is a need to find out about the candidate's sense of the community and its people rather than just determine if the candidate has job skills. Whenever possible, rural communities should include local stakeholders in the interview process. Rural residents and businesspeople add immensely to the interview process by asking questions of a "community nature" rather than of a "business nature." Moreover, lay interviewers can speak more favorably about the community and help recruit the candidate.

It is difficult to collect needed information from the candidate if the interviewer is doing most of the talking. The preferred ratio of talking time between interviewer and the interviewee should be 20% and 80%, respectively (Ralston & Kirkwood, 1995; Stewart & Cash, 1991). It is a special skill for the interviewer to be able to put the applicant at ease, ask specific questions to stimulate dialogue, and then step back and listen. Ralston and Kirkwood (1995) propose a model that essentially describes the ideal interview as an "equal opportunity." Each party (the employer and the applicant) has the equal amount of time (1) to speak, (2) to advance and test claims, (3) to disclose self, and (4) to exercise power—that is, the employer needs to soften the authoritative relationship.

Interviewers must be mindful of the AA/EO regulations that affect the interview process. There are legal guidelines that protect individuals from improper questioning. A good summary of the kinds of questions that can and cannot be asked can be found in McConnell (1999).

Checking References

Because candidates are likely to be from areas outside the rural community, reference checks are virtually always conducted over the phone. This may seem time consuming, but the entire hiring process is enhanced by conducting these interviews. Telephone conversations permit the interviewer to probe responses, ask the same question in slightly different ways, and pick up on inflections, hesitations, verbal slips, and so on, on the part of the reference. It is best to conduct telephone reference checks after the organization has interviewed the candidate. An advantage to this approach is that the organization may have some specific questions to ask that came from the candidate's interview. If reference checks are necessary prior to the interview, it may be best to have someone other than the interviewer conduct them.

Retention

Organizations attempting to recruit professionals in rural communities not only want to assure that they recruit the best candidate but also want to be certain they can retain that person. One way to increase the likelihood of retention is to present final candidates with a *realistic job preview*. The realistic job preview (RJP) is a set of written or verbal descriptions of all essential aspects of a particular job. The RJP theory proposes that if people are provided with information (both positive and negative) about the elements and expectations of their job when they are initially hired, they are less likely to leave the job (Premack & Wanous, 1985). In addition, it appears that the RJP has produced other important job-related effects, such as increasing self-selection among candidates, strengthening the new hire's organizational commitment, increasing the likelihood of job satisfaction, enhancing work performance (Premack & Wanous, 1985), and increasing the probability that newly hired employees will respond better to job stressors (Breaugh, 1983).

In rural settings where retention is very important, the realistic job preview can be an opportunity to connect job tasks to the performance appraisal system. In this way, the realistic job preview and the performance appraisal are linked to salary increases or other forms of compensation and used as a recruiting tool. Performance appraisals have long been used by organizations to measure the performance of

employees and the relationship of employee performance to desired organizational expectations and outcomes. In essence, performance appraisals are important for the following reasons.

- *Feedback and development.* Employees should be told how well they are doing, but the appraisals are also expected to identify weak areas of performance that can be improved.
- *Administrative decision making.* Employers need a mechanism to determine who to promote, who to terminate, and who to reward.
- *Program evaluation.* Program outcomes are related to performance of personnel.
- *Documentation of performance.* In instances of wrongful termination suites or other challenges to employee treatment, individual appraisals serve as a record of performance (Carson, Cardy, & Dobbins, 1993).

If done properly, performance appraisals can be an asset to the employee and the rural health agency or hospital. Performance measures tend to be most reliable if:

- The purpose of the appraisal is clear.
- Expected outcomes are simple (and measurable).
- Outcomes are predictable.
- Tasks are relatively independent.
- Task performance is observable.
- Criteria for performance are set by those who will later assess the performance.
- Appraisers feel secure in their own jobs. (Joiner & Hyde, 1998, p. 233)

The appraisal process, when implemented correctly, reinforces the employee's sense of worth, motivates the employee toward the acquisition of new skills, and increases the likelihood of retention.

Education, Training, and Development

All new employees have to go through some kind of orientation program. Employee orientations should contain some training or development, and in the case of rural organizations, should include orientation to the community as well. Training consists of planned exercises to improve performance, but more importantly, it has a positive effect on employee retention. It is a strong motivator to organizational loyalty (Goff, 1999; Olesen, 1999). Traditionally there has been a distinction made between training and development. Lower-level employees were trained, while higher-level employees were developed (Smith & Fottler, 1998). The distinction becomes somewhat meaningless in today's work environment, especially in rural settings. The organizational structure is not as deep as it might be in cities. The focus should be on preparing all employees, empowering them with a set of skills that will allow them to perform their jobs well, and providing ongoing development that will ensure retention. Hence, training and development tend to go hand in hand. Once someone assumes a new job, training and development begin.

Training Needs Assessment

Before a new employee begins a training and development program, the organization is well advised to conduct a short needs assessment to compare the new employee's training and experience to the job analysis created before the vacancy announcement was developed. There should also be a needs assessment among community stakeholders to determine training needs

that may be related to the local culture and resources.

Needs assessments are also useful for professional training outside the organization. If, for example, an organization is going to deliver training programs to hospital staff, voluntary health agencies, community coalitions, or voluntary health agencies, it should first assess the needs of the audience. Failure to do so may result in a less effective training program.

Orientation

Training and development activities can be placed on a continuum (see Table 1). The first activity is likely to be an orientation program. It doesn't matter what level of training and experience a person possesses, when in a new position, and especially in a new organization, that person will need training and orientation. Orientation introduces employees to the organization's values, mores, beliefs, behaviors, standard operating procedures, policies, and expectations (Smith & Fottler, 1998). It should also include an introduction to the rural community, its people, culture, health issues, power structures, resources, and so on. In essence, orientation prepares the new employee to function easily and properly in the organizational structure and the rural community. Issues discussed include the company benefits and how one takes advantage of them, how one submits a travel

TABLE 1. Continuum of Training and Development Activities

Strategy	Objectives	Scope of Skill	Emphasis on Personal Growth	Frequency
Orientation	Introduce employees to expectations, rules, policies.	Narrow and specific	Limited	Once
Training	Develop specific job skills and duties.			As needed
In-Service Education	Develop new skills, attitudes, etc., through company programs.			Continual
Continuing Education	Develop professional competency and currency through external programs.			Continual
Career Development	Provide opportunities to develop greater depth and breadth of professional person.	Broad	Extensive	Continual

Note: Adapted from "Training and Development," by H. L. Smith and M. D. Fottler, in M. D. Fottler, S. R. Hernandez, and C. L. Joiner (eds.), Essentials of Human Resources Management in Health Services Organizations, 1998, Boston: Delmar.

voucher, what the best mechanism for disseminating information to the community is, what the local barriers to health care delivery are, and so on. Orientation programs can be one-day long, or can take longer. It depends on the complexity of the organization and the organization's predefined objectives.

Training and Education

Training is a series of exercises designed to prepare the employee with specific skills and attitudes to perform the job better. Although training programs are often provided to employees, many organizations do not approach the process with clear planning. Like other components of planned programs, training should be approached by first developing a clear set of objectives. These objectives will arise from an assessment of pertinent factors in the rural community. Activities and training programs can then be developed and implemented. There are volumes of creative training exercises that can be used or adapted for this purpose (see Kroehnert, 1991; Newstrom & Scannell, 1980). These exercises represent creative ways of training employees (or others) in leadership skills, presentation skills, problem-solving skills, motivation, listening skills, and so on. These activities can often be adapted to education and training programs that reflect community values and standards.

Education and training are important aspects of developing a health promotion workforce. In rural areas, numerous members of the workforce practice without complete skills. These individuals may have been trained in one professional capacity and then given responsibilities that do not match their training, or perhaps community and professional needs have evolved to the point where these employees need additional skills to keep up. Kennedy's study of Texas public health organizations revealed that management and communication skills were the top training needs identified by the survey respondents (Kennedy, 1996). When a sample of Texas Department of Health employees were asked to identify areas of training needs. Community-related issues were reported most frequently. Specifically, the need for skills in community assessment, community organization, and com-

munity development were the specific areas of interest (Robinson & Griffith, 1999).

Institutions of higher education are now recognizing the importance of rural health issues and the need for increased training and education opportunities. Health care and promotion activities can no longer be confined to urban areas alone. In 1998, the first school of public health in the nation devoted specifically to public health practice in rural settings was started (Texas A&M Health Science Center, 1999). Rural public health training is also being delivered through teleconferencing to various remote sites around Texas, and a telemedicine project is being delivered to community health centers in the Lower Rio Grande Valley. The faculty of the school also work closely with the Texas Agricultural Extension Service to conduct research in and deliver programs to rural communities. One such program is Health Education and Rural Outreach (HERO). HERO has been able to deliver numerous health promotion and health screening programs to rural communities. Other academic institutions around the country will be undertaking similar activities in the years to come.

Training and education of health care personnel is one of the main objectives of area health education center (AHEC) programs. The AHECs were developed using federal support as defined by the Comprehensive Manpower Training Act of 1971. In 1998, federal AHEC funding exceeded $32 million (Ricketts, 1999). Local AHEC offices will deliver training programs via Web-based learning or local conferences. A check of the local AHEC office's Web page will reveal upcoming workshops, courses, and conferences.

Continuing Education

Continuing education programs are designed to help employees keep current in their professional competencies and standards. There are instances where professionals are required to gain continuing education credits in order to maintain their professional certification or license. Current trends are moving some of these continuing education activities online. It is now possible for professionals in remote sites to access not only training activities but entire degree programs over the Internet. The Public Health Training Network, started by the CDC in 1993, has delivered more than 1 million training opportunities through its distance learning network (Public Health Practice Program, 1999). Training and continuing education programs for health personnel are also being delivered by institutions of higher education in partnership with AHECs, as previously noted.

All training activities are designed to make the individual a better employee. In a rural area where recruitment is very important, and retention is paramount, the organization wants to attract and keep employees. "What keeps them around . . . are extensive training and career-development programs that offer benefits to both workers and employers" (Dobbs, 1999, p. 50). Organizations that promote human resource development activities are likely to see such tangible benefits as higher employee productivity, activation of employee responsibility for improving services and performance, ability to deliver optimal services and products under budgetary constraints, integration of employees that promotes organizational identity while underscoring service, and greater likelihood of engaging in teamwork (Smith & Fottler, 1998).

It is important for rural employers to use education and training as incentives to promote employee dedication.

The Psychological Environment of the Rural Workplace

Ever since the now-classic Hawthorne Studies were conducted at the Western Electric Company plant outside of Chicago in the mid to late 1920s, corporations have attended to the human relations aspects of their companies (Seta, Paulus, & Baron, 2000). The Hawthorne researchers, and those who followed, have concluded that the work environment actually consists of complex social situations that affect employee motivation. Organizational social structures will mirror the social setting of the rural area where they are located. Employers and managers are likely to obtain optimum performance and retention among their employees if they make a concerted effort to create a work environment that capitalizes on the strengths of the workforce and is responsive to the needs of the rural professional who is practicing in relative isolation with limited resources and staff.

In 1984, the Conference Board produced a research report that summarized findings from a study of 52 large American corporations. The study was designed to qualitatively measure the degree to which the companies employed innovative human resource management techniques to institute change. Among other things, the report identified characteristics or assumptions that were common among the corporations (Gorlin & Schein, 1984). Although the study included large corporations in the sample, there are implications of these findings for even small rural organizations. The study found that workers are much more productive if they have input into the work and product development, that they need to feel that their efforts are contributing to the success of the organization, and that they want to work where practices, procedures, and rules are reasonable.

Stress and the Workplace

Ever since Hans Selye's reports on stress research in the 1950s our personal and professional lives have included reference to stress in some fashion at some point in time. Stress is a state that almost becomes debilitating for some people, but for others stress and its effects are barely noticeable. The effects of stress seem to depend on the manner in which we react to stress.

The rural work environment has a unique set of stressors. Professionals find themselves working in isolation from others practicing in the same discipline. It is generally a luxury to have "same-job" colleagues working alongside them. Having to function on one's own is a challenge for many professionals, and it carries with it a certain level of stress. If the professional and his or her family are used to living in an urban environment, an adjustment to rural living is necessary. The practitioner may find that he or she has limited staff support, and the staff is likely to be less qualified and less skilled. The practitioner will need to find creative ways to deal with the unique stressors of rural practice. Likewise, rural administrators will need to help new personnel adjust to rural stressors in a healthy way.

Stress, especially if it is uncontrolled, has been linked to numerous health conditions such as heart disease, hypertension, depression, and gastrointestinal disorders (Payne & Hahn, 2000). However, some people exhibit stress-hardiness (Kobasa, 1979). Stress-hardy individuals exhibit the personal characteristics of *commitment, control,* and *challenge.*

- *Commitment:* a sense of purpose in life; a zest and an energy for wanting to engage in life activities that may be labeled as stressful to others
- *Control:* a feeling of being in control; the ability to influence the outcome of events that may be stress-producing
- *Challenge:* enjoying the excitement of the stress environment; an interest in facing new opportunities with keen interest. (Lewis, Garcia, & Jobs, 1990).

Adjustment to work demands will help reduce turnover, absenteeism, and retraining.

Burnout

Herbert Freudenberger coined the term *burnout* in 1980. He defined it this way: "To deplete oneself. To exhaust one's physical and mental resources" (Freudenberger, 1980, p. 17). Burnout is a syndrome "of emotional, physical, and mental exhaustion coupled with feelings of low self-esteem, or low self-efficacy, resulting from prolonged exposure to intense stress" (Seta *et al.,* 2000, p. 417). The characteristics of burnout include *physical exhaustion, emotional exhaustion, depersonalization,* and *low personal achievement* (Green, Walkey, & Taylor, 1991).

Burnout can be caused by a number of things in the work environment. People who take their work seriously, and experience external organizational pressures such as role ambiguity, lack of social support, work units with unclear rules and procedures, and poor opportunities for advancement in the presence of inflexible rules and procedures may be candidates for burnout. The lower a manager's concern for the welfare of the employees, the greater the likelihood of employees' experiencing burnout (Seta *et al.,* 2000).

There are ways to counter burnout. The wise and creative manager can fashion the work environment to be less stressful.

- Create as low-stress a work environment as possible.
- Encourage exercise breaks, and power naps; give permission to leave work early.
- Be flexible. For example, though there needs to be order in the workplace, letting someone go home a half-hour early once in a while can result in many more hours of productivity.
- Reward employees. Verbal praise, gifts at special times, statements of appreciation via e-mail, and having a special "staff day" are all forms of reward.

Remember that stress and burnout are strong contributors to turnover and absenteeism. If retention is important to the organization, the employee must feel comfortable in the organizational work setting.

Summary

The health needs of rural Americans are not unlike those of Americans in urban areas, but the challenges facing rural health organizations are somewhat different. The next decade is likely to be an era of increased interest in dealing with the health needs of rural individuals. As the interest in and funding for programs in rural communities increases, there will be an increased need for professionals who can manage those programs and activities. This chapter provided an overview of the basic important management functions that a rural practitioner might use when recruiting, hiring, training, and retaining personnel. Creative incentives, training programs, and appraisals will also help achieve organizational objectives.

It is likely that the rural health professional will practice in a small organization and may even function initially as the only or first administrator in the organization. This information can be used by the rural practitioner to develop managerial skills and carry out human resource development.

References

Breaugh, J. A. (1983). Realistic job previews: A critical appraisal and future research directions. *Academy of Management Review, 8*(4), 612–619.

Carson, K. P., Cardy, R. L., & Dobbins, G. H. (1993). Upgrade the employee evaluation process. *Survey of Business, 29*(1), 29–32.

Dobbs, K. (1999). Winning the retention game. *Training, 36*(9), 50–52.

Freudenberger, H. J. (1980). *Burn-out: The high cost of high achievement.* New York: Doubleday.

Gamm, L., & Kassab, C. (1982). *A survey of volunteer programs in not-for-profit human services organizations: Characteristics, conditions and outlook.* State College: Pennsylvania State University.

Gay, E. G. (1990). The rural health care market. *HealthSpan, 7*(2), 11–15.

Goff, L. (1999). Top ten retention tactics. *Computerworld, 33*(47), 48.

Gorlin, H., & Schein, L. (1984). *Innovations in managing human resources.* New York: The Conference Board.

Graham, H. T., & Bennett, R. (1998). *Human resources management.* London: Financial Times Management/Pitman Publishing.

Green, D. E., Walkey, F. H., & Taylor, A. J. W. (1991). The three-factor structure of the Maslach Burnout Inventory: A multicultural, multinational confirmatory study. *Journal of Social Behavior and Personality, 6,* 453–472.

Health Resource Services Administration. (2000). Health professional shortage areas: Database search form (March 10, 2000). http://www.bphc.hrsa.gov/databases/hpsa/hpsa.cfm.

Hernandez, S. R. (1998). Formulating organizational strategy. In M. D. Fottler, S. R. Hernandez, & C. L. Joiner (Eds.), *Essentials of human resources management in health services organizations.* Boston: Delmar.

Hernandez, S. R., Fottler, M. D., & Joiner, C. L. (1998). Integrating management and human resources. In M. D. Fottler, S. R. Hernandez, & C. L. Joiner (Eds.), *Essentials of human resources management in health services organizations.* Boston: Delmar.

Higgins, J. (1991). *The management challenge.* New York: MacMillan.

Joiner, C. L., & Hyde, J. C. (1998). Performance appraisal. In M. D. Fottler, S. R. Hernandez, & C. L. Joiner (Eds.), *Essentials of human resource management in health services organizations.* Boston: Delmar.

Kennedy, V. C. (1996). *The professional public health workforce in Texas.* Houston: University of Texas, Houston Health Science Center.

Kobasa, S. (1979). Stressful life events, personality, and health: An inquiry into hardiness. *Journal of Personality & Social Psychology, 37*(1), 1–11.

Kroehnert, G. (1991). *100 training games.* Boston: McGraw-Hill.

Landau, J., & Abelson, M. (1998). Recruitment and retention. In M. D. Fottler, S. R. Hernandez, & C. L. Joiner (Eds.), *Essentials of human resource management in health services organizations.* Boston: Delmar.

Larson, E. H., Hart, G., Goodwin, M. K., Geller, J., & Andrilla, C. (1999). Dimensions of retention: A national study of the locational histories of physician assistants. *Journal of Rural Health, 15*(4), 391–402.

LeBlanc, H.P.I.; Simon, B., & Garard, D. (1997) *Using public health data to guide the recruitment, training, and placement of certified nurse midwives in rural areas of Illinois and Indiana* (March 17, 2000); http://www.siu.edu/~crhssd/crbriefs/vol3 no2.htm.

Lewis, C. T., Garcia, J. E., & Jobs, S. M. (1990). *Managerial skills in organizations.* Boston: Allyn & Bacon.

McArdle, G.E.H. (1996). Conducting a needs assessment for your work group. *Supervisory Management, 41*(3), 6.

McClelland, S. B. (1994). Training needs assessment data-gathering method: Part 3. Focus groups. *Journal of European Industrial Training, 18*(3), 29–32.

McConnell, Charles R. (1999). A working manager's guide to effective and legal employee selection interviewing. *Health Care Supervisor, 17*(4), 77–89.

Morgan, D. L. (1997). *Focus groups as qualitative research* (2nd ed.). Thousand Oaks, CA: Sage Publications.

Newman, M. A. (1997). Sex, race, and affirmative action: An uneasy alliance. *Public Productivity & Management Review, 20*(3), 295–307.

Newstrom, J. W., & Scannell, E. E. (1980). *Games trainers play.* New York: McGraw-Hill.

Olesen, M. (1999). What makes employees stay. *Training and Development, 53*(10), 48–52.

Payne, W. A., & Hahn, D. B. (2000). *Understanding your health* (6th ed.). Boston: McGraw-Hill.

Premack, S. L., & Wanous, J. P. (1985). A meta-analysis of realistic job preview experiments. *Journal of Applied Psychology, 70*(4), 706–719.

Public Health Practice Program Office. (April 28, 2000); *About PHPPO* http://www.phppo.cdc.gov/about.asp.

Rabin, J., Teasley, C. E., Finkle, A., & Carter, L. F. (1985). *Personnel: Managing human resources in the public sector.* New York: Harcourt Brace Jovanovich.

Ralston, S. M., & Kirkwood, W. G. (1995). Overcoming managerial bias in employment interviewing. *Journal of Applied Communication Research, 23*(1), 75–92.

Ricketts, T. C. (1999). Federal programs and rural health. In T. C. Ricketts (Ed.), *Rural health in the United States.* New York: Oxford University Press.

Ricketts, T. C., Johnson-Webb, K. D., & Randolph, R. K. (1999). Rural populations and places in rural America. In T. C. Ricketts (Ed.), *Rural health in the United States.* New York: Oxford University Press.

Robinson, J., & Griffith, J. M. (1999). *Survey of public health training needs among Texas Department of Health employees.* College Station, TX: Texas A&M University System Health Science Center School of Rural Public Health.

Rosenblatt, R. A., & Hart, G. L. (1999). Physicians in rural America. In T. Ricketts (Ed.), *Rural health in the United States.* New York: Oxford University Press.

Seta, K. E., Paulus, P. B., & Baron, R. A. (2000). *Effective human relations: A guide to people at work* (4th ed). Boston: Allyn & Bacon.

Shur, C. L., & Franco, S. J. (1999). Access to health care. In T. Ricketts (Ed.), *Rural health in the United States.* New York: Oxford University Press.

Skrentny, J. D. (1996). *The ironies of affirmative action.* Chicago: University of Chicago Press.

Slifkin, R. (1999). State laws and programs that affect rural health delivery. In T. Ricketts (Ed.), *Rural*

health in the United States. New York: Oxford University Press.

Smith, H. L., & Fottler, M. D. (1998). Training and development. In M. D. Fottler, S. R. Hernandez, & C. L. Joiner (Eds.), *Essentials of human resources management in health services organizations .* Boston: Delmar.

Stewart, C. J., Cash, W. B. (1991). *Interviewing: Principles and practices* (6th ed.). Dubuque, IA: W. C. Brown.

Texas A&M Health Science Center. (1999). *School of rural public health* (April 1, 2000). http:// tamushsc.tamu.edu/SRPH.

U.S. Equal Opportunity Commission. (1997) *Facts about the Americans with disabilities act* (January 5, 2000); http://www.eeoc.gov/facts/fs-ada.html.

U.S. Department of Justice. (1992). *The Americans with Disabilities Act: Questions and answers* (March 4, 2000); http://www.usdoj.gov/crt/ada/ada.html.

Index

The letter f after a page number indicates a figure. The letter t indicates a table.

CPSIA information can be obtained at www.ICGtesting.com
Printed in the USA
LVOW100540190412

278260LV00004BB/6/P